THE 16-BIT 8096 PROGRAMMING, INTERFACING, APPLICATIONS.

122 HANDS-ON EXPERIMENTS WITH INTEL'S iSBE-96 EMULATOR

by
RON KATZ
(AT&T BELL LABORATORIES)
and
HOWARD BOYET
(MICROPROCESSOR TRAINING INC.)

MTI PUBLICATIONS

MICROPROCESSOR TRAINING INC.

14 East 8th Street, NYC 10003
(212) 473-4947

DEDICATIONS:

To that special SFR, my daughter Gigi Rebecca Boyet,

To Linda and Vanessa Katz—the sparkles of my life,

and

To the Intel Troika: Andy Grove, Gordon Moore, and Bob Noyce.

Printing 10, 9, 8, 7, 6, 5, 4, 3, 2 1991

Library of Congress Catalog Card Number: 85-61954

Printed in the United States of America

FOREWORD

Since the introduction of 8048 (MCS®-48) Microcontroller in 1976, Intel has continued to drive the evolution of single chip microcontrollers. In 1980, Intel introduced the 8051 (MCS-51) the second generation of microcontrollers integrating more functions, features and a powerful CPU with ability to address larger memory spaces and improved overall performance. The 8048 and 8051 have since become the industry standard 8 bit microcontrollers.

In recent years, parallel to the advances in circuit design the process technologies have continued to evolve allowing more complex circuits to be fabricated on a single piece of silicon. Microcontroller designers at Intel have exploited the most advanced process technologies and forged a third generation of single chip microcontrollers called the 8096. (MCS-96 family of microcontrollers). The 8096 offers the highest level of system integration every achieved on a single chip microcontroller. It uses over 120,000 transistors to implement a high performance, powerful 16 bit CPU, 8K bytes of program memory, 232 bytes of RAM and analog, digital and serial I/O subsystems. The 8096 executes most instructions in 1 to 1.5us with the 16 x 16 multiply and 32 x 16 divide taking 6.25 usec.

The members of the MCS-96 microcontroller family (8396 ROM version, 8096 ROMless version and 8796 EPROM version) contain an oscillator and clock circuitry, full duplex serial port, watchdog timer, pulse width modulated output, 16 bit timer, 16 bit counter, high speed I/O (HSIO) subsystem, and 20 interrupt sources. In addition, versions are available with three or five 8-bit ports and 10 bit A/D converter. ROM options include 8K bytes of ROM or 8K bytes of EPROM. The package offerings include a 48 pin DIP, 68 pin grid array and a 68 pin plastic lead chip carrier.

This book provides a hands-on-experience with the MCS-96 system. Howard and Ron have made enormous efforts to provide experiments on using every aspect of this powerful single chip system. Included are experiments using the comprehensive instruction set, external and internal interrupt structure, the special function registers, PWM, A/D converters, Serial port, the high speed I/O units, arithmetic applications, the timer/counters, WDT, and signal processing.

There is an extensive range of development support tools available for the 8096 including macro assembler, PL/M, SBE-96 (Single Board Emulator) and VLSiCE-96. The authors have provided extensive hands-on working knowledge with these tools especially the SBE-96 which is a low cost, stand-alone emulator board.

I believe that this book will provide invaluable assistance to engineers, scientists, students and all others needing to learn the 8096 and to design 8096-based applications. Intel highly recommends this book.

Manmohan S. Passi
Product Marketing Manager
Microcontroller Operation
INTEL Corporation, Chandler, AZ

As part of Intel's new open development environment, the iSBE-96 Single Board Emulator can now be used on a wide variety of Intel development systems and PC-DOS compatible machines.

This low cost, easy to use tool may be run, along with the experiments in this book, on Intel's Intellec Series III and Series IV development systems. The SBE96SKIT includes an iSBE-96 emulator and Intel's assembler ASM-96 (Series III/Series IV version).

For those engineers who have an IBM PC AT, IBM PC XT, or compatible system running DOS Version 3.0 or greater, Intel offers the SBE96DKIT containing Intel's DOS version of ASM-96, all host communcation software, and cables needed to run on these systems. Intel's ASM-96 high quality assembler (both the DOS and Series III/IV versions) runs with RL-96, (linker and relocater) makes this a complete symbolic relocatable assembler supporting full macro capabilities. Intel also offers the PL/M-96 high-level language which runs on all of the above systems and complements Intel's ASM-96.

For those engineers who have an Intel iPDS system or Series II development system, iSBE-96 host communication software (ATOP-96) and cross assembler may be purchased from U.S. Software Corporation. This software can be used with either of the two kits SBE96SKIT or SBE96DKIT available from Intel.

Intel highly recommends this book on the 8096. All of the experiments may be run using any of the above host systems. This excellent hands-on applications book will quickly propel engineers, scientists, designers, technicians and all those with a need to know, into the technologically advanced world of the 8096 microcontroller. This book makes an excellent supplement to the Intel Microcontroller Handbook and any other Intel literature.

Stephen Isacoff
Product Manager
Development Systems
INTEL CORP. Hillsboro, Oregon

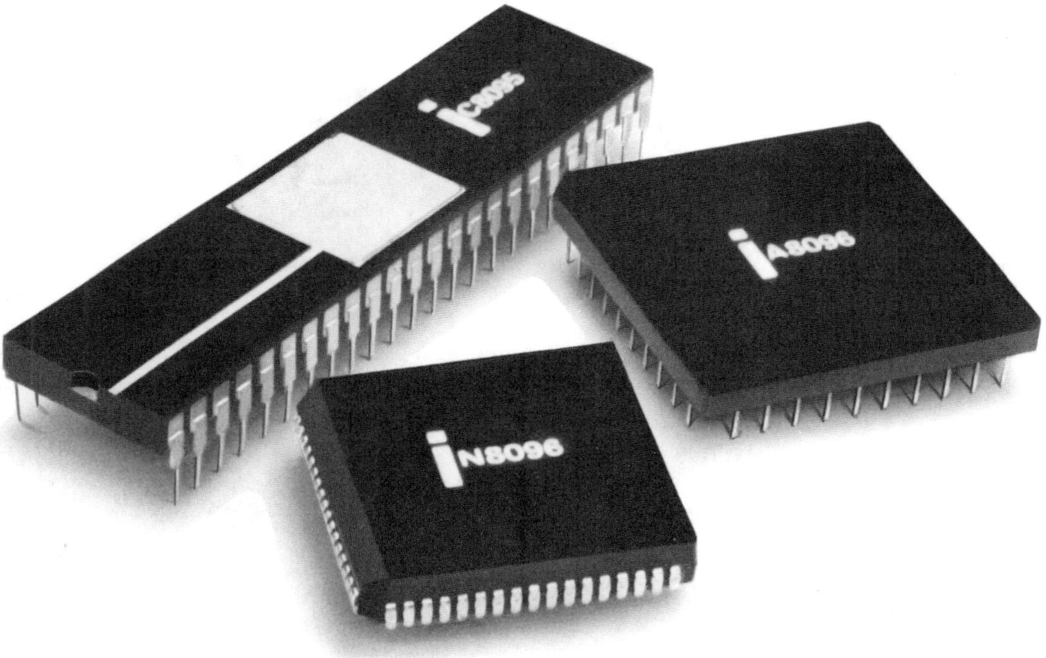
C8095
A8096
N8096

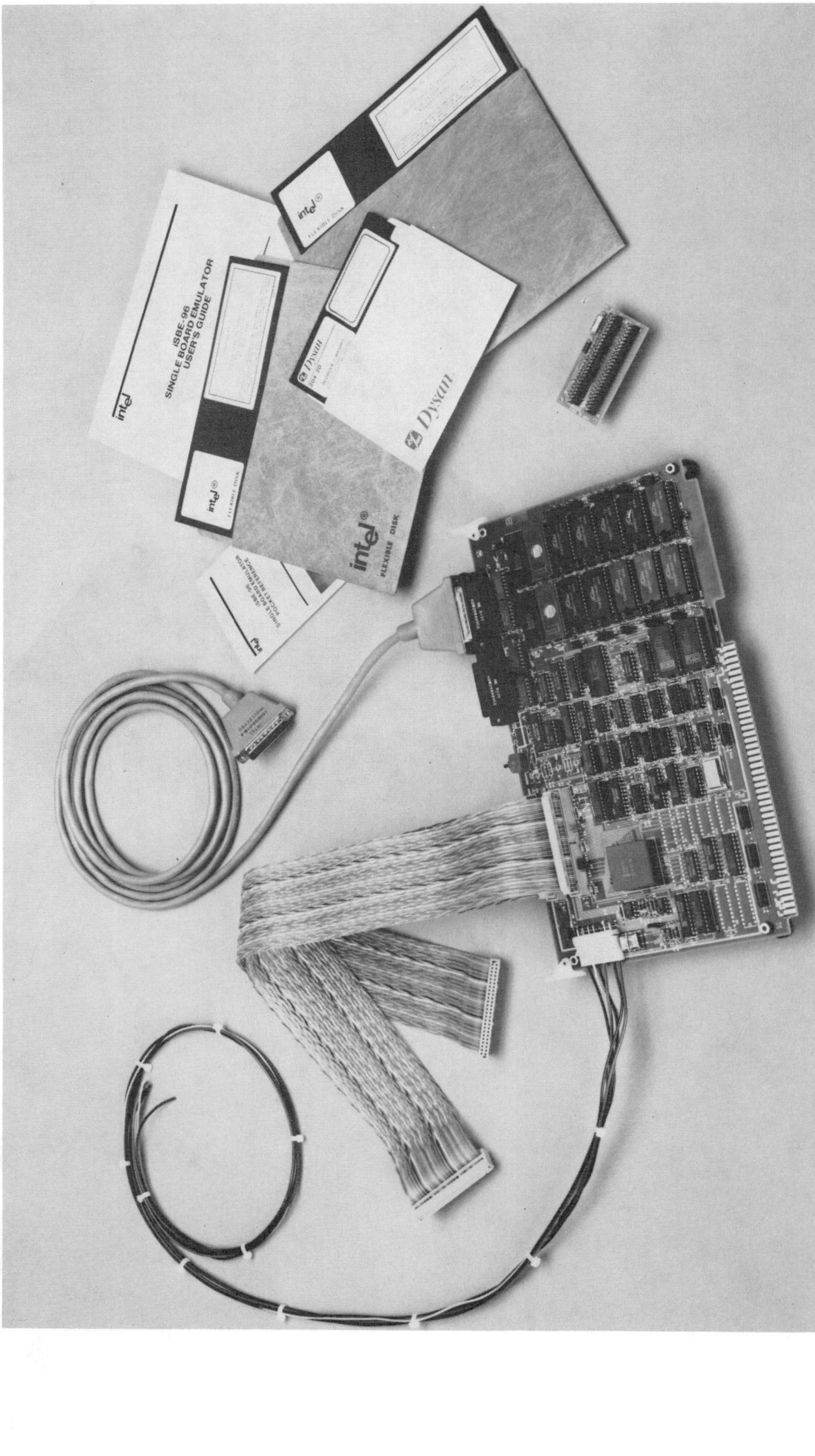
intel
iSBE-96
SINGLE BOARD EMULATOR
USER'S GUIDE
intel
FLEXIBLE DISK
Dysan
intel
FLEXIBLE DISK

CONTENTS

CHAPTER 5:

CHAPTER 9:

IMPORTANT REMARKS TO THE USER OF THIS BOOK

SEE THE FOREWORD AND PP. 59-61 FOR A DISCUSSION AND LISTING OF HOST SYSTEMS, INCLUDING PERSONAL COMPUTERS AND INTEL DEVELOPMENT SYSTEMS, ON WHICH THE EXPERIMENTS IN THIS BOOK MAY BE RUN WHEN USED IN CONJUNCTION WITH THE iSBE-96 (D OR S KIT VERSIONS) AND ASM-96. ALSO, SEE P. 52 REGARDING KEEPING POSTED ON UPDATED INFORMATION FROM INTEL ON THE 8096. THE EXPERIMENTS IN THIS BOOK WERE PERFORMED ON THE iSBE-96, MONITOR VERSION V1.1, COPYRIGHT 1984. EXCEPT FOR CHAPTER 10, ALL EXPERIMENTS USED ASM-96 IN THE PROGRAMMING. THE PROGRAM PRINT-OUTS PRESENTED IN EACH EXPERIMENT SHOW ASM-96 MNEMONICS AND ASSEMBLED HEX CODE, AS WELL AS COMMENTARY. THE INSTRUCTION SET WITH ALL ASSOCIATED INFORMATION CAN BE FOUND ON PP. 44-48, AS NEEDED.

PREFACE

In a word, a powerhouse of a single-chip microcomputer/microcontroller and a milestone in I/O controls!

The 16-bit 8096 is a complex chip with enormous power, functionality, versatility, and far-ranging, industry-wide applications capability. In the opinion of the authors, no other chip, as of this writing, can match it in the area of microcontroller applications.

And yet, it is also a powerful general purpose microcomputer which excels in areas aside from the purely microcontroller domain. It rivals, and even surpasses in a number of areas, other well-known 16-bit microprocessors.

At this point it is desirable to present a preview of some of the advanced features of the 8096, so that the reader may gain insight and perspective as to what this book is about, why it is needed, and what it will accomplish for the user. In what follows, we occasionally refer to the 8096 by its family designation MCS-96 (Intel trademark), as there are presently a number of versions of the chip (68 pin, 48 pin, ROMLESS, ROM, EPROM, Digital I/O only, analog and digital I/O).

The 8096, 68-pin versions with analog and digital I/O on-chip, has a 16-bit CPU (register to register architecture) with 8K bytes of on-chip ROM (8397) or 8K bytes of on-chip EPROM (8797), 232 bytes of RAM (registers), 38 Special Function Registers (SFRs), 8 A/D input channels (10-bit conversion), pulse width modulation capability (PWM) with programmable duty cycle for motor control and D/A conversion, and five 8-pin I/O ports, one with alternate function capability. It has on-chip a full duplex serial communications port that is also capable of implementing I/O port expansion. This serial port also allows efficient realization of interprocessor (master-slave) communications. The versatile A/D inputs (22 usec. conversion time, sample and hold) and D/A output (PWM) allow for efficient on-chip signal processing capability, motor and closed loop control. 232 registers mean less Push/Pop, more pointers, etc.

A "watchdog Timer" (WDT) on-chip allows the programmer to take precautions against possible software/hardware malfunctions. Available to the programmer is the option of selecting at run-time the external bus width, 8-bits or 16-bits, to offer the user a choice that best adapts to his/her existing peripherals.

A 16-bit, free-running, real-time timer (2 usec. intervals) and a 16-bit event counter (with the unusual feature of two possible event sources and four software/hardware reset sources), each with overflow interrupt capability, are on-chip and can be read as Special Function Registers. The event counter can record 0 to 1 and 1 to 0 transitions that are separated in time by 2 usec. or more.

The interrupt system is extremely versatile and highly suited to the multitasking requirements of a microcontroller environment. There are 8 interrupt vectors (2 external and 6 internal) with each vector having 1 or more sources (for a total of 24 different interrupt sources). All activities (related or independent) are tied together and kept humming, in a manner transparent to the user, by the 8096's powerful interrupt system. The main program and its background/foreground activities perform in a "well-oiled" manner.

A truly remarkable and advanced feature of the MCS-96 family are the High Speed Output (HSO) and High Speed Input (HSI) units. The HSO unit on the chip can be programmed to create events (transitions) at any one or more of 6 HSO output lines at any specified times (or to generate interrupts at any programmed times from four independent "Software Timers", or to reset the event counter at any event value, or to start an A/D conversion at any desired time). The times referred to can be any multiple of 2 usec. Delay loops are thus circumvented. The HSI unit can be programmed to record the times of incoming events (and the nature of those transitions) that may appear at any one or more of 4 HSI input lines. The recorded times will be some multiple of 2 usec. The HSO and HSI pins are in addition to the 40 pins at the 5 I/O ports mentioned earlier. The resulting vastly increased I/O through-put and extremely accurate I/O control and monitoring is impressive. The HSI/O units form an independent subsystem that can be programmed to generate interrupts when their current activity is over. Thus, they may be commanded to engage in a sequence of independent I/O control and monitoring activities that significantly helps alleviate software overhead and speeds up execution time.

The HSO unit, as mentioned, contains four "Software Timers". They, too, can be programmed to provide up to four independent and, importantly, concurrent time delays of specified amount without the need to write software loops. When the specified time(s) expire(s), the software timer(s) can generate interrupts(s) to vector the program flow from "other activity" to the Software Timer Interrupt Routine where action appropriate to that expiration time is programmed. Again, the effect on I/O through-put is considerable. Times can be programmed to 2 usec.

resolution (12 MHz clock) ensuring unusual accuracy.

The many aspects and novel features of the powerful 8096 instruction set will be brought out in the experiments where they are used and explained. Some of those unusual features follow. 6 addressing modes (with two variants), allows the programmer to deal with both internal and external memory in a flexible and general manner. The ease this affords in operating on any register or memory location overcomes the bottleneck often associated with accumulator-based processors. Another powerful attribute is the ease of establishing pointers with the indirect addressing mode (with or without auto-increment). This allows the use of any on-chip word register location (116 of them) as a pointer to anywhere in memory, providing an extremely powerful tool for manipulation of data. Other features are the availability of 3-operand instructions (usually associated only with minicomputers or main frames) which make the programmer's task easier; inclusion of 16 x 16 (or 8 x 8) multiply and 32 x 16 (or 16 x 8) divide instructions (both signed and unsigned); a very versatile and complete set of multiple shift instructions; a normalization instruction (valuable in floating point arithmetic); the existence of the "sticky bit" and "overflow trap" flags (useful in rounding, truncation, and precision arithmetic); "sign extend" and "load extend" instructions (for ease in matching 8-bit to 16-bit quantities); the flexibility and accuracy to be had with the availabilty of byte, word, and doubleword operand instructions -- these are just some of the features that allow the 8096's instruction set to go beyond some of the more powerful 16-bit microprocessors, let alone microcontrollers. Its arithmetic processing power is formidable, accurate and fast. Average execution time of the multiply and divide instructions is about 6.5 usec. Most of the 8096's instructions execute in 1 to 1.5 usec. (12 MHz clock).

These are just some of the advanced and powerful features and attractions of the MCS-96 family of microcontrollers that over 120,000 transistors on-chip have implemented. And that makes a lot to learn and master.

All these features and functionality in the 8096 make the task of learning and mastering the 8096 by oneself a formidable one, even for the experienced microprocessor designer or user.

The purpose of this book is to get you through all aspects of the 8096 in the quickest and, yet, most thorough manner. We do this by a logical step-by-step, chapter-by-chapter approach from ground up. 122 hands-on experiments, programmed in ASM-96 (and assembled in 8096 HEX code) are presented, using Intel's iSBE-96 emulator as the learning and applications vehicle. All the fundamentals behind the 8096 are stressed and investigated, and a large number and variety of applications experiments are presented, either in conjunction with the presentation of the fundamentals, or separately (but always based on them).

The 8096 and this book are not for beginners. While no prior 8096 background is assumed, it is assumed that the reader has a solid classical microprocessor background (architecture, assembly language, a thorough working facility with HEX and binary, interfacing/digital logic, and programming). While not necessary, previous exposure to microcontrollers (e.g. the 8051) might be helpful (see the book "The 8051: Programming, Interfacing, Applications. 81 Hands-On Experiments with Intel's SDK-51" by the authors of this book). Except for their serial ports, the 8051 and 8096 are completely different microcontrollers.

The keys to understanding and mastering the 8096 are: 1) its Special Function Registers, through which efficient control of all 8096 I/O (or its monitoring) is accomplised, 2) its versatile interrupt system which makes possible the transparent execution of a large number of related or unrelated tasks, 3) its ultra-fast independent HSI/O input/output units, and 4) the unique and powerful features of its instruction set. Keep that in mind as you go through this book and as you read the descriptions of the various chapters which follow.

The experienced user may find that chapters 2 and 3 can be skipped or given brief attention. In that case the reader can go directly to chapter 4. All the experiments in this book were entered in ASM-96 assembly language, with the program print-outs showing both ASM-96 mnemonics and HEX object code (chapter 10 gives examples using the high level language PL/M-96).

Chapter 1 presents the relevant 8096 information, gathered in one place for the convenience of the user. It is to be referred to, as necessary, when the experiments are studied. A list of Intel references, from which the information was taken, and others, are presented, should the reader need additional 8096 information.

Chapter 2 is concerned with the iSBE-96 emulator. Relevant and necessary information on it is presented. We then discuss our approach in downloading programs to the iSBE-96 in HEX format object code from ASM-96 assembly language input to an IBM PC. A listing of other host systems and PCs on which the experiments in this book can be performed is given (see also the FOREWORD to the book). After the interfacing requirements needed to do the experiments are given, 9 experiments are performed demonstrating the use of the iSBE-96, its relevant commands, and the important features of the iSBE-96 monitor's stack that the user should be alerted to. Debugging techniques (single-step, breakpoints, etc.) using the SBE's commands are covered. The first I/O experiment involving ports P0 and P1 is presented, as well as one on the Watchdog Timer.

Chapter 3 focuses on the 8096 instruction set and its capabilities. 18 experiments demonstrate all the addressing modes, the flags, the shift instructions, the "sticky bit", the "overflow trap", the load/extend, the normalization, and the multiply and divide instructions. Also covered are the indirect branch and generic branch instructions, the conditional jumps, the PUSHF, POPF, PUSH, and POP instructions, the System Reset instruction, the CALL and JUMP instructions (of various kinds), use of 3-operand instructions, and more.

Chapter 4 on the 8096's interrupt system is a key chapter in coming to grips and working with the 8096. 10 experiments are presented covering every facet of the 8096's interrupt structure. While the experiments center on the 8096's two external interrupts (to more easily and conveniently demonstrate the interrupt facilities), their understanding will lead to a direct understanding of the 8096's six internal interrupt vectors (and their sources). The fundamentals are identical. (The internal interrupts are introduced in Chapter 5 and used in all their aspects thereafter through-out the book). Conditions for interrupt servicing (immediate or pending) are established. The interplay among the pending interrupt, interrupt mask, and global interrupt bits in the relevant SFRs is thoroughly investigated. Both hardware and software-generated interrupts are explored. Nesting of interrupts with the 8096 is thoroughly covered. A powerful user option available with the 8096 is the possibility of establishing one's own priority interrupt structure among the 8 interrupt vectors. This is covered in two experiments.

Chapter 5 is extremely important to understanding and applying the 8096. It involves a study of all the 8096's SFRs (except the serial I/O SFRs that are deferred until chapter 8). To this end, 25 experiments are presented in which all SFR bits are examined as they relate to I/O control and status or data monitoring. A good number of these experiments already project a strong applications orientation. It should be kept in mind that the 8096 on-chip devices (A/D, PWM, WDT, HSI/O, serial I/O, timers, counters, digital I/O ports) and interrupt facilities are controlled and monitored by means of on-chip (RAM) register-mapped I/O through the SFRs. This reduces software overhead and results in extremely efficient I/O processing. Half the experiments in this chapter deal with the HSI/O SFRs.

Chapter 6 covers 26 applications experiments centered around the SFRs. Half are devoted to the HSI/O units. In several examples the applications are purposely implemented first the "classical way", to point out the major software and hardware I/O advantages the HSI/O units afford. A glance at the table of contents will reveal the broad scope of this important chapter. A mastery of this chapter is essential to working successfully with, and applying, the 8096's SFRs and HSI/O units.

Chapter 7 is devoted to a discussion of the important arithmetic features of the 8096 that give it its extraordinary arithmetic processing capability where speed, accuracy, versatility, and reductions in software overhead are essential. In particular, the normalization instruction (very useful in floating point arithmetic), the sign-extend and load-extend instructions, the "sticky bit", "overflow trap", and "negative" flags are all discussed and used to illustrate the 8096's efficiency and power in the arithmetic realm. Three experiments involving sign extension, the sticky bit (in rounding operations), and the negative flag are presented to illustrate some of the points brought out in the chapter. More extended arithmetic is cound in ch. 9.

Chapter 8 deals with the 8096's serial port. Serial communications is the medium employed in many real world applications. A thorough discussion and explanation of the relevant SFRs and how to program them to achieve desired transmission/reception characteristics in the various serial modes are first presented. Six applications experiments are then studied demonstrating serial communciations via the TXD and RXD pins on the 8096. The first two are concerned with I/O port expansion (most important for a microcontroller), and are implemented in serial mode 0. Reception from, and transmission back (echo) to a CRT terminal involving mode 1 is next covered in three experiments. Two involve polling of the serial port's status SFR and the other is based on the serial port's interrupt vector. All three illustrate either a simple echo or the processing of the received data before re-transmission (in the latter case processed data buffer tables are created). Finally, an experiment on interprocessor communciations between master and slave(s) is presented (here an iSBE-96 master and another iSBE-96 slave). Serial modes 2 and 3 and serial interrupts are involved.

Chapter 9, in a sense, is the culmination point of the book. It presents applications with the 8096 in a broad range of areas beyond those covered in previous chapters. The vehicle is again the iSBE-96. As always, we attempt to emphasize the unique features of the 8096 that make it the microcontroller of choice in the applications covered (or suggested in the problems). It is not our intent (nor within our capability) to focus on everyone's areas of interest, or to implement the reader's specific problem(s) and needs with the 8096. In this chapter we endeavor to present a series of broad applications in various areas with the purpose of suggesting ideas and methods of implementation, and of illustrating the far-ranging capabilities, power, versatility, and efficiency of the 8096. The chapter puts to use everything learned in the previous chapters. The applications presented may themselves be of direct interest and use to the reader. They span a wide range from areas involving frequency measurement and control, to serial (remote) control of I/Os, to high speed manufacturing operations, to materials handling, to closed loop control, to digital filters, to smoothing, and more-much more (consult the table of contents under chapter 9). We could go on and on with a microcomputer like the 8096.

Chapter 10, the final one of the book, attempts to make the reader aware, albeit in a small way, of some of the Intel software/hardware development tools available for the 8096 besides the iSBE-96 emulator board that we have been working with. Thus, 2 applications using the high level language PL/M-96 are offered (one of which is a PL/M-96 version of a previous experiment from chaper 6 that used ASM-96 assembly language). FPAL-96 routines are used. Also presented is some information on the Intel VLSiCE-96P (Intel trademark): In-Circuit Emulator for the MCS-96 Family of Microcontrollers. These software/hardware development tools are often indispensable in achieving quicker and more economical solutions to specific applications.

We should like to bring to your attention that a large number of problems have been added in the book. They appear at the end of various experiments and suggest either other ways of accomplishing the same application with the 8096 and/or new or further applications to explore based on that experiment. We believe these problems will add significant value to the book.

Also to be kept in mind is the fact that in many experiments we have ended the main program part of the application in a self loop, simulating "other tasks" rather than a mere "halt". The various interrupt sources employed in the particular experiment then achieve multitasking over and above the main activity, as various interrupt routines are alternately entered and serviced. The multitasking capability of the 8096 is impressive.

The various applications and programs represented in the numerous experiments can themselves possibly serve as a library of modules in building more encompassing programs for still larger applications.

ACKHOWLEDGEMENTS

The undertaking of this book was originally suggested by Alex Toth and Martin Pawloski of the Intel Microcontroller Operation, Chandler, Az. The final decision rested with Mohan Passi, product marketing manager of 16-bit operations in the Microcontroller group. We are indebted for his confidence and continued solid support, encouragement, and total cooperation. He made the book possible and did everything to ease our task.

The authors would like to single out two individuals who played key roles in helping to expedite the book's progress both from a technical and time stand-point: Ira Horden, Applications Engineer in the Microcontroller Operation was outstanding for his prompt assistance on a number of technical questions relating to the 8096 raised by the authors. Some of the mysteries of the 8096 began to unravel as Ira showed the way. This led to important break-throughs. We greatly appreciate all the time he took, on top of a very busy schedule, to go through the manuscript from beginning to end. His comments and suggestions were invaluable. Errors of any sort are the responsibility of the authors. Steve Isacoff, Product manager, Development Systems, Intel (Hillsboro, Oregon) was indispensable. His prompt, concerned, and enthusiastic cooperation in contributing several iSBE-96 emulator boards at various stages of iSBE-96 hardware and monitor updating (and in expediting a prompt repair at a critical time in the book's undertaking) was instrumental to the smooth, uninterrupted flow of progress that would otherwise not have been possible. The master-slave and master-remote controller experiments would not be in this book were it not for Steve's help in supplying boards. He was also responsible for supplying latest information on VLSiCE-96 that appears in chapter 10 and on iSBE-96 emulators that appears in chapter 2.

We would also like to express our thanks to Randy Wilhelm, Dennis Regimbal, Dave Ryan, and Lionel Smith of the Intel Microcontroller Operation for their help in many different and important ways. Dennis was instrumental in getting updated 8096 information to us at a number of critical times. Mohan, Denis, and Dave also made valuable suggestions regarding the manuscript. Tom Geletka of Intel's Customer Training division in Schaumburg, IL was responsible for duplicating one of our experiments, and for contributing another, both in PL/M-96, which then became part of chapter 10. Tom was another example of cooperation with personal effort over and above a busy work load. We thank him for his timely contribution.

The Intel Sales Office in Hauppauge, NY helped in providing updated Intel manuals on a number of crucial occasions. (With the 8096 you've got to have manuals and you've got to read them like a hawk. We think you've also got to have this book).

One of us (R.K.) wishes to express thanks to his management at AT&T Bell Laboratories, Whippany, NJ for their encouragement and support of his independent effort in this important project.

The word-processing of the manuscript was a tedious, long and difficult undertaking. "A Personal Touch Word Processing Service Bureau" of 550 Durie Avenue, Closter, NJ was outstanding in its service and promptness. President (Pauline Carroll) and Office Manager (Linda Jackle) came through during many a crunch. They're real pros. (Mike Carroll also helped out).

Another real pro is Frank Moore who has done many covers, and title/copyright pages for MTI Publications. His work on the mechanicals has always been outstanding.

The manuscript for this book was written in many near and far-off places: airlines, parks, restaurants, busses, subways, vans, taxis, trains, pubs, libraries, in bed, dance and acting studios (daughter Gigi) - wherever a table, desk, or prop of any kind was available. One of us (H.B.) wishes to thank MaryLou's and Viva Pancho's restaurants in Greenwich Village, NY for providing a conducive atmosphere where ideas and experiments fermented through various stages of the book.

The 8096 was a BIG challenge from beginning (January 1985) to end (January 1986) - more so than any of the other microprocessors and microcomputers on which the authors have written books. We hope we have met that challenge and that this book will succeed in quickly helping others conquer this complex chip of great versatility and awesome, but beautiful, power. We are indebted to Migdalia and Linda for their unswerving patience and understanding during this period of almost total immersion.

January, 1986
New York, NY

Ron Katz
(AT&T Bell Laboratories)

Howard Boyet
(Microprocessor Training Inc.)

CHAPTER 1

INTRODUCTION AND 8096 REFERENCE MATERIAL

INTRODUCTION

The Intel 8096 single-chip microcontroller is, in all likelihood, the most powerful 16 bit single-chip microcomputer/microcontroller in the field of controls as of this writing. And yet, its versatility and power extend beyond controls into many other areas such as telecommunications, serial I/O, modems, image processing, graphics, floating point arithmetic, video recorders, signal processing, laser disc drives, and more. In the area of controls, per se, it probably suprasses any other microcontroller extant in applications dealing with servos, motor or engine control, robotics, discrete and continuous process control (numeric controls, quality control, automation, programmable controllers), manufacturing, guidance, testing/monitoring, instrumentation, and in the many areas of the automotive and aerospace industries (end products and production) and other industrial environments.

What are the features that make the 8096 so powerful and so well suited for applications cutting across so many market areas? (Note that we are using 8096 as the generic part number for the MCS-96 family that includes other configurations: 8094, 8396, 8394, 8097, 8095, 8397, 8395 - see section B later in this chapter). The 8096 uses over 120,000 transistors to implement a high performance microcontroller system on a chip with the following major features: a powerful 16-bit CPU and associated instruction set, 38 I/O Special Function Registers, 8 K bytes of program memory (ROM), 232 bytes of data memory (RAM) in the form of on-chip registers (the "internal register file"), a 16-bit timer, a 16-bit counter, 5 parallel I/O ports (each 8 lines), a full duplex serial I/O port, 8 input A/D channels (10 bit results), pulse width modulation (PWM) capability which can implement D/A conversion and generate a programmably variable duty cycle on an output pulse train, and a powerful interrupt system consisting of 24 sources (8 vectors with priority: 2 external, 6 internal, with a third external interrupt possible). In connection with the latter, the user can create his/her own interrupt priority structure by means of software. Further, there is a "watchdog timer" (WDT) which is extremely useful in preventing hardware malfunction as a result of any software upset. The WDT forces a reset of the 8096 and any other components connected to the reset line if the software does wander off to "unknown territory" where periodic clearing of the WDT no longer occurs. This reset prevents unwanted and possibly dangerous responses.

The instruction set is versatile and powerful for I/O control applications and in areas where arithmetic and data or signal processing are important. There are hardware multiply (MUL) and divide (DIV) instructions for signed and unsigned arithmetic. 16 bit quantities can be multiplied with 32 bit results; 8 bit quantities can be multiplied with 16 bit results; 32 bit quantities can be divided by 16 bit quantities with 16 bit quotient and 16 bit remainder results; 16 bit quantities can be divided by 8 bit quantities with 8 bit quotient and 8 bit remainder results - all in either signed or unsigned operations. There are 6 different addressing modes which avails the user of powerful programming flexibility for either I/O or data manipulation (register direct, register indirect, register indirect with autoincrement, immediate, short indexed, and long indexed). If one includes ZERO register addressing (a form of long indexed) and Stack Pointer register addressing (a form of indirect or short indexed) then 8 different addressing modes are possible.

With a 12 MHz input clock most of the instructions execute in 1 or 2 usec. If the operands are in external memory, the times are slightly longer. The MUL and DIV instructions execute in anywhere from 4 to 10 usec (depending on the exact instruction, the addressing mode, and on whether the operand(s) is fetched from internal or external memory). High speed math processing, number crunching, and signal processing (through 8 on-chip A/D lines) are thus readily implemented with the 8096. 8-channel analog processing with high speed number crunching make for a powerful combination.

The 8096 instruction set has several other powerful and welcome features for the programmer. The introduction of two new flags is but one. The VT flag (overflow trap bit) allows for testing of a possible overflow condition at the end of a sequence of related arithmetic operations, rather than testing the overflow flag (V) after each arithmetic instruction. In the same way, the ST flag (sticky bit) is introduced so that, when used with the carry flag (C), rounding after a number of right shifts can be more conveniently accomplished (e.g. as in multiplying two 8-bit quantities and then scaling the result down to 12 bits).

Another feature of the instruction set that is significant for the programmer is the existence of 3-operand versions of the ADD, ADDB, SUB, SUBB, MULU, MULUB, MUL, MULB, AND, and ANDB instructions. Thus, for example, two operands can be added and the result placed in a completely different destination operand. The original two operands remain intact. Not having to deal with temporary storage and retrieval of operands is an advantage as it relates to software overhead. An instruction that is very useful in floating point arithmetic is the "Normalization" instruction, in which a 32-bit double word is shifted left as many times as necessary till its most significant bit is 1.

One of the major features and advances of the 8096 has to do with the High Speed I/O units on board the chip (HSO for output event control and HSI to record input events). Briefly, the HSO output unit, for example, can be programmed to set up events (pulses) on any one or more of 6 HSO output pins at any desired times (to within 2 usec. resolution). Further, it can be programmed, if desired, to generate an "HSO Interrupt" when an event, or a number of events, start or end, allowing the user program to concentrate on "other tasks". The interrupt routine could then ask for new or additional HSO-created events. Not only can the HSO unit do the above, but it can also be programmed, ADDITIONALLY AND INDEPENDENTLY, to start an A/D conversion at a specified time; or to reset the Timer 2 event counter; or to have it engage any one or more of four "Software Timers", each of which can provide a specified amount of time delay and, if desired, provide an interrupt at the end of the delay, with vectoring to a "Software Timer" interrupt routine. 14 different kinds of actions can be asked of the HSO.

Up to 8 requests for various actions of the types described above can be programmed and pending (in the "HSO CAM File") at any one time and, as they eventually execute, new requests can be programmed into the File. A 9th can be waiting in the Holding Register if the CAM is full. All the while, your program is off doing "other things". And, since the HSO unit can create pulses of programmable on-times, it, too, can generate analog signals just as the PWM facility can - hence, if you like, the availability of 7 D/A converters on the chip (PWM plus 6 HSO output pins).

What about the HSI input unit? It can be programmed to record the time and nature of incoming events on any one of four HSI input pins. The user can program the unit to record incoming events on either positive-going or negative-going transitions only, or on either kind of transition, or only after 8 positive transitions occur. Again, one can program the HSI unit to generate an "HSI Data Available Interrupt" when it has recorded a single event or after recording a number of events. In the service routine, user can query the status of the pin (i.e. the nature of the event) and the exact time of the occurrence of the event (to within 2 usec). As with the HSO unit, the HSI unit allows the user's program to take care of many "other tasks" while the HSI unit monitors incoming events, interrupting "other tasks" only when a specified event occurs. Measurement of events and times becomes a simple software task.

What is the significance of the High Speed I/O Units in the 8096? It is simply this: a drastic reduction in software overhead; a significant enhancement of multi-tasking capability, and speed of execution; and a powerful, accurate, and high speed I/O capability, in addition to all the I/O features on-chip previously mentioned and discussed. We treat the HSO and HSI Units quite thoroughly in this book.

Keys to understanding and working with the 8096 are the powerful and intricate interrupt system, the High Speed I/O Units, and the Special Function Registers (SFRs). The many I/O devices on board the 8096 (serial and parallel ports, A/D converters, PWM (D/A), HSO and HSI units, WDT, software timers, timers 1 and 2, the interrupt facilities, and the I/O control and status registers) are all either polled or controlled by means of SFR register-mapped I/O. Those 8-and 16-bit SFRs have designated addresses in the register file. There are 38 of them (if one counts an SFR twice when it can be written to and read). Writing to the "writeable" ones controls events; reading the "readable" ones polls the status of 8096 hardware. And just about every bit within these 38 SFRs has a special meaning and significance in the I/O operation of the 8096. Hence, if we are to master the 8096 and have it implement our needs, it is essential that we come to grips with the SFRs in great detail - to understand them and to be able to manipulate their bits for whatever purposes we have in mind. Which we do in great detail in this book, in addition to doing many other things related to the 8096. WE LEAVE NO SFR BIT UNTURNED.

It should be mentioned that there are 48 pin (DIP) and 68 pin (Plastic Leaded Chip Carrier, Pin Grid Array) versions of the 8096. The MCS-96 options consist of 1) purely digital I/O versions: 8096, 68 pin ROMless; 8094, 48 pin ROMless; 8396, 68 pin ROM; and 8394, 48 pin ROM; and 2) versions containing digital I/O and Analog I/O capabilities: 8097, 68 pin ROMless; 8095, 48 pin ROMless; 8397, 68 pin ROM; and 8395, 48 pin ROM.

How does one go about learning, mastering, and applying the 8096? We think by going through all the hands-on experiments in this book using the Intel iSBE-96 Emulator. We start from ground up and proceed very far, trying to tap as many features and possibilities with the 8096 as possible, within the scope and purpose of our undertaking. We attempt to build up our knowledge and mastery of the 8096 in a very logical, systematic, and methodical way, covering as many aspects as possible. Fundamentals and Applications are stressed throughout. After completing this book we would strongly suggest that you continue by reading the excellent Intel Application Notes on the 8096 listed in the references below. And of course, the Intel 8096 manuals, handbooks, and User's Guides are always necessary where additional information is needed. Again, see references below.

The authors have found with their book on the 8051 ("The 8051: Programming, Interfacing, Applications. 81 Hands-On Experiments With Intel's SDK-51") that a convenient assembling of the relevant chip information in one place was very popular with the reader. You are spared the "agony" of consulting various pages in 4 or 5 manuals strewn all over the desk, floor, and lap. With that in mind, we devote the rest of Chapter 1 to presenting in one place the relevant 8096 information, particularly as it relates to the needs of the experiments in this book. We have endeavored to compile that information in a logical, easily accessible order. The information, while plentiful, is by no means exhaustive. The Intel Manuals, Guides, and Microcontroller Handbook listed in the references below should be consulted where additional information may be necessary or desirable.

Relevant and helpful information on the iSBE-96 single board emulator, on which the experiments are done, is presented separately in Chapter 2.

All the experiments in this book were performed with the iSBE-96, monitor version V1.1, copyright 1984, Intel Corp. We should like to thank the Intel Corporation for their permission to reproduce information from their literature on the 8096 in both chapters 1 and 2. That information was taken and compiled from the first seven references listed in the section that follows.

REFERENCES

1. Microcontroller Handbook, 1985. (Copyright Intel Corp., 1984).

2. MCS-96 User's Manual, 1984. (Copyright Intel Corp., 1983).

3. MCS-96 Macro Assembler User's Guide. (Copyright Intel Corp., 1983).

4. iSBE-96 Single Board Emulator User's Guide. (Copyright Intel Corp., 1984).

5. MCS-96 Macro Assembler and Utilities Pocket Reference. (Copyright Intel Corp., 1983).

6. iSBE-96 Pocket Reference. (Copyright Intel Corp., 1984).

7. MCS-96 809X-90, 839X-90 (Preliminary). (Dated 1/29/85, Copyright Intel Corp., 1984).

8. Application Note 248. Using the 8096. Ira Horden. Intel, 1985.

9. 8096 Examples. Ref. 1 above (pp. 3-16 through 3-22).

10. PL/M-96 User's Guide. (Copyright Intel Corp., 1983).

11. MCS-96 Utilities User's Guide. (Copyright Intel Corp., 1983).

12. 8096 Floating-Point Arithmetic Library User's Guide (order number 122133).

13. Intel FPAL96 Library.

14. VLSiCE-96: In-Circuit Emulator for the MCS-96 Family of Microcontrollers, Sept. 1985. (Copyright Intel Corp., 1985. #280140-001).

IMPORTANT NOTE TO USER OF THIS BOOK

SEE PP. 59-61 FOR A LISTING OF HOST SYSTEMS, INCLUDING PCs AND INTEL DEVELOPMENT SYSTEMS, ON WHICH THE EXPERIMENTS IN THIS BOOK IN ASM-96 MAY BE RUN.

A. 8096 ARCHITECTURAL BLOCK DIAGRAM, MEMORY MAP, AND RALU BLOCK DIAGRAM.

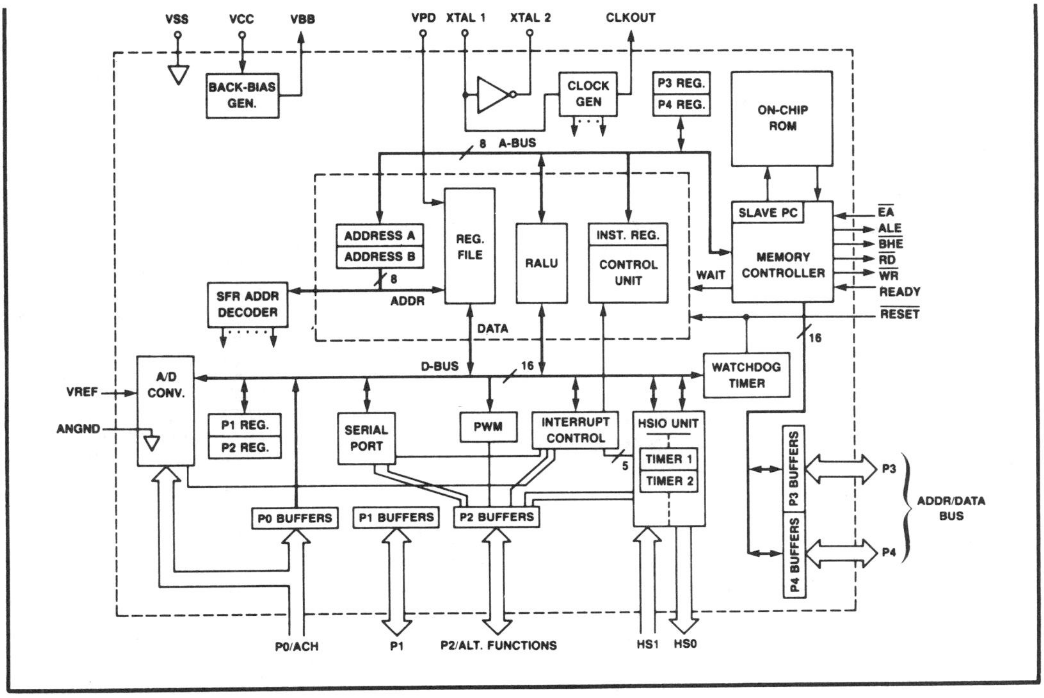

Figure 2-1. Block Diagram (For simplicity, lines connecting port registers to port buffers are not shown.)

Hardware Overview

The 8096 microcontroller features include

- 8K of on-chip ROM (in the 8396)
- High-speed pulse I/O
- 10-bit A/D converter
- Eight interrupt sources
- Pulse-width modulated output
- Four 16-bit software timers
- 232-byte register file
- Memory-to-memory architecture
- Full duplex serial port
- Five 8-bit I/O ports
- Watchdog timer

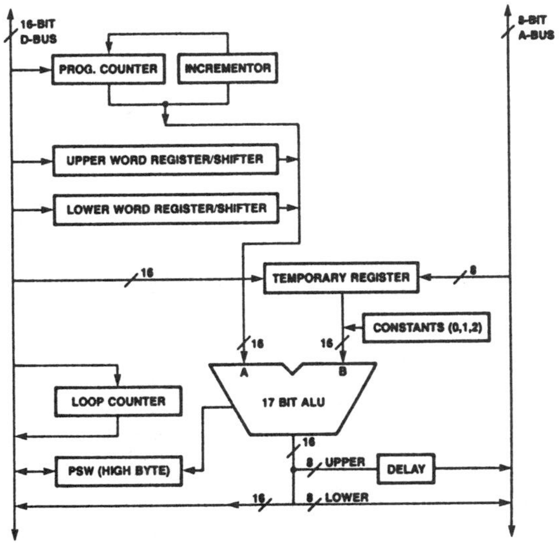

Figure 2-2. RALU Block Diagram

2.3. MEMORY SPACE

The addressable memory space on the 8096 consists of 64K bytes, most of which is available to the user for program or data memory. Locations which have special purposes are 0000H through 00FFH and 1FFEH through 2010H. All other locations can be used for either program or data storage or for memory mapped peripherals. A memory map is shown in figure 2-5.

2.3.1. Register File

Locations 00H through 0FFH contain the Register File and SFRs. Complete information on this section of memory space can be found in section "RAM SPACE". No code can be executed from this internal RAM section. If an attempt to execute instructions from locations 000H through 0FFH is made, the instructions will be fetched from *external* memory. This section of external memory is reserved for use by Intel development tools. Execution of a nonmaskable interrupt (NMI) will force a call to external location 0000H, therefore, the NMI instruction is also reserved for Intel development tools.

2.3.2. Reserved Memory Spaces

Locations 1FFEH and 1FFFH are reserved for Ports 3 and 4 respectively. This is to allow easy reconstruction of these ports if external memory is used in the system. An example of reconstructing the I/O ports is given in section 4.6.7. If ports 3 and 4 are not going to be reconstructed then these locations can be treated as any other external memory location.

The 9 interrupt vectors are stored in locations 2000H through 2011H. The 9th vector is used by Intel development systems, as explained in section 2.5. Internal locations 2012H through 2077H are reserved for Intel's factory test code. These locations may be used in external memory.

Resetting the 8096 causes instructions to be fetched starting from location 2080H. This location was chosen to allow a system to have up to 8K of RAM continuous with the register file. Further information on reset can be found in section 2.15.

2.3.3. Internal ROM

When a ROM part is ordered, the internal memory locations 2080H through 3FFFH are user specified as are the interrupt vectors in locations 2000H through 2011H. Instruction and data fetches from the internal ROM occur only if the part has a ROM, $\overline{EA}$ is tied high, and the address is between 2000H and 3FFFH. At all other times data is accessed from either the internal RAM space or external memory and instructions are fetched from external memory.

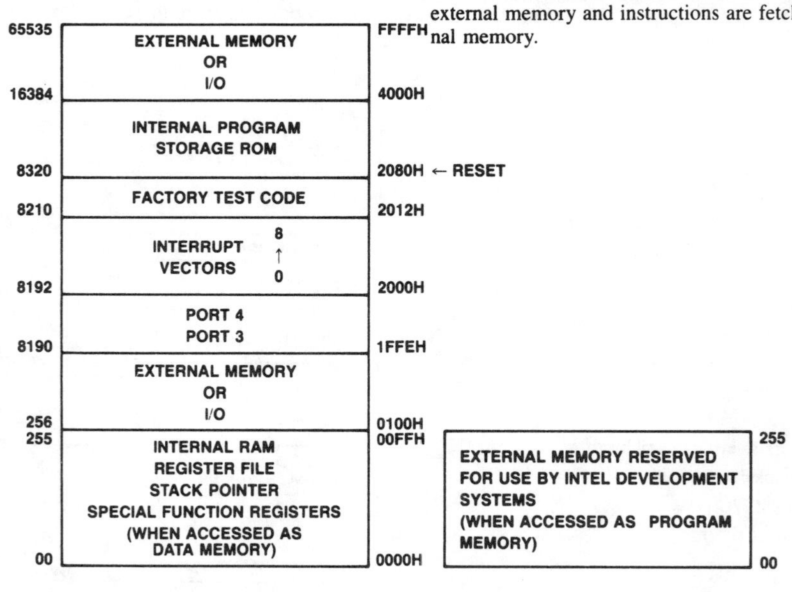

Figure 2-5. Memory Map

Memory Space

The 8096 uses the same address space for both program and data memory. It can execute instructions from any memory address. (Instructions cannot, however, be fetched from internal RAM. Instruction fetches from locations 0000H through 00FFH are automatically directed to external memory. These locations in external memory should be reserved for future Intel developments.)

Internal locations 0000H through 0017H are special function registers (ports, control registers, etc.). Locations 0018H through 00FFH access the register file, of which the top 16 bytes (addresses 00F0H through 00FFH) are preserved during power down if a backup supply is available. Locations 0018H and 0019H contain the stack pointer.

The 8396 carries 8K bytes of on-chip ROM, occupying addresses 2000H through 3FFFH. Addresses 2000H through 200FH contain the interrupt vectors. Addresses 2010H through 207FH contain a factory test code. Reset commences execution from location 2080H.

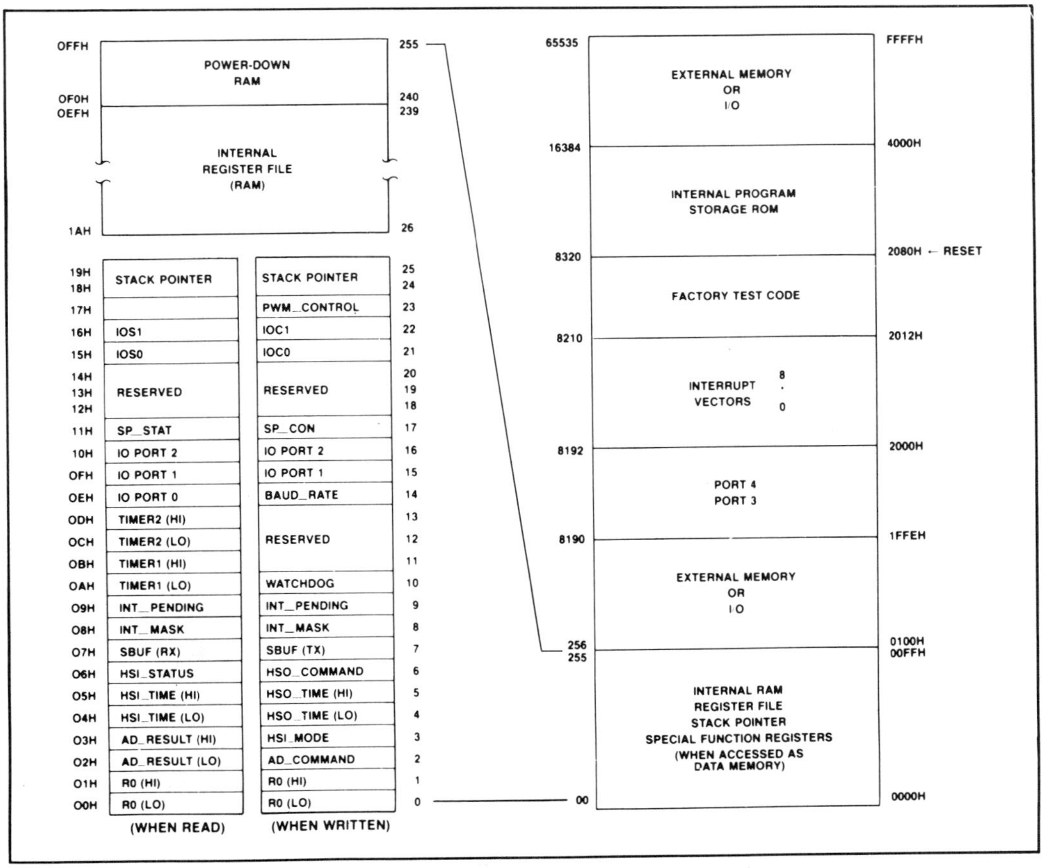

Figure 5. Memory Map

B. 8096 FAMILY PIN-OUTS, PIN LIST, PIN DESCRIPTION (SEE P. 52 FOR MCS-96 68-PIN PLCC PIN-OUT)

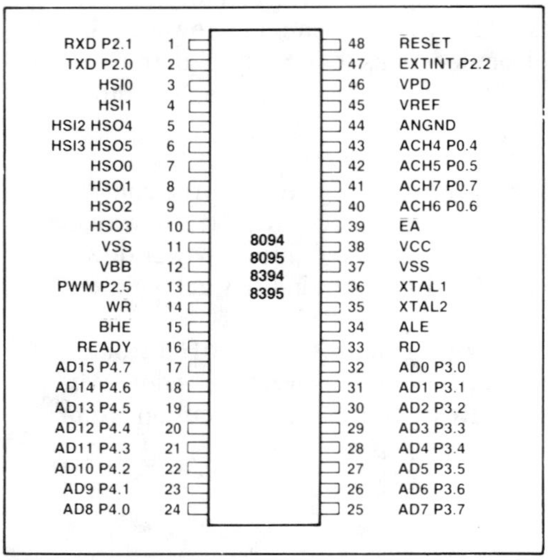

Figure 2. 48-Pin Package

The 48-pin version is offered in Dual-In-Line package while the 68-pin version comes in a Plastic Leaded Chip Carrier and a Pin Grid Array.

OPTIONS		68 PIN	48 PIN
DIGITAL I/O	ROMLESS	8096	8094
	ROM	8396	8394
ANALOG AND DIGITAL I/O	ROMLESS	8097	8095
	ROM	8397	8395

Figures 2, 3 & 4 show the pinouts for the 48- and 68-pin packages. The 48-pin version is offered in Dual-In-Line package while the 68-pin version comes in a Flat-pack and a Pin Grid Array.

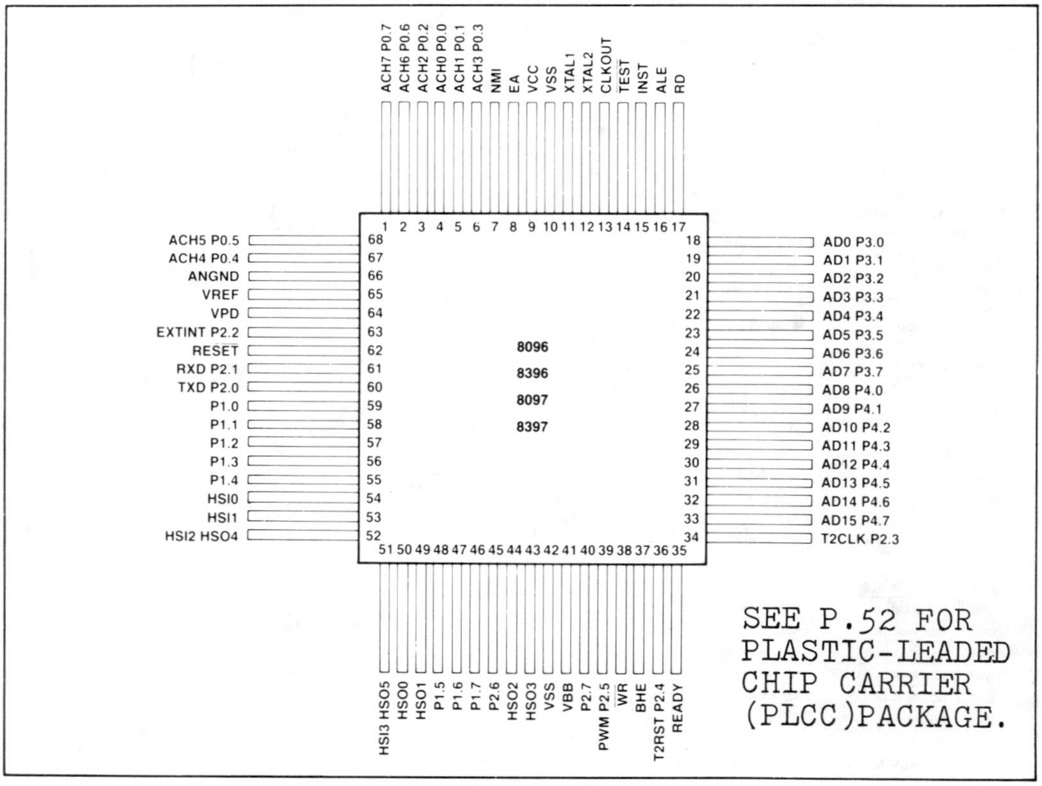

Figure 3. 68-Pin Package (Flat Pack-Top View)

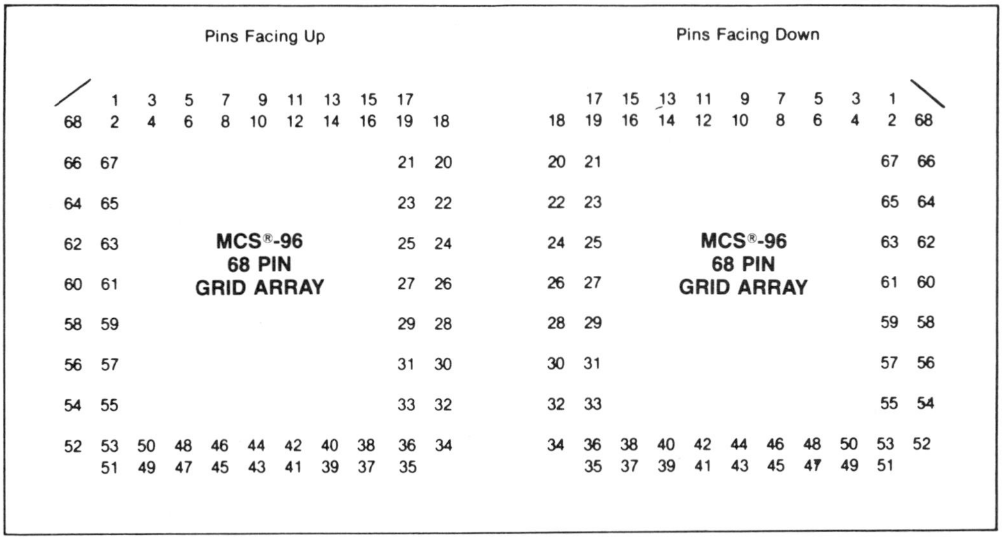

Figure 4. Pin Grid Array

Note

1. When the pin grid array package is mounted on the PC board, the pins are numbered counterclockwise as seen from the component side of the board, just like the flatpack when it's mounted in the contactor. Consequently, the PC board layout for pin grid array is compatible with the flat pack in a contactor except for the footprint size. The pin functions (from -1 to -68) on both packages are identical. Refer to Intel's Microcontroller handbook for mechanical dimensions on these packages.

2.16. PIN DESCRIPTION

VCC
Main supply voltage (5V).

VSS
Digital circuit ground (0V).There are two VSS pins, both must be tied to ground.

VPD
RAM standby supply voltage (5V). This voltage must be present during normal operation. See section 2.4.2 and 4.1.

VREF
Reference voltage and power supply for the analog portion of the A/D converter. Nominally at 5 volts. See section 2.9.1 and 4.1.

ANGND
Reference ground for the A/D converter. Should be held at nominally the same potential as VSS. See section 2.9.1 and 4.1.

VBB
Substrate voltage from the on-chip back-bias generator. This pin should be connected to ANGND through a 0.01 uf capacitor (and not connected to anything else). The capacitor is not required if the A/D convertor is not being used.

XTAL1
Input of the oscillator inverter and input to the internal clock generator. See sections 2.2 and 4.1.

XTAL2
Output of the oscillator inverter. See section 2.2.

CLKOUT
Output of the internal clock generator. The frequency of CLKOUT is ⅓ the oscillator frequency. It has a 33% duty cycle. CLKOUT can drive one TTL input. See section 2.2.

$\overline{\text{RESET}}$
Reset input to the chip, also output to other circuits. Input low for at least 2 state times to reset the chip. $\overline{\text{RESET}}$ has a strong internal pullup. See section 2.15 and 4.1.

$\overline{\text{TEST}}$
Input low enables a factory test mode. The user should tie this pin to VCC for normal operation.

NMI
A low to high transition a vector to *external* memory location 0000H. Reserved for use in Intel Development systems.

INST
Output high while the address is valid during an external read indicates the read is an instruction fetch. See section 2.3.5 and 4.6.

$\overline{\text{EA}}$
Input for memory select (External Access). $\overline{\text{EA}}$ = 1 causes memory accesses to locations 2000H through 3FFFH to be directed to on-chip ROM. $\overline{\text{EA}}$ = 0 causes accesses to these locations to be directed to off-chip memory. $\overline{\text{EA}}$ has an internal pulldown, so it goes to 0 unless driven to 1. See section 2.3.4.

ALE
Address Latch Enable output. ALE is activated only during external memory accesses. It is used to latch the address from the multiplexed address/data bus. See section 2.3.5 and 4.6.

$\overline{\text{RD}}$
Read signal output to external memory. $\overline{\text{RD}}$ is activated only during external memory reads. See section 2.3.5 and 4.6.

$\overline{\text{WR}}$
Write signal output to external memory. $\overline{\text{WR}}$ is activated only during external memory writes. See section 2.3.5 and 4.6.

$\overline{\text{BHE}}$
Bus High Enable signal output to external memory. $\overline{\text{BHE}}$ (0/1) selects/deselects the bank of memory that is connected to the high byte of the data bus. See section 2.3.5 and 4.6.

READY
The READY input is used to lengthen external memory bus cycles up to the time specified in the data sheet. It has a weak internal pullup. See section 2.3.5 and 4.6.

HSI
High impedance inputs to HSI Unit. Four HSI pins are available: HSI.0, HSI.1, HSI.2, and HSI.3. Two of them (HSI.2 and HSI.3) are shared with the HSO Unit. See section 2.7.

HSO
Outputs from HSO Unit. Six HSO pins are available: HSO.0, HSO.1, HSO.2, HSO.3, HSO.4, and HSO.5. Two of them (HSO.4 and HSO.5) are shared with the HSI Unit. All HSO pins are capable of driving one TTL input. See section 2.8.

PORT 0/ANALOG CHANNEL
High impedance input-only port. These pins can be used as digital inputs and/or as analog inputs to the on-chip A/D converter. See sections 2.9 and 2.12.1.

PORT 1
Quasi-bidirectional I/O port. All pins of P1 are capable of driving one LS TTL input. See section 2.1.2.

PORT 2
Multi-functional port. Six of its pins are shared with other functions in the 8096, as shown below.

Port	Function	Alternate Function	Reference section
P2.0	output	TXD (serial port transmit)	2.11.3
P2.1	input	RXD (serial port receive)	2.11.3
P2.2	input	EXTINT (external interrupt)	2.5
P2.3	input	T2CLK (Timer 2 input)	2.6.2
P2.4	input	T2RST (Timer 2 reset)	2.6.2
P2.5	output	PWM (pulse-width modulator)	2.10
P2.6	quasi-bidirectional		
P2.7	quasi-bidirectional		

The multi-functional inputs are high impedance. See section 2.1.3.

PORTS 3 AND 4
8-bit bidirectional I/O ports. These pins are shared the multiplexed address/data bus when accessing external memory, with the Port 3 pins accessing the low byte and Port 4 pins accessing the high byte. They are open drain except when being used as system bus pins. See section 2.3.5.

2.17. PIN LIST : PGA(PLCC ON P.52)

The following is a list of pins in alphabetical order. Where a pin has two names it has been listed under both names, except for the system bus pins, AD0-AD15, which are listed under Port 3 and Port 4.

Name	68-Pin	48-Pin
ACH0/P0.0	4	—
ACH1/P0.1	5	—
ACH2/P0.2	3	—
ACH3/P0.3	6	—
ACH4/P0.4	67	43
ACH5/P0.5	68	42
ACH6/P0.6	2	40
ACH7/P0.7	1	41
ALE	16	34
ANGND	66	44
BHE	37	15
CLKOUT	13	—
EA		39
EXTINT/P2.2	63	47
HSI.0	54	3
HSI.1	53	4
HSI.2/HSO.4	52	5
HSI.3/HSO.5	51	6
HSO.0	50	7
HSO.1	49	8
HSO.2	44	9
HSO.3	43	10
HSO.4/HSI.2	52	5
HSO.5/HSI.3	51	6
INST	15	—
NMI	7	—
PWM/P2.5	39	13
P0.0/ACH0	4	—
P0.1/ACH1	5	—
P0.2/ACH2	3	—
P0.3/ACH3	6	—
P0.4/ACH4	67	43
P0.5/ACH5	68	42
P0.6/ACH6	2	40
P0.7/ACH7	1	41
P1.0	59	—
P1.1	58	—
P1.2	57	—
P1.3	56	—
P1.4	55	—
P1.5	48	—
P1.6	47	—
P1.7	46	—
P2.0/TXD	60	2
P2.1/RXD	61	1
P2.2/EXTINT	63	47
P2.3/T2CLK	34	—
P2.4/T2RST	36	—
P2.5/PWM	39	13
P2.6	45	—
P2.7	40	—
P3.0/AD0	18	32
P3.1/AD1	19	31
P3.2/AD2	20	30
P3.3/AD3	21	29
P3.4/AD4	22	28
P3.5/AD5	23	27
P3.6/AD6	24	26
P3.7/AD7	25	25
P4.0/AD8	26	24
P4.1/AD9	27	23
P4.2/AD10	28	22
P4.3/AD11	29	21
P4.4/AD12	30	20
P4.5/AD13	31	19
P4.6/AD14	32	18
P4.7/AD15	33	17
RD	17	33
READY	35	16
RESET	62	48
RXD/P2.1	61	1
TEST	14	—
TXD/P2.0	60	2
T2CLK/P2.3	34	—
T2RST/P2.4	36	—
VBB	41	12
VCC	9	38
VPD	64	46
VREF	65	45
VSS	10	11
VSS	42	37
WR	38	14
XTAL1	11	36
XTAL2	12	35

The Following pins are not bonded out in the 48-pin package:

P1.0 through P1.7, P0.0 through P0.3, P2.3, P2.4, P2.6, P2.7 CLKOUT, INST, NMI, TEST, T2CLK(P2.3), T2RST(P2.4).

Note: Pin # for EA in 68 pin version should be 8.

C. PROGRAM STATUS WORD (FLAGS)

3.3 PROGRAM STATUS WORD

The program status word (PSW) is a collection of Boolean flags which retain information concerning the state of the user's program. The format of the PSW is shown in figure 3-1. The information in the PSW can be broken down into two basic categories; interrupt control and condition flags. The PSW can be saved in the system stack with a single operation (PUSHF) and restored in a like manner (POPF).

15	14	13	12	11	10	09	08	07	06	05	04	03	02	01	00
Z	N	V	VT	C	—	I	ST	<Interrupt Mask Reg>							

Figure 3-1. PSW Register

3.3.1. Interrupt Flags

The lower eight bits of the PSW are used to individually mask the various sources of interrupt to the 8096. A logical '1' in these bit positions enables the servicing of the corresponding interrupt. These mask bits can be accessed as an eight bit byte (INT_MASK — address 8) in the on-board register file. Bit 9 in the PSW is the global interrupt enable. If this bit is cleared then all interrupts will be locked out except for the Non Maskable Interrupt (NMI). Note that the various interrupts are collected in the INT_PENDING register even if they are locked out. Execution of the corresponding service routines will procede according to their priority when they become enabled. Further information on the interrupt structure of the 8096 can be found in sections 2.5 and 3.6.

3.3.2. Condition Flags

The remaining bits in the PSW are set as side effects of instruction execution and can be tested by the conditional jump instructions.

Z. The Z (Zero) flag is set to indicate that the operation generated a result equal to zero. For the add-with-carry (ADDC) and subtract-with-borrow (SUBC) operations the Z flag is cleared if the result is non-zero but is never set. These two instructions are normally used in conjunction with the ADD and SUB instructions to perform multiple precision arithmetic. The operation of the Z flag for these instructions leaves it indicating the proper result for the entire multiple precision calculation.

N. The N (Negative) flag is set to indicate that the operation generated a negative result. Note that the N flag will be set to the algebraically correct state even if the calculation overflows.

V. The V (oVerflow) flag is set to indicate that the operation generated a result which is outside the range that can be expressed in the destination data type.

VT. The VT (oVerflow Trap) flag is set whenever the V flag is set but can only be cleared by an instruction which explicitly operates on it such as the CLRVT or JVT instructions. The operation of the VT flag allows for the testing for a possible overflow condition at the end of a sequence of related arithmetic operations. This is normally more efficient than testing the V flag after each instruction.

C. The C (Carry) flag is set to indicate the state of the arithmetic carry from the most significant bit of the ALU for an arithmetic operation or the state of the last bit shifted out of the operand for a shift. Arithmetic Borrow after a subtract operation is the complement of the C flag (i.e. if the operation generated a borrow then C=0).

ST. The ST (STicky bit) set to indicate that during a right shift a 1 has been shifted first into the C flag and then been shifted out. The ST flag is undefined after a multiply operation. The ST flag can be used along with the C flag to control rounding after a right shift. Consider multiplying two eight bit quantities and then scaling the result down to 12 bits:

```
MULUB    AX,CL,DL    ; AX:=CL*DL
SHR      AX,#4       ; Shift right 4 places
```

If the C flag is set after the shift it indicates that the bits shifted off the end of operand were greater-than or equal-to one half the least significant bit (LSB) of the result. If the C flag is clear after the shift it indicates that the bits shifted off the end of the operand were less than half the LSB of the result. Without the ST flag, the rounding decision must be made on the basis of this information alone. (Normally the result would be rounded up if the C flag is set.) The ST flag allows a finer resolution in the rounding decision:

C ST	Value of the bits shifted off
0 0	Value = 0
0 1	0 < Value < ½ LSB
1 0	Value = ½ LSB
1 1	Value > ½ LSB

Figure 3-2. Rounding Alternatives

Imprecise rounding can be a major source of error in a numerical calculation; use of the ST flag improves the options available to the programmer.

D. THE SPECIAL FUNCTION REGISTERS (SFRs): DESCRIPTION, MEMORY MAP, ADDRESSES.

2.4.1. Special Function Registers

All of the I/O on the 8096 is controlled through the SFRs. Many of these registers serve two functions; one if they are read from, the other if they are written to. Figure 2-7 shows the locations and names of these registers. A summary of the capabilities of each of these registers is shown in Figure 2-8, with complete descriptions reserved for later

Register	Description	Chapter
R0	Zero Register — Always reads as a zero, useful for a base when indexing and as a constant for calculations and compares.	3.2.7
AD_RESULT	A/D Result Hi/Low — Low and high order Results of the A/D converter (byte read only)	2.9.3
AD_COMMAND	A/D Command Register — Controls the A/D	2.9.2
HSI_MODE	HSI Mode Register — Sets the mode of the High Speed Input unit.	2.7.1
HSI_TIME	HSI Time Hi/Lo — Contains the time at which the High Speed Input unit was triggered. (word read only)	2.7.4
HSO_TIME	HSO Time Hi/Lo — Sets the time for the High Speed Output to execute the command in the Command Register. (word write only)	2.8.3
HSO_COMMAND	HSO Command Register — Determines what will happen at the time loaded into the HSO Time registers.	2.8.2
HSI_STATUS	HSI Status Registers — Indicates which HSI pins were detected at the time in the HSI Time registers.	2.7.4
SBUF (TX)	Transmit buffer for the serial port, holds contents to be outputed.	2.11
SBUF (RX)	Receive buffer for the serial port, holds the byte just received by the serial port.	2.11
INT_MASK	Interrupt Mask Register — Enables or disables the individual interrupts.	2.5.2 3.6.2
INT_PENDING	Interrupt Pending Register — Indicates when an interrupt signal has occurred on one of the sources.	2.5.2 3.6.2
WATCHDOG	Watchdog Timer Register — Written to periodically to hold off automatic reset every 64K state times.	2.14
TIMER1	Timer 1 Hi/Lo — Timer 1 high and low bytes. (word read only)	2.6.1 2.7-8
TIMER2	Timer 2 Hi/Lo — Timer 2 high and low bytes. (word read only)	2.6.2 2.7-8
IOPORT0	Port 0 Register — Levels on pins of port 0.	2.12.1
BAUD_RATE	Register which contains the baud rate, this register is loaded sequentially.	2.11.4
IOPORT1	Port 1 Register — Used to read or write to Port 1.	2.12.2
IOPORT2	Port 2 Register — Used to read or write to Port 2.	2.12.3
SP_STAT	Serial Port Status — Indicates the status of the serial port.	2.11.3
SP_CON	Serial port control — Used to set the mode of the serial port.	2.11.1
IOS0	I/O Status Register 0 — Contains information on the HSO status.	2.13.4
IOS1	I/O Status Register 1 — Contains information on the status of the timers and of the HSI.	2.13.5 3.7.2
IOC0	I/O Control Register 0 — Controls alternate functions of HSI pins, Timer 2 reset sources and Timer 2 clock sources.	2.13.2
IOC1	I/O Control Register 1 — Controls alternate functions of Port 2 pins, timer interrupts and HSI interrupts.	2.13.3
PWM_CONTROL	Pulse Width Modulation Control Register — Sets the duration of the PWM pulse.	2.10

Figure 2-8. SFR Summary

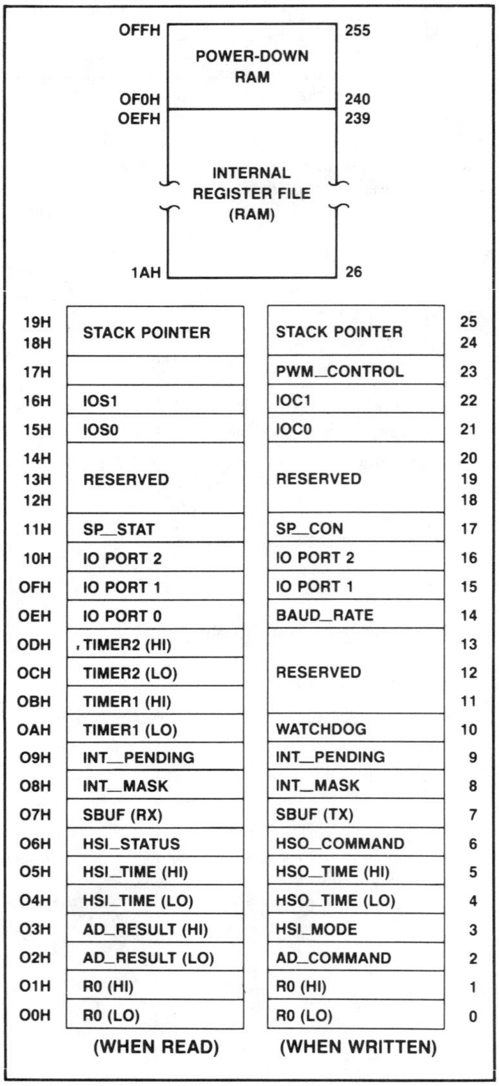

Figure 2-7. Register File Memory Map

2.4. RAM SPACE

The internal register locations on the 8096 are divided into two groups, a register file and a set of Special Function Registers (SFRs). The RALU can operate on any of these 256 internal register locations. Locations 00H through 17H are used to access the SFRs. Locations 18H and 19H contain the stack pointer. The stack pointer must be initialized by the user program and can point anywhere in the 64K memory space. The stack builds down. There are no restrictions on the use of the remaining 230 locations except that code cannot be executed from them.

Within the SFR space are several registers labeled as ''RESERVED''. These registers are reserved for future expansion or test purposes. Reads or writes of these registers may produce unexpected results. For example, writing to location 000CH will set both timers to 0FFFXH, this feature is for use in testing the part and should not be used in programs.

2.4.2. Power Down

The upper 16 RAM locations (0F0H through 0FFH) receive their power from both the VCC pin and the VPD pin. If it is desired to keep the memory in these locations alive during a power down situation, one need only keep voltage on the VPD pin. The current required to keep the RAM alive is approximately 1 milliamp (refer to the data sheet for the exact specification).

To place the 8096 into a power down mode, the $\overline{\text{RESET}}$ pin is pulled low. Two state times later the part will be in reset. This is necessary to prevent the part from writing into RAM as the power goes down. The power may now be removed from the VCC pin, the VPD pin must remain within specifications. The 8096 can remain in this state for any amount of time and the 16 RAM bytes will retain their values.

To bring the 8096 out of power down, $\overline{\text{RESET}}$ is held low while VCC is applied. Two state times after the oscillator and the back bias generator have stabilized (~1 millisecond), the $\overline{\text{RESET}}$ pin can be pulled high. The 8096 will begin to execute code at location 02080H 10 state times after $\overline{\text{RESET}}$ is pulled high. Figure 2-9 shows a timing diagram of the power down sequence. To ensure that the 2 state time minimum reset time (synchronous with CLKOUT) is met, it is recommended that 10 XTAL1

E. 8096 INTERRUPTS: INTERRUPT MASK AND INTERRUPT PENDING SFRs, GLOBAL INTERRUPT BIT, INTERRUPT SOURCES, PRIORITIES, INTERRUPT VECTOR LOCATIONS.

Please note that the global interrupt enable bit PSW.9 (I) overrides all other interrupt considerations. If it is set (I=1) in the program (EI instruction), interrupts will be honored provided one is pending and the interrupt source's mask bit is set. If it is disabled (I=0) in the program (DI instruction) interrupts will not be honored but become pending and will be serviced when I is made 1 (EI), provided the interrupt source's mask bit was set to 1. Their servicing follows a priority ordering as indicated below. (See also section C on the Program Status Word and Interrupt Flags).

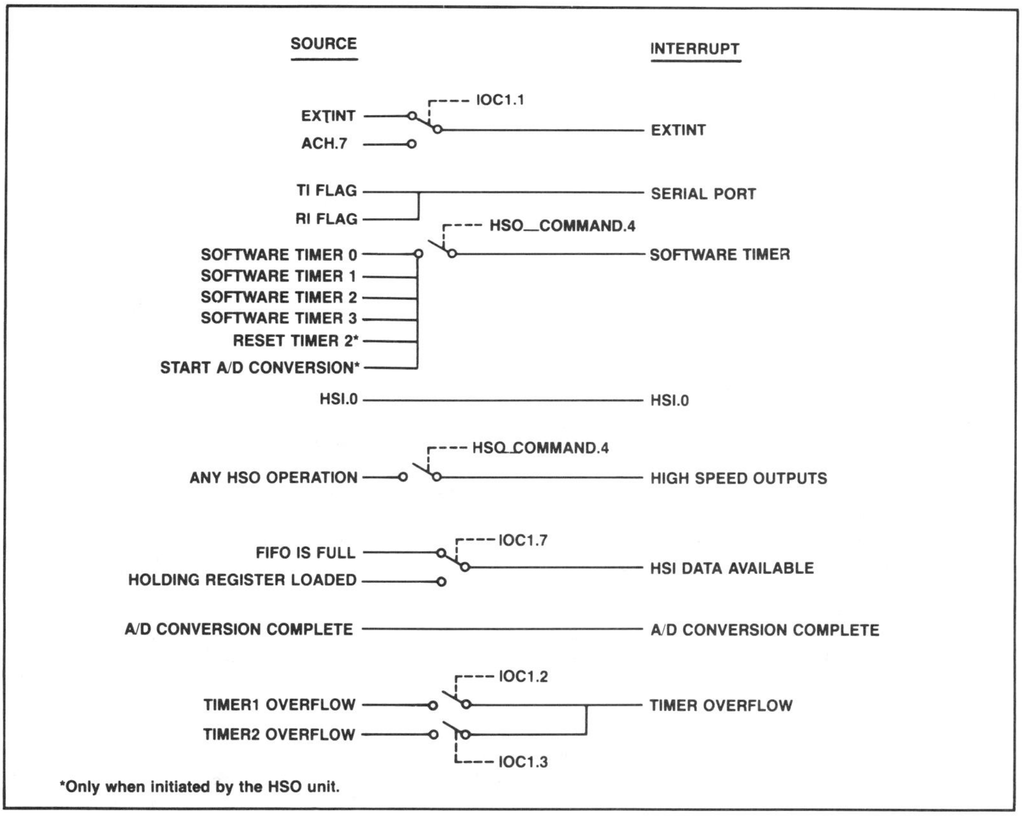

Figure 2-11. All Possible Interrupt Sources

Enabling and disabling of individual interrupts is done through the Interrupt Mask Register, located at 0008H. If the bit in the mask register is a 1 then the interrupt is enabled, otherwise it is disabled. Even if an interrupt is masked it may still become pending. It may, therefore, be desirable to clear the pending bit before unmasking an interrupt.

The Interrupt Mask Register is also the low byte of the PSW. All of the interrupts may be enabled and disabled simultaneously by using the "EI" (Enable Interrupt) and "DI" (Disable Interrupt) instructions. EI and DI set and clear PSW.9, the interrupt enable bit, they do not effect the contents of the mask register.

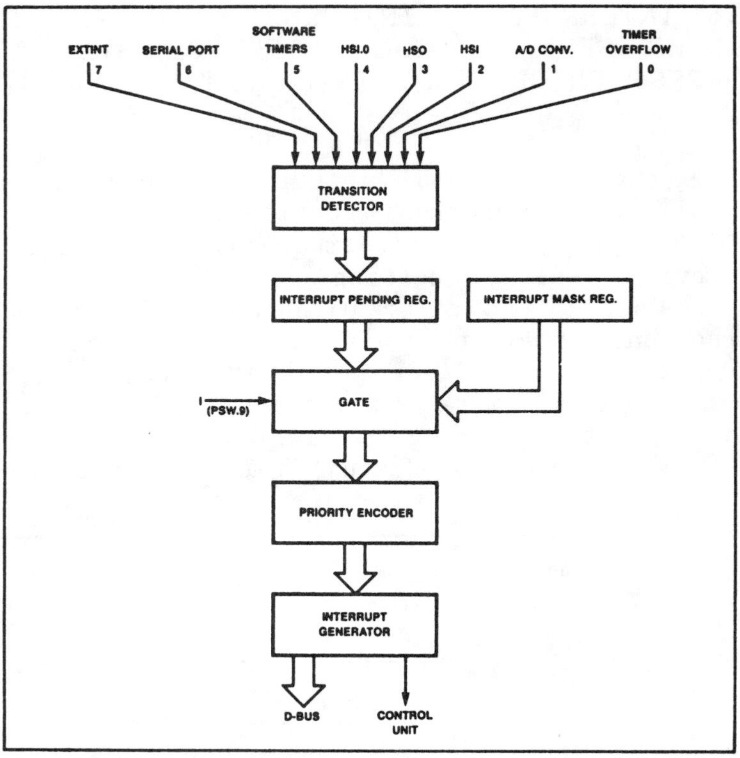

Figure 2-12. Block Diagram of Interrupt System

2.5.1. Interrupt Sources

Eight interrupt sources are available on the 8096. When enabled, an interrupt occurring on any of these sources will force a call to the location stored in the vector location for that source. The interrupt sources and their respective vector locations are listed in Figure 2-10. In addition to the 8 standard interrupts, there is a TRAP instruction which acts as a software generated interrupt. This instruction is not currently supported by the MCS-96 Assembler and is reserved for use by Intel development systems. Many of the interrupt sources can be activated by several methods, Figure 2-11 shows all of the possible sources for interrupts.

Source	Vector Location		Priority
	(High Byte)	(Low Byte)	
Software	2011H	2010H	Not Applicable
Extint	200FH	200EH	7 (Highest)
Serial Port	200DH	200CH	6
Software Timers	200BH	200AH	5
HSI.0	2009H	2008H	4
High Speed Outputs	2007H	2006H	3
HSI Data Available	2005H	2004H	2
A/D Conversion Complete	2003H	2002H	1
Timer Overflow	2001H	2000H	0 (Lowest)

Figure 2-10. Interrupt Vector Locations

2.5.2. Interrupt Control

A block diagram of the interrupt system is shown in Figure 2-12. Each of the interrupt sources is tested for a 0 to 1 transition. If this transition occurs, the corresponding bit in the Interrupt Pending Register, located at 0009H, is set. The bit is cleared when the vector is taken to the interrupt routine. Since this register can be written to, it is possible to generate software interrupts by setting bits within the register, or remove pending interrupts by clearing the bits in this register. The pending register can be set even if the interrupt is disabled.

Caution must be used when writing to the pending register to clear interrupts. If the interrupt has already been acknowledged when the bit is cleared, a 4 state time ''partial'' interrupt cycle will occur. This is because the 8096 will have to fetch the next instruction of the normal instruction flow, instead of proceeding with the interrupt processing as it was going to. The effect on the program will be essentially that of an extra NOP. This can be prevented by clearing the bits using a 2 operand immediate logical, as the 8096 holds off acknowledging interrupts during these ''read/modify/write'' instructions.

2.5.3. Interrupt Priority Programming

The priority encoder looks at all of the interrupts which are *both pending and enabled,* and selects the one with the highest priority. The priorities are shown in Figure 2-10 (7 is highest, 0 is lowest.) The interrupt generator then forces a call to the location in the indicated vector location. This location would be the starting location of the Interrupt Service Routine (ISR).

3.6.1. Global Lockout

The processing of interrupts can be enabled or disabled by setting or clearing the I bit in the PSW. This is accomplished by the EI (Enable Interrupts) and DI (Disable Interrupts) instructions. Note that the I bit only controls the actual servicing of interrupts; interrupts that occur during periods of lockout will be held in the pending register and serviced on a prioritized basis when the lockout period ends.

3.6.2. Pending Interrupt Register

When the hardware detects one of the eight interrupts it sets the corresponding bit in the pending interrupt register (INT_PENDING-register 09H). This register, which has the same bit layout as the interrupt mask register (see next section), can be read or modified as a byte register. This register can be read to determine which of the interrupts are pending at any given time or modified to either clear pending interrupts or generate interrupts under software control. Any software which modifies the INT_PENDING register should ensure that the entire operation is indivisible. The easiest way of doing this is to use the logical instructions in the two or three operand format, as examples:

```
ANDB    INT_PENDING,#11111101B
ORB     ; Clears the A/D interrupt
        INT_PENDING,#00000010B
        Sets the A/D interrupt
```

If the required modification to INT_PENDING cannot be accomplished with one instruction then a critical region should be established and the INT_PENDING register modified from within this region (see section 3.6.5).

3.6.3. Interrupt Mask Register

Individual interrupts can be enabled or disabled by setting or clearing bits in the interrupt mask register (INT_MASK-register 08H). The format of this register is shown in figure 3-4.

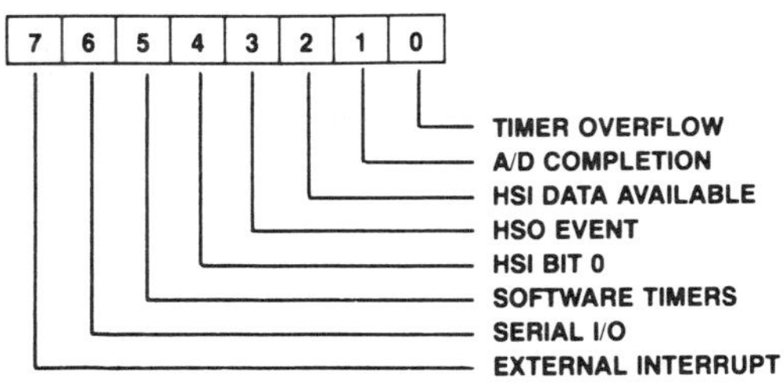

Figure 3-4. Interrupt Mask Register

The INT_MASK register can be read or written as a byte register. A one in any bit position will enable the corresponding interrupt source and a zero will disable the source. The individual masks act like the global lockout in that they only control the servicing of the interrupt; the hardware will save any interrupts that occur in the pending register even if the interrupt mask bit is cleared. The INT_MASK register also can be accessed as the lower eight bits of the PSW so the PUSHF and POPF instructions save and restore the INT_MASK register as well as the global interrupt lockout and the arithmetic flags.

3.6.4. Interrupt Vectors

The 8096 has eight sources of hardware interrupt, each with its own priority and interrupt vector location. Table 3-6 shows the interrupt sources, their priority, and their vector locations. See section 2.5 for a discussion of the various interrupt sources.

Table 3-5. Interrupt Vector Information

Source	Priority	Vector
Timer Overflow	0-Lowest	2000H
A/D Completion	1	2002H
HSI Data Available	2	2004H
HSO Excution	3	2006H
HSI.O	4	2008H
Software timers	5	200AH
Serial I/O	6	200CH
External Interrupt	7-Highest	200EH

The programmer must initialize the interrupt vector table with the starting addresses of the appropriate interrupt service routine. It would be a good idea to vector any interrupts that are not used in the system to an error handling routine.

The priorities given in the table give the *hardware* enforced priorities for these interrupts. This priority controls the order in which pending interrupts are passed to the software via interrupt-calls. The software can implement its own priority structure by controlling the mask register (INT_MASK-register 08H). To see how this is done consider the case of a serial I/O service routine which must run at a priority level which is lower than the HSI data available interrupt but higher than any other source. The "preamble" and exit code for this interrupt service routine would look like this:

```
serial_io_isr:
    PUSHF                       ; Save the PSW
                                  (Includes INT_MASK)
    LDB   INT_MASK,#00000100B
    EI                          ; Enable interrupts again
    ;
    ;
    ;
    ;      Service the interrupt
    ;
    ;
    ;
    POPF                        ; Restore the PSW
    RET
```

Note that location 200CH in the interrupt vector table would have to be loaded with the value of the label serial_io_isr and the interrupt be enabled for this routine to execute.

F. PULSE WIDTH MODULATION: THE PWM SFR.

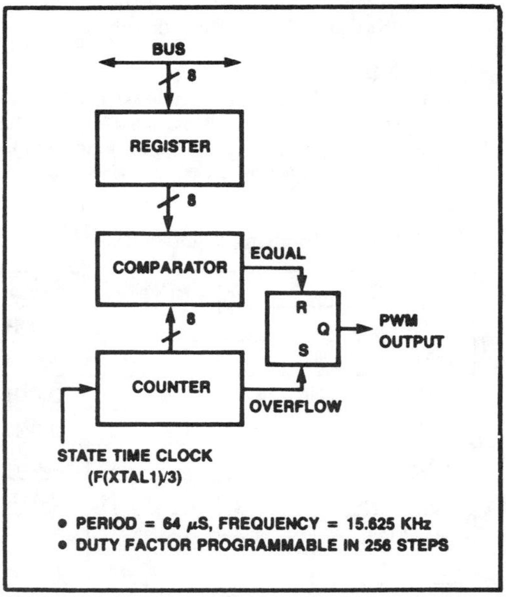

Figure 2-21. Pulse Width Modulated (D/A) Output

2.10. PULSE WIDTH MODULATION OUTPUT (D/A)

Digital to analog conversion can be done with the pulse width modulation output; a block diagram of the circuit is shown in Figure 2-21. The 8-bit counter is incremented every state time. When it equals 0, the PWM output is set to a one. When the counter matches the value in the PWM register, the output is switched low. When the counter overflows, the output is once again switched high. A typical output waveform is shown in Figure 2-22. Note that when the PWM register equals 00, the output is always low.

The output waveform is a variable duty cycle pulse which repeats every 256 state times (64 μS at 12MHz). Changes in the duty cycle are made by writing to the PWM register at location 17H. There are several types of motors which require a PWM waveform for most efficient operation. Additionally, if this waveform is integrated it will produce a DC level which can be changed in 256 steps by varying the duty cycle.

Details about the hardware required for smooth, accurate D/A conversion can be found in section 4.3.2. Typically, some form of buffer and integrator are needed to obtain the most usefulness from this feature.

The PWM output shares a pin with Port 2, pin 5 so that these two features cannot be used at the same time. IOC1.0 equal to 1 selects the PWM function instead of the standard port function. More information on IOC1 is in section 2.13.3.

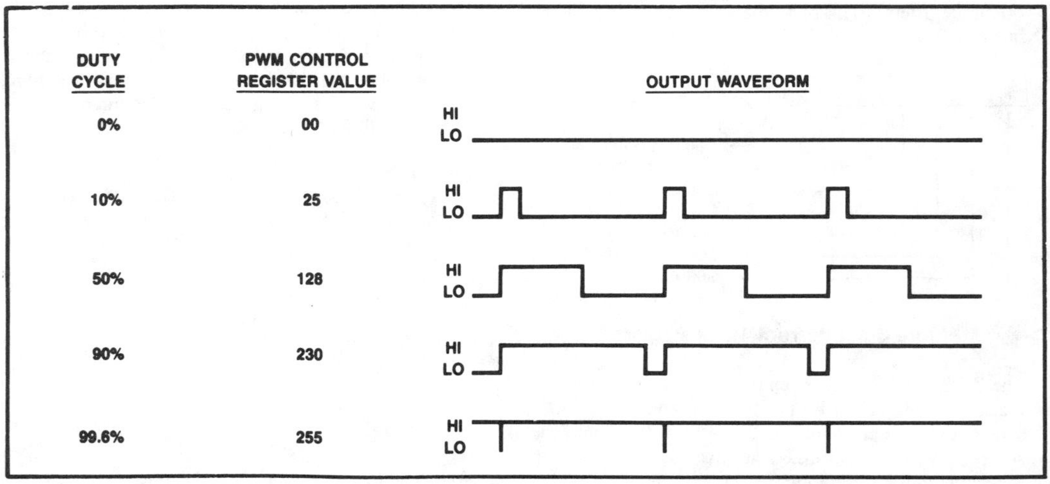

Figure 2-22. Typical PWM Outputs

4.3.2. Analog Output Suggestions

Analog outputs can be generated by two methods, either by using the PWM output or the HSO. Either device will generate a rectangular pulse training that varies in duty cycle and (for the HSO only) period. If a smooth analog signal is desired as an output, the rectangular waveform must be filtered.

In most cases this filtering is best done after the signal is buffered to make it swing from 0 to 5 volts since both of the outputs are guaranteed only to TTL levels. A block diagram of the type of circuit needed is shown in Figure 4-11. By proper selection of components, accounting for temperature and power supply drift, a highly accurate 8-bit D to A converter can be made using either the HSO or the PWM output. If the HSO is used the accuracy could be theoretically extended to 16-bits, however the temperature and noise related problems would be extremely hard to handle.

When driving some circuits it may be desirable to use unfiltered Pulse Width Modulation. This is particularly true for motor drive circuits. The PWM output can be used to generate these waveforms if a fixed period on the order of 64 uS is acceptable. If this is not the case then the HSO unit can be used. The HSO can generate a variable waveform with a duty cycle variable in up to 65536 steps and a period of up to 131 milliseconds. Both of these outputs produce TTL levels.

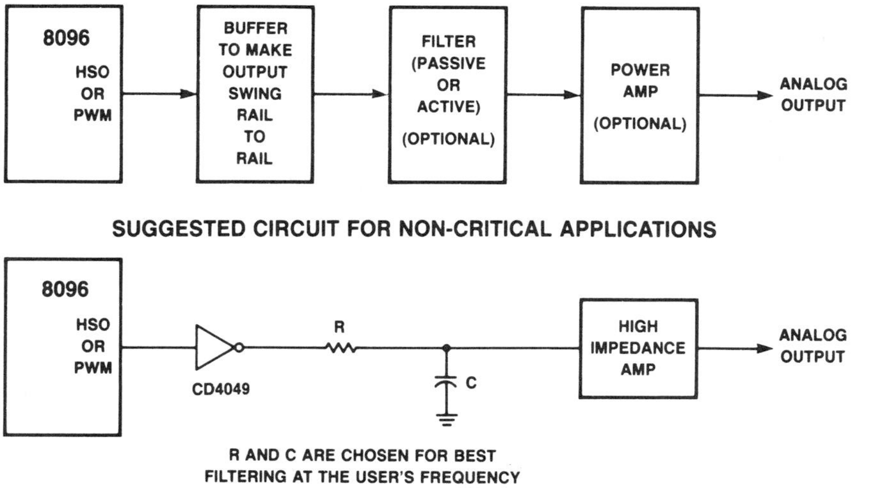

Figure 4-11. D/A Buffer Block Diagram

G. A/D CONVERSION AND RELEVANT SFRs.

2.9. ANALOG INPUTS

The A to D converter on the 8096 provides a 10-bit result on one of 8 input channels. Conversion is done using successive approximation with a result equal to the ratio of the input voltage divided by the analog supply voltage. If the ratio is 1.00, then the result will be all ones. The A/D converter is available on the 8097, 8397, 8095 and 8395 members of the MCS®-96 family.

2.9.1. A/D Accuracy

Each conversion requires 168 state-times (42μS at 12 MHz) independent of the accuracy desired or value of input voltage. The input voltage must be in the range of 0 to VREF, the analog reference and supply voltage. For proper operation, VREF (the reference voltage and analog power supply) must be held at VCC ± 0.3V with VREF = 5.0 ± 0.5V. The A/D result is calculated from the formula:

$$1023 \times (\text{input voltage-AVGND}) \,/\, (\text{VREF-AVGND})$$

It can be seen from this formula that changes in VREF or AVGND effect the output of the converter. This can be advantageous if a ratiometric sensor is used since these sensors have an output that can be measured as a proportion of VREF.

If high absolute accuracy is needed it may be desirable to use a separate power supply, or power traces, to operate the A/D converter. There is no sample and hold circuit internal to the chip, so the input voltage must be held constant for the entire 168 state times. Examples of connecting the A/D converter to various devices are given in section 4.3.

2.9.2. A/D Commands

Analog signals can be sampled by any one of the 8 analog input pins (ACH0 through ACH7) which are shared with Port 0. ACH7 can also be used as an external interrupt if IOC1.1 is set (see section 2.5). The A/D Command Register, at location 02H, selects which channel is to be converted and whether the conversion should start immediately or when the HSO (Channel #14) triggers it. A to D commands are formatted as shown in Figure 2-19.

The command register is double buffered so it is possible

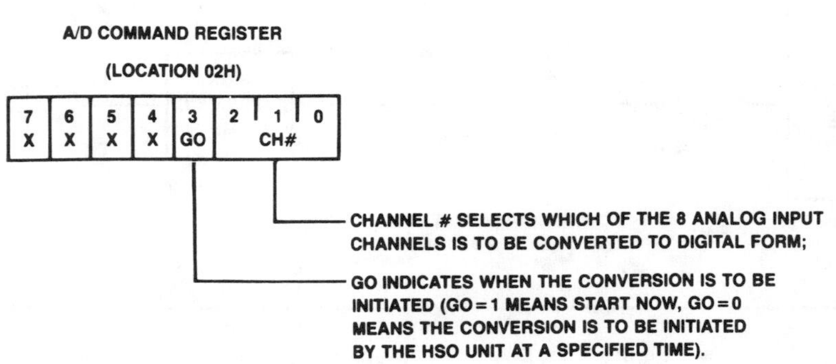

Figure 2-19. A/D Command Register

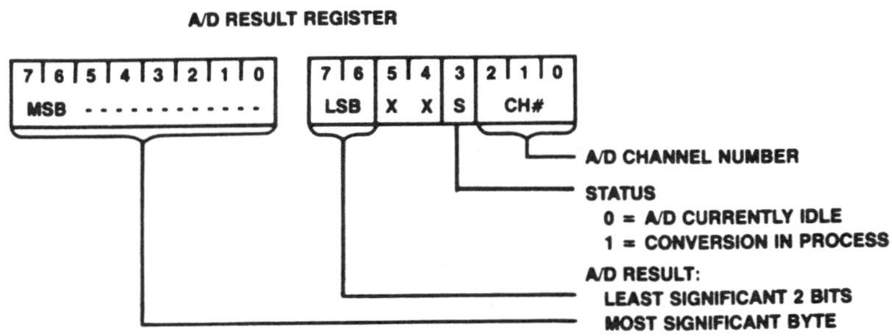

Figure 2-20. A/D Result Register

to write a command to start a conversion triggered by the HSO while one is still in progress. Care must be taken when this is done since if a new conversion is started while one is already in progress, the conversion in progress is cancelled and the new one is started. When a conversion is started, the result register is cleared. For this reason the result register must be read before a new conversion is started or data will be lost.

2.9.3. A/D Results

Results of the analog conversions are read from the A/D Result Register at locations 02H and 03H. Although these addresses are on a word boundary, they must be read as individual bytes. Information in the A/D Result register is formatted as shown in Figure 2-20. Note that the status bit may not be set until 8 state times after the go command. Information on using the HSO is in section 2.8.

4.3. ANALOG INTERFACE

Interfacing the 8096 to analog signal can be done in several ways. If the 8096 needs to measure an analog signal the A to D converter can be used. Creation of analog outputs can be done with either the PWM output or the HSO unit.

4.3.1. Analog Inputs

The 8096 can have 8 analog inputs and can convert one input at a time into a digital value. Each conversion takes 42 microseconds with a 12 MHz signal on XTAL1. The input signal is applied to one of the Port 0/Analog Channel inputs. Since there is no sample and hold on the A to D, the input signal must remain constant over the sampling period.

Whan a conversion takes place, the 8096 compares the external signal to that of its internal D to A. Based on the result of the comparison it adjusts the D to A and compares again. Each comparison takes 8 state times.

20 comparisons are made during a conversion, two times for each bit of resolution. An additional 8 states are used to load and store values. The total number of state times required is 168 for a 10-bit conversion. Attempting to do other than a 10-bit conversion is not recommended.

Since the capacitance of the comparator input is around 0.5pf, the sample and hold circuit must be able to charge a 10pf (20*0.5pf) capacitor without a significant voltage change. To keep the effect of the sample and hold circuit below ±½ lsb on a 10-bit converter, the voltage on the sample and hold circuit may vary no more than 0.05% (1/2048).

The effective capacitance of the sample and hold must, therefore, be at least 20000pf or 0.02 uf. If there is external leakage on the capacitor, its value must be increased to compensate for the leakage. At 10μA leakage, 2.5 mV (5/2048) will be lost from a 0.17 uf capacitor in 42 μS. The capacitor connected externally to the pin should, therefore, be at least 0.2 uf for best results. If the external signal changes slowly relative to 42 μS, then a larger capacitor will work well and also filter out unwanted noise.

The converter is a 10-bit, successive approximation, ratiometric converter, so the numerical value obtained from the conversion will be:

1023 * (VIN-ANGND) / (VREF-ANGND)

It can be seen that the power supply levels strongly influence the absolute accuracy of the conversion. For this reason, it is recommended that the ANGND pin be tied to a clean ground, as close to the power supply as possible. VREF should be well regulated and used only for the A to D converter. If ratiometric information is derived, VREF can be connected to VCC, but this should be done at the power supply not at the chip. It needs to be able to source around 15 milliamps. Bypass capacitors should be used between VREF and ANGND. ANGND should be within about a tenth of a volt of VSS and VREF should be within a few tenths of a volt of VCC. A 0.01 uf capacitor should be connected between the ANGND and VBB pins to reduce the noise on VBB and provide the highest possible accuracy. Figure 4-5 shows all of these connections.

H. SERIAL COMMUNICATIONS: MODES AND THE SERIAL PORT'S CONTROL/STATUS SFRs. BAUD AND SBUF SFRs.

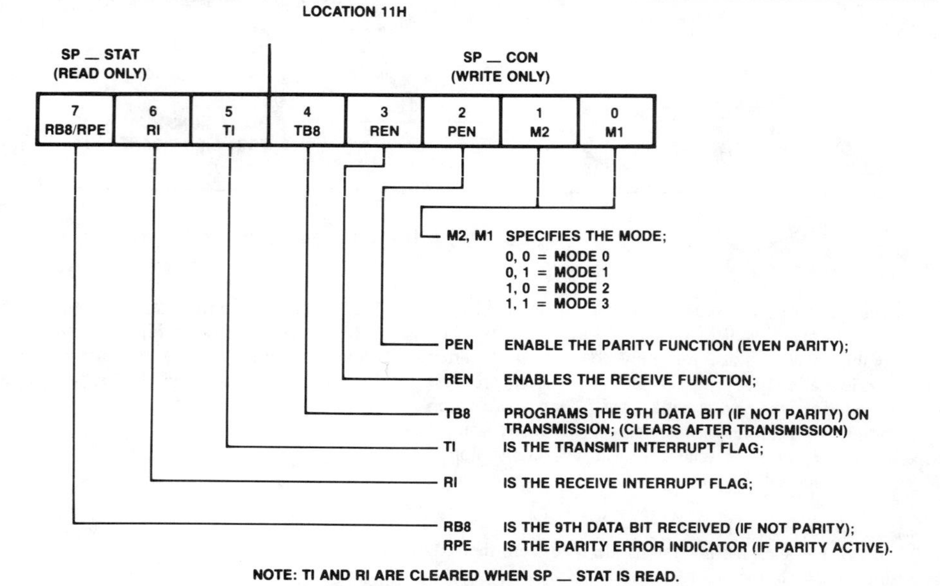

Figure 2-27. Serial Port Control/Status Register

2.11. SERIAL PORT

The serial port is compatible with the MCS-51 serial port. It is full duplex, meaning it can transmit and receive simultaneously. It is also receive-buffered, meaning it can commence reception of a second byte before a previously received byte has been read from the receive register. The serial port registers (SBUF) are both accessed at location 07H. A write to this location accesses the transmit register, and a read accesses a physically separate receive register.

The serial port can operate in 4 modes (explained below). Selection of these modes is done through the Serial Port Status/Control register at location 11H, shown in Figure 2-27.

2.11.1. Serial Port Modes

MODE 0

Mode 0 is a shift register mode. The 8096 outputs a train of 8 shift pulses to an external shift register to clock 8 bits of data into or out of the register from or to the 8096. Serial data enters and exits the 8096 through RXD. TXD outputs the shift clock. 8 bits are transmitted or received, LSB first. A timing diagram of this mode is shown in Figure 2-24. This mode is useful as an I/O expander in which application external shift registers can be used as additional parallel I/O ports. An example of using the port in this mode is given in section 4.5.

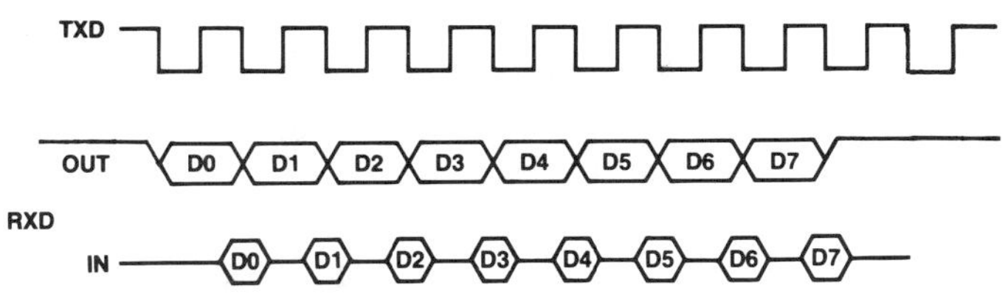

Figure 2-24. Serial Port Mode 0 Timing

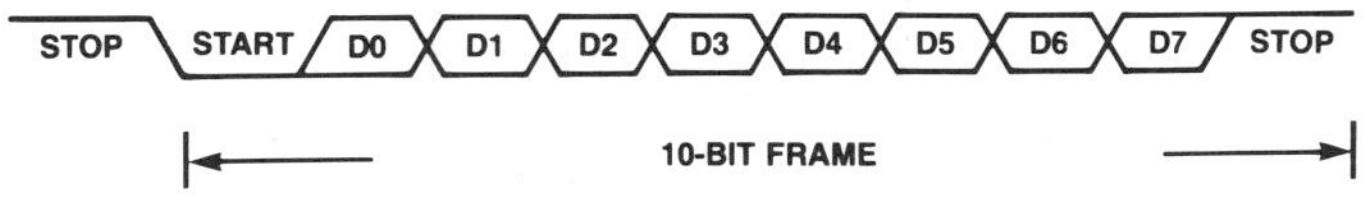

Figure 2-25. Serial Port Frame — Mode 1

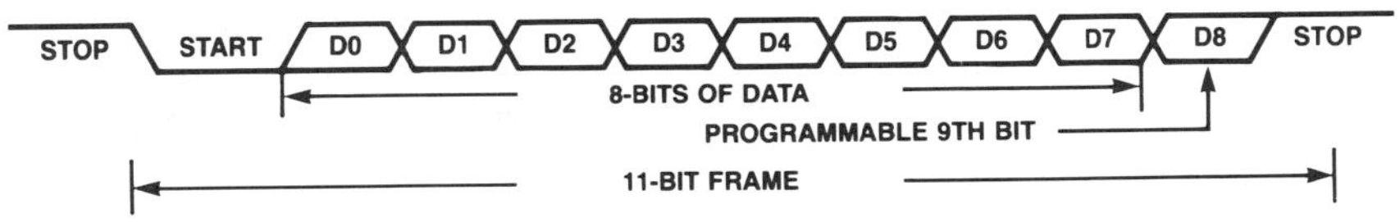

Figure 2-26. Serial Port Frame Modes 2 and 3

MODE 1
10-bit frames are transmitted through TXD, and received through RXD: a start bit (0), 8 data bits (LSB first), and a stop bit (1). If PEN = 1 then an even parity bit is transmitted instead of the eighth data bit. This mode is the one commonly used for CRT terminals. The data frame for Mode 1 is shown in Figure 2-25.

MODE 2
11-bit frames are transmitted through TXD and received through RXD: a start bit (0), 8 data bits (LSB first), a programmable 9th data bit, and a stop bit (1). On transmit, the 9th data bit can be assigned the value of 0 or 1 using the TB8 bit. This bit is cleared on each transmission. On receive, the serial port interrupt is not activated unless the received 9th data bit is 1. Parity cannot be enabled in this mode. This mode is commonly used along with mode 3 in a multiprocessor environment.

MODE 3
11-bit frames are transmitted through TXD and received through RXD: a start bit (0), 8 data bits (LSB first), a programmable 9th data bit, and a stop bit (1). On transmit, the 9th data bit can be assigned the value of 0 or 1 using the TB8 bit. If PEN = 1 the 9th bit will be parity. On receive, the received 9th data bit is stored and the serial port interrupt is activated regardless of its value. The data frame for Modes 2 and 3 is shown in Figure 2-26.

2.11.2. Multiprocessor Communications

Mode 2 and 3 are provided for multiprocessor communications. In mode 2 if the received 9th data bit is not 1, the serial port interrupt is not activated. The way to use this feature in multiprocessor systems is described below.

When the master processor wants to transmit a block of data to one of several slaves, it first sends out an address frame which identifies the target slave. An address frame will differ from a data frame in that the 9th data bit is 1 in an address frame and 0 in a data frame. No slave in mode 2 will be interrupted by a data frame. An address frame, however, will interrupt all slaves so that each slave can examine the received byte and see if it is being addressed. The addressed slave switches to mode 3 to receive the coming data frames, while the slaves that were not addressed stay in mode 2 and go on about their business.

2.11.3. Controlling the Serial Port

Control of the Serial Port is done through the Serial Port Control/Status register. The format for the control word is shown in Figure 2-27. Note that reads access only part of the byte, as do writes, and that TB8 is cleared after each byte is transmitted.

In Mode 0, if REN=0, writing to SBUF will start a transmission. Causing a rising edge on REN, or clearing RI with REN=1, will start a reception. Setting REN=0 will stop a reception in progress, and inhibit further receptions. To avoid a partial or complete undesired reception, REN must be set to zero before clearing RI. This can be handled in an interrupt environment by using software flags, or in a straight-line code environment by using the Interrupt Pending register to signal the completion of a receive. In any mode, it is necessary to set IOC1.5 to a 1 to enable the TXD pin. Some examples of the software involved in using the serial port can be found in section 3.8. More information on IOC1 is in section 2.13.3.

2.11.4. Determining Baud Rates

Baud rates in all modes are determined by the contents of a 16-bit register at location 000EH. This register must be loaded sequentially with 2 bytes (least significant byte first). The MSB of this register selects one of two sources for the input frequency to the baud rate generator. If it is a 1, the frequency on the XTAL1 pin is selected, if not, the external frequency from the T2CLK pin is used. It should be noted that the maximum speed of T2CLK is one transition every 2 state times, with a minimum period of 16 XTAL1 cycles.

The unsigned integer represented by the lower 15 bits of the baud rate register defines a number B, where B has a maximum value of 32767. The baud rate for the four serial modes using either XTAL1 or T2CLK as the clock source is given by:

Using XTAL1:

$$\text{Mode 0: } \text{Baud Rate} = \frac{\text{XTAL1 frequency}}{4*(B+1)};\ B \neq 0$$

$$\text{Others: } \text{Baud Rate} = \frac{\text{XTAL1 frequency}}{64*(B+1)}$$

Using T2CLK:

$$\text{Mode 0: } \text{Baud Rate} = \frac{\text{T2CLK frequency}}{B};\ B \neq 0$$

$$\text{Others: } \text{Baud Rate} = \frac{\text{T2CLK frequency}}{16*B};\ B \neq 0$$

Note that B cannot equal 0, except when using XTAL1 in other than mode 0.

Common baud rate values, using XTAL1 at 12MHz, are shown below.

Baud Rate	**Baud Register** Mode 0	**Value** Others
9600	8137H	8013H
4800	8270H	8026H
2400	84E1H	804DH
1200	89C3H	809BH
300	A70FH	8270H

The maximum asynchronous baud rate is 187.5 Kbaud, with a 12MHz clock.

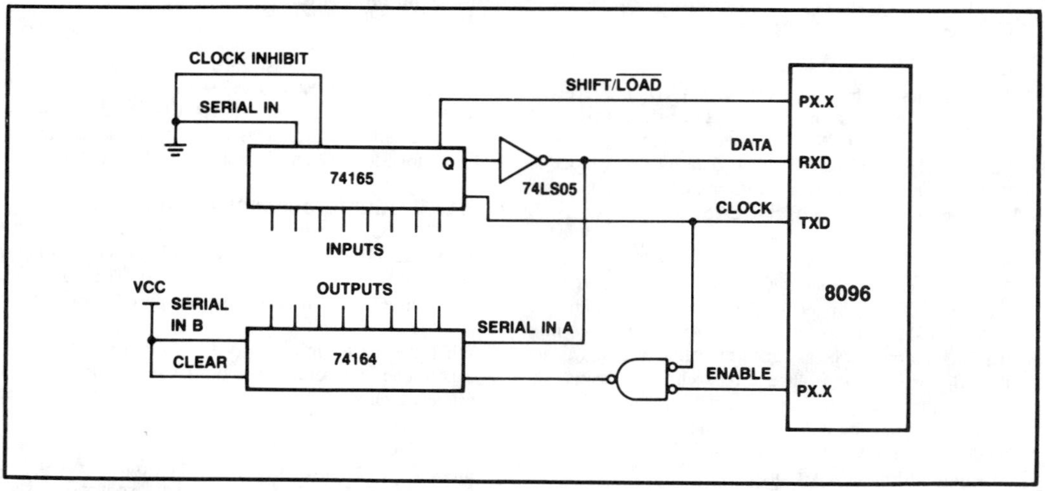

Figure 4-13. Mode 0 Serial Port Example

Reader: Consult also Fig. 4-12, p. 4-10 of your Microcontroller Handbook for serial port timings in mode 0.

I. TIMER 2 SFR (EVENT COUNTING): CLOCK AND RESET OPTIONS. TIMER 1. TIMER INTERRUPTS. RELATION TO HSI/HSO UNITS.

2.6. TIMERS

Two 16-bit timers are available for use on the 8096. The first is designated "Timer 1", the second, "Timer 2". Timer 1 is used to synchronize events to real time, while Timer 2 can be clocked externally and synchronizes events to external occurences.

2.6.1. Timer 1

Timer 1 is clocked once every eight state times and can be cleared only by executing a reset. The only other way to change its value is by writing to 000CH but this is a test mode which sets both timers to 0FFFXH and should not be used in programs.

2.6.2. Timer 2

Timer 2 can be incremented by transitions (one count each transition, rising *and* falling) on either T2CLK or HSI.1. The multiple functionality of the timer is determined by the state of I/O Control Register 0, bit 7 (IOC0.7). To ensure that all CAM entries are checked each count of Timer 2, the maximum transition speed is limited to once per eight state times. Timer 2 can be cleared by: executing a reset, by setting IOC0.1, by triggering HSO channel 0EH, or by pulling T2RST or HSI.0 high. The HSO and

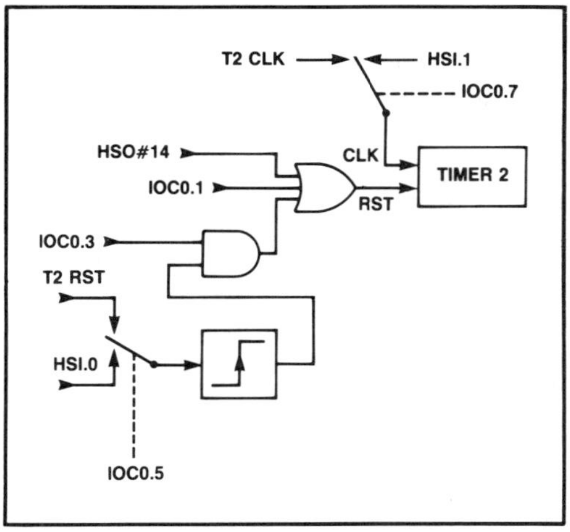

Figure 2-13. Timer 2 Clock and Reset Options

CAM are described in section 2.8. IOC0.3 and IOC0.5 control the resetting of Timer 2. Figure 2-13 shows the different ways of manipulating Timer 2.

2.6.3. Timer Interrupts

Both Timer 1 and Timer 2 can be used to trigger a timer overflow interrupt and set a flag in the I/O Status Register 1 (IOS1). The interrupts are controlled by IOC1.2 and IOC1.3 respectively. The flags are set in IOS1.5 and IOS1.4, respectively.

Caution must be used when examining the flags, as any access (including Compare and Jump on Bit) of IOS1 clears the whole byte, including the software timer flags. It is, therefore, recommended to write the byte to a temporary register before testing bits. The general enabling and disabling of the timer interrupts are controlled by the Interrupt Mask Register bit 0. In all cases, setting a bit enables a function, while clearing a bit disables it.

2.6.4. Timer Related Sections

The High Speed I/O unit is coupled to the timers in that the HSI records the value on Timer 1 when transitions occur and the HSO causes transitions to occur based on values of either Timer 1 or Timer 2. The Baud rate generator can use the T2CLK pin as input to its counter. A complete listing of the functions of IOS1, IOC0, and IOC1 are in section 2.13.

High-Speed Input/Output Unit

Timers

The high-speed input/output unit contains two 16-bit timer registers. The timer 1 register free-runs; that is, it is automatically incremented every eight state times (every 2.0 μs, if the oscillator frequency is 12 MHz). It is cleared only by RESET.

The timer 2 register, also 16 bits, can be programmed to count transitions on either T2CLK or HSI.1. The selected input to timer 2 is sampled every state time, and the count is incremented when the sample train shows a transition (*any* transition: 0-to-1 or 1-to-0) to have occurred. Timer 2 is cleared by RESET and also by software, and can be programmed to be cleared by signals from either T2RST or HSI.0.

Either timer register can be programmed to generate an interrupt on overflow.

J. THE HIGH SPEED INPUT UNIT AND ITS SFRs. THE HSI's FIFO AND HOLDING REGISTER.

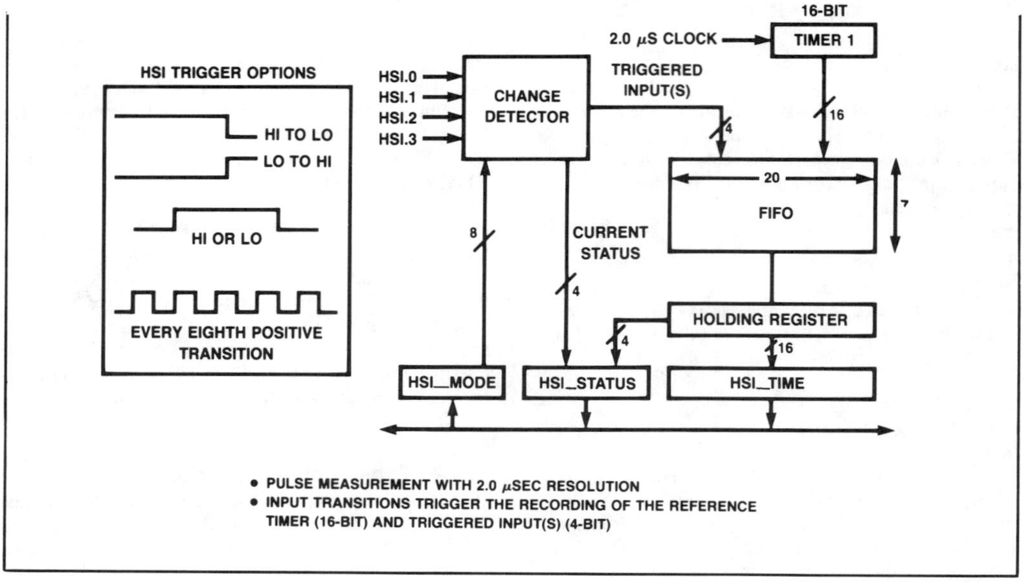

Figure 2-14. High Speed Input Unit

2.7. HIGH SPEED INPUTS

The High Speed Input Unit (HSI), can be used to record the time at which an event occurs with respect to Timer 1. There are 4 lines (HSI.0 through HSI.3) which can be used in this mode and up to a total of 8 events can be recorded. HSI.2 and HSI.3 share pins with HSO.4 and HSO.5. The I/O Control Registers (IOC0 and IOC1) are used to determine the functions of these pins. A block diagram of the HSI unit is shown in Figure 2-14.

2.7.1. HSI Modes

There are 4 possible modes of operation for each of the HSI. The HSI mode register is used to control which pins will look for what type of events. The 8-bit register is set up as shown in Figure 2-15.

High and low levels each need to be held for at least 1 state time to ensure proper operation. The maximum input speed is 1 event every 8 state times except when the 8 transition mode is used, in which case it is 1 transition per state time.

The HSI lines can be individually enabled and disabled using bits in IOC0, at location 0015H. Figure 2-16 shows the bit locations which control the HSI pins. If the pin is disabled, transitions will not be entered in the FIFO.

High Speed Inputs

The HSI unit looks for transitions in any of its input lines, and when it sees one it records the time (from timer 1) and which input line made the transition. This information is stored in an eight-deep FIFO. The unit can be programmed to look for either positive or negative transitions, and can be programmed to activate the HSI data available interrupt either when the first entry to the FIFO has been made or when the seventh entry has been made.

The HSI unit has four input lines. HSI.0 through HSI.3. Two of these lines are shared with the high-speed output unit. Each input line can be individually enabled or disabled to the HSI unit by software.

2.7.2. HSI FIFO

When an HSI event occurs, a 7x20 FIFO stores the 16 bits of Timer 1 and the 4 bits indicating the state of the 4 HSI lines at the time the status is read. It can take up to 8 state times for this information to reach the holding register. When the FIFO is full, one additional event can be stored by considering the holding register part of the FIFO. If the FIFO and holding register are full any additional events will not be recorded.

2.7.3. HSI Interrupts

Interrupts can be generated from the HSI unit in one of two ways, determined by IOC1.7. If the bit is a 0, then an interrupt will be generated every time a value is loaded into the holding register. If it is a 1, an interrupt will only be generated when the FIFO, (independent of the holding register), has six entries in it. Since all interrupts are rising edge triggered, if IOC1.7 = 1, the processor will not be re-interrupted until the FIFO first contains 5 or less records, then contains six or more. Interrupts can also be generated by pin HSI.0, which has its own interrupt vector.

There are also two interrupts associated with the HSI unit. The HSI data available interrupt (vector = (2004H)) is generated if there is data in the HSI FIFO that the program should read. The other HSI related interrupt is the HSI.0 interrupt which occurs whenever High Speed Input pin 0 makes a zero-to-one transition. This interrupt will become pending in the INT_PENDING register even if the HSI unit is programmed to ignore changes on HSI.0 or look for a one-to-zero transition.

2.7.4. HSI Status

Bits 6 and 7 of the I/O Status register 1 (IOS1) indicate the status of the HSI FIFO. If bit 6 is a 1, the FIFO contains at least six entries. If bit 7 is a 1, the FIFO contains at least 1 entry and the holding register has been loaded. The FIFO may be read after verifying that it contains valid data. Caution must be used when reading or testing bits in IOS1, as this action clears the entire byte, including the software and hardware timer overflow flags. It is best to store the byte and then test the stored value. See Section 3.7.2.

Reading the HSI is done in two steps. First, the HSI Status register is read to obtain the current state of the HSI pins and which pins had changed at the recorded time. The format of the HSI_STATUS Register is shown in Figure 2-17. Second, the HSI Time register is read. Reading the Time register unloads one word of the FIFO, so if the Time register is read before the Status register, the information in the Status register will be lost. The HSI Status register is at location 06H and the HSI Time registers are in locations 04H and 05H.

If the HSI_TIME and Status register are read without the holding register being loaded, the values read will be undeterminate.

It should be noted that many of the Status register conditions are changed by a reset, see section 2.15.2. A complete listing of the functions of IOS0, IOS1, and IOC1 can be found in section 2.13.

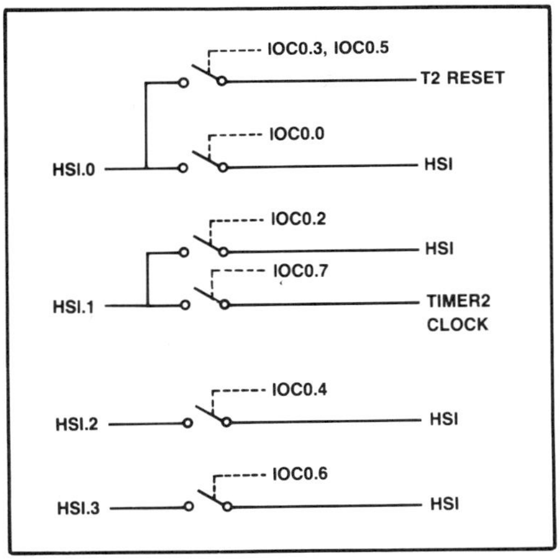

Figure 2-16. IOC0 Control of HSI Pin Functions

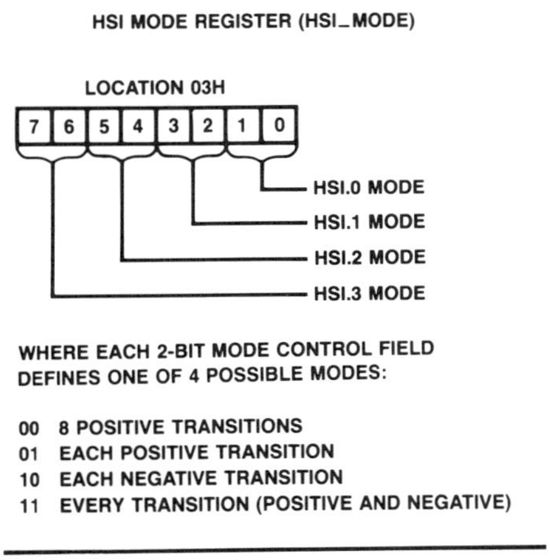

Figure 2-15. HSI Mode Register Diagram

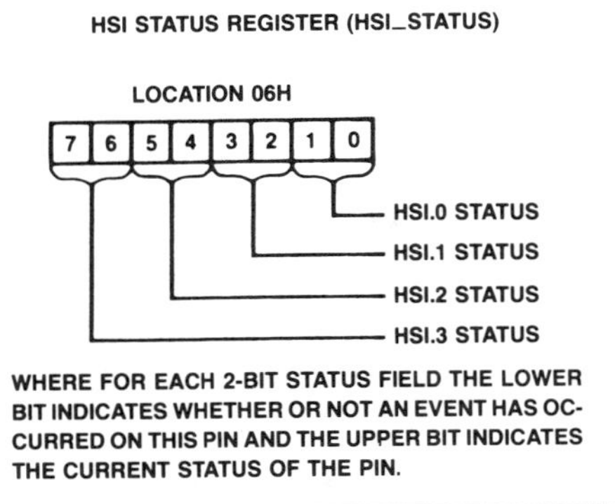

Figure 2-17. HSI Status Register Diagram

K. THE HIGH SPEED OUTPUT UNIT AND ITS RELATED SFRs. ITS CAM FILE, HOLDING REGISTER, COMPARATOR, SOFTWARE TIMERS.

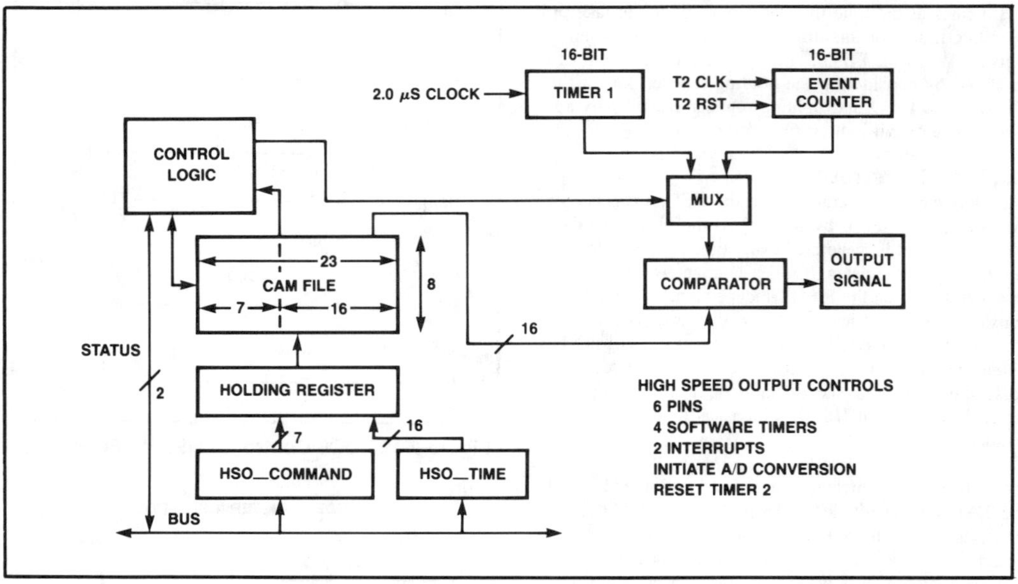

Figure 2-18. High Speed Output Unit

High Speed Outputs

The high-speed output (HSO) unit (figure 1-6) can be programmed to cause transitions on any of its output lines at specified times. The HSO unit has six output lines, HSO.0 through HSO.5. HSO.4 and HSO.5 are shared with the HSI unit as HSI.2 and HSI.3. These two outputs can be individually enabled or disabled by software.

The HSO unit can be programmed to set or clear any of its output lines, or reset timer 2, or trigger an A/D conversion at the preset time. Either timer 1 or timer 2 can be selected to be the reference timer for this purpose. Up to eight such preset actions can be in storage at any one time. As each action is carried out at its preset time, its command line is deleted from storage.

Storage of HSO commands is an eight-deep content addressable memory (CAM) file. Each CAM register is 23 bits wide. Sixteen bits specify the time at which the action is to be carried out; seven bits specify the nature of the action and whether timer 1 or timer 2 is the reference.

To enter a command into the CAM file, write the seven-bit "command tag" into location 0006H and the time at which the action is to be carried out into word address 0004H. Writing to these addresses accesses the HSO holding register. The command does not actually enter the CAM file until an empty CAM register rotates around the holding register (see figure 1-6).

The CAM file rotates one register position per state time. Thus it takes eight state times for the holding register to have had access to all eight CAM registers. Similarly, it takes eight state times for the comparator to have had access to all eight CAM registers. This defines the time-resolution of the HSO unit to be eight state times (2.0μs, if the oscillator frequency is 12 MHz).

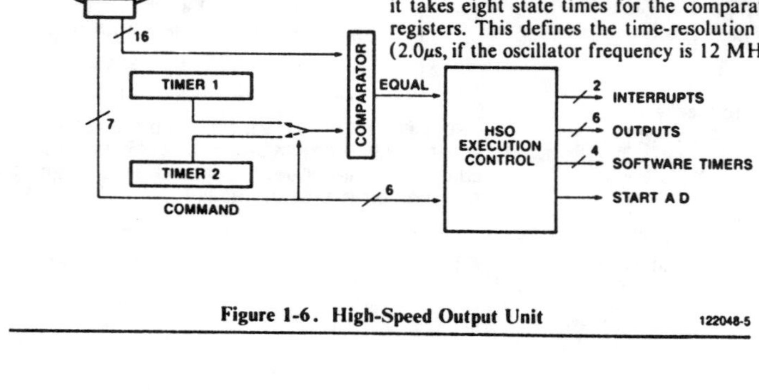

Figure 1-6. High-Speed Output Unit 122048-5

2.8. HIGH SPEED OUTPUTS

The High Speed Output unit (HSO) is used to trigger events at specific times with minimal CPU overhead. These events include: starting an A to D conversion, resetting Timer 2, setting 4 software flags, and switching up to 6 output lines. Interrupts can be generated whenever one of these events is triggered. Up to 8 events can be pending at any one time.

2.8.1. HSIO Shared Pins

Two of the 6 output lines (HSO.0 through HSO.5) are shared with the High Speed Input (HSI) lines. HSO.4 and HSO.5 are shared with HSI.2 and HSI.3, respectively. Bits 4 and 6 of the I/O Control Register 1 (IOC1) are used to enable HSO.4 and HSO.5 as outputs.

2.8.2. HSIO CAM

A block diagram of the HSO unit is shown in Figure 2-18. The Content Addressable Memory (CAM) file is the center of control. One CAM register is compared with a time value every state time. Therefore, it takes 8 state times to compare all CAM registers with a timer.

Each CAM register is 23 bits wide. Sixteen bits specify the time at which the action is to be carried out and 7 bits specify both the nature of the action and whether Timer 1 or Timer 2 is the reference. The format of the command to the HSO unit is shown in Figure 2-19.

To enter a command into the CAM file, write the 7-bit "Command Tag" into location 0006H followed by the time at which the action is to be carried out into word address 0004H. Writing the time value loads the HSO Holding Register with both the time and the last written command tag. The command does not actually enter the CAM file until an empty CAM register becomes available. It can take up to 8 state times for a command to enter the CAM. For this reason, if Timer 1 is being used as the reference, the minimum time that can be loaded is Timer 1 + 1. A similar restriction applies if Timer 2 is used as the reference.

Care must be taken when writing the command tag for the HSO. If an interrupt occurs during the time between writing the command tag and loading the time value, and the interrupt service routine writes to the HSO time register, the command tag used in the interrupt routine will be written to the CAM at both the time specified by the interrupt routine and the time specified by the main program. The command tag from the main program will not be executed. One way of avoiding this problem would be to disable interrupts when writing commands and times to the HSO unit. See also Section 3.7.3.

3.7.4. High Speed I/O Interrupts

The HSO unit can generate two types of interrupts. The HSO execution interrupt (vector = (2006H)) is generated (if enabled) for HSO commands which operate on one of the six HSO pins. The other HSO interrupt is the Software Timer interrupt (vector = (200AH)) which is generated (if enabled) for any other HSO command (e.g. triggering the A/D, resetting Timer2 or generating a software time delay).

2.8.3. HSO Status

Before writing to the HSO, it is desirable to ensure that the Holding Register is empty. If it is not, writing to the HSO will overwrite the value in the Holding Register. I/O Status Register 0 (IOS0) bits 6 and 7 indicate the status of the HSO unit. This register is described in section 2.13.4. If IOS0.6 equals 0, the holding register is empty and at least one CAM register is empty. If IOS0.7 equals 0, the holding register is empty.

One location in the CAM file is checked each state-time. Thus, it takes 8 state-times for the Holding Register to have had access to all 8 CAM registers. Similarly, it takes 8 state-times for the comparator to have had access to all 8 CAM registers. This defines the time-resolution of the HSO unit to be 8 state-times (2.0 μsec, if the oscillator frequency is 12 MHz). Note that the comparator does not look at the holding register, so instructions in the holding register do not execute.

2.8.4. Clearing The HSO

All 8 CAM locations of the HSO are compared before any action is taken. This allows a pending external event to be cancelled by simply writing the opposite event to the CAM. However, once an entry is placed in the CAM, it cannot be removed until either the specified timer matches the written value or the chip is reset. Internal events are not synchronized to Timer 1, and therefore cannot be cleared. This includes events on HSO channels 8 through F and all interrupts. Since interrupts are not synchronized it is possible to have multiple interrupts at the same time value.

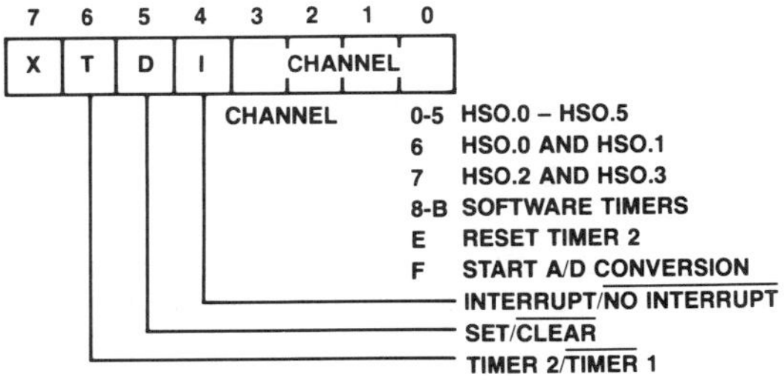

Figure 2-19. HSO Command Tag Format

2.8.5. Using Timer 2 With The HSO

Timer 1 is incremented only once every 8 state-times. When it is being used as the reference timer for an HSO action, the comparator has a chance to look at all 8 CAM registers before Timer 1 changes its value. Following the same reasoning, Timer 2 has been synchronized to allow it to change at a maximum rate of once per 8 state-times. Timer 2 increments on both edges of the input signal.

When using Timer 2 as the HSO reference, caution must be taken that Timer 2 is not reset prior to the highest value for a Timer 2 match in the CAM. This is because the HSO CAM will hold an event pending until a time match occurs, if that match is to a time value on Timer 2 which is never reached, the event will remain pending in the CAM until the part is reset.

Additional caution must be used when Timer 2 is being reset using the HSO unit, since resetting Timer 2 using the HSO is an internal event and can therefore happen at any time within the eight-state-time window. For this reason, any events scheduled to occur at the same time as a Timer 2 reset should be logged into the CAM with a Timer 2 value of zero. When using this method to make a programmable modulo counter, the count will stay at the maximum Timer 2 value only until the Reset T2 command is recognized. The count will stay at zero for the transition which would have changed the count from "N" to zero, and then change to a one on the next transition.

2.8.6. Software Timers

The HSO can be programmed to generate interrupts at preset times. Up to four such "Software Timers" can be in operation at a time. As each preprogrammed time is reached, the HSO unit sets a Software Timer Flag. If the interrupt bit in the command tag was set then a Software Timer Interrupt will also be generated. The interrupt service routine can then examine I/O Status register 1 (IOS1) to determine which software timer expired and caused the interrupt. When the HSO resets Timer 2 or starts an A to D conversion, it can also be programmed to generate a software timer interrupt but there is no flag to indicate that this has occurred. See also Section 3.7.4.

If more than one software timer interrupt occurs in the same time frame it is possible that multiple software timer interrupts will be generated.

Each read or test of any bit in IOS1 will clear the whole byte. Be certain to save the byte before testing it unless you are only concerned with 1 bit. See also Section 3.2.2.

A complete listing of the functions of IOS0, IOS1, and IOC1 can be found in section 2.13. The Timers are described in section 2.6 and the HSI is described in section 2.7.

3.7.3. Sending Commands to the HSO Unit

Commands are sent to the HSO unit via a byte and then a word write operation:

```
LDB     HSO_COMMAND,#what_to_do
ADD     HSO_TIME,TIMER1,#when_to_do_it
```

The command is actually accepted when the HSO_TIME register is written. It is important to ensure that this code piece is not interrupted by any interrupt service routine which might also send a command to the HSO unit. If this happens the HSO will know when to do it but not know what to do when it's time to do it. In many systems this becomes a null problem because HSO commands are only issued from one place in the code. If this is not the case then a critical region must be established and the two instructions executed from within this region (see section 3.6.5).

Commands in the holding register will not execute even if their time tag is reached. Commands must be in the CAM for this to occur. Flags are available in IOS0 which indicate the holding register is empty (IOS0.7) or that both the holding register is empty *and* the CAM is not full (IOS0.6). The programmer should carefully decide which of these two flags is the best to use for each application.

It is possible to enter commands into the CAM which never execute. This occurs if TIMER2 has been set up as a variable modulo counter and a command is entered with a time tag referenced to TIMER2 which has a value that TIMER2 never reaches. The inaccessible command will never execute and continue to take up room in the CAM until either the system is reset or the program allows TIMER2 increment up to the value stored in the time tag. Note that commands cannot be flushed from the CAM without being executed but that they can be cancelled. This is accomplished by setting the opposite command in the CAM to execute at the same time tag as the command to be cancelled. Since internal events are not synchronized to Timer 1, it is not possible to cancel them. If, as an example, a command has been issued to set HSO.1 when TIMER1 = 1234 then entering a second command which clears HSO.1 when TIMER1 = 1234 will result in a no-operation on HSO.1. Both commands will remain in the CAM until TIMER1 = 1234.

L. THE CRUCIAL CONTROL AND STATUS SFRs: IOC0, IOC1, IOS0, IOS1.

2.13. STATUS AND CONTROL REGISTERS

2.13.1. I/O Control Registers

There are two I/O Control registers, IOC0 and IOC1. IOC0 controls Timer 2 and the HSI lines. IOC1 controls some pin functions, interrupt sources and 2 HSO pins.

Whenever input lines are switched between two sources, or enabled, it is possible to generate transitions on these lines. This could cause problems with respect to edge sensitive lines such as the HSI lines, Interrupt line, and Timer 2 control lines.

2.13.2. I/O Control Register 0 (IOC0)

IOC0 is located at 0015H. The four HSI lines can be enabled or disabled to the HSI unit by setting or clearing bits in IOC0. Timer 2 functions including clock and reset sources are also determined by IOC0. The control bit locations are shown in Figure 2-28.

2.13.3. I/O Control Register 1 (IOC1)

IOC1 is used to select some pin functions and enable or disable some interrupt sources. Its location is 0016H. Port pin P2.5 can be selected to be the PWM output instead of a standard output. The external interrupt source can be selected to be either EXTINT (same pin as P2.2) or Analog Channel 7 (ACH7, same pin as P0.7). Timer 1 and Timer 2 overflow interrupts can be individually enabled or disabled. The HSI interrupt can be selected to activate either when there is 1 FIFO entry or 7. Port pin P2.0 can be selected to be the TXD output. HSO.4 and HSO.5 can be enabled or disabled to the HSO unit. More information on interrupts is available in section 2.5. The positions of the IOC1 control bits are shown in Figure 2-29.

2.13.4. I/O Status Register 0 (IOS0)

There are two I/O Status registers, IOS0 and IOS1. IOS0, located at 0015H, holds the current status of the HSO lines and CAM. The status bits of IOS0 are shown in Figure 2-30.

2.13.5. I/O Status Register 1 (IOS1)

IOS1 is located at 0016H. It contains status bits for the timers and the HSI. Every access of this register clears all of the timer overflow and timer expired bits. It is, therefore, important to first store the byte in a temporary location before attempting to test any bit unless only one bit will ever be of importance to the program. The status bits of IOS1 are shown in Figure 2-31.

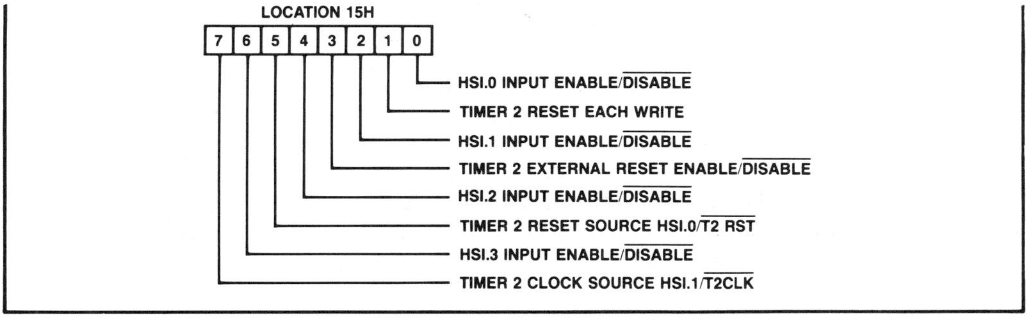

Figure 2-28. I/O Control Register 0 (IOC0)

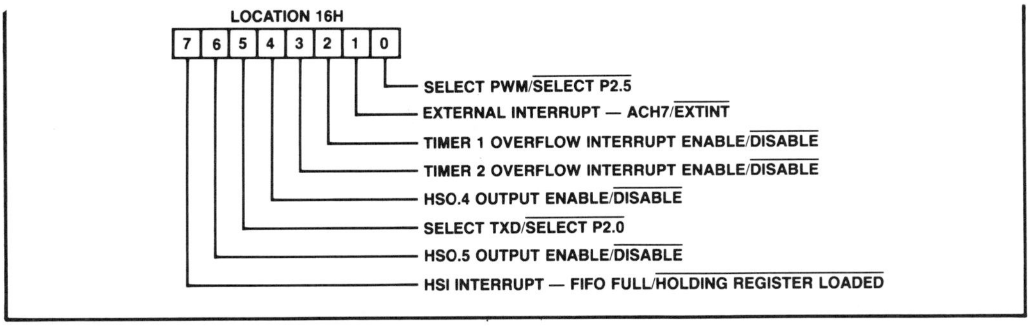

Figure 2-29. I/O Control Register 1 (IOC1)

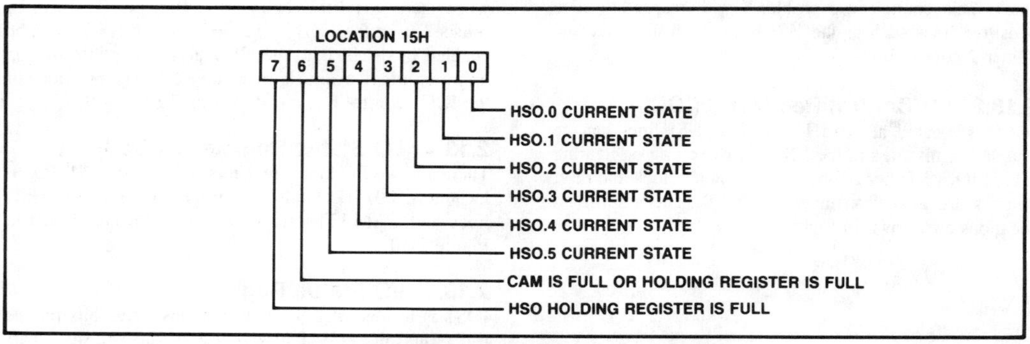

Figure 2-30. I/O Status Register 0 (IOS0)

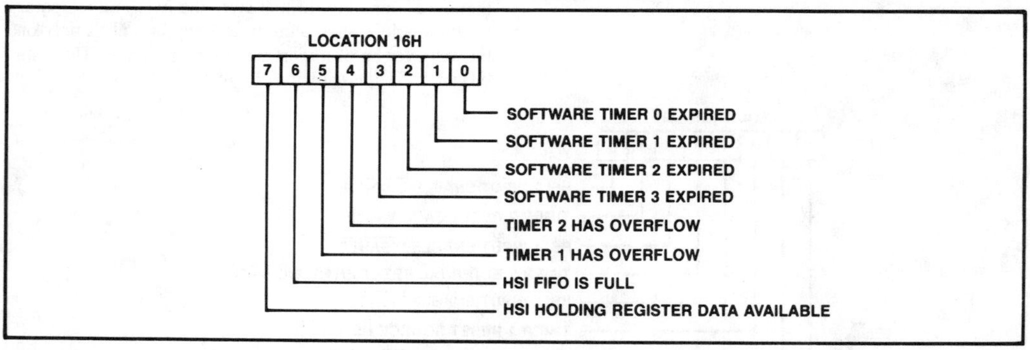

Figure 2-31. HSIO Status Register 1 (IOS1)

M. I/O PORTS 0, 1, 2 (SFRs) AND I/O PORTS 3, 4.

2.12. I/O PORTS 0, 1, 2, 3, AND 4

There are five 8-bit I/O ports on the 8096. Some of these ports are input only, some output only, some bidirectional and some have alternate functions. Input ports connect to the internal bus through an input buffer. Output ports connect through an output buffer to an internal register that holds the output bits. Bidirectional ports consist of an internal register, an output buffer, and an input buffer.

When an instruction accesses a bidirectional port as a source register, the question often arises as to whether the value that is brought into the CPU comes from the internal port register or from the port pins through the input buffer. In the 8096, the value always comes from the port pins, never from the internal register.

2.12.1. Port 0

Port 0 is an input only port which shares its pins with the analog inputs to the A/D Converter. One can read Port 0 digitally, and/or, by writing the appropriate control bits to the A/D Command Register, select one of the lines of this port to be the input to the A/D Converter.

2.12.2. Port 1

Port 1 is a quasi-bidirectional I/O port. ''Quasi-bidirectional'' means the port pin has a weak internal pullup that is always active and an internal pulldown which can either be on (to output a 0) or off (to output a 1). If the internal pulldown is left off (by writing a 1 to the pin), the pin's logic level can be controlled by an external pulldown which can either be on (to input a 0) or off (to input a 1). From the user's point of view the main distinction is that a quasi-bidirectional input will source current while being externally held low and will pull itself high if left alone.

In parallel with the weak internal pullup, is a much stronger internal pullup that is activated for one state time when the pin is internally driven from 0 to 1. This is done to speed up the 0-to-1 transition time. See also Sections 3.7.1 and 4.2.2.

2.12.3. Port 2

Port 2 is a multi-functional port. Six of its pins are shared with other functions in the 8096, as shown below.

Port	Function	Alternate Function	Controlled by
P2.0	output	TXD (serial port transmit)	IOC1.5
P2.1	input	RXD (serial port receive)	N/A
P2.2	input	EXTINT (external interrupt)	IOC1.1
P2.3	input	T2CLK (Timer 2 input)	IOC0.7
P2.4	input	T2RST (Timer 2 reset)	IOC0.5
P2.5	output	PWM (pulse-width modulation)	IOC1.0
P2.6	quasi-bidirectional		
P2.7	quasi-bidirectional		

2.12.4. Ports 3 and 4

Ports 3 and 4 have two functions. They are either bidirectional ports with open-drain outputs or System Bus pins which the memory controller uses when it is accessing off-chip memory. If the $\overline{EA}$ line is low, the pins always act as the System Bus. Otherwise they act as bus pins only during a memory access. If these pins are being used as ports and bus pins, ones must be written to them prior to bus operations.

Strong internal pullups are used during external memory read or write cycles when the pins are used as address or data outputs. At any other time, the internal pullups are disabled. The port pins and their system bus functions are shown below:

Port Pin	System Bus Function
P3.0	AD0
P3.1	AD1
P3.2	AD2
P3.3	AD3
P3.4	AD4
P3.5	AD5
P3.6	AD6
P3.7	AD7
P4.0	AD8
P4.1	AD9
P4.2	AD10
P4.3	AD11
P4.4	AD12
P4.5	AD13
P4.6	AD14
P4.7	AD15

N. THE WATCHDOG TIMER SFR

2.14. WATCHDOG TIMER (WDT)

This feature is provided as a means of graceful recovery from a software upset. Once the watchdog is initialized, if the software fails to reset the watchdog at least every 64K state times, a hardware reset will be initiated.

The watchdog is initialized by the first write of the clear WDT code to the WDT register. Once the watchdog is initialized it cannot be disabled by software. On reset the watchdog is not active.

The software can be designed so that the watchdog times out if the program does not progress properly. The watchdog will also time-out if the software error was due to ESD (Electrostatic Discharge) or other hardware related problems. This prevents the controller from having a malfunction for longer than 16 mS if a 12 MHz oscillator is used.

The watchdog timer is a 16-bit counter which is incremented every state time. When it overflows it pulls down the RESET pin for at least two state times, resetting the 8096 and any other chips connected to the reset line. To prevent the timer from overflowing and resetting the system, it must be cleared periodically. Clearing the timer is done by writing a "01EH" followed by an "0E1H" to the WDT register at location 000AH.

Use of a large reset capacitor on the RESET pin will increase the length of time required for a watchdog initiated reset. This is because the capacitor will keep the RESET pin from responding immediately to the internal pull-ups and pull-downs. A large capacitor on the RESET pin may also interfere with the reset of other parts connected to the RESET pin. Under some circumstances, it may be desirable to use an open collector circuit. See section 4.4.

2.14.1. Disabling The Watchdog

The watchdog should be disabled by software not initializing it. If this is not possible, such as during program development, the watchdog can be disabled by holding the RESET pin at 2.0 to 2.5 volts. Voltages over 2.5 volts on the pin could quickly damage the part. Even at 2.5 volts, using this technique for other than debugging purposes is not recommended, as it may effect long term reliability. It is further recommended that any part used in this way for more than several seconds, not be used in production versions of products.

It should be stressed that writing 01EH, followed by 0E1H, into the WDT register at 0AH does two things: enables the WDT AND clears it.

O. 8096 RESET CONDITIONS

2.15. RESET

2.15.1. Reset Signal

As with all processors, the 8096 must be reset each time the power is turned on. To complete a reset, the RESET pin must be held active (low) for at least 2 state times after VCC, the oscillator, and the back bias generator have stabilized (~1.0 milliseconds). Then when RESET is brought high again, the 8096 executes a reset sequence that takes 10 state times. (It initializes some registers, clears the PSW and jumps to address 2080H.)

The 8096 can be reset using a capacitor, 1-shot, or any other method capable of providing a pulse of at least 2 state times longer than required for VCC and the oscillator to stabilize.

For best functionality, it is suggested that the reset pin be pulled low with an open collector device. In this way, several reset sources can be wire ored together. Remember, the RESET pin itself can be a reset source (see section 2.14). Details of hardware suggestions for reset can be found in section 4.4.

2.15.2. Reset Status

The I/O lines and control of the 8096 will be in their reset state within 2 state times after reset is low, with VCC and the oscillator stabilized. Prior to that time, the status of the I/O lines is indeterminate. After the 10 state time reset sequence, the Special Function Registers will be set as follows:

SFR	reset value
Port 1	11111111B
Port 2	110XXXX1B
Port 3	11111111B
Port 4	11111111B
PWM Control	00H
Serial Port (Transmit)	undefined
Serial Port (Receive)	undefined
Baud Rate Register	undefined
Serial Control/Status	undefined
A/D Command	undefined
A/D Result	undefined
Interrupt Pending	undefined
Interrupt Mask	00000000B
Timer 1	0000H
Timer 2	0000H
Watchdog Timer	0000H
HSI Mode	11111111B
HSI Status	undefined
IOS0	00000000B
IOS1	00000000B
IOC0	X0X0X0X0B
IOC1	X0X0XXX1B

Other conditions following a reset are:

Register	reset value
HSI FIFO	empty
HSO CAM	empty
HSO lines	000000B
PSW	0000H
Stack Pointer	undefined
Program Counter	2080H
RD	high
WR	high
ALE	low
BHE	low
INST	high

2.15.3. Reset Sync Mode

The RESET line can be used to start the 8096 at an exact state time to provide for synchronization of test equipment and multiple chip systems. RESET is active low. To synchronize parts, RESET is brought high on the rising edge of XTAL1. Complete details on synchronizing parts can be found in section 4.1.5.

It is very possible that parts which start in sync may not stay that way. The best example of this would be when a "jump on I/O bit" is being used to hold the processor in a loop. If the line changes during the time it is being tested, one processor may see it as a one, while the other sees it as a zero. The result is that one processor will do an extra loop, thus putting it several states out of sync with the other.

P. 8096 SOFTWARE AND PROGRAMMING INFORMATION

P(a). DEFINITIONS, NOTATION, ADDRESSING MODES.

MCS®-96 SOFTWARE DESIGN INFORMATION

3.0. INTRODUCTION

This section provides information which will primarily interest those who must write programs to execute in the 8096. Several other sources of information are currently available which will also be of interest:

MCS®-96 MACRO ASSEMBLER USER'S GUIDE
Order Number 122048-001

MCS-96 UTILITIES USER'S GUIDE
Order Number 122049-001

MCS-96 MACRO ASSEMBLER AND UTILITIES POCKET REFERENCE
Order Number 122050-001

Throughout this chapter short segments of code are used to illustrate the operation of the device. For these sections it has been assumed that a set of temporary registers have been predeclared. The names of these registers have been chosen as follows:

AX, BX, CX, and DX are 16 bit registers.

AL is the low byte of AX, AH is the high byte.

BL is the low byte of BX

CL is the low byte of CX

DL is the low byte of DX

These are the same as the names for the general data registers used in 8086. It is important to note, however, that in the 8096, these are not dedicated registers but merely the symbolic names assigned by the programmer to an eight byte region within onboard register file.

3.1. OPERAND TYPES

The MCS®-96 architecture provides support for a variety of data types which are likely to be useful in a control application. In the discussion of these operand types that follows, the names adopted by the PLM-96 programming language will be used where appropriate. To avoid confusion the name of an operand type will be capitalized. A "BYTE" is an unsigned eight bit variable; a "byte" is an eight bit unit of data of any type.

3.1.1. Bytes

BYTES are unsigned 8-bit variables which can take on the values between 0 and 255. Arithmetic and relational operators can be applied to BYTE operands but the result must be interpreted in modulo 256 arithmetic. Logical operations on BYTES are applied bitwise. Bits within BYTES are labeled from 0 to 7 with 0 being the least significant bit. There are no alignment restrictions for BYTES so they may be placed anywhere in the MCS-96 address space.

3.1.2. Words

WORDS are unsigned 16-bit variables which can take on the values between 0 and 65535. Arithmetic and relational operators can be applied to WORD operands but the result must be interpreted modulo 65536. Logical operations on WORDS are applied bitwise. Bits within words are labeled from 0 to 15 with 0 being the least significant bit. WORDS must be aligned at even byte boundaries in the MCS-96 address space. The least significant byte of the WORD is in the even byte address and the most significant byte is in the next higher (odd) address. The address of a word is the address of its least significant byte.

3.1.3. Short-Integers

SHORT-INTEGERS are 8-bit signed variables which can take on the values between −128 and +127. Arithmetic operations which generate results outside of the range of a SHORT-INTEGER will set the overflow indicators in the program status word. The actual numeric result returned will be the same as the equivalent operation on BYTE variables. There are no alignment restrictions on SHORT-INTEGERS so they may be placed anywhere in the MCS-96 address space.

3.1.4. Integers

INTEGERS are 16-bit signed variables which can take on the values between −32,768 and 32,767. Arithmetic operations which generate results outside of the range of an INTEGER will set the overflow indicators in the program status word. The actual numeric result returned will be the same as the equivalent operation on WORD variables. INTEGERS conform to the same alignment and addressing rules as do WORDS.

3.1.5. Bits

BITS are single-bit operands which can take on the Boolean values of true and false. In addition to the normal support for bits as components of BYTE and WORD operands, the 8096 provides for the direct testing of any bit in the internal register file. The MCS-96 architecture requires that bits be addressed as components of BYTES or WORDS, it does not support the direct addressing of bits that can occur in the MCS-51 architecture.

3.1.6. Double-Words

DOUBLE-WORDS are unsigned 32-bit variables which can take on the values between 0 and 4,294,967,295. The MCS-96 architecture provides direct support for this operand type only for shifts and as the dividend in a 32 by 16 divide and the product of a 16 by 16 multiply. For these operations a DOUBLE-WORD variable must reside in the on-board register file of the 8096 and be aligned at an address which is evenly divisible by 4. A DOUBLE-WORD operand is addressed by the address of its least significant byte. DOUBLE-WORD operations which are not directly supported can be easily implemented with two WORD operations. For consistency with INTEL provided software the user should adopt the conventions for addressing DOUBLE-WORD operands which are discussed in section 3.5.

3.1.7. Long-Integers

LONG-INTEGERS are 32-bit signed variables which can take on the values between −2,147,483,648 and 2,147,483,647. The MCS-96 architecture provides direct support for this data type only for shifts and as the dividend in a 32 by 16 divide and the product of a 16 by 16 multiply.

LONG-INTEGERS can also be normalized. For these operations a LONG-INTEGER variable must reside in the onboard register file of the 8096 and be aligned at an address which is evenly divisible by 4. A LONG-INTEGER is addressed by the address of its least significant byte.

LONG-INTEGER operations which are not directly supported can be easily implemented with two INTEGER operations. For consistency with Intel provided software, the user should adopt the conventions for addressing LONG operands which are discussed in section 3.5.

3.2. OPERAND ADDRESSING

Operands are accessed within the address space of the 8096 with one of six basic addressing modes. Some of the details of how these addressing modes work are hidden by the assembly language. If the programmer is to take full advantage of the architecture, it is important that these details be understood. This section will describe the addressing modes as they are handled by the hardware. At the end of this section the addressing modes will be described as they are seen through the assembly language. The six basic addressing modes which will be described are termed register-direct, indirect, indirect with auto-increment, immediate, short-indexed, and long-indexed. Several other useful addressing operations can be achieved by combining these basic addressing modes with specific registers such as the ZERO register or the stack pointer.

3.2.1. Register-direct References

The register-direct mode is used to directly access a register from the 256 byte on-board register file. The register is selected by an 8-bit field within the instruction and register address must conform to the alignment rules for the operand type. Depending on the instruction, up to three registers can take part in the calculation.

```
Examples
   ADD     AX,BX,CX        ; AX:=BX+CX
   MUL     AX,BX           ; AX:=AX*BX
   INCB    CL              ; CL:=CL+1
```

3.2.2. Indirect References

The indirect mode is used to access an operand by placing its address in a WORD variable in the register file. The calculated address must conform to the alignment rules for the operand type. Note that the indirect address can refer to an operand anywhere within the address space of the 8096, including the register file. The register which contains the indirect address is selected by an eight bit field within the instruction. An instruction can contain only one indirect reference and the remaining operands of the instruction (if any) must be register-direct references.

```
Examples
   LD      AX,[AX]       ; AX:=MEM_WORD(AX)
   ADDB    AL,BL,[CX]    ; AL:=BL+MEM_BYTE(CX)
   POP     [AX]          ; MEM_WORD(AX):=MEM_WORD(SP); SP:=SP+2
```

3.2.3. Indirect with Auto-increment References

This addressing mode is the same as the indirect mode except that the WORD variable which contains the indirect address is incremented *after* it is used to address the operand. If the instruction operates on BYTES or SHORT-INTEGERS the indirect address variable will be incremented by one, if the instruction operates on WORDS or INTEGERS the indirect address able will be incremented by two.

```
Examples
   LD      AX,[BX]+       ; AX:=MEM_WORD(BX); BX:=BX+2
   ADD     AL,BL,[CX]+    ; AL:=AL+BL+MEM_BYTE(CX); CX:=CX+1
   PUSH    [AX]+          ; SP:=SP-2;
                          ;   MEM_WORD(SP):=MEM_WORD(AX)
                          ;   AX:=AX+2
```

MCS®-96 SOFTWARE DESIGN INFORMATION

3.2.4. Immediate References

This addressing mode allows an operand to be taken directly from a field in the instruction. For operations on BYTE or SHORT-INTEGER operands this field is eight bits wide, for operations on WORD or INTEGER operands the field is 16 bits wide. An instruction can contain only one immediate reference and the remaining operand(s) must be register-direct references.

```
Examples
  ADD   AX,#340   ; AX: = AX + 340
  PUSH  #1234H    ; SP: = SP – 2; MEM _ WORD(SP): = 1234H
  DIVB  AX,#10    ; AL: = AX/10; AH: = AX MOD 10
```

3.2.5. Short-indexed References

In this addressing mode an eight bit field in the instruction selects a WORD variable in the register file which is assumed to contain an address. A second eight bit field in the instruction stream is sign-extended and summed with the WORD variable to form the address of the operand which will take part in the calculation. Since the eight bit field is sign-extended the effective address can be up to 128 bytes before the address in the WORD variable and up to 127 bytes after it. An instruction can contain only one short-indexed reference and the remaining operand(s) must be register-direct references.

```
Examples
  LD      AX,12[BX]     ; AX: = MEM _ WORD(BX + 12)
  MULB    AX,BL,3[CX]   ; AX: = BL*MEM _ BYTE(CX + 3)
```

3.2.6. Long-indexed References

This addressing mode is like the short-indexed mode except that a *16-bit* field is taken from the instruction and added to the WORD variable to form the address of the operand. No sign extension is necessary. An instruction can contain only one long-indexed reference and the remaining operand(s) must to register-direct references.

```
Examples
  AND   AX,BX,TABLE[CX]      ; AX: = BX AND MEM _ WORD(TABLE + CX)
  ST    AX,TABLE[BX]         ; MEM _ WORD(TABLE + BX) : = AX
  ADDB  AL,BL,LOOKUP[CX]     ; AL: = BL + MEM _ BYTE(LOOKUP + CX)
```

3.2.7. ZERO Register Addressing

The first two bytes in the register file are fixed at zero by the 8096 hardware. In addition to providing a fixed source of the constant zero for calculations and comparisons, this register can be used as the WORD variable in a long-indexed reference. This combination of register selection and address mode allows any location in memory to be addressed directly.

```
Examples
  ADD   AX,1234[0]   ; AX: = AX + MEM _ WORD(1234)
  POP   5678[0]      ; MEM _ WORD(5678): = MEM _ WORD(SP)
                     ;   SP: = SP + 2
```

3.2.8. Stack Pointer Register Addressing

The system stack pointer in the 8096 can be accessed as register 18H of the internal register file. In addition to providing for convenient manipulation of the stack pointer, this also facilitates the accessing of operands in the stack. The top of the stack, for example, can be accessed by using the stack pointer as the WORD variable in an indirect reference. In a similar fashion, the stack pointer can be used in the short-indexed mode to access data within the stack.

```
Examples
  PUSH   [SP]        ; DUPLICATE TOP _ OF _ STACK
  LD     AX,2[SP]    ; AX: = NEXT _ TO _ TOP
```

3.2.9. Assembly Language Addressing Modes

The 8096 assembly language simplifies the choice of addressing modes to be used in several respects:

Direct Addressing. The assembly language will choose between register-direct addressing and long-indexed with the ZERO register depending on where the operand is in memory. The user can simply refer to an operand by its symbolic name; if the operand is in the register file, a register-direct reference will be used, if the operand is elsewhere in memory, a long-indexed reference will be generated.

Indexed Addressing. The assembly language will choose between short and long indexing depending on the value of the index expression. If the value can be expressed in eight bits then short indexing will be used, if it cannot be expressed in eight bits then long indexing will be used.

The use of these features of the assembly language simplifies the programming task and should be used wherever possible.

Table 3-1. Abbreviations and Notations Used in Instruction Pages

Abbreviation, Notation	Meaning
baop	byte address moded operand
BEA	bytes of effective address
bitno	bit number
breg	byte register
cadd	code address
CEA	cycles of effective address
cnt	count
DEST	destination
disp	displacement
disp-hi	high order byte of displacement
disp-low	low order byte of displacement
lreg	long word register
offs.hi	value of high order byte
offs.lo	low order byte of offset
PC	program counter
SP	stack pointer
SRC	source
val-hi	value of high order byte
val-lo	value of low order byte
waop	word address moded operand
wreg	word register
AND	logical AND
NOT	logical complement
OR	logical OR
XOR	logical exclusive OR
+	plus
−	minus
/	divide
*	multiply
X	the contents of X
(X)	the contents of the contents of X
=	equal to
<>	not equal to
<	less than
>	greater than
←	is replaced by

MCS®-96 SOFTWARE DESIGN INFORMATION

3.13. DETAILED INSTRUCTION SET DESCRIPTION

This section gives a description of each instruction recognized by the 8096 sorted alphabetically by the mnemonic used in the assembly language for the 8096. Note that the effect on the program counter (PC) is not always shown in the instruction descriptions. All instructions increment the PC by the number of bytes in the instruction. Several acronynms are used in the instruction set descriptions which are defined here:

aa. A two bit field within an opcode which selects the basic addressing mode user. This field is only present in those opcodes which allow address mode options. The encoding of the field is as follows:

aa	Addressing mode
00	Register direct
01	Immediate
10	Indirect
11	Indexed

The selection between indirect and indirect with auto-increment or between short and long indexing is done based on the least significant bit of the instruction byte which follows the opcode. This type selects the 16-bit register which is to take part in the address calculation. Since the 8096 requires that words be aligned on even byte boundaries this bit would be otherwise unused.

breg. A byte register in the internal register file. When confusion could exist as to whether this field refers to a source or a destination register it will be prefixed with an "S" or a "D."

baop. A byte operand which is addressed by any of the address modes discussed in section 3.2.

bitno. A three bit field within an instruction op-code which selects one of the eight bits in a byte.

wreg. A word register in the internal register file. When confusion could exist as to whether this field refers to a source register or a destination register it will be prefixed with an "S" or a "D."

waop. A word operand which is addressed by any of the address modes discussed in section 3.2.

Lreg. A 32-bit register in the internal register file.

BEA. Extra bytes of code required for the address mode selected.

CEA. Extra state times (cycles) required for the address mode selected.

cadd An address in the program code.

Flag Settings. The modification to the flag setting is shown for each instruction. A checkmark (√) means that the flag is set or cleared as appropriate. A hyphen means that the flag is not modified. A one or zero (1) or (0) indicates that the flag will be in that state after the instruction. An up arrow (↑) indicates that the instruction may set the flag if it is appropriate but will not clear the flag. A down arrow (↓) indicates that the flag can be cleared but not set by the instruction. A question mark (?) indicates that the flag will be left in an indeterminant state after the operation.

Generic Jumps and Calls. The assembler for the 8096 provides for generic jumps and calls. For all of the conditional jump instructions a "B" can be substituted for the "J" and the assembler will generate a code sequence which is logically equivalent but can reach anywhere in the memory. A JH can only jump about 128 locations from the current program counter; a BH can jump anywhere in memory. In a like manner a BR will cause a SJMP or LJMP to be generated as appropriate and a CALL will cause a SCALL or LCALL to be generated. The assembler user guide (see section 3.0) should be consulted for the algorithms used by the assembler to convert these generic instructions into actual machine instructions.

P(b). FLAG CONSIDERATIONS AND INFORMATION

Table 3-2. Program Status Word Flags

Bits	Flag	Description
0-7		Interrupt Mask.
8	ST	STICKY BIT—Indicates whether any 1's were lost due to right shift. It is cleared at the start of any right shift. It is then set if at any time during the shift a 1 is shifted first into the carry (i.e., the bit shifted out of LSB position) and a further shift cycle occurs (another bit shifted into the carry). After multiply this bit is undefined.
9	I	INTERRUPT ENABLE BIT—If this bit is 0, all interrupts are ignored. If 1, interrupts are processed according to the interrupt enable mask and interrupt level.
10	–	Unused.
11	C	CARRY BIT—Set when an arithmetic carry occurs or bit is shifted out in a shift instruction. Borrow is complement of carry. This bit is cleared before any right shift instruction is executed.
12	VT	OVERFLOW TRAP BIT—Set each time the V bit has been set; and is cleared only on the completion of the CLRVT, JVT, or JNVT instructions.
13	V	OVERFLOW BIT—Set after arithmetic operations in which the magnitude of the algebraically correct result is too large to be represented in the available space.
14	N	NEGATIVE BIT—Shows the algebraically correct sign in case the sign bit of the result of an operation is incorrect due to an overflow.
15	Z	ZERO BIT—For the ADDC and SUBC instructions, the zero condition of the result is ANDed with the previous Z bit before it is saved.

Program Status Word

The low byte of the program status word (PSW) is the interrupt mask register. The high byte is as follows:

Bit:	15	14	13	12	11	10	9	8
	Z	N	V	VT	C	(X)	I	ST

Z — Zero bit. Z = 1 means the result of the previous operation was zero. (ADDC and SUBC can clear Z, but they cannot set it.)

N — Negative bit. N = 1 means the algebraically correct result is negative. (The actual result as stored may have an incorrect sign due to an overflow, but N reflects the algebraically correct sign.)

V — Overflow bit. V = 1 means the magnitude of the algebraically correct result is too large to be correctly represented in the available space.

VT — Overflow Trap bit. Anytime V gets set, VT gets set too. Subsequent operations may clear V, but VT can be cleared only by software.

C — Carry bit. This is the carry out of the MSB of the result of any arithmetic operation. During left-shifts, the MSB moves into C and a 0 moves into the LSB. During right-shifts, the LSB moves into C and a 0 moves into the MSB.

(X) — Unused. (Reads 0.)

I — Interrupt enable bit. I = 0 disables all interrupts.

ST — Sticky bit. During right-shifts the LSB moves into C. If the previous value C was 1, ST gets set (see SHR and SHRA instructions).

P(c). INSTRUCTION SET SUMMARY

MCS®-96 SOFTWARE DESIGN INFORMATION

Table 3-1. Instruction Summary

Mnemonic	Operands	Operation (Note 1)	Flags						Notes
			Z	N	C	V	VT	ST	
ADD/ADDB	2	D ← D+A	√	√	√	√	↑	—	
ADD/ADDB	3	D ← B+A	√	√	√	√	↑	—	
ADDC/ADDCB	2	D ← D+A+C	↓	√	√	√	↑	—	
SUB/SUBB	2	D ← D − A	√	√	√	√	↑	—	
SUB/SUBB	3	D ← B − A	√	√	√	√	↑	—	
SUBC/SUBCB	2	D ← D − A + C − 1	↓	√	√	√	↑	—	
CMP/CMPB	2	D − A	√	√	√	√	↑	—	
MUL/MULU	2	D, D + 2 ← D * A	—	—	—	—	—	?	2
MUL/MULU	3	D, D + 2 ← B * A	—	—	—	—	—	?	2
MULB/MULUB	2	D, D + 1 ← D * A	—	—	—	—	—	?	3
MULB/MULUB	3	D, D + 1 ← B * A	—	—	—	—	—	?	3
DIV/DIVU	2	D ← (D, D + 2)/A D + 2 remainder	—	—	—	√	↑	—	2
DIVB/DIVUB	2	D ← (D, D + 1)/A D + 1 remainder	—	—	—	√	↑	—	3
AND/ANDB	2	D ← D and A	√	√	0	0	—	—	
AND/ANDB	3	D ← B and A	√	√	0	0	—	—	
OR/ORB	2	D ← D or A	√	√	0	0	—	—	
XOR/XORB	2	D ← D (excl. or) A	√	√	0	0	—	—	
LD/LDB	2	D ← A	—	—	—	—	—	—	
ST/STB	2	A ← D	—	—	—	—	—	—	
LDBSE	2	D ← A; D + 1 ← SIGN(A)	—	—	—	—	—	—	3,4
LDBZE	2	D ← A; D + 1 ← 0	—	—	—	—	—	—	3,4
PUSH	1	SP ← SP − 2; (SP) A	—	—	—	—	—	—	
POP	1	A ← (SP); SP ← SP + 2	—	—	—	—	—	—	
PUSHF	0	SP ← SP − 2; (SP) ← PSW; PSW ← 0000H I ← 0	0	0	0	0	0	0	
POPF	0	PSW ← (SP); SP ← SP + 2 I ← √	√	√	√	√	√	√	
SJMP	1	PC ← PC + 11-bit offset	—	—	—	—	—	—	5
LJMP	1	PC ← PC + 16-bit offset	—	—	—	—	—	—	5
BR(indirect)	1	PC ← (A)	—	—	—	—	—	—	
SCALL	1	SP ← SP − 2; (SP) ← PC; PC ← PC + 11-bit offset	—	—	—	—	—	—	5
LCALL	1	SP ← SP − 2; (SP) ← PC; PC ← PC + 16-bit offset	—	—	—	—	—	—	5
RET	0	PC ← (SP); SP ← SP + 2	—	—	—	—	—	—	
J(conditional)	1	PC ← PC + 8-bit offset	—	—	—	—	—	—	5
JC	1	Jump if C = 1	—	—	—	—	—	—	5
JNC	1	Jump if C = 0	—	—	—	—	—	—	5

Note

1. If the mnemonic ends in "B", a byte operation is performed, otherwise a word operation is done. Operands D, B, and A must conform to the alignment rules for the required operand type. D and B are locations in the register file; A can be located anywhere in memory.
2. D, D + 2 are consecutive WORDS in memory; D is DOUBLE-WORD aligned.
3. D, D + 1 are consecutive BYTES in memory; D is WORD aligned.
4. Changes a byte to a word.
5. Offset is a 2's complement number.

MCS®-96 SOFTWARE DESIGN INFORMATION

Table 3-2. Instruction Summary

Mnemonic	Oper-ands	Operation (Note 1)	Flags Z	N	C	V	VT	ST	Notes
JE	1	Jump if Z = 1	—	—	—	—	—	—	5
JNE	1	Jump if Z = 0	—	—	—	—	—	—	5
JGE	1	Jump if N = 0	—	—	—	—	—	—	5
JLT	1	Jump if N = 1	—	—	—	—	—	—	5
JGT	1	Jump if N = 0 and Z = 0	—	—	—	—	—	—	5
JLE	1	Jump if N = 1 or Z = 1	—	—	—	—	—	—	5
JH	1	Jump if C = 1 and Z = 0	—	—	—	—	—	—	5
JNH	1	Jump if C = 0 or Z = 1	—	—	—	—	—	—	5
JV	1	Jump if V = 1	—	—	—	—	—	—	5
JNV	1	Jump if V = 0	—	—	—	—	—	—	5
JVT	1	Jump if VT = 1; Clear VT	—	—	—	—	0	—	5
JNVT	1	Jump if VT = 0; Clear VT	—	—	—	—	0	—	5
JST	1	Jump if ST = 1	—	—	—	—	—	—	5
JNST	1	Jump if ST = 0	—	—	—	—	—	—	5
JBS	3	Jump if Specified Bit = 1	—	—	—	—	—	—	5,6
JBC	3	Jump if Specified Bit = 0	—	—	—	—	—	—	5,6
DJNZ	1	D ← D − 1; if D ≠ 0 then PC ← PC + 8-bit offset	—	—	—	—	—	—	5
DEC/DECB	1	D ← D − 1	√	√	√	√	↑	—	
NEG/NEGB	1	D ← 0 − D	√	√	√	√	↑	—	
INC/INCB	1	D ← D + 1	√	√	√	√	↑	—	
EXT	1	D ← D; D + 2 ← Sign (D)	√	√	0	0	—	—	2
EXTB	1	D ← D; D + 1 ← Sign (D)	√	√	0	0	—	—	3
NOT/NOTB	1	D ← Logical Not (D)	√	√	0	0	—	—	
CLR/CLRB	1	D ← 0	1	0	0	0	—	—	
SHL/SHLB/SHLL	2	C ← msb — — — — — lsb ← 0	√	?	√	√	↑	—	7
SHR/SHRB/SHRL	2	0 → msb — — — — — lsb → C	√	0	√	0	—	√	7
SHRA/SHRAB/SHRAL	2	msb → msb — — — — — lsb → C	√	√	√	0	—	√	7
SETC	0	C ← 1	—	—	1	—	—	—	
CLRC	0	C ← 0	—	—	0	—	—	—	
CLRVT	0	VT ← 0	—	—	—	—	0	—	
RST	0	PC ← 2080H	0	0	0	0	0	0	8
DI	0	Disable All Interrupts (I ← 0)	—	—	—	—	—	—	
EI	0	Enable All Interrupts (I ← 1)	—	—	—	—	—	—	
NOP	0	PC ← PC + 1	—	—	—	—	—	—	
SKIP	0	PC ← PC + 2	—	—	—	—	—	—	
NORML	2	Normalize (See sec 3.13.66)	√	1	0	—	—	—	7
TRAP	0	SP ← SP − 2; (SP) ← PC; PC ← (2010H)	—	—	—	—	—	—	9

Note

1. If the mnemonic ends in "B", a byte operation is performed, otherwise a word operation is done. Operands D, B and A must conform to the alignment rules for the required operand type. D and B are locations in the register file; A can be located anywhere in memory.
5. Offset is a 2's complement number.
6. Specified bit is one of the 2048 bits in the register file.
7. The "L" (Long) suffix indicates double-word operation.
8. Initiates a Reset by pulling RESET low. Software should re-initialize all the necessary registers with code starting at 2080H.
9. The assembler will not accept this mnemonic.

MCS®-96 SOFTWARE DESIGN INFORMATION

Table 3-3. Opcode and State Time Listing

MNEMONIC	OPERANDS	DIRECT			IMMEDIATE			INDIRECT⊛ NORMAL			INDIRECT⊛ AUTO-INC.		INDEXED⊛ SHORT			INDEXED⊛ LONG	
		OPCODE	BYTES	STATE TIMES	OPCODE	BYTES	STATE TIMES	OPCODE	BYTES	STATE① TIMES	BYTES	STATE① TIMES	OPCODE	BYTES	STATE① TIMES	BYTES	STATE① TIMES
ARITHMETIC INSTRUCTIONS																	
ADD	2	64	3	4	65	4	5	66	3	6/11	3	7/12	67	4	6/11	5	7/12
ADD	3	44	4	5	45	5	6	46	4	7/12	4	8/13	47	5	7/12	6	8/13
ADDB	2	74	3	4	75	3	4	76	3	6/11	3	7/12	77	4	6/11	5	7/12
ADDB	3	54	4	5	55	4	5	56	4	7/12	4	8/13	57	5	7/12	6	8/13
ADDC	2	A4	3	4	A5	4	5	A6	3	6/11	3	7/12	A7	4	6/11	5	7/12
ADDCB	2	B4	3	4	B5	3	4	B6	3	6/11	3	7/12	B7	4	6/11	5	7/12
SUB	2	68	3	4	69	4	5	6A	3	6/11	3	7/12	6B	4	6/11	5	7/12
SUB	3	48	4	5	49	5	6	4A	4	7/12	4	8/13	4B	5	7/12	6	8/13
SUBB	2	78	3	4	79	3	4	7A	3	6/11	3	7/12	7B	4	6/11	5	7/12
SUBB	3	58	4	5	59	4	5	5A	4	7/12	4	8/13	5B	5	7/12	6	8/13
SUBC	2	A8	3	4	A9	4	5	AA	3	6/11	3	7/12	AB	4	6/11	5	7/12
SUBCB	2	B8	3	4	B9	3	4	BA	3	6/11	3	7/12	BB	4	6/11	5	7/12
CMP	2	88	3	4	89	4	5	8A	3	6/11	3	7/12	8B	4	6/11	5	7/12
CMPB	2	98	3	4	99	3	4	9A	3	6/11	3	7/12	9B	4	6/11	5	7/12
MULU	2	6C	3	25	6D	4	26	6E	3	27/32	3	28/33	6F	4	27/32	5	28/33
MULU	3	4C	4	26	4D	5	27	4E	4	28/33	4	29/34	4F	5	28/33	6	29/34
MULUB	2	7C	3	17	7D	3	17	7E	3	19/24	3	20/25	7F	4	19/24	5	20/25
MULUB	3	5C	4	18	5D	4	18	5E	4	20/25	4	21/26	5F	5	20/25	6	21/26
MUL	2	②	4	29	②	5	30	②	4	31/36	4	32/37	②	5	31/36	6	32/37
MUL	3	②	5	30	②	6	31	②	5	32/37	5	33/38	②	6	32/37	7	33/38
MULB	2	②	4	21	②	4	21	②	4	23/28	4	24/29	②	5	23/28	6	24/29
MULB	3	②	5	22	②	5	22	②	5	24/29	5	25/30	②	6	24/29	7	25/30
DIVU	2	8C	3	25	8D	4	26	8E	3	28/32	3	29/33	8F	4	28/32	5	29/33
DIVUB	2	9C	3	17	9D	3	17	9E	3	20/24	3	21/25	9F	4	20/24	5	21/25
DIV	2	②	4	29	②	5	30	②	4	32/36	4	33/37	②	5	32/36	6	33/37
DIVB	2	②	4	21	②	4	21	②	4	24/28	4	25/29	②	5	24/28	6	25/29

Notes:

⊛ Long indexed and Indirect + instructions have identical opocodes with Short indexed and Indirect modes, respectively. The second byte of instructions using any indirect or indexed addressing mode specifies the exact mode used. If the second byte is even, use Indirect or Short Indexed. If it is odd, use Indirect + or Long indexed. In all cases the second byte of the instruction always specifies an even (word) location for the address referenced.

① Number of state times shown for internal/external operands.

② The opcodes for signed multiply and divide are the opcodes for the unsigned functions with an "FE" appended as a prefix.

MCS®-96 SOFTWARE DESIGN INFORMATION

Table 3-3. Continued

MNEMONIC	OPERANDS	DIRECT			IMMEDIATE			INDIRECT⑥					INDEXED⑥				
								NORMAL			AUTO-INC.		SHORT			LONG	
		OPCODE	BYTES	STATE TIMES	OPCODE	BYTES	STATE TIMES	OPCODE	BYTES	STATE① TIMES	BYTES	STATE① TIMES	OPCODE	BYTES	STATE① TIMES	BYTES	STATE① TIMES
LOGICAL INSTRUCTIONS																	
AND	2	60	3	4	61	4	5	62	3	6/11	3	7/12	63	4	6/11	5	7/12
AND	3	40	4	5	41	5	6	42	4	7/12	4	8/13	43	5	7/12	6	8/13
ANDB	2	70	3	4	71	3	4	72	3	6/11	3	7/12	73	4	6/11	5	7/12
ANDB	3	50	4	5	51	4	5	52	4	7/12	4	8/13	53	5	7/12	6	8/13
OR	2	80	3	4	81	4	5	82	3	6/11	3	7/12	83	4	6/11	5	7/12
ORB	2	90	3	4	91	3	4	92	3	6/11	3	7/12	93	4	6/11	5	7/12
XOR	2	84	3	4	85	4	5	86	3	6/11	3	7/12	87	4	6/11	5	7/12
XORB	2	94	3	4	95	3	4	96	3	6/11	3	7/12	97	4	6/11	5	7/12
DATA TRANSFER INSTRUCTIONS																	
LD	2	A0	3	4	A1	4	5	A2	3	6/11	3	7/12	A3	4	6/11	5	7/12
LDB	2	B0	3	4	B1	3	4	B2	3	6/11	3	7/12	B3	4	6/11	5	7/12
ST	2	C0	3	4	—	—	—	C2	3	7/11	3	8/12	C3	4	7/11	5	8/12
STB	2	C4	3	4	—	—	—	C6	3	7/11	3	8/12	C7	4	7/11	5	8/12
LDBSE	2	BC	3	4	BD	3	4	BE	3	6/11	3	7/12	BF	4	6/11	5	7/12
LDBZE	2	AC	3	4	AD	3	4	AE	3	6/11	3	7/12	AF	4	6/11	5	7/12
STACK OPERATIONS (internal stack)																	
PUSH	1	C8	2	8	C9	3	8	CA	2	11/15	2	12/16	CB	3	11/15	4	12/16
POP	1	CC	2	12	—	—	—	CE	2	14/18	2	14/18	CF	3	14/18	4	14/18
PUSHF	0	F2	1	8													
POPF	0	F3	1	9													
STACK OPERATIONS (external stack)																	
PUSH	1	C8	2	12	C9	3	12	CA	2	15/19	2	16/20	CB	3	15/19	4	16/20
POP	1	CC	2	14	—	—	—	CE	2	16/20	2	16/20	CF	3	16/20	4	16/20
PUSHF	0	F2	1	12													
POPF	0	F3	1	13													

JUMPS AND CALLS

MNEMONIC	OPCODE	BYTES	STATES	MNEMONIC	OPCODE	BYTES	STATES
LJMP	E7	3	8	LCALL	EF	3	13/16⑤
SJMP	20-27④	2	8	SCALL	28-2F④	2	13/16⑤
BR[ ]	E3	2	8	RET	F0	1	12/16⑤
				TRAP③	F7	1	

Notes:

① Number of state times shown for internal/external operands.

③ The assembler does not accept this mnemonic.

④ The least significant 3 bits of the opcode are concatenated with the following 8 bits to form an 11-bit, 2's complement, offset for the relative call or jump.

⑤ State times for stack located internal/external.

⑥ The assembler uses the generic jump mnemonic (BR) to generate this instruction.

MCS®-96 SOFTWARE DESIGN INFORMATION

Table 3-4. CONDITIONAL JUMPS

All conditional jumps are 2 byte instructions. They require 8 state times if the jump is taken, 4 if it is not.

MNEMONIC	OPCODE	MNEMONIC	OPCODE	MNEMONIC	OPCODE	MNEMONIC	OPCODE
JC	DB	JE	DF	JGE	D6	JGT	D2
JNC	D3	JNE	D7	JLT	DE	JLE	DA
JH	D9	JV	DD	JVT	DC	JST	D8
JNH	D1	JNV	D5	JNVT	D4	JNST	D0

JUMP ON BIT CLEAR OR BIT SET

These instructions are 3-byte instructions. They require 9 state times if the jump is taken, 5 if it is not.

	BIT NUMBER							
MNEMONIC	0	1	2	3	4	5	6	7
JBC	30	31	32	33	34	35	36	37
JBS	38	39	3A	3B	3C	3D	3E	3F

LOOP CONTROL

DJNZ OPCODE EO; 3 BYTES; 5/9 STATE TIMES (NOT TAKEN/TAKEN)

SINGLE REGISTER INSTRUCTIONS

MNEMONIC	OPCODE	BYTES	STATES	MNEMONIC	OPCODE	BYTES	STATES
DEC	05	2	4	EXT	06	2	4
DECB	15	2	4	EXTB	16	2	4
NEG	03	2	4	NOT	02	2	4
NEGB	13	2	4	NOTB	12	2	4
INC	07	2	4	CLR	01	2	4
INCB	17	2	4	CLRB	11	2	4

SHIFT INSTRUCTIONS

INSTR	WORD		INSTR	BYTE		INSTR	DBL WD		
MNEMONIC	OP	B	MNEMONIC	OP	B	MNEMONIC	OP	B	STATE TIMES
SHL	09	3	SHLB	19	3	SHLL	0D	3	7 + 1 PER SHIFT⑦
SHR	08	3	SHRB	18	3	SHRL	0C	3	7 + 1 PER SHIFT⑦
SHRA	0A	3	SHRAB	1A	3	SHRAL	0E	3	7 + 1 PER SHIFT⑦

SPECIAL CONTROL INSTRUCTIONS

MNEMONIC	OPCODE	BYTES	STATES	MNEMONIC	OPCODE	BYTES	STATES
SETC	F9	1	4	DI	FA	1	4
CLRC	F8	1	4	EI	FB	1	4
CLRVT	FC	1	4	NOP	FD	1	4
RST	FF	1	16	SKIP	00	2	4

NORMALIZE

NORML	0F	3	11 + 1 PER SHIFT

Notes:

⑥ This instruction takes 2 states to pull RST low, then holds it low for 2 states to initiate a reset. The reset takes 12 states, at which time the program restarts at location 2080H.

⑦ Execution will take at least 8 states, even for 0 shift.

Q. SFR AND OTHER GENERAL PRECAUTIONS AND RESTRICTIONS

Table 3-7 Special Function Register Restrictions

Address	Function	Restrictions
1-0	Zero register	Read only
3-2	A/D control/result	Byte access only
5-4	HSI/HSO time	Word access only
06	HSI stat/HSO command	Byte read only
07	Serial IN/OUT	Byte access only
08	Interrupt mask	Byte access only
09	Interrupt pending	Byte access only
B-A	Timer 1	Word read only
D-C	Timer 2	Word read only
0E	Port0/baud	Byte access only
0F	Port1	Byte access only
10	Port2	Byte access only
11	Serial control	Byte access only
12	Reserved	No access allowed
13	Reserved	No access allowed
14	Reserved	No access allowed
15	HSI status/control	Byte access only
16	HSI status/control	Byte access only
17	PWM control	Byte write only

3.7.5. Accessing Register Mapped I/O

The on-board I/O devices such as the serial port or the A/D converter are controlled as register mapped I/O. This allows convenient and efficient I/O processing. The implementation of the current members of the MCS-96 family place some restrictions on how these registers can be accessed. While these restrictions are not severe, the programmer must be aware of them. A complete listing of these registers is shown in figure 2-7 and 2-8. The restrictions are as follows:

a). TIMER1, TIMER2 and HSI_TIME are *word read only*. They cannot be read as bytes or written to in any format.

b). HSO_TIME is *word write only*. It cannot be written to as individual bytes or read in any format.

c). R0 (the ZERO register) is byte or word read or write but writing to it will not change its' value.

d). All of the other I/O registers can be accessed only as bytes. This applies even to the AD_RESULT which is logically a word operand.

Other information that may prove helpful follows:

1. Do not use SFR space (00 - 17H in RAM Register File) to write programs or store results or stack information. This space is dedicated to be used as SFRs in register mapped I/O. The SFRs are used to control I/Os. In that connection you will note in all the SHR and SHL instructions (and their variants) that the Intel manuals state: "the count may be specified either as an immediate value in the range 0 to 15 inclusive, or as the content of any register, the address of which is 16 to 255." A glance at the SFR map indicates that the above should read "the address of which is 24 to 255" (noticing that location 24 is the Stack Pointer which can not be used if stack operations are performed).

2. PUSHF causes PSW to be placed on the stack and the PSW is then left with 0000.

3. Reading IOS1 (16H) or any of its bits clears IOS1.

4. TI and RI bits in SPSTAT (11H) are cleared when SPSTAT is read.

5. The instructions JVT, CLRVT, JNVT, PUSHF, and RST all clear the VT flag (the only ways it can be cleared).

6. After reading HSI-TIME (04, 05H), information in HSI-STATUS (06H) is lost as one entry from the FIFO is unloaded into the holding register. Hence, read HSI-STATUS before reading HSI-TIME. Make sure at least 8 state times exist between reading of successive FIFO entries out of the HSI-TIME portion of the holding register. The Microcontroller Handbook states "it can take up to 8 state times for this information (i.e. HSI-STATUS and HSI-TIME) to reach the holding register" (i.e. from the FIFO) for it to be read from there.

7. To BOTH enable and clear the WDT, one must write LDB WDT, #01EH followed by LDB WDT, #0E1H where WDT = 0AH.

8. The quasi directional port pins are P1.0 - P1.7 (all) and P2.7, P2.6. P0 is an input port. P2.0, 2.5 are output pins, P2.1, 2.2, 2.3, 2.4 are input pins. Ports 3 and 4 are either bi-directional ports with open drain outputs or system bus pins which the memory controller uses when it is accessing off-chip memory.

9. Word boundaries start at even addresses with low order byte on the even address and high order byte in the next higher odd address.

10. Between writing to the GO bit in the A/D COMMAND register (02H) and a read of the conversion status bit S in the A/D RESULT register (02H), place two NOPs for the necessary 8 state times before A/D conversion starts.

11. Make sure at least 8 state times exist between writing successive commands into the HSO CAM File.

12. Even if HSI.0 is disabled (IOC0.0 = 0), it can still be used to reset T2. Even if HSI.1 is disabled (IOC0.2 = 0), it can still be used to clock timer T2. Even if HSI.0 is disabled (IOC0.0 = 0) it can still be used as an interrupt source (if its mask bit, #4, is set and the global bit, I, in PSW is set).

13. The example on p. 3-2 (paragraph 3.2.3) in the Microcontroller Handbook, 1985 (see our previous section P(a)) is in error. ADD should be ADDB and the right side of the equation should have AL + deleted. Also, the Normalization (NORML) instruction does not set the N flag. It is indeterminate.

14. In doing the experiments, it is always a good idea to clear all pending interrupts by typing in BY 09 = 00 on the iSBE-96 before executing. Likewise, in any experiments dealing with HSI and HSO, it is a good idea to make sure that HSI FIFO and HSO CAM are empty by resetting the iSBE-96 before executing.

15. For inputting at ports or pins, or for external interrupts, always use DEBOUNCED switches, except where noted. See Fig 2-2 in next chapter.

16. 8096 addressing modes are again summarized:

DIRECT — The operand is specified by an 8-bit address field in the instruction. The operand must be in the Register File or SFR space (locations 0000H through 00FFH).

IMMEDIATE — The operand itself follows the opcode in the instruction stream as immediate data. The immediate data can be either 8-bits or 16-bits as required by the opcode.

INDIRECT — An 8-bit address field in the instruction gives the address of a word register in the Register File which contains the 16-bit address of the operand. The operand can be anywhere in memory.

INDIRECT WITH AUTO-INCREMENT — Same as Indirect, except that, after the operand is referenced, the word register that contains the operand's address is incremented by 1 if the operand is a byte, or by 2 if the operand is a word.

INDEXED — The instruction contains an 8-bit address field and either an 8-bit or a 16-bit displacement field. The 8-bit address field gives the address of a word register in the Register File which contains a 16-bit base address. The 8- or 16-bit displacement field contains a signed displacement that will be added to the base address to produce the address of the operand. The operand can be anywhere in memory.

The 8096 contains a Zero Register at word address 0000H (and which contains 0000H). This register is available for performing comparisons and for use as a base register in indexed addressing. This effectively provides direct addressing to all 64K of memory.

In the 8096, the Stack Pointer is at word address 0018H in the Register File. If the 8-bit address field in an indexed instruction contains 18H, the Stack Pointer becomes the base register. This allows direct accessing of variables in the stack.

IMPORTANT NOTE TO THE USER OF THIS BOOK

INTEL USER'S MANUALS ARE CONTINUALLY UPDATED WITH CLARIFICATIONS AND NEW INFORMATION. BEFORE DESIGNING WITH ANY PART, MAKE CERTAIN YOU HAVE THE LATEST USER'S MANUAL AND DATA SHEET.

AS THIS BOOK IS BEING WRITTEN, THE 1985 MICROCONTROLLER HANDBOOK IS BEING UPDATED FOR 1986. INFORMATION ON THE FOLLOWING TOPICS ARE AMONG THOSE TO BE UPDATED: BUS TIMINGS, A/D CONVERTER, PACKAGE TYPES, SERIAL PORT OPERATION, SHIFT INFORMATIONS, AND THE HSI/O. PLCC INFORMATION IS SHOWN BELOW.

OPTIONS		68-PIN	48-PIN
DIGITAL I/O	ROMLESS	8096	8094
	ROM	8396	8394
ANALOG AND DIGITAL I/O	ROMLESS	8097	8095
	ROM	8397	8395

Figures 2, 3 and 4 show the pinouts for the 48- and 68-pin packages. The 48-pin version is offered in Dual-In-Line package while the 68-pin version comes in a Plastic Leaded Chip Carrier and a Pin Grid Array.

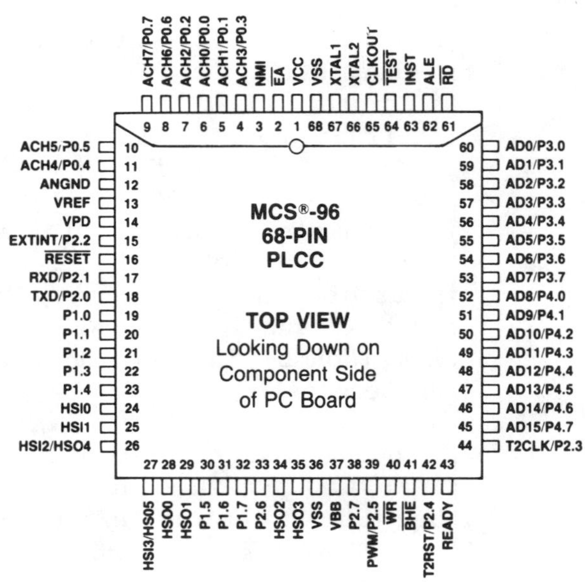

PGA	PLCC	Description	PGA	PLCC	Description	PGA	PLCC	Description
1	9	ACH7/P0.7	24	54	AD6/P3.6	47	31	P1.6
2	8	ACH6/P0.6	25	53	AD7/P3.7	48	30	P1.5
3	7	ACH2/P0.2	26	52	AD8/P4.0	49	29	HSO.1
4	6	ACH0/P0.0	27	51	AD9/P4.1	50	28	HSO.0
5	5	ACH1/P0.1	28	50	AD10/P4.2	51	27	HSO.5/HSI.3
6	4	ACH3/P0.3	29	49	AD11/P4.3	52	26	HSO.4/HSI.2
7	3	NMI	30	48	AD12/P4.4	53	25	HSI.1
8	2	EA	31	47	AD13/P4.5	54	24	HSI.0
9	1	VCC	32	46	AD14/P4.6	55	23	P1.4
10	68	VSS	33	45	AD15/P4.7	56	22	P1.3
11	67	XTAL1	34	44	T2CLK/P2.3	57	21	P1.2
12	66	XTAL2	35	43	READY	58	20	P1.1
13	65	CLKOUT	36	42	T2RST/P2.4	59	19	P1.0
14	64	$\overline{\text{TEST}}$	37	41	$\overline{\text{BHE}}$	60	18	TXD/P2.0
15	63	INST	38	40	$\overline{\text{WR}}$	61	17	RXD/P2.1
16	62	ALE	39	39	PWM/P2.5	62	16	$\overline{\text{RESET}}$
17	61	$\overline{\text{RD}}$	40	38	P2.7	63	15	EXTINT/P2.2
18	60	AD0/P3.0	41	37	VBB	64	14	VPD
19	59	AD1/P3.1	42	36	VSS	65	13	VREF
20	58	AD2/P3.2	43	35	HSO.3	66	12	ANGND
21	57	AD3/P3.3	44	34	HSO.2	67	11	ACH4/P0.4
22	56	AD4/P3.4	45	33	P2.6	68	10	ACH5/P0.5
23	55	AD5/P3.5	46	32	P1.7			

NOTE: THE LATEST ON-CHIP A/D CONVERTER INCLUDES SAMPLE AND HOLD. CONVERSION TIME IS 22 USEC. A CHIP CONFIGURATION REGISTER (CCR) CAN STORE OPERATING MODE INFORMATION: BUS CONTROL SIGNAL DEFINITIONS AND RUN-TIME SELECTION OF EXTERNAL BUS WIDTH (8 OR 16 BITS) CAN NOW BE SPECIFIED.

CHAPTER 2

HANDS-ON WITH THE iSBE-96 EMULATOR

INTRODUCTION

All the experiments in this book were performed on Intel's iSBE-96 single board emulator (monitor version V1. 1, copyright 1984 Intel Corp). It provides execution and debugging capabilities for the MCS-96 family of microcontrollers. It is a combination of hardware and software that permits MCS-96 programs to be run and debugged in the emulator's artificial environment prior to actually using those programs with the microcontroller. We refer you to your iSBE-96 Single Board Emulator User's Guide (ref. 4 in list of references at the end of the Introduction section in Chapter 1). There, on pp. 1-1 through 1-7, the purpose of emulation, its definition, the typical microcontroller development cycle before and with emulation, and a generalized emulation session, with procedures, are all discussed and described.

This chapter is divided into four sections: section A presents relevant information on the iSBE-96. (We also enclose with the book, courtesy Intel Corp., an iSBE-96 Pocket Reference card - ref. 6 in the reference list in chapter 1.) Section A and the card should give you sufficient iSBE-96 command and hardware information for the purposes of using this book. Should more be needed, consult ref. 4 (iSBE-96 Single Board Emulator User's Guide).

Section B discusses how we downloaded 8096 assembly language programs into the iSBE-96 from an IBM-PC. It also lists host systems (development systems or PCs) on which the experiments in this book may be run. Except for chapter 10, all the experiments in the book were done using the IBM-PC, 8096 cross-assembler, and a communications program to talk to the emulator via the IBM PC.

Section C presents material on the basic interfacing to the iSBE-96 with the switches, LEDs, A/D pots, the D/A filter circuit, a motor driver, and debounced switches needed to do the experiments. Where additional or special interfacing is needed for certain experiments in later chapters, it will be described at the time the experiments are done.

Section D presents the introductory hands-on experiments with the iSBE-96. Their purpose is to demonstrate the use of various relevant emulator commands in executing programs, applying breakpoints and single-stepping; to study the workings of the iSBE-96 monitor's stack operations and how they dovetail with the user's stack; and to demonstrate use of a switch bank at input port P0 and LEDs at output port P1. Monitor version V1.1 is the one used in the experiments with the iSBE-96.

NOTE

Throughout the book != stands for "not equal to". ISR stands for "interrupt service routine". H.R. stands for "Holding Register", Int. stands for "Interrupt", MINT stands for "Interrupt Mask Register", PINT stands for "Interrupt Pending Register", INVEC for "Interrupt Vector Address". HSO and HSI are the High Speed Output and Input units, respectively.

A. iSBE INFORMATION

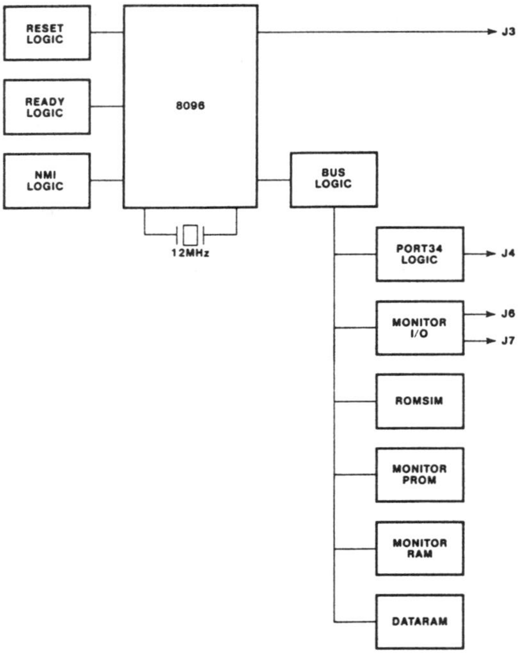

Figure 3-1 iSBE-96 Block Diagram

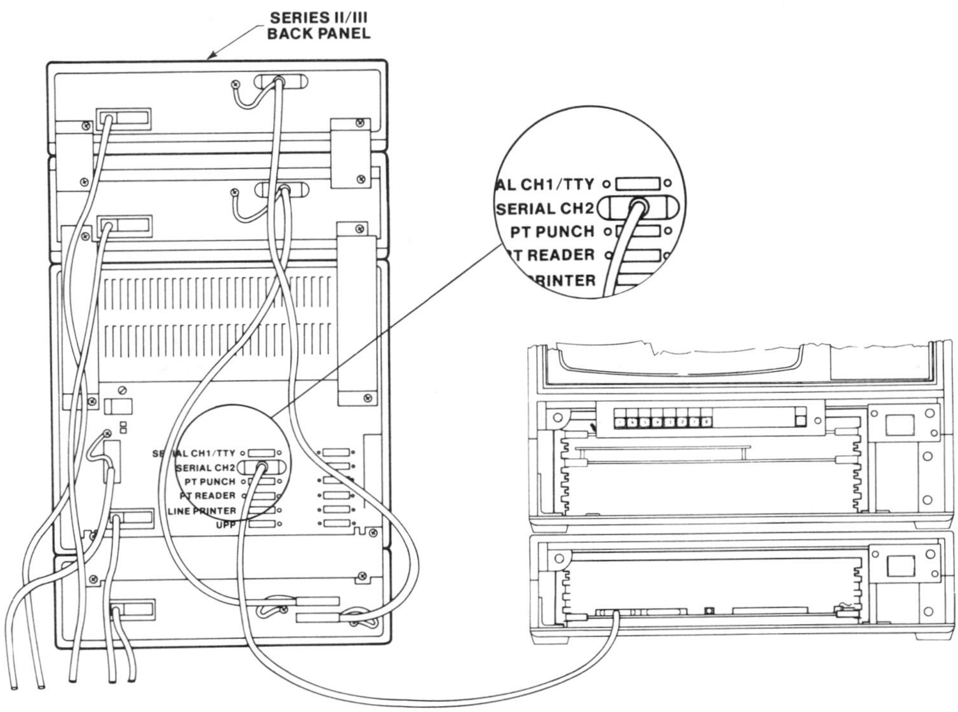

Figure 2-2 Hardware Installation (Using a Series II/III Expansion Chassis)

The iSBE-96 single board emulator does not work on the MDS-800.

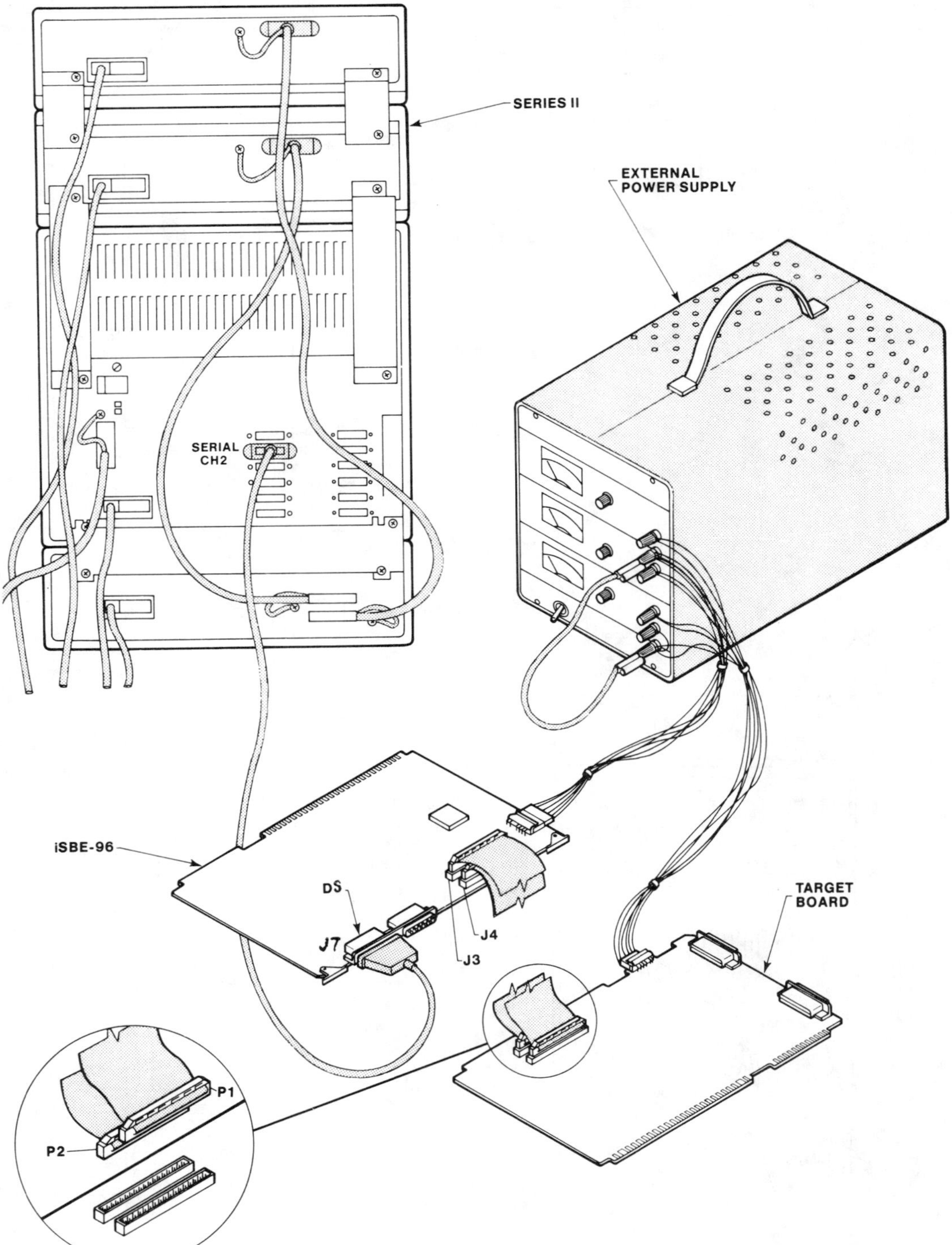

Figure 2-3 Hardware Installation (Using an External Power Supply)

Table 3-1 J3 and J4 Ribbon Cable Assignments

J3 Pin Number	Assignment		J4 Pin Number	Assignment	
1	Analog ground	(UAGND)	1	Connector key	
2	Analog channel 3	(UACH3)	2	Spare	
3	Analog channel 1	(UACH1)	3	Clock out	(UCLKOUT)
4	Analog ground	(UAGND)	4	Digital ground	
5	Analog channel 0	(UACH0)	5	INST	(UINST)
6	Analog channel 2	(UACH2)	6	Digital ground	
7	Analog ground	(UAGND)	7	ALE	(UALE)
8	Analog channel 6	(UACH6)	8	Digital ground	
9	Analog channel 7	(UACH7)	9	Read/	(UREAD/)
10	Connector key		10	Digital ground	
11	Analog channel 5	(UACH5)	11	AD0/P3.0	
12	Analog channel 4	(UACH4)	12	Digital ground	
13	Analog ground	(UAGND)	13	AD1/P3.1	
14	Analog VREF	(UVREF)	14	Digital ground	
15	Digital ground		15	AD2/P3.2	
16	External interrupt	(UEXTINT)	16	Digital ground	
17	Reset	(URESET)	17	AD3/P3.3	
18	Digital ground		18	Digital ground	
19	Received data	(URXD)	19	AD4/P3.4	
20	Transmit data	(UTXD)	20	Digital ground	
21	Digital ground		21	AD5/P3.5	
22	Port 1.0	(UP1.0)	22	Digital ground	
23	Port 1.1	(UP1.1)	23	AD6/P3.6	
24	Port 1.2	(UP1.2)	24	Digital ground	
25	Port 1.3	(UP1.3)	25	AD7/P3.7	
26	Port 1.4	(UP1.4)	26	Digital ground	
27	Digital ground		27	AD8/P4.0	
28	High speed input 0	(UHSI0)	28	Digital ground	
29	High speed input 1	(UHSI1)	29	AD9/P4.1	
30	Digital ground		30	Digital ground	
31	High speed output 4	(UHSO4)	31	AD10/P4.2	
32	High speed output 5	(UHSO5)	32	Digital ground	
33	Digital ground		33	AD11/P4.3	
34	High speed output 0	(UHSO0)	34	Digital ground	
35	High speed output 1	(UHSO1)	35	AD12/P4.4	
36	Digital ground		36	Digital ground	
37	Port 1.5	(UP1.5)	37	AD13/P4.5	
38	Port 1.6	(UP1.6)	38	Digital ground	
39	Port 1.7	(UP1.7)	39	AD14/P4.6	
40	Port 2.6	(UP2.6)	40	Digital ground	
41	Digital ground		41	AD15/P4.7	
42	High speed output 2	(UHSO2)	42	Digital ground	
43	High speed output 3	(UHSO3)	43	READY	(UREADY)
44	Digital ground		44	Digital ground	
45	Port 2.7	(UP2.7)	45	Byte high enable enable	(UBHE/)
46	PWM output	(UPWM)	46	Digital ground	
47	Digital ground		47	Write	(UWRITE/)
48	Timer 2 reset	(UT2RST)	48	Digital ground	
49	Timer 2 clock	(UT2CLK)	49	Reserved for future use	
50	Digital ground		50	Digital ground	

Monitor PROM

The monitor PROM on the iSBE-96 board consists of two EPROMs that contain the monitor routines that operate the iSBE-96. This memory is mapped between locations 02000H and 09FFFH. This monitor PROM is not directly accessible, so attempts to access this memory are made to ROMSIM.

Monitor RAM

The monitor RAM consists of 2K bytes of on-board static RAM mapped to locations 0800H to 0FFFH. The monitor RAM is only accessible to the monitor and is not available for application code or to the monitor commands.

DATARAM

Locations 100 to 7FFH are designated as the DATARAM space. Note that in mode 1 this area is extended to include 100H to 1EFFH provided that positions U48 and U56 on the iSBE-96 board contain 8K x 8 static RAMs. In modes 4-7, DATARAM can be expanded by locating RAM on the user's prototype in the USER address space from 100H to 1EFFH (see Figure 3-3). Any memory mapped as I/O in the user's prototype should be placed in these partitions.

Monitor I/O Page

Locations 1F00H to 1FFFH are reserved by the monitor for iSBE-96 I/O devices. Part of this I/O is a reconstruction of ports 3 and 4 (addresses 1FFEH and 1FFFH) of an 839X. Table 3-3 shows the memory mapped I/O address assignments.

ROMSIM

The on-board RAMS become the area where a user program is loaded for execution. Locations 2000H to 5FFFH contain this RAM and are called ROMSIM. ROMSIM is available at these locations when modes 1, 2, 3, 4, or 5 of the MAP command are selected (see Chapter 4 for the MAP command syntax).

The ROMSIM partition may be expanded to locations 2000H to 0FFFFH if 8K by 8 static RAMs are used in this space. See Figure 3-3 and Appendix B, Figure B-1 for details on reconfiguring the iSBE-96 system.

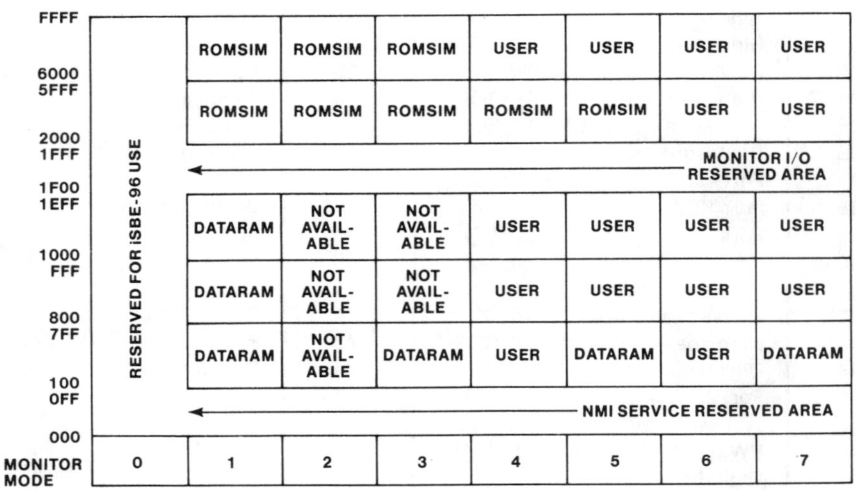

Figure 3-3 iSBE-96 Memory Map and Monitor Modes

B. USING THE IBM-PC TO DOWNLOAD TO THE iSBE-96. RUNNING THE EXPERIMENTS ON OTHER HOST SYSTEMS.

The Intel 8096 Single Board Emulator (iSBE-96) is a tool available to designers for developing systems based on the 8096 microcontroller. Throughout this book we will be using the iSBE-96 to execute the various programs used to demonstrate hardware and software features and applications of the 8096 device. Before describing the way the iSBE-96 is used in this book, we would like to present a typical 8096 development environment built around the iSBE-96.

A typical development environment for designing and proto-typing a microprocessor or microcontroller based product consists of the following facilities:

A) Firmware generation system - the means of writing, translating (assembling/compiling), linking, loading and debugging microcontroller code.

B) Hardware emulation system - the means of duplicating the hardware and firmware operation of the microcontroller. The emulator also allows the designer to read and write internal and external memory/registers of the microcontroller and its associated prototype hardware.

With the above facilities the designer can build a prototype of the target product, develop firmware for it, and debug and test its operation prior to the product entering the manufacturing stage. Once into that phase, the emulator may serve as an in-line test facility to catch failed components.

While this latter use of the emulator is a slow and expensive means of automated factory testing, it is sometimes necessary when complexity of the product is high.

The iSBE-96 provides a hardware emulation system but does not allow the development of firmware for the 8096. Typically, the iSBE-96 is coupled with an Intellec Series II, III or IV system. The latter provides an environment for writing, translating, linking and downloading 8096 firmware. An example scenario would go as follows:

Using the editor, the user would enter a program(s) into a file(s) on disk. The user would then run the assembler or compiler, depending on the nature of the source code. The output of either of these translators is relocatable object code. The user would then use the linker/loader facility to generate an object module which contained absolute addresses based on the target address space. This object module would then be converted to a hexadecimal format which could then be downloaded to the target system via the iSBE-96.

The specific environment used in this book is modeled after the above description and procedure. An IBM-PC is used for both firmware development and as an interface to the iSBE-96 emulator. An 8096 cross-assembler available from 2500ADSOFTWARE Inc. was used for assembly, linking/loading and hexadecimal format preparation (8096 XASM for MSDOS, CP/M86, version 3.00, 2500ADSOFTWARE, 17200 E. Ohio Drive, Aurora, CO 80017). The text editor available with the PC-DOS operating system was used to enter programs on the IBM-PC. After the file containing the assembly language program was edited, the X8096 command (see above reference re: 2500ADSOFTWARE Inc.) was used to translate the file.asm (containing the assembly language program) to a file.obj (containing the relocatable object code). The final processing of the program requires the use of the LINK2 command to link and load the program and convert the output to hexadecimal format. Once in that format, the program can then be downloaded using the LOAD HEXFILE command of our SBEIPC communications program. This program allows the IBM-PC to communicate with the iSBE-96 via the serial communication port of the IBM-PC and the DT serial port of the iSBE-96. The SBEIPC program operates in the same manner as the iSBE-96 routines provided by Intel for their Intellec Series of Microprocessor Development Systems.

The iSBE-96 monitor supports the following command to allow the downloading of 8096 programs: LOAD HEXFILE: this command will respond with "Enter HEX File to be Downloaded". Once the file .hex is entered, the program contained will be loaded into the appropriate memory locations specified in the Link/Loading phase of program translation.

With the executable code downloaded, the user can begin the emulation/debugging session. This phase makes extensive use of the GO, BR, STEP, BYTE, WORD, CHANGE, etc. commands acknowledged by the iSBE-96 monitor (see the experiments in section D of this chapter). (We are not emphasizing iSBE-96 commands unless they play a role in the implementation and execution of the experiments in this book.)

The above procedure is used in downloading the programs for each experiment in the book. A complete user's guide for the SBEIPC program is provided with a supplemental experiment diskette containing all the experiments in this book. It is available from Microprocessor Training Inc., 14 East 8th Street, New York, NY 10003 (212-473-4947).

It should be noted that even though we have described the use of the X8096 cross assembler and the SBEIPC programs, all of the experiments in the book can be performed using equivalent 8096 tools on the Intel Intellec Series MDS systems. Also, user can always enter the programs in object (machine) code via a terminal/iSBE-96 hook-up. The print-outs of the programs for all experiments in the book give the HEX as well as ASM code.

The physical hook-up of the iSBE-96 is described in the iSBE-96 User's Guide, pp. 2-1 through 2-6 (see our section A this chapter). As mentioned, the IBM-PC COM1:port is used to connect to the DT(J6) port of the iSBE-96. We mention again that all experiments were performed on the V1.1 version of the iSBE-96 monitor program.

IMPORTANT NOTE TO THE USER OF THIS BOOK

Recent developments at Intel now allow the iSBE-96 to be used on a wide variety of Intel systems and on PC-DOS compatible machines. The SBE96SKIT now includes an iSBE-96 and Intel's ASM-96 assembler: Series III/Series IV versions of Intel's Intellec Development System. Thus the experiments in this book can be run on the latter.

For those who have an IBM PC/AT or IBM PC/XT, or other compatible system running DOS Version 3.0 or greater, Intel's SBE96 DKIT contains the Intel DOS version of ASM-96 with the necessary host communication software and cables needed to run on these systems. Further, the Intel ASM-96 assembler (both DOS and Series III/IV versions) runs with the RL-96 linker/relocator, thus supporting full macro capability as a symbolic relocatable assembler. PLM-96 also runs on all the above systems and is compatible with the Intel ASM-96.

In addition, for those who have an Intel iPDS or Series II Development System, iSBE-96 host communication software (ATOP 96) and cross assembler (XASM-96) are available from U.S. Software Corp., along with the SBE96SKIT or SBE96DKIT mentioned above from Intel.

ALL THE EXPERIMENTS IN THIS BOOK MAY BE RUN ON ANY OF THE ABOVE HOST SYSTEMS.

C. THE BASIC INTERFACING TO THE PORTS AND PINS ON THE iSBE-96 NEEDED TO DO THE EXPERIMENTS. EQUIPMENT REQUIRED.

The circuitry needed to have a bank of 8 switches input their data to port 0 of the 8096 and to have port P1 output a byte to 8 LEDs is shown in Fig. 2-1. (Additional components or equipment needed for special experiments are described in those experiments as they come up.)

We also used LEDs at port pins P2.6 and P2.7 for outputting purposes. The circuits to accomplish that are exactly as for any of the LEDs interfaced to P1 in Fig. 2-1. Note that P2.6 and P2.7 are J3 pin numbers 40 and 45, respectively, on the iSBE-96.

LEDs were also used at HSO output pins HSO.0, .1, .2, .3 (J3 pin numbers 34, 35, 42, 43). Again the same circuitry as in Fig. 2-1 was employed.

Debounced switches were always used to input to T2CLK (J3 pin 49), T2RST (J3 pin 48), HSI.1 (J3 pin 29), HSI.0 (J3 pin 28), EXTINT (J3 pin 16), HSI.2, .3 (J3 pins 31, 32), and to ACH.7 (J3 pin 9, when it was used as a source of external interrupts). In some cases a debounced switch was also needed at one of the inputs to port P0, replacing a switch from the switch bank. We indicate in the experiments where that became necessary. A circuit for a debounced switch is shown in Fig. 2-2.

The R, C values we used in the filter circuit at the PWM output to smooth out the pulse response to an analog output (see Fig. 4-11, p. 4-8 Microcontroller Handbook, or section F, chapter 1) were R = 3K, C = .3 uf for a frequency around 1100 Hz. The buffer used in that Fig. 4-11 was the CD 4049, as shown. We did a double inversion to see positive swings on the scope. This filter circuit was used at the output pin P2.5 (PWM, J3, pin 46) and again at output pin HSO.0 (J3, pin 34) when the latter was used to generate D/A. Where the PWM output was used to drive a simple 5V DC motor, the filter circuit was not used. Instead a transistor driver shown in Fig. 2-3 was employed at the PWM output before the motor.

Pots were used to provide 0-5V analog levels to the A/D input channels at port 0. They were 1K pots driven by the +5V available on the iSBE-96 board. No more than three are needed. When additional channels were needed to illustrate an experiment, they were simply connected to ground or to +5V to provide 00 or FF after conversion to confirm the point of the experiment.

In certain experiments, the need arises to observe and measure waveforms and pulses at the PWM, HSO, and port 1 outputs. The use of an oscilloscope is desirable in those cases. Its calibrated 1KHz output is also useful as an input source to the HSI unit in other experiments.

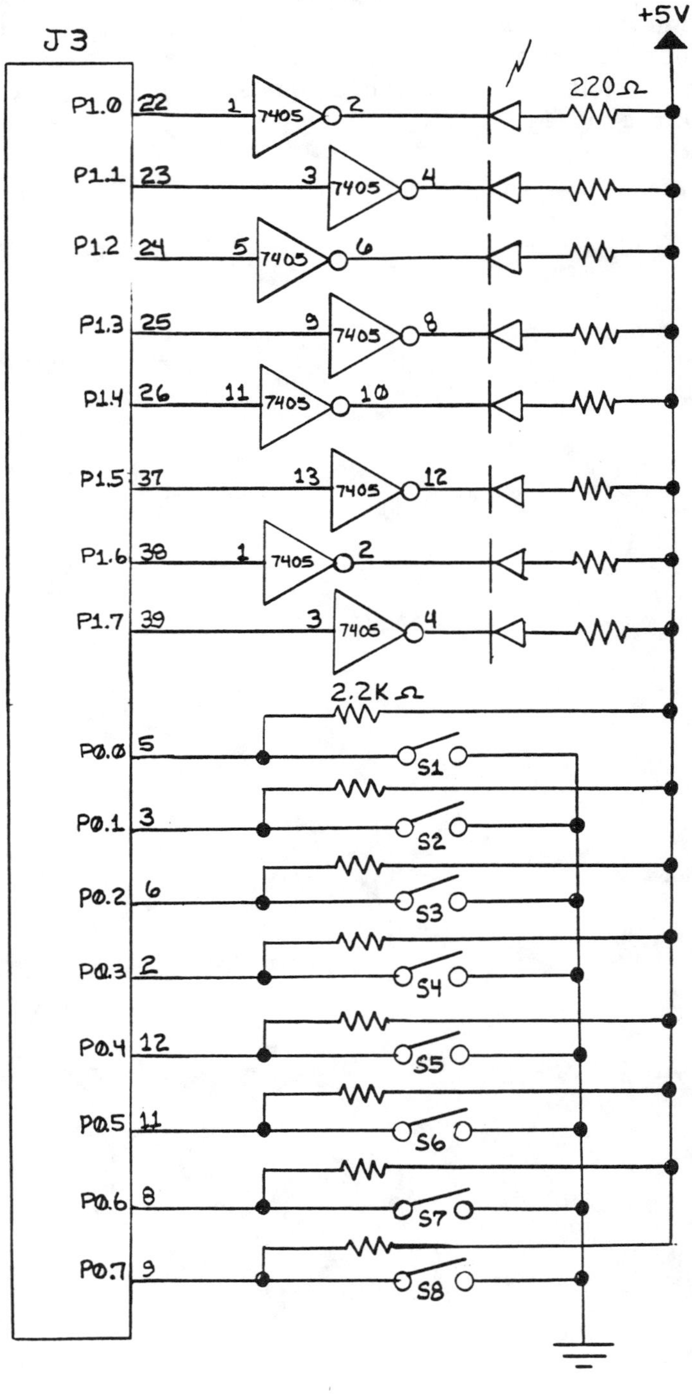

FIGURE 2-1: Switch and LED connections to ports 0 and 1, respectively.

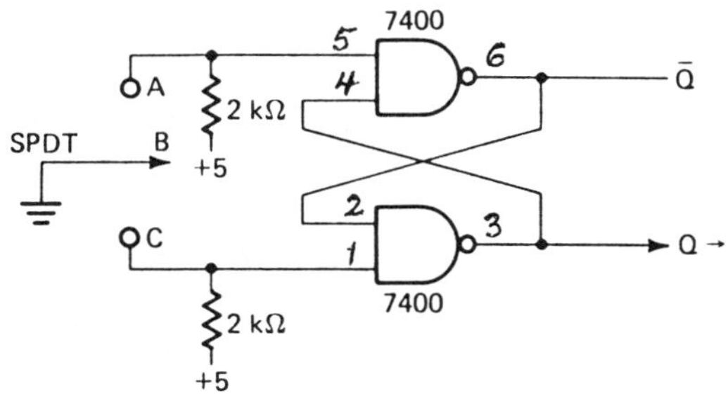

FIGURE 2-2: Circuitry for a debounced switch. 1K resistors will do just as well.

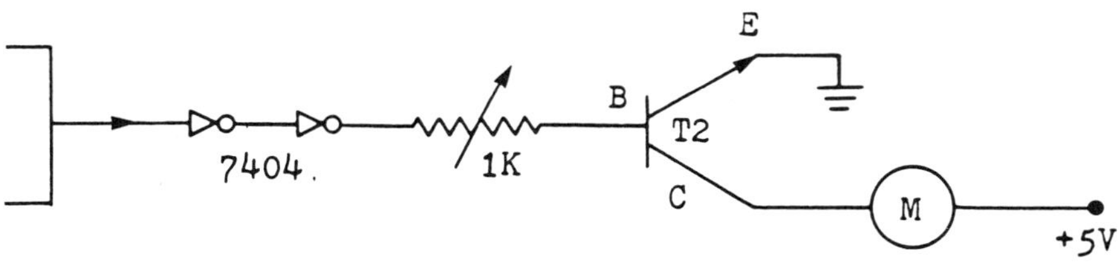

FIGURE 2-3: Transistor driver circuit for 5V DC motor M at the PWM (unfiltered) output. A diode (IN4001) across the motor in the collector circuit (with cathode at collector and anode at ground) is advised. That would prevent inductive spikes. Transistor T2 could be a TIP 31 or 2N3724A.

D. INTRODUCTORY EXPERIMENTS WITH THE iSBE-96.

EXPERIMENT 2-1

INPUTTING THROUGH PORT 0 AND OUTPUTTING TO PORT 1.

The program at 2100 below reads the byte value on the switch bank at port 0 (Fig. 2-1) into register 50 in the internal RAM register file. Port 0 is SFR 0EH. To execute the program, the user enters GO FROM 2100 FOREVER or simply G FR 2100 FO or just G FR 2100, followed in each case by a carriage return. The FOREVER (or FO) is needed if there are breakpoints that have been set and one wishes to have emulation proceed beyond the breakpoints i.e. disabling them. You then set the switches to some byte value. Enter BYTE 50 carriage return. The screen will then show 0050:"value", where "value" is the HEX byte of the switch setting. On the fly, change the switch setting. Again enter BYTE 50 carriage return, and see 0050:"new value" on the screen, where "new value" is the new HEX byte at the switch port. Repeat for other settings of the switch bits. Note that the SJMP THERE back to 2100 keeps polling P0 for any changes.

In the next program at 2105, we input the switch byte at port 0 directly to SFR 0FH (port 1 i.e. P1). Port 1 is here being used as an output port with LEDs connected (see Fig. 2-1). The SJMP HERE back to 2105 polls P0 continuously. The LEDs at P1 mirror the value of the switch byte at P0 immediately. Enter G FR 2105 carriage return. Vary the switch settings and observe the LEDs at P1 change and match the byte at P0 as the settings change.

```
        50 00          REG     EQU     50H
        18 00          SP      EQU     18H
        0E 00          PORT0   EQU     0EH
        0F 00          PORT1   EQU     0FH
                       ;
2100                           ORG     2100H
                       ;
                       ;
2100    B0 0E 50       THERE:  LDB     REG,PORT0        ;Read in the switch data.
2103    27 FB                  SJMP    THERE            ;Loop back and repeat.
```

```
2105                       ORG     2105H
                  ;
2105   B0 0E 0F   HERE:    LDB     PORT1,PORT0     ;Output switch data to LEDs.
2108   27 FB               SJMP    HERE            ;Loop back to repeat.
                  ;
                  ;
210A                       END
```

EXPERIMENT 2-2

PROGRAM EXECUTION WITH THE VARIOUS FORMS OF THE GO COMMAND. EXAMINING REGISTERS, MEMORY, STACK POINTER, PROGRAM COUNTER

The program at 3000 on the next page anticipates working with some of the instructions in the 8096 instruction set. We can explain them right here so that the experiment will make sense. Please note again that iSBE-96 with monitor version V1.1 was used throughout the book.

```
        50 00       REG1    EQU     50H
        60 00       REG2    EQU     60H
        70 00       REG3    EQU     70H
        18 00       SP      EQU     18H
                    ;
                    ;
3000                        ORG 3000H
                    ;
3000    A1 30 00 18         LD SP,#0030H        ;Initialize SP to 0030H.
3004    A1 00 00 50         LD REG1,#0000H      ;Initialize REG1 to 0000H.
3008    A1 1E 30 60         LD REG2,#301EH      ;Initialize REG2 to address 301EH.
300C    C2 60 50            ST REG1,[REG2]      ;Store contents of REG1 at address
                                                ;pointed to by REG2.
300F    A2 60 70    THERE:  LD REG3,[REG2]      ;Load contents of memory pointed
                                                ;by REG2 into REG3.
3012    07 70               INC REG3            ;Increment REG3.
3014    C2 60 70            ST REG3,[REG2]      ;Store contents of REG3 into
                                                ;memory location pointed to by REG2.
3017    27 F6               SJMP THERE          ;Loop to THERE.
                    ;
                    ;
3019                        END
```

The first instruction sets the stack pointer to 0030H. Please note that in doing so, the iSBE-96 monitor takes the first 6 bytes (3 words) of the stack at 002F, 2E, 2D, 2C, 2B, 2A for itself (to save the state of the user program during emulation e.g. the user's PSW and PC, among other things). Hence the SP command to read the value of the stack pointer will show 002A in this case, because the monitor has stacked information vital to it at the 6 bytes 002F to 002A, leaving the stack pointer at 002A. But, as Expt. 2-6 will show, when the user is going to use the stack to save his/her information, that information gets pushed, as hoped for, to 002F, 2E, 2D, etc. (assuming our program had set SP to 0030) and the monitor's 6 byte stack RECEDES, always using the 6 bytes BELOW the LATEST information pushed by user. Then, when user starts popping back the information from the stack, user's SP starts going back toward 0030 with the monitor's stack of 6 bytes trailing right behind to fill any void, so that user's stack information is lost after the popping. Expt. 2-6 will demonstrate all this very well.

The second instruction loads REG1 (50H) with 0000 and the third instruction loads REG2 (60H) with 301EH. The fourth instruction stores the value of REG1 at the address pointed to by the contents of REG2 i.e. 0000 is stored at word address 301E in this indirect addressing mode of the ST instruction. The fifth instruction takes the word value at location 301E and loads it into REG3 (70H). The next instruction increments that value while the instruction after that stores the incremented value back at word address 301E. [ ] indicates indirect addressing. SJMP THERE will have the effect of constantly incrementing the word contents at address 301E in memory. Please note that THIS program is treating REG1, REG2 and REG3 as word registers because of the use of the LD, ST and INC forms of the load, store, and increment instructions. The ST form of Store also guarantees that a word will be stored at addresses 301E,301F (low byte at 301E, high byte at 301F). Thus, REG1 is the word register 0050,51 (low byte in 50, high byte in 51), REG2 is the word register 0060,61 (high byte in 61, low byte in 60), and similarly for REG3 and 0070,71. 301E is a word address here.

Note also that we could NOT directly increment memory location 301E as we might have wished. The INC and INCB instructions increment only word or byte registers in the internal register file. Hence the three instructions at 300F,3012,3014.

PROCEDURE

1. Enter G FR 3000 FO carriage return (we'll no longer specify carriage return. It is, of course, necessary at the end of all commands entered). Then strike the ESC key and examine the PC (program counter). PC = 3017 is what we observed. Type in SP. We observed SP = 002A, as discussed before. Enter WO 50 and see 0050:0000 on the screen. Then WO 60 gives 0060:301E. We then found that WO 70 gave 0070:AB78 and WO 301E gave AB78, all in keeping with expectations. At most, WO 70 and WO 301E will differ by 1, depending where in the SJMP loop we were at the time of ESC. AB78 was the value in both, after the numerous increments in the loop at the time we did an ESC. Execute again and read out the various registers and the memory location as above. A few will be different. Why?
2. Escape and enter G FR 3000 TILL 300F. The screen should show "program break at 300F." Type in PC, then SP, then WO 50, then WO 60, then WO 70, then WO 301E. You should observe respectively: PC = 3012; SP = 002A; 0050:0000; 0060:301E; 0070:0000; 301E:0000. PC = 3012 is pointing to the next instruction after 300F, but not executing it.
3. Escape and enter G FR 3000 TILL 3012. Observe "program break at 3012." Enter PC and see PC = 3014 as expected i.e. PC is now pointing to the next instruction (at 3014), but not executing it. SP reveals 002A, WO 50 shows

0050:0000, WO 60 displays 0060:301E, WO 70 shows 0070:0001 (as expected) and WO 301E gives 301E:0000 (as expected).

4. ESC. G FR 3000 TILL 3014. See "program break at 3014". Enter "PC". Observe PC = 3017 as expected. "SP" should reveal 002A. WO 50 shows 0000, WO 60 301E, WO 70 0001, and WO 301E 0001, as we'd expect.
5. Without striking the ESC key, enter G TILL 3017. Observe "program break at 3017". "PC" shows 300F i.e. address of the next instruction to be executed is now at 300F. SP, WO 50, WO 60, WO 70, and WO 301E are exactly the same as in 4 above.
6. No ESC. Enter G TILL 3017 (again). See "program break at 3017". "PC" again shows 300F (another SJMP loop has been done). Therefore, you'll now record WO 70:0002; WO 301E: 0002, as expected. SP, WO 50, and WO 60 are unchanged in values.
7. No ESC. Enter G TILL 3012. See "program break at 3012". "PC" reveals 3014, pointing to next instruction. This time WO 70 shows 0003 and WO 301E has 0002, as expected, The other word values are unchanged.
8. No ESC. Enter G TILL 3017. See "program break at 3017". "PC" reveals PC = 300F. This time WO 70 shows 0003 (as before) but WO 301E now reveals 0003, as expected. The other parameters are unchanged.
9. Finally, without ESC, enter G TILL 3017 once more. See "program break at 3017" and "PC" = 300F. Another loop has been made and you should observe WO 70 = 0004 and WO 301E = 0004, with the other parameters unchanged.

EXPERIMENT 2-3

USING BREAKPOINTS IN EXPERIMENT 2-2.

There is no new program in this experiment. We still work with the program of Expt. 2-2.

Strike ESC key and set up breakpoints as follows: enter BR = 300F, 3012, 3014, 3017 then a carriage return. Check that these breakpoints were set up by entering BR followed by carriage return. You should see

BR 0 = 300F DISABLED
BR 1 = 3012 DISABLED
BR 2 = 3014 DISABLED
BR 3 = 3017 DISABLED
BR 4 = 0000 DISABLED
BR 5 = 0000 DISABLED
BR 6 = 0000 DISABLED
BR 7 = 0000 DISABLED

These breakpoints are enabled when the "G TILL BR" command is used, as the following procedure details.

PROCEDURE

1. Escape and enter G FR 3000 TILL BR0. Observe "program break at 300F" on the screen. Enter "PC" and see PC = 3012. SP reveals 002A; WO 50 gives 0000; WO 60 gives 301E; WO 70 0000 and WO 301E 0000. 300F executed, PC is at 3012.
2. Without ESC, enter G TILL BR1 and observe "program break at 3012". PC = 3014; SP = 002A; WO 50 0000; WO 60 301E; WO 70 0001; WO 301E 0000, as expected. 3012 executed.
3. Without ESC, enter G TILL BR2 and see "program break at 3014". Then PC = 3017; SP = 002A; WO 50 0000; WO 60 301E; WO 70 0001; WO 301E 0001, as expected. Enter BYTE 301E and observe 301E:01 on the screen.
4. No ESC. Enter G TILL BR 3 and observe "program break at 3017". PC reveals 300F; SP 002A; WO 50 0000; WO 60 301E; WO 70 0001; WO 301E 0001. Nothing new except PC. Enter BYTE 70 and observe 0070:01.
5. Without ESC, enter G FR 3000 TILL BR. We find "program break at 300F" i.e. at BR = 300F, the FIRST breakpoint. PC shows 3012; SP 002A; WO 50 = 0000; WO 60 = 301E; WO 70 = 0000; WO 301E = 0000, all as expected. Enter BYTE 60 and see 0060:1E.
6. No ESC. Enter G and carriage return. The program executes from the last PC (3012 above) until the first break encountered (at 3012). So we find "program break at 3012", PC = 3014; SP 002A; WO 50 = 0000; WO 60 = 301E; WO 70 = 0001; WO 301E = 0000.
7. Again enter G and carriage return. Observe "program break at 3014", PC = 3017; WO 70 = 0001; WO 301E = 0001; the other values the same as in 6.
8. Enter G and carriage return again. See "program break at 3017" with PC = 300F. All other values are as in 7.
9. Enter G and carriage return again. See "program break at 300F" and PC = 3012. All other values are as in 7.
10. Another G and carriage return reveals "program break at 3012", PC at 3014, WO 70 = 0002, WO 301E = 0001 and the other parameters unchanged.

11. G carriage return now shows "program break at 3014", PC = 3017, WO 70 = 0002, WO 301E = 0002, other values unchanged.
12. Another G carriage return reveals "program break at 3017", PC = 300F, all parameters unchanged.
13. G carriage return once more reveals "program break at 300F", PC = 3012, all other values unchanged.
14. G carriage return this time shows "program break at 3012", PC = 3014, WO 70 = 0003, WO 301E = 0002, other values unchanged. All as expected.
15. Finally, enter G FR 3000 FO without a previous ESC. This disables all breakpoints and the program of Expt. 2-2 keeps looking. ESC and query WO 70 and WO 301E. What do you now find? (0003, 0002 highly unlikely).

EXPERIMENT 2-4

USING BREAKPOINTS IN A PROGRAM WITH SUBROUTINES.

The use of breakpoints can be very valuable in debugging programs involving subroutines of one sort or another (such as interrupt routines). The question frequently arises: "did the program get to the subroutine in question? If not, what prevented it from getting there?" The program below illustrates how breakpoints can be used in such cases. Switches at port 0 and LEDs at port 1 are used in the experiment to help illustrate the method. The subroutines labeled "HERE" at 3120, "THERE" at 3130 and "YON" at 3140 simulate any general subroutine of a main program.

In this experiment (see program at 3100 below), we ask that the subroutine HERE execute if the switch byte at port 0 is equal to 01; that subroutine THERE execute if the switch byte equals 03; and that subroutine YON execute if the switch byte equals 07. The comparisons are made in the main program. The NOPs at 3120, 3130, and 3140 are placed there just to see if the program executes the NOP when the breakpoints placed at 3120 or 3130 or 3140 are reached. If the program gets to the relevant breakpoint, we'll know it from the screen read-out "program break at 3120", or "break at 3130", or "break at 3140" with the LEDs at port 1 reading 01, or 03, or 07, respectively. If the switch byte is not 01 or 03 or 07 (00 instead), the LEDs at P1 will be 00 and we will NOT see the "break" message on the screen. REMEMBER, REACHING A BREAKPOINT MEANS THAT THE INSTRUCTION AT THE BREAKPOINT EXECUTES.

```
          0F 00      PORT1   EQU    0FH
          0E 00      PORT0   EQU    0EH
                     ;
                     ;
3100      B0 0E 0F   BEGIN:  LDB    PORT1,PORT0     ;Read switches and output data to LEDs.
3103      99 01 0F           CMPB   PORT1,#01H      ;Compare PORT1 with 01H.
3106      DF 18              JE     HERE            ;If equal jump to HERE.
3108      99 03 0F   CMP3:   CMPB   PORT1,#03H      ;Else compare P1 with 03H.
310B      DF 23              JE     THERE           ;If P1 = 03H, jump to THERE.
310D      99 07 0F   CMP7:   CMPB   PORT1,#07H      ;Else compare P1 with 07H.
3110      DF 2E              JE     YON             ;If P1 = 07H, jump to YON.
3112      27 EC              SJMP   BEGIN           ;Else loop back to BEGIN.
                     ;
3120                         ORG 3120H
3120      FD         HERE:   NOP                    ;No operation.
3121      27 E5              SJMP CMP3              ;Jump back to CMP3.
                     ;
                     ;
3130                         ORG 3130H
3130      FD         THERE:  NOP                    ;No operation.
3131      27 DA              SJMP CMP7              ;Jump back to CMP7.
                     ;
                     ;
3140                         ORG 3140H
3140      FD         YON:    NOP                    ;No operation.
3141      27 BD              SJMP BEGIN             ;Jump back to BEGIN.
```

PROCEDURE

1. Set breakpoints as follows: BR = 3120, 3130, 3140.
2. Set the switch bank to 00000000 at port 0.
3. Enter G FR 3100 TILL BR. See all LEDs at port 1 off. The program is looping (SJMP BEGIN).
4. Set the switch bank to 01H. Immediately observe on the screen "program break at 3120" with the LEDs at 01. Enter PC and see PC = 3121.
5. Change the switch byte to 00 again. Enter G followed by a carriage return. LEDs go out. The main program is looping again.
6. Set the switches to 03. The screen now reads "program break at 3130" and the LEDs read 03. Enter PC and read PC = 3131.
7. Change switch byte to 00. Enter G and carriage return. LEDs go off. Main program loops again.
8. Set switch byte to 07. Screen reads "program break at 3140". LEDs read 07. Enter PC and read PC = 3141.
9. Set switch byte back to 00. Enter G and carriage return. LEDs go out and program loops again (SJMP BEGIN).

10. Set switch byte to 03. See "program break at 3130". PC reads 3131. LEDs read 03.
11. Set switch byte to 00 again. Enter G and carriage return. LEDs read 00 and no breakpoint is reached.

The above example and procedure illustrates how breakpoints help in tracing the program flow, which in this case revealed no flaws.

PROBLEM

Modify the program in a simple way so that the subroutine at "THERE" is never reached even when the switch byte is 03. Show how the above use of breakpoints reveals that THERE is not reached and how the error in the main program (your modification) is thereby discovered and remedied.

EXPERIMENT 2-5

USING THE STEP COMMAND IN EXPT. 2-2 AND THE BYTE COMMAND TO LOAD REGISTERS

We shall apply the STEP command to trace the program flow in Expt. 2-2. The STEP command, like the BR (BREAK) command used in Expt. 2-3 and Expt. 2-4, is useful in debugging.

We first load the following bytes using the BY command into registers in the internal register file of on-chip RAM (each command is followed by a carriage return):

```
BY 08 = 0BB
BY 18 = 80
BY 19 = 00
BY 1A TO 3F = 0FF
BY 80 = 00, 01, 02 .... 0F
BY 90 TO 00FF = 0AA
```

Verify the bytes just entered by entering:

```
BY 08.See 0008:BB
BY 18.See 0018:80
BY 19.See 0019:00
BY 1A TO 3F.See FF FF FF .... FF
BY 80 TO 8F.See 00 01 .... 0F
BY 90 TO 00FF.See AA AA .... AA
```

Or, simply enter BY 18 TO 00FF and see all of the above (except BY 08). Note that we have loaded the stack pointer SP (word register 18) with 0080, over-riding the 0030 that the first instruction of Expt. 2-2 would have loaded into SP IF we ran or stepped from address 3000 there. Note, also, that if we tried to read BY 08 TO 00FF in one span, we'd have a syntax error message displayed because Special Function Registers TIMER1 (at 0A, 0B) and TIMER2 (at 0C, 0D) can not be byte-read, but only word-read. That's why we could read BY 18 TO 00FF in one span, if we wished, but only separately could we read BY 08.

PROCEDURE

1. Enter STEP FROM 3004 DISPLAY STATUS (or briefly STE FR 3004 DI STA). We are asking for a step from the second instruction of Expt. 2-2. After several steps we struck the space bar and found PC = 3012, PSW = 48BB, STACK (0086) = (0706 0908 0B0A 0D0C 0F0E AAAA AAAA AAAA). We have stepped from 3004 through, but not including, the instruction at 3012. Hence we see PC = 3012. The value PSW = 48BB observed is in keeping with the BB we placed into the interrupt mask register (i.e. BY 08 = 0BB) and the 48 is the flag byte (Z, N, V, VT, C, -, I, ST) from some previous operation (left over probably from Expt. 2-4). Information on the stack from 0086 on up to 0095 is also displayed. It is in perfect keeping with the data we entered into the registers before stepping i.e. 06 at 86, 07 at 87,....0F at 8F and AA from 90 on to 00FF. Notice that the read-out of 16 bytes of stack information occurs in word formation 0706, 0908, etc. meaning that 06 is in 86 and 07 in 87, 08 in 88, 09 in 89 etc. (low byte in even lower address and high byte in next higher odd address).
2. Striking the space bar twice in quick succession took us to PC = 300F (stepping to, but not including, address 300F). We evidently stepped through 3012, 14, 17 to, but not including, 300F in the SJMP THERE loop of Expt. 2-2. We now saw PC = 300F, PSW = 00BB, STACK (0086) = (0706 0908 .... AAAA AAAA AAAA). The stack information is as before, but PSW = 00BB i.e. the flag byte is now 00 in keeping with the INC REG3 instruction at 3012 which affects flags (in this case resetting them all to 0 since REG3 was 0000 before the INC).
3. Again enter the space character twice. This time we saw PC = 3014, the instructions at 300F and 3012 being executed. Again we found PSW = 00BB displayed (plausible). The stack information was exactly as before.
4. ESC and enter STE FR 3004 DI A (to display all). We saw PC 3008, PSW = 00BB (flags left over from steps 2 and 3 above). The stack information is as in 1 above i.e. Stack

(0086) = (0706 0908 etc). But now, in addition we see the contents of the whole register file from 0018 on up to 00FF. What we observed was:

```
0018:80 00 FF FF FF ............... FF (at 003F)
0040:DD 58 07 ..................... 00 (at 007F)
0080:FF FF BB 00 09 30 06 07 08 .... 0F (at 008F)
0090:AA AA AA ..................... AA (at 00FF)
```

This is in perfect keeping with the bytes we previously entered into parts of the register file. We entered nothing between 0040 and 007F and that is reflected in the "garbage" displayed above at those addresses. A very interesting and significant aspect of the above display is the data shown at 0080 through 008F. We had previously loaded those locations with 00, 01, 02, ... 0F and indeed we see 06, 07, ... 0F from 0086 through 008F. However, the 00, 01, ... 05 from 0080 through 0085 are gone, being replaced by FF, FF, BB, 00, 09, 30. This tells us that the iSBE-96 monitor "snuck in" with 6 bytes into our stack area. In fact, four of the six stack bytes it saves are user PC +1 (3009) and PSW (00BB) i.e. an important aspect of the state of the USER program. The next experiment goes into some detail on the weaving in and out of the iSBE-96 monitor's stack with respect to user's stack.

EXPERIMENT 2-6

USER'S STACK VS iSBE-96 MONITOR'S STACK. USING BREAKPOINTS AND THE BYTE COMMAND TO QUERY THEIR CONTENTS.

The following program at 2200 was used to investigate the "mysteries" of the stack insofar as how the iSBE-96 monitor's use of it may or may not interfere with the user's stack. The experiment will show that the user's stack does everything expected of it in pushing and popping information, but that the information is lost after all POPs have been executed corresponding to the original PUSHs. The iSBE-96 monitor's stack "gives ground" just behind the user's pushed stack information, always saving its "sacred" 6 bytes (four of them being user's PC+1 and PSW). It then follows the user's stack right back behind it with its 6 bytes as the user's stack pointer returns to its original address after successive POPs.

```
2200                           ORG 2200H
                      ;
                      ;
      08 00           REG1     EQU 0008H
      18 00           REG2     EQU 0018H
      60 00           REG3     EQU 0060H
                      ;
                      ;
2200  B1 BB 08                 LDB    REG1,#0BBH    ;Load interrupt mask REG1 with 0BBH.
2203  A1 40 00 18              LD     REG2,#0040H   ;Set REG2 (SP) to 0040H.
2207  A1 55 AA 60              LD     REG3,#0AA55H  ;Load word 0AA55H into REG3.
220B  65 FF FF 60              ADD    REG3,#0FFFFH  ;Add 0FFFFH to REG3. Flags effected.
220F  28 2F                    SCALL  THERE         ;Call subroutine THERE (short call).
2211  27 FE           HERE:    SJMP   HERE          ;Loop here.
                      ;
                      ;
2240                           ORG 2240H
                      ;
2240  F2              THERE:   PUSHF                ;Push flag and Int. mask bytes onto
                                                    ;stack, PSW is now 0.
2241  C8 60                    PUSH   REG3          ;Push REG3 contents onto stack.
2243  A1 00 00 60              LD     REG3,#0000H   ;Load REG3 with 0000H.
2247  B1 12 08                 LDB    REG1,#12H     ;Load Int. mask REG1 with 12H.
224A  CC 60                    POP    REG3          ;Pop top of stack back into REG3.
224C  F3                       POPF                 ;Restore flags and Int. mask back
                                                    ;into PSW.
224D  F0                       RET                  ;Return to main program.
```

The above program is simple enough. Let's first analyze it with the aim of trying to predict what to expect on the stack after each CALL or PUSH. The first four instructions have the effect of loading BB into the low byte (mask register) of PSW, setting SP to 0040, and leaving AA54 in REG3 (60) after FFFF is added to AA55. The flag byte in the PSW after execution of the fourth instruction should be 48 (Z, N, V, VT, C, -, I, ST) inasmuch as the addition in this case sets the N flag (signed arithmetic where the MSB of each 16 bit quantity is a 1 indicating adding negative numbers) and also sets the C flag since there is a carry out of the 16th bit when the addition is made. Hence PSW to this point should be 48BB. The SCALL (short call) to the routine THERE should save the next address (2211) on the stack. Thus we'd expect to find 22 at address 003F (SP-1) and 11 at address 003E (SP-2) with SP now at 003E.

The PUSHF at 2240 saves the PSW on the stack and leaves PSW loaded with 0000 afterwards. Hence we should find 48 at 0030 and BB at 003C on the stack. PUSH REG3 at 2241 should store AA54 on the stack i.e. AA at 003B and 54 at 003A. The instruction at 2247 loads 12 into the interrupt mask so that PSW should now be 0012. We are now going to see if all this comes about.

PROCEDURE

1. Using the break (BR) command, set breakpoints at BR0 = 2207, BR1 = 220B, BR2 = 220F, BR3 = 2247, BR4 = 224A, BR5 = 224C, and BR6 = 2211. This is simply done by entering BR = 2207, 220B, 220F, 2247, 224A, 224C, 2211 carriage return. Verify that these breakpoints are in.
2. Enter the GO command G FR 2200 TILL BR. The screen will show "program break at 2207". Type in PC. See 220B (PC is pointing to the next instruction). Using the SP and PSW commands reveals "SP = 003A" (see below) and "PSW = 40BB (Z=0 N=1 V=0 T=0 C=0 I=0 S=0 INTR=BB)". 40 is the flag byte left over from some previous operation. WO 60 reveals AA55 as expected i.e. 55 in 60 and AA in 61 (BYTE 60 and BYTE 61 commands confirm this). BYTE 08 reveals BB, as expected. WO 18 (stack pointer registers at 18, 19) reveals 003A (as did the SP command). Finally BYTE 30 TO 40 showed us the following register contents at 30 to 40: FD 9F 0C 00 00 10 AA AA 00 08 12 40 BB 40 0C 22 DD. This is significant. The SP is currently at 003A because the SBE monitor saved the words 220C, 40BB, 4012 on the stack at locations 3F, 3E, 3D, 3C, 3B, 3A, repsectively (starting, as expected, at SP-1 i.e. our program set user's SP to 0040). 220C is recognized as user's PC+1 (220B+1) while 40BB is user's PSW. We set the SP, and the monitor used 6 bytes of the stack starting at SP-1 for its purposes.
3. Enter the GO command G followed by carriage return. This will cause execution to the next breakpoint at 220B. See "break at 220B". Then confirm PC = 220F, PSW = 48BB (Z=0 N=1 V=0 T=0 C=1 I=0 S=0 INTR=BB), SP = 003A, WO 60 : AA54, WO 18 : 003A, and BYTE 30 TO 40 : FD 9F 0C 00 00 10 AA AA 00 08 12 40 BB 48 10 22 DD. Also BYTE 08 reveals BB, as expected. SP is still at 003A, but the 6 bytes saved by the monitor at 003F down to 003A are slightly altered. 2210 now indicates user PC+1 while PSW of user is now 48BB (48 after the addition at 220B). The monitor saves this user status in those 6 bytes in the stack.
4. Enter G and carriage return. Execution proceeds till the next breakpoint at 220F. See "break at 220F". PC reveals 2240 (pointing to the next instruction after SCALL). PSW shows 48BB with same flag bit readout as before. SP is now revealed to be 0038, WO 60 : AA54, WO 18 : 0038, BYTE 08 : BB, and BYTE 30 TO 40 shows FD 9F 0C 00 00 10 AA AA 12 40 BB 48 41 22 11 22 DD. Notice what's happened: SCALL did indeed save the return address (next instruction) 2211 on the stack where the user would expect to find it i.e. at 003F, 3E (SP-1, SP-2). The monitor gives ground and saves its 6 bytes 2241, 48BB, 4012 at 003D, 3C, 3B, 3A, 39, 38 leaving SP at 0038. Again 2241 represents PC+1 of user and 48BB is user's PSW (so far unchanged).

5. G followed by carriage return leads to "break at 2247" on the screen, as expected. PC reveals 224A, PSW = 0012 (Z=0 N=0 V=0 T=0 C=0 I=0 S=0 INTR=12). (Remember PUSHF leaves 0000 in PSW and the instruction at 2247 loads 12 into the interrupt mask register.) SP now reveals 0034. WO 60 is now 0000 (from the instruction at 2243), WO 18 gives 0034, BYTE 08 now shows 12 in keeping with the instruction at 2247. Finally BYTE 30 TO 40 comes up with FD 9F 0C 00 12 40 12 00 4B 22 54 AA BB 48 11 22 DD. The PUSHF at 2240 saves PSW (48BB) on the user's stack at 003D, 3C as expected, and the PUSH REG3 instruction saved AA54 on the user's stack at 003B, 3A, as expected. The monitor's stack area recedes and it saves 224B (PC+1) at 0039, 38 and 0012 (current PSW of the user after the instruction at 2247 was executed) at 0037, 36 on the stack. After saving 4012 at 0035, 34, its SP should be at 0034, and that was previously revealed above.
6. Another G command followed by carriage return gets us to the next breakpoint and we see "break at 224A". PC shows 224C and PSW = 0012, with same flag bit display as in 5 above. SP reveals 0036, WO 60 : AA54 (the POP REG3 at 224A did that), WO 18 : 0036, BYTE 08 : 12, and BYTE 30 TO 40 now shows FD 9F 0C 00 12 40 12 40 12 00 4D 23 BB 48 11 22 DD. The POP REG3 not only popped back AA54 from the stack to REG3 but the monitor "filled the void" by sneaking right behind our stack to save 234D (PC+1) at 003B, 3A and PSW (0012) at 0039, 38, and its other two bytes 40 12 at 0037, 36 leaving SP at 0036. Notice that 4012 at 0035, 34 is still there from the previous save of the monitor's 6 bytes.
7. Again enter G followed by carriage return. The next breakpoint is revealed: "break at 224C". PC shows 224D, SP is 0038, PSW is 48BB (Z=0 N=1 V=0 T=0 C=1 I=0 S=0 INTR=BB). The POPF at 224C restores 48BB, saved on the stack, to the PSW. Also WO 60 : AA54 as expected, WO 18 : 0038, BYTE 08 : BB (because of POPF), and we now have BYTE 30 TO 40 : FD 9F 0C 00 12 40 12 40 12 40 BB 48 4E 22 11 22 DD. The POPF popped back 48BB into PSW and the monitor rushed in to remove our 48BB from the stack, moving in with its 6 bytes 224E (PC+1) at 003D, 3C, 48BB (user PSW) at 003B, 3A, and 4012 at 0039, 38 leaving SP at 0038. Again, note the two previous saves of 4012 are still there.
8. And finally a last G carriage return brings us to the final breakpoint at 2211 as revealed by "break at 2211". PC now shows 2211 (SJMP HERE), PSW = 48BB (same flag bits), SP = 003A, WO 60 : AA54, WO 18 : 003A, BYTE 08 : BB (all as expected). BYTE 30 TO 40 now reveals: FD 9F 0C 00 12 40 12 40 12 40 12 40 BB 48 12 22 DD. The RET instruction popped the return address 2211 from the stack into the PC

to get us back to SJMP. The monitor's famous 6 bytes move up and are stored at 003F, 3E (2212 = PC+1), at 003D, 3C (48BB = PSW), and at 003B, 3A (4012). Thus the SP is now at 003A where it all started (see step 2 above). Note the four times that 4012 is left in user's stack "wake" as SP climbs back to 003A.

CONCLUSION: All user stack operations go as expected starting from SP-1, where SP is set by the user in the program. But the SBE monitor stores 6 bytes just below user's stack and thus shows an SP value 6 locations lower than where user thinks his latest SP is. When POPs or RET occur, all user information gets restored correctly, but the monitor's 6 bytes move up along with SP to "fill the void". Thus user stack information is lost. Hence don't do data acquisition in the stack area. It can be retrieved just once!

We should like to point out that we originally, and mistakenly, wrote the program in this experiment at 2000. After scratching our heads to understand the results of our debugging session, the appearance of F7 (TRAP) made us realize that addresses 2010, 11 are reserved for the software TRAP interrupt i.e. 2010, 11 are loaded by the SBE-96's monitor with the address to which the TRAP instruction vectors, over-writing any information placed there by user. The program, therefore, did not work. Write programs only at 2080 and higher.

STACK WARNING

This experiment also points out the necessity for setting one's own SP, preferably as far away from the SP registers and the SFRs as possible. If you don't, the iSBE-96 will set it for you at 0020 (verify that at power-up) and save the "sacred" 6 bytes starting at 001F down to 001A (perilously close to 0019, 18 - the SP registers - and to 0017, the beginning of the SFR region down to 00). If, then, you save your data in the monitor's stack area beginning at 001F, the monitor backs away and starts saving its 6 bytes from 0019 down, destroying SP and your SFR values so necessary to the I/O work you will be doing, in which user controlled manipulation of the SFRs is involved. The only (few) times we don't set our own SP are when user stack operations are not involved. In all other cases we set SP to 00C0 in the register file. It's a good idea to ALWAYS set your SP at the beginning of the program.

EXPERIMENT 2-7

THE WATCHDOG TIMER DISABLE SWITCH S2 USED IN A WDT EXPERIMENT (SEE SECTION N, CHAPTER 1).

In the program shown below at 2300, the WDT (SFR 0AH) is loaded first with 1EH (enabling it) and then with 0E1H (clearing it). These two LDB instructions are part of a loop in which the switch byte at input port 0 is read out at the LEDs of port 1. The rest of the loop consists of decrementing REG (previously loaded with FFFF) and jumping back to THERE where the WDT is cleared again before it times out and causes a reset (which would occur in 16 msec if it were not periodically cleared). This jump back to THERE occurs as long as REG is not 0. You can verify that one pass in the loop requires 24 state times (6 usec) so that after about 0.4 sec (65,536 x 6 usec) the loop is exited. In part (A) of the experiment the fall-through lands on SJMP HERE. No further clearing of the WDT in the program takes place. Thus if P0 was originally set at, for example, AA, we should observe the LEDs at P1 stay at AA for about 0.4 sec. and, then, 16 msec after the fall-through, the WDT overflows pulling down the RESET pin on the 8096. On reset, P1 comes up as FF, so we should see the LEDs change from AA to FF at the end of 0.4 sec (+16 msec).

In part (B) of the experiment SJMP HERE is changed to SJMP THERE so that the WDT is ALWAYS being cleared before 16 msec expire. Hence we should see AA at the LEDs always. Note that DEC REG has the effect of reloading REG with FFFF each time SJMP THERE takes effect.

```
        0A 00          WDT      EQU     0AH
        0F 00          PORT1    EQU     0FH
        0E 00          PORT0    EQU     0EH
        60 00          REG      EQU     60H
                       ;
                       ;
2300    A1 FF FF 60             LD      REG,#0FFFFH    ;Load Time REG with 0FFFFH.
                       ;
2304    B1 1E 0A       THERE:   LDB     WDT,#01EH      ;Enable watchdog timer.
2307    B1 E1 0A                LDB     WDT,#0E1H      ;Clear watchdog timer.
230A    B0 0E 0F                LDB     PORT1,PORT0    ;Read switch byte at PORT0
                                                       ;out to LEDs at PORT1.
230D    05 60                   DEC     REG            ;Decrement REG for time.
230F    D7 F3                   JNE     THERE          ;If REG != 0, jump to THERE.
2311    27 FE          HERE:    SJMP    HERE           ;Else loop here.
```

PROCEDURE

With WDT Disable Switch S2 on during power-up, and following any hardware reset, execute Expt. 2-7(A), above, from 2300, with the switches at port 0 set to e.g. AA. You should observe the LEDs at port 1 display AA for about 0.4 sec and then change to FF and stay that way.

In part (B) of the experiment you need only change the byte FE at 2312 to F1 by entering the command BY 2312 = 0F1. This causes SJMP to THERE at 2304, rather than to HERE at 2311. Executing this modified program will cause AA to be displayed at port 1's LEDs at all times. Switch S2 should be turned off when the experiment is over.

EXPERIMENT 2-8

SUMMARY OF CORRECT USAGE OF THE BYTE, WORD, AND CHANGE COMMANDS; MORE ON THE SP COMMAND.

1. THE BYTE COMMAND

We have been using the BYTE command to load registers and memory as well as to read out their contents. For the sake of completeness and clarity we are adding this section.

Type in the command BY 4900 = 90, 91, 92, 93 carriage return. Then enter BY 4900 to 4904 carriage return and observe the read-out on the display, namely 4900:90 91 92 93 XY (where XY is the random byte in 4904).

Next enter BY 50 TO 53 = 0FF carriage return. Then enter BY 50 TO 54 carriage return and observe 0050:FF FF FF FF XY where, again, XY is random.

Finally, enter BY 60 = 60 carriage return. Query register 60 by entering BY 60 carriage return. You'll see 0060:60 on the display.

The situation where the BYTE command is to be entered DURING EMULATION is very important. We've dealt with that situation during the experiments but re-iterate it again here. To illustrate the situation, consider the trivial program 27 0FE entered at address 2400 (enter BY 2400 = 27, 0FE carriage return). 27 FE is machine code for SJMP, with the jump looping back to 2400 i.e. a constant looping on itself. Run the program by entering G FR 2400 carriage return. Now try to change a register value by entering e.g. BY 70 = 07 carriage return. Then query register 70's contents by entering BYTE 70 carriage return. You'll see 0070:07 - all this being done and observed while the program 27 FE is executing from 2400. Note BY 70 won't work on the run, BYTE 70 is necessary to read 70H.

2. THE WORD COMMAND

We have also been using the WORD command in the experiments to load words into register or memory locations and also to read contents of word registers or locations.

Enter WO 4900 = 8180, 8382, 8584 carriage return. Then enter WO 4900 TO 4906 carriage return. Observe 4900:8180 8382 8584 XYUV where XYUV is the random word at location 4906. Next enter BY 4900 TO 4906 carriage return and observe 4900:80 81 82 83 84 85 UV i.e. the low byte of each word (80 or 82 or 84) resides in the low even address and the high byte (81 or 83 or 85) resides in the next higher odd address (ditto for the random byte UV - part of the random word XYUV).

Now try WO 4900 = 81, 82, 83, 84, 85 carriage return. Then enter WO 4900 TO 490A carriage return and observe 4900:0081 0082 0083 0084 0085 XYUV. Thus the 81, 82, etc in the original word loading is interpreted as words 0081, 0082, etc. Now try BY 4900 TO 490A carriage return and observe 4900:81 00 82 00 83 00 84 00 85 00 UV, again in keeping with low byte of word residing in even address and hi byte in next higher odd address.

As another example, enter WO 4900 TO 4908 = 1234 carriage return. Then enter WO 4900 TO 4908 carriage return. Observe 4900:1234 1234 1234 1234 1234. Then enter BY 4900 TO 490A carriage return and see 4900:34 12 34 12 34 12 34 12 34 12 UV. Everything is consistent.

Finally, execute the program 27 FE at 2400 (SJMP) previously placed there. DURING EXECUTION enter WO 4900 = 4321 carriage return. Then enter WO 4900 carriage return and observe 4900: 4321. Next enter BYTE 4900 TO 4901 carriage return and observe 4900:21 43. Now enter WO 4900 TO 4904 = 49 carriage return. Then try WO 4900 TO 4904 carriage return and observe 4900:0049 0049 0049. Enter BY 4900 TO 4905 and observe 4900:49 00 49 00 49 00. Querying register 70 during emulation required BYTE 70 carriage return. BY 70 carriage return won't work.

3. THE CHANGE COMMAND

This command changes memory beginning at the address specified. Here are some examples. But first, load in WO 4900 TO 4950 = 0FFFF carriage return. Then examine, by entering WO 4900 TO 4950 carriage return, and see FFFF FFFF .... FFFF (at 4950).

Now enter CHA BY 4900 carriage return. See 4900:FF/. Type in 01 and carriage return. See 4901:FF/. Type in 02 carriage return. See 4902:FF/. Type in 03 carriage return. See 4903:FF/.

Type in 04 carriage return. See 4904:FF/. Type in DONE carriage return. Now enter BY 4900 TO 4906 carriage return and observe 4900:01 02 03 04 FF FF FF.

Now try CHA WO 4940 carriage return. See 4940:FFFF/. Enter 0AAAA carriage return. Observe 4942:FFFF/. Enter 0BBBB carriage return. See 4944:FFFF/. Enter 0CCCC carriage return and observe 4946:FFFF/. Type in DONE carriage return, (or enter the ESC character). Now enter WO 4940 TO 4950 carriage return and observe 4940:AAAA BBBB CCCC FFFF FFFF .... through 4950.

Finally, run the 27 FE (SJMP) program at 2400 (G FR 2400 carriage return). Now try CHA BY 4920 carriage return. Observe 4920:FF/. Enter 99 carriage return. See 4921:FF/. Enter DONE carriage return (or strike the ESC key). Now enter BYTE 4920 carriage return. Observe 4920:99. Next enter CHA WO 4930 carriage return. Observe 4930:FFFF/. Enter 5555 carriage return. See 4932:FFFF/. Type DONE and carriage return. Enter WO 4930 carriage return. See 4930:5555.

IMPORTANT NOTE

In employing the BY, WO or CHA commands, when dealing with the SFRs (00 to 17H), be sure to consult section Q of chapter 1. Certain SFRs can only be word-read, others only word-written, all others can be accessed only as bytes. Section Q in chapter 1 tells you which are which. Also consult section D, chapter 1 for those SFRs that are read-only, others that are write-only, and their addresses and meanings.

4. MORE ON THE SP COMMAND AND THE SBE-96 MONITOR'S STACK

Entering the command SP = 0060 carriage return, to set the stack pointer, immediately brings forth the following message on the screen: "SP = 0060, adjusted to 005A to allow for monitor use". The monitor has taken possession of locations 005F, 5E, 5D, 5C, 5B, 5A to store its 6 bytes having to do with user program status (see Expt. 2-6). That leaves the SP at 005A. If, and when, user needs to save data on the stack, it gets stored at 005F, 5E, ... as you'd expect, with monitor's 6 bytes (changed) backing off deeper into the stack, always trailing user's stack. Entering WO 18 carriage return reveals 0018:005A as expected since word registers 0018, 19 are the SP.

In another aspect of this stack matter, if you execute the program LD SP, #0080 SJMP HERE at 2410 (G FR 2410) (entered there by simply using the byte command BY 2410 = A1, 80, 00, 18, 27, 0FE carriage return), and then query SP on the run (SP carriage return), you'll find "SP = 007A" displayed on the screen for the same reason as above. Examining word register 18 by entering WO 18 will also show 0018:007A on the display.

Now execute the program 27 FE entered at 2400 (G FR 2400). While it's running, set the SP to 00D0 by means of the command SP = 0D0 carriage return. This immediately results in the following display on the screen: "SP = 0D0 adjusted to 00CA to allow for monitor use". WO 18 shows 0018:00CA, as expected. Now query SP directly with the command SP carriage return (all the while the program is running). You'll see SP = 00CA on the screen. Now try to set SP = 90 carriage return. It does not take! Strike the ESC key. Again G FR 2400. This time set SP = 0090 carriage return. Immediately see "SP = 0090 adjusted to 008A to allow for monitor use". Try SP = 0B0 carriage return. See "SP = 0B0 adjusted to 00AA to allow for monitor use". Enter SP carriage return. See "SP = 00AA". Evidently, the best advice is to enter WORD DATA as the complete two bytes in all cases. You could run into trouble if you don't, as the above indicates.

Finally, it is important to re-iterate that if you don't set your own SP in the program, the monitor will at 0020 on power-up. (Verify this by entering SP carriage return on power-up.) Then when saving data in your own stack operations you'll be down into the SP (0019, 18) and the SFRs (0017 down to 00) before you know it - with devastating results for the I/O control you are attempting.

EXPERIMENT 2-9

THE ASM, DASM COMMANDS

With DOS 3.0 or greater, enter the following program using the ASM command: ASM 2500H = LD SP, #00C0H (CR) LDB 40H, #AAH (CR) LDB IOPORT1, 40H (CR) SJMP 250AH (CR)(CR). Here (CR) stands for "carriage return". Note how the entry of (CR) after each mnemonic causes the next address after the mnemonic instruction just entered to be displayed as the prompt to enter the next mnemonic. The (CR)(CR) will cause the iSBE-96 to stop prompting after the last mnemonic was entered.

Now verify that the MCS-96 assembler mnemonics entered were converted to machine code by entering BY 2500 TO 2510 (CR). The screen should display the machine code HEX program: A1 C0 00 18 B1 AA 40 B0 40 0F 27 FE - - - - -. where - are random data.

Disassemble the machine code back to ASM-96 mnemonics by entering the DASM command: DASM 2500H TO 2510H (CR). You should see the complete program mnemonics in agreement with the mnemonics entered with the ASM command at the beginning of the first paragraph above. You'll also see added "mnemonics" corresponding to the random data at 250C through 2510.

CHAPTER 3

USING THE 8096 INSTRUCTION SET

INTRODUCTION

In this chapter we present examples of the use of the various instructions in the 8096 set, as well as examples employing all its addressing modes. The examples are not yet intended to show much in the way of applications - that is stressed in the following chapters - but rather emphasize the use of the instructions, and their significance. Not all the instructions are covered, but most are. We skip over those that are either rather obvious and similar to those employed by the reader in his/her experience with other microprocessors, or which will be employed, anyway, in the many experiments to be presented after chapter 3. We have tried to concentrate on those that are new and unique to the 8096. Naturally, in constructing the experiments in this chapter, other instructions in the 8096 set had to be used also, unique or not. They are all explained as they are used. Where our treatment was not exhaustive [for example, in two experiments dealing with MUL (multiply) and DIV (divide)], we come back later in the book to deal with the subject or instruction in much greater depth e.g. the multiply and divide are treated in more detail in the chapter on arithmetic (ch. 7). Also note that a number of instructions have been used, and explained, already in chapter 2's various experiments. We'll meet them again here.

EXPERIMENT 3-1

EXAMPLES OF ALL THE 8096's ADDRESSING MODES

A. DIRECT AND IMMEDIATE ADDRESSING

```
        UE 00          REG     EQU    OEH           ;PORTO switches
        OF 00          P1      EQU    OFH           ;PORT1 LEDs
        00 00          RO      EQU    OOH           ;Just OOH value
        50 00          REG1    EQU    50H
        60 00          REG2    EQU    60H
        70 00          REG3    EQU    70H
        80 00          REG4    EQU    80H
        18 00          SP      EQU    18H
        00 10          TABLE   EQU    1000H
                    ; EXPT. 3-1.
                    ; Part A): Direct and Immediate Addressing
3200  A1 34 12 60          LD      REG2,#1234H     ;Load REG2 with word 1234H.
3204  A0 60 50             LD      REG1,REG2       ;Load REG1 with contents of REG2.
3207  C0 70 50             ST      REG1,REG3       ;Store contents of REG1 into REG3.
320A  27 FE         HERE:  SJMP    HERE            ;Loop here.
                    ;
                    ; Then try the following program:
                    ;
3210                       ORG 3210H
                    ;
3210  B1 AA 60             LDB     REG2,#OAAH      ;Load OAAH into REG2.
3213  B0 60 50             LDB     REG1,REG2       ;Load contents of REG2 into REG1.
3216  C4 70 50             STB     REG1,REG3       ;Store contents of REG1 into REG3.
3219  27 FE         THERE: SJMP    THERE           ;Loop here.
```

In the first of the above programs, #1234 is loaded into word REG2 (immediate addressing), then loaded into word REG1 from REG2 (LD direct addressing), and then stored in word REG3 from REG1 (ST direct addressing). The program halts on the loop at HERE. Immediate addressing involves a number as one of the operands (the last) while direct addressing involves register to register content transfer, with the registers being any from among the 256 in the on-board register file (RAM). Execute the program (G FR 3200) and then examine registers as follows: WO 60, then WO 50, then WO 70. In each case you should observe 1234. If you examine bytes e.g. enter BYTE 60 TO 61, then BYTE 50 TO 51, then BYTE 70 TO 71 you will observe 34 12 in each case, as expected (low byte goes to even address).

In the first part of the program REG1, REG2, and REG3 were treated as word registers. The nature of the Op. Code took care of that i.e. LD and ST are word oriented instructions. The second part of the program treats those same registers as byte registers by employing the byte forms of the instructions LDB and STB. If you execute the program at 3210 (G FR 3210) and then query BYTE 50 TO 51, BYTE 60 TO 61, and BYTE 70 TO 71, respectively, you'll find AA 12 in each case, the 12 remaining from the results of the previous experiment. There, 34 went to the even byte address and 12 went to the odd (higher) byte address as word 1234 was loaded into REG1 = 50, REG2 = 60, and REG3 = 70. This time AA is loaded into each of those BYTE registers.

B. INDIRECT ADDRESSING

```
3220                         ORG 3220H
                     ;
3220  A1 AA 55 50            LD     REG1,#55AAH     ;Load WORD 55AAH into REG1.
3224  A1 50 42 60            LD     REG2,#4250H     ;Load WORD 4250H into REG2.
3228  C2 60 50               ST     REG1,[REG2]     ;Store contents of REG1 into memory
                                                    ;pointed to by REG2 (4250H).
322B  A2 60 70               LD     REG3,[REG2]     ;Load contents of memory pointed to
                                                    ;by REG2 (4250H) into REG3.
322E  27 FE          CADD:   SJMP   CADD            ;Loop here.
                     ;
                     ; Then try the following program:
                     ;
3230                         ORG 3230H
                     ;
3230  B1 FF 50               LDB    REG1,#0FFH      ;Load BYTE FFH into REG1.
3233  A1 60 43 60            LD     REG2,#4360H     ;Load WORD 4360H into REG2.
3237  C6 60 50               STB    REG1,[REG2]     ;Store BYTE contained in REG1 into
                                                    ;memory pointed to by REG2 (4360H).
323A  B2 60 70               LDB    REG3,[REG2]     ;Load the byte contents of memory
                                                    ;pointed to by REG2 into REG3.
323D  27 FE          NOW:    SJMP   NOW             ;Loop here
```

In the first of the above programs (at 3220) the word number 55AA is loaded into word REG1 (immediate), word number 4250 is loaded into word REG2 (immediate), then 55AA is stored at address 4250 (i.e. at the address pointed to by the contents of REG2), and finally the word contents 55AA of address 4250 (i.e. the contents of the memory location pointed to by the contents of REG2) are loaded into word REG3 before the program ends on a self loop. This is an example of indirect addressing wherein a register in the RAM file is loaded with a value and that value becomes the address in memory to which access is made for storing or retrieving data. In this case [REG2] signifies that REG1's contents are not to be stored in REG2, but rather in the location in memory pointed to by the CONTENTS of REG2. If you G FR 3220 and then examine WO 50, WO 60, WO 4250, and WO 70, you'll find, respectively 55AA, 4250, 55AA, and 55AA.

The byte-oriented counterpart program to the one discussed above is written at 3230. This time byte REG1 is loaded with FF, word REG2 is loaded with 4360, FF is stored at 4360 (STB REG1, [REG2]), and finally the byte contents of 4360 (FF) are loaded (LDB REG3, [REG2]) into byte REG3. Execute from 3230 and enter BYTE 50 TO 51. Observe FF 55 (the 55 is at 0051 from the previous experiment). Then query BYTE 60 TO 61 and observe 60 43 (why?). Next enter WO 4360 and observe XYFF (where XY is random at 4361 but FF is at 4360 as a result of program execution). Then try BYTE 4360 and observe, indeed, FF. WO 70 should reveal 55FF (where 55 is the remains at 71 from the previous experiment) and BYTE 70 will show FF, as expected. BYTE 70 TO 71 should give FF 55.

C. INDIRECT ADDRESSING WITH AUTO INCREMENT. APPLICATION TO BLOCK TRANSFER.

```
3240                          ORG 3240H
                    ;
3240  A1 00 44 80             LD     REG4,#4400H    ;Load DESTINATION address into
                                                    ;REG4.
3244  A1 00 43 60             LD     REG2,#4300H    ;Load SOURCE address into REG2.
3248  B1 08 50                LDB    REG1,#08H      ;Load number of WORDS to be
                                                    ;transfered into REG1.
324B  A2 61 70      READ:     LD     REG3,[REG2]+   ;Load WORD pointed to by REG2 into
                                                    ;REG3 and double increment REG2.
324E  C2 81 70                ST     REG3,[REG4]+   ;Store WORD contained in REG3 into
                                                    ;memory location pointed to by REG4
                                                    ;and double increment REG4.
3251  E0 50 F7                DJNZ   REG1,READ      ;Decrement WORD count register REG1,
                                                    ;if not = 0, then jump to READ.
3254  27 FE         HALT:     SJMP   HALT           ;Loop here.
                    ;
```

Then try the following program:

```
                          ;
3280                           ORG    3280H
                          ;
3280   A1 00 44 80             LD     REG4,#4400H     ;Load DESTINATION address into
                                                      ;REG4.
3284   A1 00 43 60             LD     REG2,#4300H     ;Load SOURCE address into REG2.
3288   B1 04 50                LDB    REG1,#04H       ;Load number of BYTES to be
                                                      ;transfered into REG1.
328B   B2 61 70       FETCH:   LDB    REG3,[REG2]+    ;Load BYTE pointed to by REG2 into
                                                      ;REG3 and increment REG2.
328E   C6 81 70                STB    REG3,[REG4]+    ;Store BYTE contained in REG3 into
                                                      ;memory location pointed to by REG4
                                                      ;and increment REG4.
3291   E0 50 F7                DJNZ   REG1,FETCH      ;Decrement BYTE count register REG1,
                                                      ;if not = 0, then jump to FETCH.
3294   27 FE          STOP:    SJMP   STOP            ;Loop here.
```

The programs above are good examples of block transfer. The one at 3240 transfers words and that at 3280 transfers bytes, each from a source block to a destination block. Here the auto-increment version of indirect addressing greatly facilitates matters. In the auto-increment indirect addressing mode LD REG3, [REG2]+, for example, loads REG3 with the word at the location pointed to by the contents of REG2, and then increments the contents of REG2 TWICE, so that [REG2] is now pointing to the word in the very next word location. ST REG3, [REG4]+ stores the contents of REG3 onto the memory location pointed to by the contents of REG4 and then increments REG4 twice. Similarly, LDB REG3, [REG2]+ loads REG3 with the byte at the location whose address is the contents of REG2 and then increments the contents of REG2 ONCE, so that [REG2] is now pointing to the byte in the very next byte location.

In the first of the above programs REG1 is loaded with 08 to signify that 8 words are to be transfered from source block at base address 4300 (loaded previously into REG2) to a destination block starting at base address 4400 (loaded previously into REG4). The transfer of each word is accompanied by a double increment of source pointer REG2 and a double increment of destination pointer REG4 to get ready for the transfer of the very next word in the source table. The process ends when counter REG1 is 0, as it will be after 8 decrements as a result of the DJNZ REG1,READ instruction. Execution then halts at SJMP (self loop). Notice that the transfer from source to destination takes place through a "middleman", REG3, as it must, because of the nature of the LD and ST instructions and the role of the "waop" operands. Waop and baop operands are the RIGHTMOST operands when involved in an instruction. They occur only ONCE in an instruction, when involved. [REG2]+ and [REG4]+ are examples of waops in the first program above, and [REG2]+ is a baop in the second program.

Before executing the program at 3240 enter the source block as follows: BY 4300 = 00, 01, 02, 03, 04, 05, ..., 0F. Then "obliterate" the destination block with BY 4400 TO 440F = 0AA. G FR 3240 executes the program. Now query BYTE 4300 TO 430F and see 00 01 02....0F as expected. Then examine the destination block BYTE 4400 TO 440F and observe 00 01 02....0F. The block has been transferred. Enter WO 60 and observe 4310 which is indeed what REG2 should be after 8 double auto-increments from 4300. Further, WO 80 should reveal 4410 since REG4 has also been double auto-incremented 8 times from its original value 4400.

In the same way, before executing the second of the above experiments, enter BY 4300 = FF, EE, DD, CC, BB, AA, 99, 88,....,00 as our new source block. Execute (G FR 3280). Query BYTE 4300 TO 430F and observe FF EE DD.....00. Next enter BYTE 4400 TO 440F and see FF EE DD CC 04 05....0F. The four bytes FF EE DD CC from the source, starting at 4300, were transferred - no more - in keeping with LDB REG1, #04 in the program. They went, as required, to 4400, 01, 02, 03. The bytes 04 05.....0F observed after 4403 in the destination block are the remains from the block transfer of words done in the previous part of the experiment. Examining WO 60 should show 4304 (i.e. 4 single auto-increments on REG2 were now accomplished starting from 4300). Likewise, WO 80 reveals 4404 in keeping with 4 single auto-increments on REG4 starting from 4400.

D. BASED OR INDEXED ADDRESSING MODE.

```
                        ;       1) Short Indexed Addressing.
                        ;
                        ;
3500                            ORG     3500H
                        ;
3500  A1 20 45 50               LD      REG1,#4520H     ;Load WORD 4520H into REG1.
3504  A3 50 04 60               LD      REG2,4[REG1]    ;Load WORD pointed to by REG1 + 4
                                                        ;(4524H) into REG2.
3508  07 50                     INC     REG1            ;Increment REG1.
350A  A3 50 05 70               LD      REG3,5[REG1]    ;Load WORD pointed to by REG1 + 5
                                                        ;(4526H) into REG3.
350E  27 FE             FINIS:  SJMP    FINIS           ;Loop here.
```

```
                      ;       2) Long Indexed Addressing.
                      ;
3540                          ORG    3540H
                      ;
3540  A1 60 45 50             LD     REG1,#4560H      ;Load WORD 4560H into REG1.
3544  A1 FE FF 60             LD     REG2,#0FFFEH     ;Load WORD 0FFFEH into REG2.
3548  C3 51 00 10 60          ST     REG2,TABLE[REG1];Store contents of REG2 at location
                                                      ;pointed to by REG1 + TABLE (5560H).
354D  27 FE           FINITO: SJMP   FINITO           ;Loop here
```

The first of the two programs above (at 3500) illustrates the "short indexed" addressing mode. In this form 4[REG1] adds the 8 bit byte 04 (sign extended) to the contents of REG1 (4520). The new contents of REG1 are now 4524, so that LD REG2, 4[REG1] will load REG2 with the word pointed to by REG1 + 4 (= 4524) i.e. the pointer is now [REG1 + 4]. Hence if address 4524 has the word 2524, it will be loaded into REG2. Similarly, after REG1 is incremented (to 4521) in the program, LD REG3, 5[REG1] will load REG3 with the word at address REG1 + 5 = 4526. If that word is 2726, it will be loaded into REG3.

Before executing the program at 3500, enter the table: BY 4520 = 20, 21, 22, 23, 24, 25, 26, 27,....2F. Then execute with a G FR 3500 command. Query WO 50 and see 4521, as expected of REG1 after one increment. Query WO 60 (REG2) and observe 2524, in keeping with the fact that the word in the table at 4524 is indeed 2524 (25 at 4525 and 24 at 4524). WO 70 should show 2726 i.e. REG3 gets loaded with the word contents of 4526 which are 2726, since 5[REG1] = [4526] after one increment of REG1. Finally, BYTE 60 TO 61 and BYTE 70 TO 71 should show 24 25 and 26 27, respectively.

The second program above (at 3540) illustrates the long indexed mode. It stores the FFFE word in REG2 at the memory address TABLE [REG1], where TABLE equates to 1000 and REG1 has been loaded previously with the value 4560. Thus FFFE should appear at (4560 + 1000] i.e. at memory location 5560. Execute the program (G FR 3540) and then enter WO 50, WO 60, WO 5560 in turn. You will observe 4560 at 50, FFFE at 60, and FFFE at 5560. Short indexed can reach out to within -128 or +127 locations whereas long indexed can access any location in memory.

E. ZERO REGISTER ADDRESSING AND THE ZERO REGISTER.

Zero Register Addressing is really another form of long indexed addressing. It is based on the fact that the "ZERO Register", (SFR 00, Register R0) is ALWAYS loaded with the word 0000 at locations 00, 01. This leads to DIRECT ADDRESSING TO ANYWHERE IN MEMORY if the indexed addressing mode is employed with R0, as the following example at 3560 shows. Please understand that [0] really stands for [R0].

```
3560                            ORG     3560H
                        ;
3560   A3 01 44 44 50           LD      REG1,4444H[0]   ;Load REG1 with word contents of
                                                        ;location 0 + 4444H.
3565   27 FE            NOMOR:  SJMP    NOMOR           ;Loop here.
                        ;
```

Executing the above program from 3560 should result in REG1 (50) being loaded with the word located at 0 + 4444 i.e. a DIRECT access of memory location 4444 is accomplished in this way. Before executing, enter the word AABB at 4444 i.e. WO 4444 = 0AABB. Then G FR 3560. Query WO 50 (REG1). You should find AABB stored there. We employ this form of direct addressing extensively through-out the book.

The program below employs the Zero Register R0 and has nothing to do with Zero Register Addressing used in direct addressing discussed above.

```
3570   98 00 0E    COMP:   CMPB   REG,R0     ;Compare switches on PORT0 to 00H.
3573   DF 05               JE     LEDS1      ;If they are equal,  jump to
                                             ;LEDS1 and observe 55H at PORT1 LEDS.
3575   B1 AA 0F    LEDS2:  LDB    P1,#0AAH   ;If NOT, observe AAH at PORT1 LEDS.
3578   27 F6               SJMP   COMP       ;Loop back to poll the switches
357A   B1 55 0F    LEDS1:  LDB    P1,#55H    ;Switch BYTE VALUE equals 00H,
                                             ;output 55h to PORT1 LEDs.
357D   27 F1               SJMP   COMP       ;Loop back to poll switches
```

In the above program at 3570, the value of the switch byte at port 0 (REG is defined as 0EH which is port 0) is compared with the value 00 (i.e. with contents of R0). If the switch byte is 0, 55 is output to the LEDs at port 1, otherwise AA is output there. Executing the program from 3570 and varying the switch byte at P0 should confirm the above.

F. STACK POINTER REGISTER ADDRESSING

Stack Pointer Register Addressing is a variant on either indirect addressing or short indexed addressing, in both of which [SP] is involved. It allows easy access of the top of the stack or access of data anywhere within the stack, thereby facilitating the access of operands within the stack. Both forms of this addressing mode are illustrated in the program at 3590 below. Easy manipulation of the stack pointer results.

```
3590                      ORG     3590H
                    ;
3590  A1 3A 00 18         LD      SP,#003AH      ;Load Stack Pointer with 003AH.
3594  CA 18               PUSH    [SP]           ;Pushes the word pointed to by
                                                 ;SP onto the top of the stack. SP=0038
                                                 ;Top of stack has been duplicated.
3596  CC 50               POP     REG1           ;Pop word from stack into REG1.
                                                 ;SP = 003AH.
3598  CC 60               POP     REG2           ;Pop word from stack into REG2.
                                                 ;SP = 003CH
359A  A3 18 02 70         LD      REG3,2[SP]     ;Load REG3 with word pointed to by
                                                 ;SP + 2 (003CH + 2 = 003EH).
                                                 ;SP unchanged.
359E  27 FE         LAST: SJMP    LAST           ;Loop here.

35A0                      END
```

Before explaining and executing this program, enter BY 38 = 0FF, 0FF, 00, 01, 02, 03, 04, 05 (at 003F). Thus we have:

```
         38 : FF
         39 : FF
SP at 003A : 00
         3B : 01
         3C : 02
         3D : 03
         3E : 04
         3F : 05
```

The first instruction sets user SP at 003A. The next instruction pushes the values pointed to by 003A i.e. the word at 003A, 003B, namely 0100, on top of the stack at 0039, 0038. Thus 01 will reside at 0039 and 00 at 0038 (hi byte of word pushed goes to odd address and lo byte goes to lower even address). SP after PUSH is now at SP-2 i.e. at 0038. The POP REG1 instruction should pop the top of the stack i.e. the word 0100 at SP-2, into REG1 (50). SP is now back at 003A after that pop. POP

REG2 should now pop the word at 003A, which is ALSO 0100, into REG2 (60). SP is now at 003C after that pop. Finally, the LD REG3, 2[SP] instruction should load REG3 (70) with the contents of address SP + 2 i.e. with the word at location 003C + 2 = 003E. That word is 0504 at 003E, 3F. So REG3 will have 0504. But SP itself does not change. It is still at 003C!

Execute the above program from 3590. ESC and examine WO 50 (REG1). Find 0100 as expected. Examine WO 60 (REG2) and observe 0100, as predicted. Now examine WO 70 (REG3) and find 0504, again as expected. Finally, enter SP or WO 18 and observe 0036. Why? The actual MONITOR'S SP is 6 below user's SP 003C, and that gives 0036 (remember Expt. 2-6?). Examine BYTE 36 TO 3F. Account for what you see in light of Expt. 2-6. Can you spot the monitor's 6 bytes at 0036, 37, 38, 39, 3A, and 3B?, and 02, 03, 04, 05 still at 003C (user's current SP), 3D, 3E, 3F? Remember, PSW comes up as 0000 at reset.

EXPERIMENT 3-2

CARRY VS. BORROW WITH THE 8096.

With the 8096, a borrow in a subtract or compare instruction shows up in the C flag as C = 0, while if no borrow was necessary, the C flag shows a 1. The program at 3600 below will verify that.

```
      0E 00      P0      EQU    0EH      ;PORT0 switches
      0F 00      P1      EQU    0FH      ;PORT1 LEDs
                 ;
                 ;
3600                     ORG    3600H
                 ;
3600  99 01 0E   COMP:   CMPB   P0,#01H          ;Compare switch BYTE VALUE with 01H.
3603  DB 05              JC     LEDS1            ;If C = 1 (no borrow), then jump to
                                                 ;LEDS1.
3605  B1 88 0F   LEDS2:  LDB    P1,#88H          ;C = 0 (yes borrow), output 88H TO
                                                 ;LEDs.
3608  27 F6              SJMP   COMP             ;GO back to poll switch VALUE.
360A  B1 11 0F   LEDS1:  LDB    P1,#11H          ;Output 11H TO LEDs.
360D  27 F1              SJMP   COMP             ;Loop back to poll and compare.
```

Execute the above program. Set the switches to 00. The CMPB instruction does a subtract of 01 from 00 necessitating a borrow. You'll see 88 appear at P1's LEDs verifying that the C flag is 0, so that we fall through the JC instruction. Now, on the fly, change the switches to anything greater than 00. This time CMPB does not produce a borrow. This should result in C = 1, which is verified by the fact that you'll see 11 at P1 i.e. JC is obeyed and causes a jump to LEDS1. Keep varying the switches in and out of 00 and observe 88, 11, etc. alternate.

EXPERIMENT 3-3

THE GENERIC FORM OF THE CONDITIONAL BRANCH VS. THE CONDITIONAL JUMP INSTRUCTIONS.

It is suggested that you first look at p. 3-18 through 3-37 in the MCS-96 MACRO ASSEMBLER USER'S GUIDE for information on the generic forms of the conditional branch instructions and, in particular, as to what the assembler does in choosing the nature of the instruction sequence depending on the distance to the referenced address. If that distance is "short" (-128 to +127 bytes away), then a simple JC, JE, JBS, etc. is chosen, depending on which conditional branch we are talking about. If the distance is "medium" (-1024 to +1023 bytes away), then the assembler chooses the form JNE followed by SJMP (or JNC followed by SJMP or JBC followed by SJMP, etc.) since SJMP can reach out to -1024 to +1023 bytes away. If the distance is "long" i.e. to anywhere, the assembler chooses the form JNE followed by LJMP (or JNC followed by LJMP or JBC followed by LJMP, etc.) since LJMP can reach out to anywhere in memory. In every case the JE or JNE, etc. forms employed by the assembler can only reach out to -128 to +127 bytes away. The result of all this is that if you wish to conditionally branch to medium or long distances away, you should employ the conditional BRANCH instruction in which the assembler chooses the correct sequence of conditional JUMP and SJMP or LJMP instructions. If you want to conditionally jump a short distance, you can either choose the conditional BRANCH form or the conditional JUMP form. In the former case, the assembler chooses the conditional jump form anyway.

The experiment below illustrates all the above with the generic conditional BBS instruction (Branch on Bit Set) and then with the conditional JBS instruction (Jump on Bit Set). Study the object code assembled in each case that a BBS is employed. In parts A-1, 2, and 3 below we employ the BBS in short, medium, and long ranges, respectively. All works as it should. In part B below, we employ JBS in short range. When we tried to employ JBS for the medium and long range cases, the assembler gave out the message "Relative Jump Too Large" (which we did not include in the printouts below). It could not assemble the JBS in those cases.

```
                        ;       PART A) - 1
                        ;
                        ;
      0E 00             P0      EQU     0EH     ;PORT0 switches.
      0F 00             P1      EQU     0FH     ;PORT1 LEDs.
                        ;
3610                            ORG     3610H
                        ;
3610  35 0E 03 E7 2A HERE1:     BBS     P0,5,CADD1       ;If BIT 5 of switch = 1, branch
      00
                                                         ;to CADD1
3616  B1 AA 0F                  LDB     P1,#0AAH         ;Else, output AAH at LEDs
3619  27 F5                     SJMP    HERE1            ;Loop back to poll BIT 5 of switches.
                        ;
3640                            ORG     3640H
                        ;
3640  B1 55 0F          CADD1:  LDB     P1,#55H          ;BIT 5 was set = 1, output 55H.
3643  E7 CA FF                  LJMP    HERE1            ;Long jump to HERE1 to poll BIT 5.
                        ;
                        ;
                        ;       EXPT. 3-3.
                        ;
                        ;       PART A) - 2
                        ;
3650                            ORG     3650H
                        ;
3650  35 0E 03 E7 FA HERE2:     BBS     P0,5,CADD2       ;If BIT 5 of switch = 1, branch
      01
                                                         ;to CADD2
3656  B1 AA 0F                  LDB     P1,#0AAH         ;Else, output AAH at LEDs
3659  27 F5                     SJMP    HERE2            ;Loop back to poll BIT 5 of switches.
                        ;
3850                            ORG     3850H
                        ;
3850  B1 55 0F          CADD2:  LDB     P1,#55H          ;BIT 5 was set = 1, output 55H.
3853  E7 FA FD                  LJMP    HERE2            ;Long jump to HERE2 to poll BIT 5.
```

```
                        ;       PART A) - 3
                        ;
                        ;
3900                            ORG     3900H
                        ;
3900    35 0E 03 E7 FA HERE3:   BBS     P0,5,CADD3      ;If BIT 5 of switch = 1, branch
        06
                                                        ;to CADD3
3906    B1 AA 0F                LDB     P1,#0AAH        ;Else, output AAH at LEDs
3909    27 F5                   SJMP    HERE3           ;Loop back to poll BIT 5 of switches.
                        ;
4000                            ORG     4000H
                        ;
4000    B1 55 0F        CADD3:  LDB     P1,#55H         ;BIT 5 was set = 1, output 55H.
4003    E7 FA F8                LJMP    HERE3           ;Long jump to HERE3 to poll BIT 5.

                        ;       PART B)
                        ;
3700                            ORG     3700H
                        ;
3700    3D 0E 1D        THERE:  JBS     P0,5,LABEL      ;If BIT 5 of switches = 1,jump to
                                                        ;LABEL.
3703    B1 AA 0F                LDB     P1,#0AAH        ;Else output AAH to LEDs.
3706    27 F8                   SJMP    THERE           ;Loop back to poll BIT 5 of switches.
                        ;
3720                            ORG     3720H
                        ;
3720    B1 55 0F        LABEL:  LDB     P1,#55H         ;Output 55H to LEDs since BIT 5 is set.
3723    E7 DA FF                LJMP    THERE           ;Long jump to THERE to poll BIT 5.
```

In each of the experiments in parts A-1, A-2, A-3, bit 5 of switch port P0 is tested. If it is set (high) a branch to CADD1 (in the short range case) or CADD2 (in the medium range case) or CADD3 (in the long range case) is made, respectively, where 55 is outputted to the LEDs at port 1. The subsequent LJMP back to HERE1 or HERE2 or HERE3, respectively, in each case, continues to poll bit 5 of P0. If you throw S5 at P0 low from its previous hi state, you fall through the BBS instruction and in each case 55 changes to AA at P1. The subsequent SJMP back to HERE1, 2, or 3 continues the polling of P0.5. Execute from 3610 and throw S5 hi/lo/hi.... and verify 55/AA/55 etc. at P1. Then execute from 3650 and verify, then from 3900 and verify. Note that part A-1 involves a BBS from 3610 to 3640 (short), part A-2 a BBS from 3650 to 3850 (medium), and part A-3 a BBS from 3900 to 4000 (long). Study the object code in the print-outs above. Our particular assembler (XASM-96 from 2500ADSOFTWARE Inc.) ALWAYS translated the BBS (in EACH range case) to 35 0E 03 (JBC P0, 5, 03) followed by E7 -- (LJMP to CADD), where 03 is the jump JBC takes around the LJMP if bit clear.

Now execute the program in part B above. Here the JBS will jump to LABEL if S5 (P0.5) is high and cause 55 to appear at P1.LJMP THERE polls P0.5 again. If it now goes low, AA will be observed at P1. Verify this by executing from 3700. Note that JBS spans the short range 3700 to 3720 when it is obeyed. As we indicated before, when LABEL was changed to LABEL1 (ORG 3900) or to LABEL2 (ORG 4100) to attempt a JBS to a medium or long distance, the assembler gave the message "Relative Jump Too Large" and did not translate JBS. In the short range case, the print-out shows that JBS is translated correctly to 3D 0E 1D (1D jump to LABEL).

EXPERIMENT 3-4

THE INDIRECT BRANCH OR JUMP INSTRUCTION: BR (OR INDJUMP)

There are no indirect jumps employing SJMP or LJMP. The BR instruction is used for that. The "branch indirect" instruction has the assembly language format BR [wreg], where wreg is a word register in the internal register file. The instruction will cause a jump to the address contained in wreg. The program below at 4025 loads REG with 5000H, then branches to 5000 (BR [REG]) where AA is output to the LEDs at port 1. Execute the progıam (G FR 4025) and see that it happens. Clearly, this indirect branch can span the whole address space, as it is based on a word in wreg. The instruction is sometimes referred to as INDJMP by Intel (with the same Op. Code E3).

We are not bothering with the "branch direct" instruction (format BR CADD). The SJMP or LJMP instructions take care of that (the assembler translates BR to one of these anyway).

```
4025                          ORG     4025H
                      ;
4025   A1 00 50 50            LD      REG,#5000H      ;Load REG with WORD 5000H.
4029   E3 50                  BR      [REG]           ;Branch to address pointed to by REG.
                      ;
                      ;
5000                          ORG     5000H
                      ;
5000   B1 AA OF               LDB     P1,#0AAH        ;Output 0AAH to LEDs.
5003   27 FE          STOP:   SJMP    STOP            ;Loop here.

                            50 00         REG     EQU     50H
                            OF 00         P1      EQU     OFH
```

EXPERIMENT 3-5

THE ADDCB INSTRUCTION. EFFECT ON Z FLAG.

We wish to study the effect that execution of the ADDCB instruction (and by extension the ADDC instruction) has on the Z flag. The program at 4030 follows.

```
        50 00          REG1     EQU     50H
        60 00          REG2     EQU     60H
        00 00          ZEROREG  EQU     00H
        0F 00          P1       EQU     0FH
        0E 00          P0       EQU     0EH
                       ;
                       ;
4030                            ORG     4030H
                       ;
4030    90 0E 0E       BEGIN:   ORB     P0,P0          ;OR switch byte at P0 with itself.
                                                       ;This will clear C flag and clear
                                                       ;or set Z flag.
4033    B0 50 60                LDB     REG2,REG1      ;Load REG2 with the contents of REG1.
4036    B4 00 60                ADDCB   REG2,ZEROREG   ;Add 00 to REG2 with C flag = 0 from
                                                       ;previous ORB operation.
4039    DF 05                   JE      CADD           ;Test and jump to CADD if 'Z' = 1.
403B    B1 00 0F                LDB     P1,#00H        ;Else output 00H to LEDs at P1 (Z=0).
403E    27 F0                   SJMP    BEGIN          ;Loop to BEGIN to repeat.
4040    B1 AA 0F       CADD:    LDB     P1,#0AAH       ;Output 0AAH to LEDs since 'Z' = 1.
4043    27 EB                   SJMP    BEGIN          ;Loop to BEGIN to repeat.
```

The first instruction ORs the switch byte at port 0 with itself. This clears the C flag and sets or clears the Z flag depending on whether P0 is 00 or not, respectively. The second instruction loads REG2 with the byte from REG1 (entered into REG1 (50) at run time). The ADDCB instruction adds 00 (from R0) to REG2 with carry (which is 0 in this experiment). If the result of this addition is 0 (Z = 1), JE CADD jumps to CADD where AA is output to the LEDs at P1. If the result is not zero (Z = 0), we fall through JE to output 00 to the LEDs. In either case SJMP BEGIN polls P0 again in case it has changed.

Let us try two cases:

1. a). Enter BY 50 = 00 and set the switches at P0 to 00. Execute (G FR 4030). ORB sets Z to 1 and C to 0. ADDCB gives a 0 result so Z remains set. Hence JE CADD is taken and we observed AA.

b). On the fly, change P0 to 01 at the switches. This makes Z = 0 initially, and C is still 0. The addition still gives 0, so Z changes from its initial 0 value to 1. Again JE CADD is taken and AA is still observed.

2. a). ESC. Enter BY 50 = 01. Reset the switches at P0 to 00. Execute. Z is initially 1 due to ORB and C is 0. The ADDCB gives a non-zero result so Z changes from 1 to 0. JE is not taken. Hence we should, and did, observe 00 at the LEDs.

b). On the fly, change the switch setting to 01. Z is initially 0 from ORB, as is C. The addition gives a non-zero result. So Z remains at 0 and JE is not taken. 00 is still seen at the LEDs.

CONCLUSION

Some earlier manuals, or your Microcontroller Handbook, indicate that ADDC and ADDCB can ONLY clear the Z flag, but not SET it. This experiment shows that may not be true on some of the earlier parts.

EXPERIMENT 3-6

CONDITIONAL JUMPS BASED ON FLAG SETTINGS. THE PUSHF AND POPF INSTRUCTIONS.

A. EXAMINING FLAGS BY MEANS OF THE PUSHF INSTRUCTION

```
50 00        REG1    EQU   50H
60 00        REG2    EQU   60H
70 00        REG3    EQU   70H
80 00        REG4    EQU   80H
90 00        REG5    EQU   90H
71 00        REG3HI  EQU   71H
0E 00        P0      EQU   0EH          ;Switches
0F 00        P1      EQU   0FH          ;LEDs
18 00        SP      EQU   18H
```

```
                           ;       PART A)
                           ;
4050                               ORG     4050H
                           ;
4050    B1 80 50                   LDB     REG1,#80H      ;Load REG1 with BYTE 80H.
4053    74 60 50                   ADDB    REG1,REG2      ;Add contents of REG1 TO REG2.
                                                          ;Place the result in REG1.
4056    F2                         PUSHF                  ;Save FLAGS on stack.
4057    CC 70                      POP     REG3           ;Move FLAGS into REG3 from stack.
4059    B0 71 0F                   LDB     P1,REG3HI      ;Output FLAGS to LEDs.
405C    27 FE              HERE:   SJMP    HERE           ;Loop here.
```

In the above program at 4050, 80 is loaded into byte REG1 (50H). Then byte REG2 (entered at 60H at run time) is added to REG1 with the result remaining in REG1, ADDB affects all flags except ST and can only set, but never clear, the VT flag. (Note that we have not initialized SP; we are using the monitor's SP initialization for a program in which the stack is used. No harm here - but not to be repeated). To see the effect of ADDB on the flags, we push the PSW on to the stack (PUSHF), which leaves the PSW containing all 0s. The high byte of PSW is the flag byte, so that if we pop the top of the stack into word REG3 (70H) we should expect to find the flag byte in the high byte of REG3 i.e. in REG3HI = 71H. That being so, LDB P1, REG3HI loads the LEDs at byte SFR P1 (port 1) with the flag settings for inspection.

We examined 3 cases (remember flags = Z, N, V, VT, C, - I, ST).

1. Before executing, enter BY 60 = 05, then G FR 4050. We observed 01000000 on the LEDs. 80 + 05 = 85, with the MSB = 1 so that N = 1. No other flag is set by the result of this addition.
2. ESC. Enter BY 60 = 80. G FR 4050. We observed 11111000 on the LEDs, in keeping with the fact that 80 + 80 = 00 with a carry of 1. Also, it must be a negative result (since MSB of each byte is 1). Hence N = 1. Overflow occurred so V must be 1. This also sets the VT flag. The result is 00 so the Z flag is set. Thus Z, N, V, VT, C are all 1s.
3. ESC. Enter BY 60 = 0FF. G FR 4050 produced 01111000 on the LEDs. FF + 80 = 7F with a carry of 1. Each byte is negative since each MSB is 1 so N must be 1 for the result. There again is overflow so V = VT = 1.

B. CONDITIONAL JUMPS BASED ON FLAG SETTINGS. PUSHF, POPF.

```
                          ;       PART B)
                          ;
4060                              ORG     4060H
                          ;
4060   A1 40 00 18                LD      SP,#40H         ;Initialize SP to 40H.
4064   99 00 0E           BEGIN:  CMPB    P0,#00H         ;Compare BYTE switch value with 00.
4067   D7 05                      JNE     ZNOT1           ;If NOT = 0, then jump to ZNOT1.
4069   B1 80 0F           ZIS1:   LDB     P1,#80H         ;Else output 80H to LEDs.
406C   28 22                      SCALL   TIME            ;Keep 80H ON LEDs for time delay.
406E   54 70 60 50        ZNOT1:  ADDB    REG1,REG2,REG3  ;Affects FLAGS depending on the values
                                                          ;of REG2 and REG3 at run time.
4072   D5 05                      JNV     VNOT1           ;If V != 1, jump to VNOT1.
4074   B1 20 0F           VIS1:   LDB     P1,#20H         ;Else V = 1,  output 20H to LEDs.
4077   28 17                      SCALL   TIME            ;Keep 20H on LEDS for time delay.
4079   D4 05              VNOT1:  JNVT    VTNOT1          ;If VT != 1,  jump to VTNOT1.
                                                          ;This instr. automatically CLEARS VT.
407B   B1 10 0F           VTIS1:  LDB     P1,#10H         ;Else VT = 1, output 10H to LEDs.
407E   28 10                      SCALL   TIME            ;Keep 10H on LEDs for time delay.
4080   D3 05              VTNOT1: JNC     CNOT1           ;If C != 1,  jump to CNOT1.
4082   B1 08 0F           CIS1:   LDB     P1,#08H         ;Else C = 1, output 08H to LEDs.
4085   28 09                      SCALL   TIME            ;Keep 08H on LEDs for time delay.
4087   D6 05              CNOT1:  JGE     NNOT1           ;If N != 1,  jump to NNOT1.
4089   B1 40 0F           NIS1:   LDB     P1,#40H         ;Else N = 1, output 40H to LEDs.
408C   28 02                      SCALL   TIME            ;Keep 40H on LEDs for time delay.
408E   27 D4              NNOT1:  SJMP    BEGIN           ;Repeat.
                          ;
                          ;
                          ;       TIME DELAY Program.
                          ;
                          ;
4090                              ORG     4090H
                          ;
4090   F2                 TIME:   PUSHF                   ;Save flags.
4091   B1 10 80                   LDB     REG4,#10H       ;Load BYTE 10H into REG4 for outer
                                                          ;loop.
                                                          ;software.
4094   A1 FF FF 90        LOAD:   LD      REG5,#0FFFFH    ;Load WORD 0FFFFH into REG5 for inner
                                                          ;software loop.
4098   05 90              AGAIN:  DEC     REG5            ;Decrement REG5. (There is no DJNZ
                                                          ;instruction for WORD operands).
409A   D7 FC                      JNE     AGAIN           ;If REG5 != 0,  jump to AGAIN
409C   E0 80 F5                   DJNZ    REG4,LOAD       ;Else REG5 = 0. Decr. and test
                                                          ;REG4, If REG4 != 0, jump back to LOAD.
409F   F3                         POPF                    ;Else we are finished. Restore flags.
40A0   F0                         RET                     ;Return.
```

In the program at 4060 above, we use the CMPB P0, #00 instruction on the second line to affect the Z flag (it will set it if the switches at port P0 are all 0, or it will clear it if any switch at P0 is not 0). Then the JNE instruction jumps to ZNOT1 if Z = 0 or falls through to ZIS1 if Z = 1. If it falls through to ZIS1, we output 80 to the LEDs at P1 to indicate Z = 1 = P1.7, (the LEDs will represent the flags Z, N, V, VT, C, - I, ST). A call to the 3 second time delay (more about that later) at 4090 keeps 80 at P1 on for 3 seconds and then returns to ZNOT1. If Z were originally 0, the JNE instruction would have taken us to ZNOT1 without the 80 being seen at P1 i.e. P1.7 = 0 this time telling us Z = 0. There we employ the 3-operand ADDB instruction to affect all flags except ST. In it we add REG3 (70), entered at run time, to REG2 (60), also entered at run time, with the result stored in REG1 (50H), so that the REG2 value is not destroyed. It's needed again for the SJMP BEGIN go-around. We then examine the V flag by means of the JNV instruction. If V is 1, JNV falls through to VIS1 where 20 is output to P1 for 3 seconds. This will show up as P1.5 = 1 = V on the LEDs. If, however, V is not 1 due to ADDB, then JNV is taken to VNOT1 and 20 is not shown at the LEDs.

At VNOT1 we test the VT flag by means of the JNVT instruction. If VT is 1 we fall through to VTIS1 where we output 10 to P1 for 3 seconds i.e. we see P1.4 = VT = 1. If, however, VT is not 1, the JNVT is taken to VTNOT1 and 10 is not seen at P1. At VTNOT1 we test the carry, C, by means of the JNC instruction. If C is 1 we fall through to CIS1 where we output 08 to P1 for 3 sec. in keeping with C = P1.3 = 1. If C is not 1, the JNC is taken to CNOT1 and 08 is not observed. At CNOT1 we test the N flag by means of the JGE (greater than or equal) instruction which obeys the setting of the N flag. If N is 1 we fall through to NIS1 where we output 40 to the LEDs at P1 for 3 sec (in keeping with the fact that P1.6 = N should be 1 if N = 1). If N is not 1 the JGE is obeyed and we jump to NNOT1 without seeing 40 at P1. There we jump back to the beginning so that we can poll P0 (switches) again as they affect the Z flag.

The time delay at 4090 has as its first, and next to last, instructions PUSHF and POPF in order to save all flag settings, as the delay program itself affects flags. It is a delay based on outer and inner loop decrementations. REG4 (80H) is loaded with 10 for the outer loop so that 16 outer loops will be done before the DJNZ REG4, LOAD decrements it to 0. The inner loop register (REG5 = 90H) is loaded with FFFF and decremented over and over till its 0, at which time another decrement of REG4 is made and if it's not 0 REG5 is reloaded with FFFF again for another complete inner loop. Since DEC and JNE consume 12 state times (3 usec), one complete inner loop traversal will take about 0.2

sec. (65,536 x 3 usec). Since there are 16 outer loops to be made before we exit (when REG4 = 0), we should observe about 3 sec. of delay time - which we did in every case above.

PROCEDURE

1. Set the swtiches at P0 to 00. Enter BY 60 = 80, BY 70 = OFF. This causes Z=1 from the CMPB instruction and N=1, V=1, VT=1, and C=1 from the ADDB instruction. Execute from 4060 (G FR 4060). You should observe P1 = 80 for 3 sec, then 20 for 3 sec, then 10 for 3 sec, then 08, then 40, and then a repeat of these values ad infinitum. Fall-throughs the conditional jump instructions are made in all the cases in the program.
2. On the fly throw S0 (P0.0) high. All the above repeats except 80 doesn't show as Z is not 1.
3. ESC. Enter BY 60 = 70, BY 70 = 05. Set switches at P0 to 00 again. We should expect Z=1 from the switch settings. This time ADDB gives 75 so that N=V=VT=C=0. Remember also that, while VT was 1 from the last case (2 above), the very instruction JNVT itself leaves VT=0 AFTER it tests VT so that we come into this experiment with VT=0. Execute from 4060 and expect to see 80 at P1 at all times. We did.
4. On the fly throw S0 (P0.0) high. P1 now shows 00 always.
5. ESC. Enter BY 60 = 80, BY 70 = 05 and set P0 to 00 with the switches. Again Z=1, but now 80 + 05 = 85 will cause N=1 (MSB=1), but V, VT, and C will each be 0. Thus if you execute from 4060, you should observe 80 for 3 seconds followed by 40 for 3 seconds, then 80, then 40 etc.
6. On the fly, change S0 to 1. Now you should only see 40 at all times.
7. As a final case ESC and enter BY 60 = 81 and BY 70 = 81. Reset the switches at P0 to 00. Since 81 + 81 = 02 with a carry and overflow, and since the result really is negative, we should have Z=1 from the CMPB instruction and N=V=VT=C=1 from ADDB. Hence we are back to case (1) where we saw 80, 20, 10, 08, 40 over and over, each for 3 seconds. We confirmed this. If, on the fly, we set S0 to 1 so that Z is not 1, then we should, and did, see 20, 10, 08, 40 over and over.

This experiment has demonstrated in some detail the workings of a good number of the conditional jumps based on flag settings. We were careful to set our own SP since we are involved with stack operations (SCALL, RET, PUSHF, POPF).

PROBLEM

Re-write the program using JE, JV, JVT, JC, and JLT conditional jump instructions. Which way seems better? Why?

EXPERIMENT 3-7

MORE ON THE V AND VT FLAGS

The V (oVerflow) flag is set to 1 whenever the arithmetic operation generates a result that can not fit the size of the destination (double word, word, or byte). The VT (oVerflow Trap) flag is set to 1 WHENEVER the V flag is set, but won't then be cleared except by an instruction that explicitly does so (CLRVT, JVT, JNVT, PUSHF, or RST). The VT flag is helpful in that an overflow condition (V=1) in any one part of a sequence of related arithmetic operations is remembered at the end of the sequence, even though subsequent parts may have cleared the V flag. Thus a PREVIOUS overflow can be tested just ONCE (at the END of the sequence) by querying VT at the end rather than testing V after each part of the sequence. See pp. 3-4, 3-23 Microcontroller Handbook or chapter 1 sections P (b) and C in this book. V and VT will be used in the applications with arithmetic in chapter 7.

```
          18 00         SP       EQU    18H
          40 00         REG1     EQU    40H
          50 00         REG2     EQU    50H
          0E 00         P0       EQU    0EH          ;Switches
          0F 00         P1       EQU    0FH          ;LEDs
                        ;
                        ;
40B0                             ORG    40B0H
                        ;
40B0      A1 40 00 18            LD     SP,#0040H    ;Initialize SP to 0040H.
40B4      54 0E 40 50   BEGIN:   ADDB   REG2,REG1,P0 ;P0 + REG1 result placed into REG2.
                                                     ;REG1 is 0FFH at run time.
                                                     ;Flags affected. P0 switches will be
                                                     ;set at run time.
40B8      F2                     PUSHF               ;Put FLAGS onto stack. Flags now 00H.
40B9      B3 18 01 0F            LDB    P1,1[SP]     ;Output FLAGS to LEDs.
40BD      F3                     POPF                ;Restore original flags in PSW.
40BE      90 40 40               ORB    REG1,REG1    ;This makes V and C = 0 but does not
                                                     ;effect the VT flag or REG1.
40C1      F2                     PUSHF               ;Put FLAGS onto stack.
40C2      B3 18 01 0F            LDB    P1,1[SP]     ;Output FLAGS to LEDs.
40C6      F3                     POPF                ;Restore original flags in PSW.
```

```
40C7   FC            CLRVT              ;Make VT = 0.
40C8   F2            PUSHF              ;Put FLAGS onto stack.
40C9   B3 18 01 0F   LDB    P1,1[SP]    ;Output FLAGS to LEDs.
40CD   F3            POPF               ;Restore original flags in PSW.
40CE   27 E4         SJMP   BEGIN       ;Repeat.
```

In the above program at 40B0 the byte value of the switches at P0 is added to the byte value of REG1 (40H) entered at run time. The result is stored in REG2 (50H) and flags are affected, except ST. The PUSHF instruction saves the flags and interrupt mask on the stack and replaces the PSW with 0. SP is now at SP-2 i.e. at 003E in view of the first instruction in the program. The next LDB instruction outputs the value at SP + 1 in memory i.e. the value at 003F (the flag byte), to the LEDs at P1 for viewing. SP is still at 003E. Hence a breakpoint set to 40B9 should reveal the flag settings (as a result of the ADDB instruction) at P1. POPF restores the original flags to the PSW. SP is back at 0040. The ORB instruction resets C and V to 0 but does not affect the VT flag or the contents at REG1. PUSHF again saves the new flags, sets PSW to 0, and leaves SP at 003E. LDB then loads P1 with the flag byte at 003F (SP + 1), with SP still at 003E. Hence a breakpoint at 40C2 should show the effect of ORB on the flags at P1 (namely C=0, V=0 with no effect on Z (if REG1 is not 0) or N). POPF restores the flags to PSW and CLRVT resets VT to 0 (affecting no other flags). Thus, again, a breakpoint at 40C9 should have P1 show only a change in VT but not in the other flags. Finally, a breakpoint at 40CE should reveal no change in the flags as observed at P1 since SJMP affects nothing.

PROCEDURE

1. Enter BY 40 = 0FF, loading REG1 with FF. Set breakpoints at 40B9, 40C2, 40C9, 40CE. Set the switches at P0 to 80. ADDB gives FF + 80 = 7F with Z=0, N=1 (negative result), V=VT=1 (overflow occurred), C=1. Hence break at 40B9 should show 0111100- at P1. ORB REG1, REG1 causes Z=0, C=0, and V=0. N remains 1 and VT is unaffected. Hence a break at 40C2 should show 0101000- at the LEDs. CLR VT makes VT=0 and does nothing to the other flags. Hence a break at 40C9 should show 0100000- at the LEDs. Finally, a break at 40CE should reveal the same flag settings at P1. A break at 40B9 should again show 011100- at the LEDs.
2. Execute from 40B0 (G FR 40B0 TILL BR). See "break at 40B9". The LEDs should show 0111100- in view of the discussion in (1) above.
3. Enter G. See "break at 40C2". LEDs now show 0101000- in view of the discussion in (1).

4. Enter G. See "break at 40C9". LEDs show 0100000 - in keeping with (1) above.
5. Enter G. See "break at 40CE". LEDs still show 0100000 -, as they should.
6. Do another G. See "break at 40B9" and LEDs again show 0111100 -, as they should.

Thus once VT is set as a result of V=1, it stays set even when V goes back to 0. It will stay set unless explicitly or implicitly cleared by a subsequent instruction (here explicitly cleared by CLRVT).

EXPERIMENT 3-8

MORE ON THE N (NEGATIVE) FLAG

```
        50 00        REG1     EQU     50H
        60 00        REG2     EQU     60H
        61 00        REG2HI   EQU     61H              ;Switches
        0E 00        P0       EQU     0EH
        0F 00        P1       EQU     0FH              ;LEDs
                     ;
                     ;
40E0                          ORG     40E0H
                     ;
40E0    55 FF 0E 50           ADDB    REG1,P0,#0FFH    ;Add 0FFH to the value of the
                                                       ;switches and put result into REG1.
40E4    F2                    PUSHF                    ;Put flags (PSW) onto stack.
40E5    CC 60                 POP     REG2             ;Move PSW from stack into REG2.
40E7    B0 61 0F              LDB     P1,REG2HI        ;Output flags to LEDs.
40EA    27 FE        HERE:    SJMP    HERE             ;Loop here.
```

In the above program at 40E0 the byte FF is added to the byte at port 0 (switch bank) and the result is stored in REG1 (50H). Flags are affected. PUSHF saves the flags and interrupt mask on top of the stack and POP REG2 pops those bytes back into REG2 (60H), with flag byte (high byte) going to the odd register 61H. LDB P1, REG2HI outputs that flag byte to the LEDs at P1 from register 61. The program then loops on itself.

PROCEDURE

1. With P0 set to 00, execute from 40E0 and observe the LEDs. Since 00 + FF produces a non-zero result, creates no overflow or carry, but has MSB=1 (N=1), we should see a flag byte 01000-0-, and we did (-- are indeterminate. ST is not affected by ADDB).
2. ESC and set P0 to 01. ADDB now gives 00 with a carry of 1. Hence Z and C should each be 1. Execute from 40E0 and observe 10001-0- at the LEDs.
3. ESC and set P0 to 80. FF + 80 = 7F with a carry. The result must be negative (two negative numbers), there's a carry, the result is not 0, there's overflow. Hence when you execute you should see 01111-0- at P1.
4. ESC and set P0 to FF. FF + FF = FE with a carry. The result is negative. There is no overflow. Hence, on execution, we should observe 01001-0- at the LEDs.

The N flag will be used in the arithmetic applications in chapter 7.

EXPERIMENT 3-9

THE STICKY BIT AND SHIFT RIGHT INSTRUCTION

All shift right instructions (logical or arithmetic, on byte, word, or double word) affect the sticky bit. The sticky bit flag is cleared at the beginning of the instruction and set if at any time during the successive shifts right a 1 is first shifted into the carry AND A FURTHER SHIFT CYCLE OCCURS. In the logical right shifts the left bits of the result are filled with 0s and the last bit shifted out at the right end is saved in the carry. In the arithmetic right shifts the left bits of the result are filled with 0s if MSB was originally 0, otherwise 1s are shifted in at the left end. The last bit shifted out at the right end is saved in the carry.

The ST flag is useful, along with C, to control rounding after right shifts (see pp. 3-4, 3-5 Microcontroller Handbook or our chapter 1, section C) and in other arithmetic applications (see chapter 7). In the program at 4100 below, we investigate the effect on ST of the "logical right shift word" (SHR) instruction. SHR affects all flags except VT and resets V to 0. We are using SHR in the form SHR WREG, BREG in which the shifting is performed on the word WREG the number of times specified by the content of BREG (it could also be specified as an immediate value 0 to 15). The program at 4100 follows:

```
           30 00          WREG     EQU     30H
           40 00          BREG     EQU     40H              ;Count
           0F 00          P1       EQU     0FH              ;LEDs
           50 00          REG1     EQU     50H
           51 00          REG1HI   EQU     51H
                          ;
                          ;
4100                               ORG     4100H
                          ;
4100       A1 00 03 30             LD      WREG,#300H       ;Load WREG with 300H
4104       08 40 30                SHR     WREG,BREG        ;Shift the BITS in WREG right
                                                            ;the number of times specified
                                                            ;by the contents of BREG.
4107       F2                      PUSHF                    ;Put flags (PSW) onto stack.
4108       CC 50                   POP     REG1             ;Move PSW from stack into REG1.
410A       B0 51 0F                LDB     P1,REG1HI        ;Output flags (PSW) to LEDs.
410D       27 FE          HERE:    SJMP    HERE             ;Loop here.
```

Again we wish to observe the flags after the SHR instruction. We do this as we have been doing it: by a PUSHF onto stack, then retrieving PSW into REG1 and displaying high order byte of REG1 at P1's LEDs. The word chosen for shifting is 0300 = 00000011 00000000.

PROCEDURE

1. Enter BY 40 = 08 for 8 shifts, (BREG is 40H) then G FR 4100. Observe 00000-00 at the LEDs. Examine WO 30 and see 0003 (after 8 shifts on the original WREG = 0300). No carry was produced. Nor is there a 0 result. There's no overflow or negative result. Hence the flag result observed at P1 is consistent.
2. ESC. Enter BY 40 = 09 for 9 shifts. Execute from 4100. Observe 00001-00. Check WO 30 and find 0001 as expected. A 1 was shifted into the carry (9th shift) and no further shifts occurred, so ST should still be 0. The result is non-zero, non-negative, without overflow. All is consistent with the flag result at P1.
3. ESC. Enter BY 40 = 0A for 10 shifts. Execute from 4100. Observe WO 30 = 0000 as expected. The 9th shift pushed 1 into C and ANOTHER (10th) shift occurred (also pushing a 1 into C). Hence C should be 1, ST should be 1, the result is 0 so Z=1, but N, V, and VT should be 0. Indeed the LEDs displayed 10001-01.

4. ESC. Enter BY 40 = 0B for 11 shifts. Execute. Check WO 30. As expected, you'll find 0000 in WREG again. This time the 11th shift pushed a 0 into C, but since a 1 was in C from the 9th shift and further shifts occurred, ST was set to 1 AND STAYED AT 1. The result is 0 so Z=1. N=V=VT= 0. Hence we should, and did, see 10000-01 at the LEDs.

EXPERIMENT 3-10

MORE ON THE SHIFT INSTRUCTIONS

In this experiment we look into the workings of the SHL, SHRL, and SHRA instructions. The effect of SHRA on ST flag is again observed. Left shifts do not affect ST. In every case we observe the effects of the instruction on all the flags.

```
      30 00          IREG     EQU     30H
      40 00          WREG     EQU     40H
      60 00          BREG     EQU     60H
      50 00          REG1     EQU     50H
      51 00          REG1HI   EQU     51H
      0F 00          P1       EQU     0FH              ;LEDs
                     ;
                     ;
                     ;        EXPT. 3-10.
                     ;
                     ;        PART A)
                     ;
                     ;
4120                          ORG     4120H
                     ;
4120  A1 33 00 40             LD      WREG,#0033H      ;Load WREG with 0033H.
4124  09 0A 40                SHL     WREG,#0AH        ;Shift BITS in WREG left 10
                                                       ;(0AH) times. BIT shifted out
                                                       ;goes into C flag.
4127  F2                      PUSHF                    ;Put flags (PSW) onto stack.
4128  CC 50                   POP     REG1             ;Move PSW from stack into REG1
412A  B0 51 0F                LDB     P1,REG1HI        ;Output flags (PSW) to LEDs.
412D  27 FE          HERE:    SJMP    HERE             ;Loop here.
```

In the above program at 4120 we shift left 10 times on the word 0033 = 00000000 00110011. The bit shifted out on the left goes to the C flag in each case and the right bits are filled with 0s. Flags are observed at P1 as a result of the PUSHF, POP REG1, and LDB instructions. WREG is register 40H. 10 shifts left on WREG = 0033 should produce CC00 in WREG. After executing from 4120 and examining WO 40, we found the latter showed CC00, as expected. 10 shifts left did not succeed in filling the carry with a 1. The result is not 0, so Z should be 0. The flags showed 00110-00. We are at a loss to explain why V=VT=1 as a result of SHL. The manuals indicate? for the N flag after this instruction is executed.

```
                    ;       PART B)
                    ;
                    ;
4130                        ORG     4130H
                    ;
4130  A1 33 00 40           LD      WREG,#0033H     ;Load WREG with 0033H.
4134  09 60 40              SHL     WREG,BREG       ;Shift BITS in WREG left
                                                    ;the number of times specified
                                                    ;by the contents of BREG.
4137  F2                    PUSHF                   ;Put flags (PSW) onto stack.
4138  CC 50                 POP     REG1            ;Move PSW from stack into REG1
413A  B0 51 0F              LDB     P1,REG1HI       ;Output flags (PSW) to LEDs.
413D  27 FE         THERE:  SJMP    THERE           ;Loop here.
```

The above program at 4130 is exactly the same as the previous one in part (A) except the number of shifts left on WREG is determined (at run time) by the contents of BREG. Try four cases:

1. Enter BY 60 = 0B (BREG is register 60) for 11 shifts left. Execute from 4130. Query WO 40 and find 9800 in keeping with 11 shifts left on the original 0033. The flags displayed at P1 were 011110-00. C is 1 because the 11th shift does push a 1 into C. Again V=VT=1(?). This time N=1 (it's indeterminate according to the manuals).
2. ESC and enter BY 60 = 0F for 15 shifts left. Execute and check out WO 40. You should see 8000. Bit 1 of the original word was 1 and is forced into C. Hence flags show 01111-00. Again V=VT=1 is a puzzle. Z=0 and C=1 are to be expected.
3. ESC and enter BY 60 = 10 for 16 shifts left. This should give the result 0000 in WREG. Hence Z should be 1. A 1 was pushed into C on the 16th shift left (from the original bit 0 which was 1). Execute from 4130. WO 40 indeed showed 0000. The flags at P1 read 11111-00. Again V=VT= 1(?). Z=C=1, as expected.
4. Finally, ESC and enter BY 60 = 11 for 17 shifts left. We'd expect WO 40 to read 0000 after execution. Z should be 1.

This time there should be no carry as the 17th shift left forces a 0 into C. After execution we found WO 40 gave 0000 and the flags showed 10110-00 i.e. Z=1, C=0, V=VT=1(?).

```
                        ;       PART C)
                        ;
                        ;
4110                            ORG     4110H
                        ;
4110   0C 60 30                 SHRL    IREG,BREG       ;Logical right shift on double
                                                        ;word IREG.  Shift number of
                                                        ;times specified in BREG.
4113   27 FE            STOP:   SJMP    STOP            ;Loop here.
```

In the above program at 4110, double word register IREG (30H) is shifted right (logically) the number of times specified in BREG. Enter BY 60 = 18 for 24 right shifts. Also enter WO 30 = 0001 and WO 32 = 0080 so that our complete double word at 0033, 32, 31, 30 (IREG) is 00800001 (IREG are the 4 byte-registers 0033, 32, 31, 30 but is DEFINED as 30). BREG is here defined as 60. 24 shifts right should yield 00000000 (double word) in IREG and leave a 1 in C. Since a PREVIOUS 1 (bit 0) was, at an EARLIER time, shifted into C and further right shifts occurred, ST should be 1. Further, SHRL resets V and N to 0. Since the result in IREG is 0, Z should be 1.

Execute from 4110 with the above entries previously made. Then examine WO 30 and WO 32. You'll find 0000 and 0000 respectively so that IREG = 00000000 as expected. Enter PSW and find PSW = 9900. The low byte is the interrupt mask. The 99 are the flags: 10011001, showing that Z=1, N=0, V=0, VT=1 (from a previous experiment) C=1 and ST=1, which results are perfectly consistent for this case.

Now ESC and enter BY 60 = 16 (22 shifts right), WO 30 = 0001, WO 32 = 0080 (same double word 00800001). 22 shifts right should now produce 00000002 in IREG. C should be 0 as the last shift out of LSB pushed a 0 into C. A previous shift of 1 into C (from bit 0) occurred and further right shifts took place, so ST should be 1. The result is not 0 so Z=0 is expected. Execute from 4110. Examine WO 32 and find 0000. Examine WO 30 and find 0002, as expected. Examine PSW and find PSW = 1100 so the flags are 11 = 00010001: Z=0, N=0, V=0, VT=1 (from before) C=0 and ST=1, as predicted (remember SHRL resets V and N to 0).

```
                    ;       PART D)
                    ;
                    ;
4117                        ORG     4117H
                    ;
4117  0A 60 40              SHRA    WREG,BREG       ;Arithmetic right shift on word
                                                    ;WREG. Shift number of times
                                                    ;specified in BREG.
411A  27 FE         HALT:   SJMP    HALT            ;Loop here.
```

In the above program at 4117 SHRA (arithmetic shift right on a word) is investigated. The shifts are executed on WREG (40H) and the number of shifts is specified in BREG (60H). At run time enter WO 40 = 8300 as the word for WREG and BY 60 = 0C for 12 right shifts. Execute from 4117. Then examine WO 40 and find FFF8. This is so because 1s are shifted in from the left since MSB was originally 1. 12 shifts right take the leftmost nibble (8) and places it in the lowest (rightmost) nibble of the word with 1s filling in the gaps. Now examine PSW. We found PSW = 5100 so that the flags are 51 = 01010001. Z=0 because the result is not 0. N=1 is evident. V=0 since SHRA resets V. VT=1 from previous experiment. C=0 since the last bit shifted out of LSB into C was a 0. ST=1 because a previous C=1 was produced (from nibble = 3) and further shifts took place.

Now ESC and redo with WO 40 = 7300 and BY 60 = 0C again. Execute from 4117. Examine WO 40. You should find 0007 because MSB was 0 so that 0s fill in from the left as right shifts occur. This time we should find Z=0 (obvious), N=0 (MSB=0), V=0, VT=1 (leftover), C=0 (last bit shifted out of LSB into C was a 0), and ST should be 1 since the nibble 3 produced a C=1 previously and further shifts were made. Examining PSW revealed 1100 so flags = 00010001, in keeping with our expectations.

EXPERIMENT 3-11

SCALL VS LCALL. THE GENERIC CALL.

If the generic CALL (direct) instruction is used, the assembler will translate it into an SCALL or LCALL depending on the distance to the target address. The SCALL can reach anywhere from

-1024 to +1023 bytes relative to the end of that instruction. The LCALL, on the other hand, can reach anywhere in memory. The user thus has 3 options: employ the SCALL if sure that the range is within -1024 to +1023; employ the LCALL when in doubt, or when the target is out of the -1024 to +1023 range, since it can reach to anywhere; or simply employ the generic CALL and let the assembler take care of matters. If you're not sure about your assembler's relationship with CALL, then using LCALL would seem to be the best policy in all cases. SCALL requires 2 bytes of code, LCALL 3. Both consume the exact same number of state times (13 for on-chip stack and 16 for off-chip stack). No flags are affected.

PROBLEM

Call a routine that outputs AA to the LEDs at P1. The routine is to simply return to the main program which consists of nothing more than the call followed by a self loop. Write it and execute it for the following cases:

1. The main program starts at 4140 and calls the routine which is situated right at the end of the main program. Do it employing first SCALL, then LCALL, then generic CALL and observe results and the object code assembled.
2. Next, re-do (1) in which the main program starts at 4160 and the routine is written at 5100. Try it employing first SCALL, then LCALL, then generic CALL. Will it work with SCALL? What does the assembler do in that case? Will it work with LCALL? What gets assembled when you try it with the generic CALL vs. the LCALL?

EXPERIMENT 3-12

THE LDBZE AND LDBSE INSTRUCTIONS

The programs at 4170 and 4180 for part (A) (LDBZE) and for part (B) (LDBSE), respectively, are shown below. LDBZE (load word with byte zero) extends a source byte i.e. makes it into a word whose high byte is 00 and low byte is the original byte. It then loads that word into the destination word operand. LDBSE (load 16-bit signed integer with 8-bit signed short integer), on the other hand, sign extends the 8-bit signed short integer (source) into a 16-bit signed integer and loads it into the destination word operand. If MSB of the 8-bit source is 0 then 00 goes into the high byte of the destination. If it is 1, then

FF goes into high byte of destination. In either case the 8-bit source short integer is placed into the low byte of the destination. In both cases flags are not affected.

```
        60 00           WREG    EQU     60H
        70 00           BREG    EQU     70H
                        ;
                        ;       EXPT. 3-12.
                        ;
                        ;       PART A)
                        ;
4170                            ORG     4170H
                        ;
4170    A1 FF FF 60             LD      WREG,#OFFFFH    ;Load WREG with OFFFFH.
4174    AD AA 60                LDBZE   WREG,#OAAH      ;Load 00H into WREGHI, and
                                                        ;OAAH into WREGLO.
4177    27 FE           HERE:   SJMP    HERE            ;Loop here.
                        ;
                        ;
                        ;       EXPT. 3-12.
                        ;
                        ;       PART B)
                        ;
4180                            ORG     4180H
                        ;
4180    A1 55 55 60             LD      WREG,#5555H     ;Load WREG with 5555H.
4184    BC 70 60                LDBSE   WREG,BREG       ;If BREG < 80H, BREG is loaded
                                                        ;into WREGLO and 00 is loaded
                                                        ;into WREGHI.
                                                        ;Else OFFH is loaded into WREGHI.
4187    27 FE           THERE:  SJMP    THERE           ;Loop here.
```

In part (A) above, WREG (60H) is loaded with FFFF. LDBZE then zero extends the byte AA into the word 00AA and places it in WREG, replacing FFFF. Execute from 4170. Query WO 60. You should find 00AA there.

In part (B) above, WREG (60) is loaded with 5555. LDBSE then sign extends the contents of BREG and places the resulting word into WREG. We attempted 3 cases:

1. At run tme enter BY 70 = 7F for BREG (MSB=0). Execute from 4180. Examine WO 60 and find 007F. BREG in this case was a signed positive number.
2. ESC. Enter BY 70 = 80 (MSB=1 in BREG). Execute from 4180. Examine WO 60 and find FF80. BREG in this case was a signed negative number.
3. ESC. Enter BY 70 = 0AA (MSB=1 in BREG). Execute and find

WO 60 = FFAA as expected since BREG was a signed negative number.

EXPERIMENT 3-13

USING THE RST INSTRUCTION

```
        40 00         REG1    EQU     40H
        50 00         REG2    EQU     50H
        60 00         REG3    EQU     60H
        70 00         REG4    EQU     70H
        0F 00         P1      EQU     0FH              ;LEDs
                      ;
                      ;
418A                          ORG     418AH
                      ;
418A    A1 A0 00 18           LD      SP,#00A0H        ;Initialize SP to 00A0H.
418E    94 50 40              XORB    REG1,REG2        ;Exclusive OR BYTES REG2 with REG1.
4191    B0 40 0F              LDB     P1,REG1          ;Output result to LEDs.
4194    28 0A                 SCALL   TIME             ;Hold output on LEDs for several
                                                       ;seconds.
4196    B1 FF 0F              LDB     P1,#0FFH         ;Output 0FFH to LEDs.
4199    27 FE         HERE:   SJMP    HERE             ;Loop here.
                      ;
                      ;
41A0                          ORG     41A0H
                      ;
41A0    B1 10 60      TIME:   LDB     REG3,#10H        ;Load BYTE REG3 with 10H.
41A3    A1 FF FF 70   LOAD:   LD      REG4,#0FFFFH     ;Load WORD REG4 with 0FFFFH.
41A7    05 70         MORE:   DEC     REG4             ;Decrement REG4.
41A9    D7 FC                 JNE     MORE             ;If REG4 != 0, then keep looping.
41AB    E0 60 F5              DJNZ    REG3,LOAD        ;Else decrement REG3 and test.
                                                       ;If REG3 != 0, then goto LOAD.
41AE    F0                    RET                      ;Else return.
```

In the above program at 418A we attempt to have an output at P1's LEDs displayed for about 3 seconds and then change to FF as a result of the LDB P1, #0FF instruction. We use the XORB instruction on registers REG1 (40H) and REG2 (50H), whose values are entered at run-time. The result of XORB remains in REG1 and is then output to P1's LEDs before SCALL to TIME causes a 3 sec delay. The RET to LDB P1, #0FF changes the output to FF and it stays that way. Afterwards, we'll replace LDB P1, #0FF by 0FF (RST) and 0FD,0FD (two NOPs).

If you try the following cases you should find the results described:

1. Enter BY 40 = 80 and BY 50 = 01. XORB gives 81 and you should see 81 at P1 for 3 seconds before P1 changes to 0FF when you execute from 418A.
2. ESC and enter BY 40 = 80, BY 50 = 80. XORB gives 00 and that's what you'll see for 3 seconds, then FF, upon execution.
3. ESC. Enter BY 40 = 0FF, BY 50 = 0FF. Results should be exactly as in (2) above.
4. Finally, after ESC, try BY 40 = 0FF, BY 50 = 01. Execute and observe FE at P1 for 3 seconds, then FF.

After finishing the above, change the instruction LDB P1, #0FF to RST by entering BY 4196 = 0FF, 0FD, 0FD which is machine code for RST (Reset System: 0FF), followed by two NOPs (0FD). RST sets PSW to 0 and initializes PC to 2080. All registers and SFRs are set to their reset status (see chapter 1, section 0). In particular, P1 should show up as FF after RST is executed (executing RST causes a pulse to appear on the reset pin of the 8096). When we executed this modified program, with BY 40 = 80 and BY 50 = 01, entered before running, we found, as before, 81 appear at P1's LEDs for about 3 seconds, followed by FF. Thus the RST instruction indeed resets port P1 to FF as indicated in section 0 of chapter 1 (or p. 2-23 section 2.15.2 of Microcontroller Handbook 1985).

EXPERIMENT 3-14

USING THE EXTB, EXT, NEGB, NOTB AND NEG INSTRUCTIONS.

The programs for all 5 parts of this experiment (A, B, C, D, E) are shown below.

```
        30 00      WREG    EQU   30H
        40 00      REG1    EQU   40H
        50 00      IREG    EQU   50H
        60 00      REG     EQU   60H
        90 00      WREG1   EQU   90H
        A0 00      WREG2   EQU   0A0H
        0E 00      P0      EQU   0EH             ;Switches.
        0F 00      P1      EQU   0FH             ;LEDs.
                   ;
                   ;       EXPT. EX3-14.
                   ;
                   ;       PART A) EXTB Instr.
                   ;
                   ;
4200                       ORG   4200H
                   ;
4200    A0 40 30           LD    WREG,REG1       ;Load contents of REG1 into WREG.
4203    16 30              EXTB  WREG            ;Sign extend low order BYTE of
                                                 ;operand into high order BYTE.
4205    27 FE      HERE:   SJMP  HERE            ;Loop here.
                   ;
                   ;
                   ;       EXPT. EX3-14.
                   ;
                   ;       PART B) EXT Instr.
                   ;
                   ;
4210                       ORG   4210H
                   ;
4210    06 50              EXT   IREG            ;Sign extend the low order WORD of
                                                 ;operand into the high order WORD
                                                 ;of operand.
4212    27 FE      THERE:  SJMP  THERE           ;Loop here.
```

```
                        ;       EXPT. EX3-14.
                        ;
                        ;       PART C) NEGB Instr.
                        ;
4220                            ORG     4220H
                        ;
4220   B0 0E 60         BEGIN:  LDB     REG,P0          ;Load REG with value of switch.
4223   13 60                    NEGB    REG             ;Two's complement REG
4225   B0 60 0F                 LDB     P1,REG          ;Output result to LEDs.
4228   27 F6                    SJMP    BEGIN           ;Poll the switches.
                        ;
                        ;
                        ;       EXPT. EX3-14.
                        ;
                        ;       PART D) NOTB Instr.
                        ;
                        ;
4230                            ORG     4230H
                        ;
4230   B0 0E 60         START:  LDB     REG,P0          ;Load REG with value of switch.
4233   12 60                    NOTB    REG             ;One's Complement REG
4235   B0 60 0F                 LDB     P1,REG          ;Output result to LEDs.
4238   27 F6                    SJMP    START           ;Poll the switches.
                        ;
                        ;
                        ;       EXPT. EX3-14.
                        ;
                        ;       PART E) NEG Instr.
                        ;
4240                            ORG     4240H
                        ;
4240   A0 A0 90                 LD      WREG1,WREG2     ;Load contents of WREG2 into WREG1.
4243   03 90                    NEG     WREG1           ;Two's Complement WREG1
4245   27 FE            STOP:   SJMP    STOP            ;Loop here.
```

In part (A), at 4200, we investigate EXTB (sign extend short integer into integer). EXTB takes the low order byte of a 16-bit (word) register and sign extends it into its high order byte. If MSB of low order byte is 0, then 00 is placed in high byte of the word, else FF is placed there. The flags affected are Z and N; C and V both are reset to 0. At run time enter WO 40 = 0AAAA where 40 is REG1. The instruction at 4200 loads this into WREG (30H). The low byte of WREG is now AA (N=1) so that after EXTB WREG, WREG should contain FFAA. Execute from 4200, then query WO 40 and observe FFAA. Enter PSW to examine the flags. We found 5000, so flags were 01010000 i.e. Z=0, N=1, V=0, VT=1 (from a previous experiment), C=0, I=0, ST=0. This is consistent with what we'd expect. ESC and enter WO 40 = 0AA70. Since MSB of low byte is 0 we'd expect to find 0070 in WREG after execution. We did find that WO 30 gave 0070. Examination of the PSW after execution showed 1000, so that the flags were 00010000 i.e. Z=0, N=0 (as expected), V=C=0, and VT=1 from previously (it's a "trap" all right). VT and ST are not affected.

In part (B) at 4210, we work with the EXT instruction (sign extend integer into long integer). An "integer" is 16 bits long (word) while "long integer" is 32 bits long (double word) and is designated by IREG (here 50H). The effect of EXT is to sign extend the low order WORD of the double word operand IREG into the high order WORD of IREG. If MSB of low word is 0 then 0000 is placed in the high word, else FFFF is. EXT resets C and V to 0. As we'll see, it always sets Z to 1 and never sets N. Before executing, enter WO 50 = 7000 and WO 52 = 0FFFF (i.e. 32-bit double word FFFF7000 at IREG 50). Also enter PSW = 0. Execute from 4210. Then inspect WO 50 (we found 7000) and WO 52 (we found 0000), in keeping with the fact that MSB of 7000 is 0, so that the result in IREG should be 00007000. Examine PSW. We found PSW = 8000 i.e. flags = 10000000 indicating Z=1, N=0, V=C=0, VT=0 (remember, we now STARTED with PSW=0). Redo with WO 50 = 0AAAA, WO 52 = 0000. Since MSB of low order word is 1, FFFF should extend into the high order word. Executing and examining WO 50 gave AAAA, while WO 52 showed FFFF, as expected. PSW showed up as 8000 again i.e. Z=1, N=0, V=C=VT=0. Then ESC and enter PSW = 2800 (flags = 00101000). Execute and examine PSW. We found 8000, so flags became 10000000 (Z=1, V and C became 0, N stayed at 0). ESC and enter PSW = 6800 (flags = 01101000). Execute and examine PSW again. We again found PSW = 8000 so Z became 1, N became 0, V and C became 0. EVIDENTLY, EXT NEVER SETS THE N FLAG AND ALWAYS SETS THE Z FLAG. EXTB, ON THE OTHER HAND, AFFECTS THE Z AND N FLAGS IN THE NORMAL MANNER. BOTH CLEAR THE C AND V FLAGS. VT AND ST ARE NOT AFFECTED. We understand this has now been fixed.

In part (C) above, at 4220, we employ NEGB which negates a short integer (8-bit) operand in two's complement fashion. In the program we load REG (60) with the switch byte at P0, negate it with NEGB, output it from REG to P1's LEDs and then jump back to poll P0 again. Execute from 4220. Set the switches for AA. Observe 01010110 at P1's LEDs. This is in keeping with the two's complement which complements and adds 1 i.e. 10101010 becomes 01010101 + 1 = 01010110. On the fly change the switches to 55. You should see 10101010 + 1 = 10101011. Then try P0 = FF. You'll see 00 + 1 = 01. Finally, set P0 to 00. You'll see FF + 1 = 00.

In part (D) above, at 4230, we again load P0's switch byte into

REG, perform a NOTB on REG (which is a straight one's complement of the byte) and output the result to P1's LEDs. The program then jumps back to poll P0 again. Executing from 4230, vary the switches and observe the complement at P1 in every case. NOT works exactly as NOTB did here, except it complements a word.

In part (E) at 4240, we come back to NEG, this time negating a 16-bit integer in two's complement. In this program WREG1 and WREG2 are defined as internal file registers 90H and 0A0H, respectively. If, therefore, at run time we enter WO 0A0 = some value, and then execute, we should find the negated value in WREG1 (90H). Enter WO 0A0 = 0000. Execute from 4240. Examine WO 90. Find 0000, as it should be. ESC. Enter WO 0A0 = FFFF. Execute. Examine WO 90 and find 0001. ESC. Enter WO 0A0 = AAAA. Execute. Examine WO 90. Observe 5556 there. Finally, ESC and enter WO 0A0 = 5555. Execute. WO 90 should reveal AAAB.

EXPERIMENT 3-15

THE NORML INSTRUCTION

NORML (normalize long integer) shifts a 32-bit "long integer" IREG as many times to the left until its MSB is 1. If it is still 0 after 31 shifts, the shifting stops and the Z flag is set to 1. The carry flag is cleared since the previous shift left just before the first 1 appeared in MSB must have shifted a 0 into C. The N flag will be indeterminate after the operation. The number of shifts actually performed before MSB becomes 1 is stored in the second operand BREG. NORML is very useful in floating point arithmetic as chapter 7 will demonstrate. The program starts at 4248 and is shown below.

```
      30 00          IREG    EQU     30H
      40 00          BREG    EQU     40H
                     ;
                     ;
4248                         ORG     4248H
                     ;
4248  0F 40 30               NORML   IREG,BREG       ;IREG (32 bits) is shifted left
                                                     ;until its most sig. bit is a
                                                     ;1.  BREG will contain the number
                                                     ;of shifts required.
424B  27 FE          HERE:   SJMP    HERE            ;Loop here.
```

IREG is here register address 30 (actually registers 33, 32, 31, 30 for the four bytes of IREG), and BREG is here register 40. Enter WO 32 = 0000 and WO 30 = 4000, so our IREG double word is 00004000. Execute from 4248. Enter BYTE 40 and find its contents to be 11 (17 shifts were made before MSB became 1, as we'd expect). Enter WO 32 and then WO 30 and find 8000 and 0000, respectively, as expected. Query PSW. We found PSW = 1000 indicating flags = 00010000 i.e. Z=0, N=0, VT=1 (hanging in from our previous experiment).

ESC and re-do the experiment with WO 32 and WO 30 entered first as 0000 and 0000, respectively. After execution query BYTE 40 and find 1F i.e. 31 shifts were made, a 1 was not found. Enter WO 32 and WO 30 and find, as expected, 0 in both words. Now enter PSW. We found PSW = 9000 showing flags to be 10010000 i.e. Z=1 (expected) and N=0.

Finally, ESC and enter WO 30 = 2000, then WO 3200 = 0000. We would expect 18 shifts before 80000000 is reached in IREG. Execute. Enter BYTE 40 and find 12 (18 shifts). Then query WO 32 and WO 30 and find 8000, 0000, respectively. Query PSW. We found PSW = 1000 or 00010000 for the flags (Z=0, N=0). THUS N IS NOT NECESSARILY SET TO 1 BUT Z ACTS AS WE'D EXPECT. V, VT, AND ST FLAGS ARE NOT AFFECTED.

EXPERIMENT 3-16

THREE OPERAND INSTRUCTIONS WITH THE 8096

A powerful feature of the 8096 instruction set is the availability of 3-operand versions of the ADD, ADDB, AND, ANDB, MUL, MULB, SUB, SUBB, MULU, and MULUB instructions. This allows, for example, the addition or ANDing of two source words (or bytes), with the result deposited in a third, distinct word or byte destination. The contents of both sources remain intact. This spares us the trouble and software overhead of storing into another location the second source that normally might be the destination of the result, and then having to retrieve from that location the stored source for future use. We've actually made use of three-operand versions of the ADDB and ADD instructions previously in this chapter. An example employing three-operand instructions is given again in the program below at 4250.

```
        50 00         REG1    EQU     50H
        60 00         REG2    EQU     60H
        70 00         REG3    EQU     70H
        80 00         REG4    EQU     80H
                      ;
                      ;
4250                          ORG     4250H
                      ;
4250    A1 AA AA 50           LD      REG1,#0AAAAH      ;Load REG1 with 0AAAAH.
4254    A1 55 55 60           LD      REG2,#5555H       ;Load REG2 with 5555H.
4258    44 50 60 70           ADD     REG3,REG2,REG1    ;ADD REG1 to REG2 and put
                                                        ;the result into REG3.
425C    40 50 60 80           AND     REG4,REG2,REG1    ;AND REG1 with REG2 and put
                                                        ;the result into REG4.
4260    27 FE         HERE:   SJMP    HERE              ;Loop here.
```

In the above program REG1 and REG2 are first added, with result stored in REG3. The same unchanged values of REG1 and REG2 are then ANDed, with the result stored in REG4. No intermediate steps to store REG2 elsewhere were needed.

Execute (G FR 4250). Now query WO 70 (REG3) and find FFFF, as expected. Enter WO 80 (REG4) and observe 0000, as anticipated. Now enter WO 50 (REG1), then WO 60 (REG2) and find their original values intact: AAAA and 5555, respectively.

EXPERIMENT 3-17

EXAMPLE OF A MULTIPLY INSTRUCTION

We shall give a brief example of the use of one of the 8 multiply instructions with the 8096. Other forms of the multiply instructions will be treated in more detail when employed in the applications in chapters 9 and 10.

The example we've chosen below is the MUL instruction in three-operand form in which the second and third integer operands (here WREG1 and WREG2 which are 16-bit signed quantitites) are multiplied and the 32-bit signed result is stored in the destination operand (here IREG). The program at 4270 is shown below.

```
        30 00          IREG     EQU     30H
        40 00          WREG1    EQU     40H
        50 00          WREG2    EQU     50H
                       ;
4270                            ORG     4270H
                       ;
4270    FE 4C 50 40 30          MUL     IREG,WREG1,WREG2        ;Multiply the signed 16
                                                                ;bit word registers WREG1
                                                                ;and WREG2.
4275    27 FE          HERE:    SJMP    HERE                    ;Loop here.  32 bit signed
                                                                ;result is in IREG.
```

As the first of two examples, we shall multiply the words 0040 (in WREG1) and 0400 (in WREG2). Enter WO 40 = 0040 and WO 50 = 0400. Execute from 4270. Then query IREG at WO 30 and WO 32. We found WO 32 = 0001, WO 30 = 0000. Thus IREG = 00010000 which equals the decimal number 65,536; equal, of course, to 64 x 1024 (the decimal values of 0040 and 0400, respectively).

As a second example, ESC and enter WO 40 = 0400 and WO 50 = 0400. We'd expect a decimal result of 1024 x 1024 = 1,048,576. Execute the program again. Query IREG. We found WO 32 = 0010, WO 30 = 0000, so that IREG = 00100000, which equals decimal number 1,048,576, as it should. Try other cases.

EXPERIMENT 3-18

EXAMPLE OF A DIVIDE INSTRUCTION

We've chosen the DIV form of the four divide instructions with the 8096 for illustration purposes. Others will be treated in the applications in chapters 9 and 10.

The DIV instruction divides the signed 32-bit long integer that resides in a destination register (here IREG) by the contents of the 16-bit signed integer that resides in the source (here WREG). The quotient of the signed result is to be found in the low order word of IREG and the remainder resides in the high order word of IREG. The program is shown below at 4280.

```
          30 00        IREG     EQU     30H
          40 00        WREG     EQU     40H
                       ;
4280                            ORG     4280H
                       ;
4280      FE 8C 40 30           DIV     IREG,WREG     ;Divide 32 bit integer in IREG
                                                      ;by 16 bit integer in WREG.
                                                      ;(Signed arithmetic)
4284      27 FE        DONE:    SJMP    DONE          ;Loop here.  IREG contains result.
                       ;
4286                            END
```

As the first of two examples, we'll divide HEX 00020040 (placed in IREG: WO 32 and WO 30) by 0100 (placed in WREG: WO 40). If you work this out, you'll find that the expected result should be decimal 512 with a remainder of 64. Thus we'd expect to find 0200 in WO 30 and 0040 in WO 32. Enter WO 30 = 0040, WO 32 = 0002, and WO 40 = 0100. Execute from 4280 and confirm that WO 30 contains 0200 (512 dec.), and WO 32 contains 0040 (64 dec.).

ESC. Enter WO 30 = 0000, WO 32 = 0100, so that IREG contains 01000000 (= 16e6). Enter WO 40 = 1000 (= 16e3). If IREG is divided by WREG we should find 16e6/16e3 = 16e3 = 4096 = 00001000 in IREG. Thus only a quotient 4096 = 1000 and no remainder should be found in IREG. Execute from 4280. Query IREG. We found WO 32 = 0000 (no remainder) and WO 30 = 1000 = 16e3 (quotient), as expected.

This concludes chapter 3. Having covered the material in this chapter and the experiments in chapter 2, we should now be in an excellent position to move ahead into the chapters that follow. There we shall come to grips with the 8096. We'll study its interrupt system (chapter 4); its SFRs (chapter 5); its timers, its HSO/HSI high speed units, and PWM, A/D facilities (chapter 6); its arithmetic and Serial I/O capabilities (chapters 7, 8). We'll cover a broad range of applications (chapter 9) and then converse with the 8096 using several Intel development tools (chapter 10).

CHAPTER 4

THE 8096 INTERRUPT SYSTEM

INTRODUCTION

In following the discussion, it is suggested that you keep before you Fig. 2-11, p. 2-9 in the Microcontroller Handbook (1985) (also found in chapter 1, section E of this book).

The 8096 has a powerful and intricate interrupt system, as the 10 experiments in this chapter will demonstrate. There are eight interrupt vectors and six of them, in turn, can have two or more sources of their own, depending on which bits are manipulated in which SFRs, for a total of 24 interrupt sources.

The 8096 interrupts and their sources can be divided into two broad vector categories: 2 external and 6 internal. These two classes of interrupts obey the same general rules and exhibit the same general features. That being so, we feel the best approach to gaining a solid understanding and mastery of the 8096 interrupt system is to start with the EXTERNAL INTERRUPTS. Working with them allows us to be in a better position "to make things happen" through the use of switches as sources of the EXTINT or ACH.7 or HSI.0 external interrupts. Once having studied the external interrupts by means of the experiments in this chapter, our understanding of the 6 INTERNAL INTERRUPTS will be immediately apparent, as the same rules and features hold for them as for the external interrupts. We'll then be in an excellent position to work with external AND internal interrupts in Chapters 5 and 6, and beyond.

Working with the external interrupts in this chapter will, of necessity, bring us into contact with certain Special Function Registers even before the detailed study of all of them (except Serial I/O SFRs - reserved for Chapter 8) is made in the 25 experiments of Chapter 5. The SFRs needed in this chapter are 08H (Interrupt Mask Register), 09H (Interrupts Pending Register), and 16H (IOC1 : I/O Control Register 1, where bit 1 must be set or reset to choose between EXTINT and ACH.7 sources). The PSW (not an SFR) plays a role thru its bit PSW.9 (I : Global Interrupt Enable). It must be set to 1 (through an EI instruction) as a necessary (but not sufficient) condition for interrupts to be honored, or reset to 0 (through a DI instruction) as a sufficient condition to ignore interrupt requests (making them pending instead). The SFRs and PSW mentioned above are certainly also needed when working with the internal interrupt sources later on, but then, in addition, as Fig. 2-11 of the Microcontroller Handbook shows, other SFRs come into play in order to select or query the source of the internal interrupt and either to enable or disable it [i.e. SFRs IOS1 (16H), SP - STAT (11H), HSO - COMMAND (06H), and IOC1 (16H)]. That will all be gone into in Chapter 5 where ALL the SFRs (except Serial I/O reserved for ch. 8) and internal interrupts are treated in detail.

A number of 8096 interrupt "theorems" are enunciated and illustrated in the first four experiments of this chapter. They form the basis of 8096 external and internal interrupt control and behavior. An understanding of them, and how to apply them, is essential for mastery of the 8096 interrupt system. These "theorems" (A, B, C, and D) are stated and demonstrated in Expts. 4-1, 4-2, 4-3, and 4-4.

Please remember that SFR "Interrupt Mask Register" (08H) and SFR "Interrupts Pending Register" (09H) can each be read or written to, and have identical bit pattern layouts with respect to the 8 various interrupt sources as shown:

7	6	5	4	3	2	1	0
EXTINT (or ACH.7)	SERIAL PORT	SOFTWARE TIMERS	HSI.0	HSO	HSI	A/D CONV.	TIMER OVERFLOW

A study of Fig. 2-12 p. 2-10 Microcontroller Handbook (1985) (also available in ch. 1, section E in this book) is essential at this point for all that follows. It shows that A 0 TO 1 EDGE TRANSITION AT ANY OF THE ABOVE SOURCES CREATES A PENDING INTERRUPT, SETTING THE CORRESPONDING BIT IN THE "INTERRUPT PENDING" SFR (09H) REGARDLESS OF WHETHER THE GLOBAL BIT (PSW.9) WAS SET BY SOFTWARE OR WHETHER THE CORRESPONDING BIT IN THE "INTERRUPT MASK" SFR WAS SET BY SOFTWARE. The pending interrupt(s) will be serviced only when, and if, the corresponding Int. Mask bit is set to 1 (programmably) AND when, and if, PSW.9 is set to 1 (programmably); otherwise it remains just that - a pending interrupt.

Thus three conditions are necessary for interrupt servicing: a pending must have been created at the source (setting the corresponding bit in 09H) by means of a either 0 to 1 edge transition (or by setting the pending bit to 1 by software); the corresponding mask bit in 08H must be set to 1, and PSW.9 must be set to 1. The pending will "wait" if the other two conditions are not in force before being serviced - and those two can come into being at the discretion of the programmer at any time he/she chooses in the program, before or after the onset of a pending. The pending(s) can ALSO be created by SOFTWARE as opposed to a 0 to 1 hardware transition at the source, simply by writing a 1(s) out to the desired source bit(s) in 09H. This can be very useful in testing out interrupt systems before any hardware circuitry is interfaced, as one of the experiments in this chapter will demonstrate. Similarly, a pending interrupt can be removed BEFORE servicing by clearing its bit in 09 by software. However, as we shall see in Expt. 4-2, when a pending does get serviced, it is no longer pending - its bit in 09H is AUTOMATICALLY cleared.

Once the three conditions have been met for interrupt servicing (pending bit = interrupt mask bit = global bit = 1), Fig. 2-12 in the Microcontroller Handbook indicates that a priority encoder examines which interrupt sources have entered the contest for servicing. Thus, for example, it may be that several different sources have pendings, their Int. Mask bits have been set to 1 by software, but PSW.9 (global) is 0 (DI). The moment that the software makes PSW.9 = 1 (i.e. EI) those pendings all enter the servicing contest. The priority encoder will service them in the order of priority i.e. 7 (EXTINT) would be serviced first if it were pending, and 0 (Timer Overflow) last. That is accomplished by the priority encoder's outputs feeding in to the Interrupt Generator in Fig. 2-12 in the order in which those outputs are set by the encoder: 7 down to 0, with only those in the game that satisfied the three conditions discussed above. Upon return from the chosen source's service routine to the main program, the next lower priority (still pending) gets serviced, and so on.

The interrupt generator in Fig. 2-12 causes vectoring to the chosen source's Interrupt Vector Location assigned to it. Those vector locations are given in Fig. 2-10, p. 2-8 Microcontroller Handbook (1985), or section E, ch. 1 this book. Each location can accommodate a WORD which the user can insert there at program time. That WORD is the address specified by user at which the actual Interrupt Service Routine (ISR) is to be written. Thus there is a double vectoring: first to the location in Fig. 2-10 and from there to the address specified at that location by user. The interrupt vector location table is repeated here (7 to 0 priority ordering):

7	EXTINT/ACH.7	200E
6	Serial Port	200C
5	Software Timers	200A
4	HSI.0	2008
3	HSO	2006
2	HSI	2004
1	A/D Complete	2002
0	Timer Overflow	2000

We again stress that we'll work only with external interrupts EXTINT, ACH.7, and HSI.0 in this chapter and will cover all the others, except the Serial Port's, in chapter 5. Serial Port interrupts will be covered in chapter 8.

TO REITERATE

A PENDING INTERRUPT (CREATED EITHER BY A HARDWARE 0 TO 1 TRANSITION AT THE INTERRUPT SOURCE OR BY A SOFTWARE WRITE OF A 1 TO THE RELEVANT BIT IN THE INTERRUPT PENDING REGISTER) WILL BE SERVICED ONLY WHEN THE CORRESPONDING INTERRUPT MASK REGISTER AND PSW.9 (GLOBAL) BITS ARE BOTH 1. THE PENDING BIT IS CLEARED UPON ENTERING THE SERVICE ROUTINE, BUT THE INTERRUPT MASK BIT AND THE PSW.9 GLOBAL BIT ARE NOT. THE RETURN TO MAIN PROGRAM FINDS THAT SOURCE'S PENDING CLEARED BUT THE INTERRUPT MASK BIT AND GLOBAL STILL SET. REMEMBER, ALSO, SETTING A BIT IN THE INTERRUPT MASK REGISTER UNMASKS THAT INTERRUPT SOURCE.

Experiments 4-1, 4-2, and 4-3 that follow prove all the above.

NOTE ON NOTATION

ISR will always denote "Interrupt Service Routine" and != is used to represent "not equal to". MINT and PINT stand for the Interrupt Mask and Interrupt Pending registers, respectively. INVEC denotes the address in the INterrupt VECtor location table to which the interrupt vectors. H.R. stands for "Holding Register", INT stands for "Interrupt", HSO and HSI stand for "High Speed Output" and "High Speed Input" units, respectively.

EXPERIMENT 4-1

THEOREM (A): A PENDING INTERRUPT WILL BE CREATED BY A 0 TO 1 TRANSITION AT THE INTERRUPT SOURCE EVEN IF THE CORRESPONDING INTERRUPT MASK AND/OR GLOBAL ENABLE BITS ARE 0.

We shall now demonstrate that even if the pertinent interrupt mask bit in SFR 08 is not set and/or PSW.9 global bit is 0 (due to a DI instruction), a pending interrupt will be created (as evidenced by the relevant bit in pending SFR 09 having been set) if the interrupt source presents a 0 to 1 transition. We'll demonstrate this for the EXTINT, ACH.7, and HSI.0 external interrupt pins by reading the corresponding bits in the interrupt pending register 09 after the 0 to 1 transition occurs.

The program at 3000 is shown below. In it, after the SP is set to 00C0, IOC1 is loaded with the contents of address 5000 (00 or 02 entered at run time) in order to select ACH.7 (02) or EXTINT (00) as the source of interrupt line #7 (EXTINT). CLRB PINT clears all pendings in the pending register, should any exist for whatever reason. LDB MINT loads the interrupt mask 08 with the contents of address 5001 (entered at run-time) to set or clear any desired interrupt source mask bit (setting it unmasks that interrupt line). The NOP will be modified at run-time to allow us to insert EI or DI there, as we wish. LDB P1, PINT will allow us to view at P1's LEDs exactly which, if any, pendings were created when 0 to 1 transitions were made at any of the external interrupt lines EXTINT, ACH.7, HSI.0. The loop at SJMP continually polls PINT (Pending Interrupt Register 09).

```
      16 00          IOC1   EQU   16H
      09 00          PINT   EQU   09H
      08 00          MINT   EQU   08H
      0F 00          P1     EQU   0FH              ;LEDs.
      18 00          SP     EQU   18H
                     ;
                     ;
3000                        ORG   3000H
                     ;
3000  A1 C0 00 18           LD    SP,#00C0H        ;Initialize SP with 00C0H.
3004  B3 01 00 50 16        LDB   IOC1,5000H[0]    ;Load IOC1 control register with the
                                                   ;contents of memory location 5000H
                                                   ;(Select either ACH7 or EXTINT)
```

```
3009  11 09                 CLRB  PINT           ;Clear the pending interrupt register.
300B  B3 01 01 50 08        LDB   MINT,5001H[0]  ;Load interrupt mask register (MINT)
                                                 ;with the contents of memory location
                                                 ;5001H.
3010  FD                    NOP                  ;This will be modified at runtime.
3011  B0 09 0F       HERE:  LDB   P1,PINT        ;Output contents of pending register
                                                 ;(PINT) to LEDs.
3014  27 FB                 SJMP  HERE           ;Loop back to poll and display contents
                                                 ;of PINT register.
```

PROCEDURE

We treat the following cases (use only debounced switches as sources of EXTINT, ACH.7, and HSI.0 interrupts. See fig. 2-2, chapter 2):

CASE 1. At run time, enter BY 5000 = 00 to select EXTINT over ACH.7. Enter also BY 5001 = 00 to disable all sources of interrupts as far as the mask register (08) is concerned. Finally, replace NOP by entering BY 3010 = 0FA (DI: disable global bit PSW.9). Execute the program from 3000 and create two 0 to 1 transitions on HSI.0 and EXTINT in that order. You should observe 10, then 90, appear in that order at the LEDs. Two pendings, first HSI.0, then EXTINT, were created and are indicated by corresponding set bits in the pending register 09 - even though PSW.9 = 0 and their mask bits 4 and 7 were not set in the Interrupt Mask Register 08. They become candidates for future servicing (see Expt. 4-2).

CASE 2. ESC and enter BY 5000 = 02, thereby selecting ACH.7 as the source of EXTINT. Execute and create ACH.7 and then HSI.0 0 to 1 interrupts in that order. You'll see 80, then 90, on the LEDs. ACH.7 and HSI.0 became pending interrupts even though I (PSW.9) ≠ 0 and bits 4 and 7 in SFR 08 are 0.

CASE 3. ESC. Replace FA at 3010 with FB (BY 3010 = 0FB) so that EI replaces DI there. Now PSW.9 = I = 1. Execute and create ACH.7 and HSI.0 leading edge interrupts in that order. You'll again see 80 followed by 90. ACH.7 and HSI.0 pendings were created.

CASE 4. ESC. Replace FB at 3010 with FA (DI again); enter BY 5000 = 00 (EXTINT), BY 5001 = 90 (to enable the EXTINT and HSI.0 source lines in the interrupt mask register). Execute. Create edge transitions at EXTINT and HSI.0. Again observe 80, then 90, appear at the LEDs. EXTINT and HSI.0 pendings were created.

CONCLUSION

Pending interrupts will be created in the pending interrupt register, 09, whenever a 0 to 1 transition at an interrupt source occurs, even if that source's mask bit in the Interrupt Mask Register 08 is not set and/or the global bit PSW.9 = 0.

NOTE

16-bit Timer T1 is free running. It increments every 2 usec and thus should overflow every 65,536 x 2 usec. = 131 msec. If it is enabled into the internal TIMER OVERFLOW (TOV) interrupt source (see Fig. 2-11, p. 2-9 Microcontroller Handbook or section E chapter 1, this book), then it should constantly be causing TOV pendings (see Fig. 2-12, p. 2-10 Microcontroller Handbook or section E chapter 1 this book). In that case a query of bit 0 in SFR 09 (Interrupt Pending Register) should show a 1 there as that bit gives the pending status of TOV interrupt requests. Now Fig. 2-29, p. 2-21 (or chapter 1, section L this book) indicates that the two sources for possible TOV (Timer 1 and Timer 2) can be enabled or disabled together or separately by writing to control register IOC1 (16H). IOC1.2 (1 or 0) enables or disables T1's overflow interrupt and IOC1.3 (1 or 0) enables or disables T2's overflow interrupt. Hence, on power-up, if we clear all pendings by entering BY 09 = 00, and then DISABLE T1 and T2 overflow interrupts into the TOV interrupt source by entering BY 16 = 00, a subsequent query of SFR 09 should STILL reveal 00 (enter BY 09 to confirm this). If you next enter BY 16 = 08 ENABLING T2's overflow interrupt and then query BY 09, you'll find 00 STILL there (T2 is not free running, it's an event counter). Now enter BY 16 = 04 ENABLING T1's overflow interrupt. Query BY 09. You should NOW find BY 09 = 01 indicating a TOV pending from T1 overflow (bit 0 = 1). The above discussion is not related to the fact that if you queried IOS1 (16H) at power-up by entering BY 16, you'd find 20 there i.e. bit 5 = 1, indicating Timer 1 has overflowed. That may or may not cause T1 overflow interrupts into TOV depending on whether the T1 source for Timer Overflow interrupts was enabled or not i.e. IOC1.2 = 1 or 0, respectively. Regardless, IOS1.5 will ALWAYS be 1 because free running T1 always produces Timer 1 OVERFLOW.

EXPERIMENT 4-2

THEOREM (B): A 0 TO 1 TRANSITION AT AN INTERRUPT SOURCE WILL BE SERVICED ONLY WHEN 3 CONDITIONS CO-EXIST: ITS PENDING EXISTS IN 09, ITS MASK BIT IS SET IN 08, AND THE GLOBAL BIT PSW.9 IS SET. FURTHER, THE PENDING (BIT) IS CLEARED AS SOON AS THE INTERRUPT SERVICE ROUTINE IS ENTERED, BUT THE PSW.9 AND INTERRUPT MASK BITS ARE NOT AFFECTED.

A corollary to the above theorem is that if the pending was made and then cleared (by software) BEFORE the other two conditions are met, the pending interrupt will not be serviced. The theorem and its corollary will be demonstrated in this experiment for the EXTINT source first, then again for the HSI.0 source. They hold for ANY of the 8096's eight interrupt sources. The program at 3020 is shown below.

```
        16 00           IOC1    EQU     16H
        18 00           SP      EQU     18H
        09 00           PINT    EQU     09H
        08 00           MINT    EQU     08H
        0F 00           P1      EQU     0FH             ;LEDs.
        0E 20           INVEC1  EQU     200EH
        08 20           INVEC2  EQU     2008H
        50 00           TEMP    EQU     50H
                        ;
                        ;
3020                            ORG     3020H
                        ;
3020    A1 C0 00 18             LD      SP,#00C0H       ;Initialize SP register to 00C0H.
3024    A1 60 30 50             LD      TEMP,#3060H     ;Load interrupt vector table with
3028    C3 01 0E 20 50          ST      TEMP,INVEC1[0]  ;address of EXTINT service routine.
302D    A1 70 30 50             LD      TEMP,#3070H     ;Load interrupt vector table with
3031    C3 01 08 20 50          ST      TEMP,INVEC2[0]  ;address of HSI0 service routine.
3036    B3 01 00 50 16          LDB     IOC1,5000H[0]   ;Load IOC1 with the contents of
                                                        ;memory location 5000H.
                                                        ;(Selects ACH7 or EXTINT)
303B    11 09                   CLRB    PINT            ;Clear pending interrupt reg. (PINT).
303D    B3 01 01 50 08          LDB     MINT,5001H[0]   ;Load byte at 5001 into interrupt
                                                        ;mask register (MINT).
3042    FD                      NOP                     ;This will be modified at runtime.
3043    B1 FF 0F                LDB     P1,#0FFH        ;Output 0FFH to LEDs.
3046    EF B7 CF                CALL    TIME            ;Call 5 second time delay routine.
3049    FD                      NOP                     ;This will be modified at runtime.
304A    B1 AA 0F                LDB     P1,#0AAH        ;Output 0AAH to the LEDs.
304D    27 FE           THERE:  SJMP    THERE           ;Loop here.
```

```
3060                        ORG     3060H
                    ;
                    ; EXTINT SERVICE ROUTINE:
                    ;
3060  B1 0F 0F      EXTINT: LDB     P1,#0FH       ;Output 0FH to LEDs.
3063  EF 9A CF              CALL    TIME          ;Delay of 5 seconds
3066  B0 09 0F              LDB     P1,PINT       ;Output status of pendings to LEDs.
3069  27 FE         HALT:   SJMP    HALT          ;Loop here.


3070                        ORG     3070H
                    ;
                    ; HSI.0 SERVICE ROUTINE:
                    ;
3070  B1 F0 0F      HSIO:   LDB     P1,#0F0H      ;Output 0F0H to LEDs.
3073  EF 8A CF              CALL    TIME          ;Delay 5 seconds.
3076  B0 09 0F              LDB     P1,PINT       ;Output status of pendings to LEDs.
3079  27 FE         ENUF:   SJMP    ENUF          ;Loop here.



                    ;       TIME DELAY - This subroutine is used throughout the
                    ;                    remainder of the chapter.
                    ;
                            .GLOBAL TIME
                            .GLOBAL TREG1
                            .GLOBAL TREG2
                    ;
                    ;
      90 00         TREG1   EQU     90H
      A0 00         TREG2   EQU     A0H
                    ;
                    ;
3050                        ORG     3050H
                    ;
3050  B1 1A 90      TIME:   LDB     TREG1,#1AH    ;Load TREG1 (outer loop) with 1AH.
3053  A1 FF FF A0   TLOAD:  LD      TREG2,#0FFFFH ;Load TREG2 (inner loop) with 0FFFFH.
3057  05 A0         TMORE:  DEC     TREG2         ;Decrement inner loop by 1.
3059  D7 FC                 JNE     TMORE         ;If TREG2 != 0 then keep looping.
305B  E0 90 F5              DJNZ    TREG1,TLOAD   ;Else if TREG1 != 0 go back to reload
                                                  ;inner loop counter.
305E  F0                    RET                   ;Else return.
```

Let's first analyze the program. We have written EXTINT and HSI.0 interrupt service routines at 3060 and 3070, respectively. This requires loading 3060 into the interrupt vector table at 200E (INVEC 1) and 3070 into the same table at 2008 (INVEC 2). Remember 200E and 2008 are the vector entry addresses associated with the EXTINT and HSI.0 interrupt sources. This is accomplished via TEMP register 50H in the 2nd, 3rd, 4th, and 5th lines of code. LDB IOC1 again permits choosing either EXTINT or ACH.7, depending on the byte entered in 5000 at run-time. CLRB PINT is needed to avoid an undesired interrupt that could result from a possible pending still residing in 09 (created in a previous experiment). LDB MINT sets or clears desired interrupt mask bits in 08, as determined by the byte entered in 5001 at run-time. The NOP at 3042 will be changed at run-time to either FA (DI) or FB (EI). The main activity is the outputting of FF at P1's LEDs for about 5 seconds (see the time delay at TIME, 3050, previously analyzed in Expt. 3-6; it's now 5 sec. as a result of loading 1AH in TREG1). The return from TIME to 304A results in FF changing to AA at P1, staying that way forever, UNLESS an interrupt was serviced. The NOP at 3049 will either remain that way or be changed at run-time to FA (DI) or FB (EI). SJMP THERE represents "other tasks".

If an interrupt is serviced (which it will be if the three conditions of Theorem (B) are met, as we'll see) then, depending on whether the source was EXTINT or HSI.0, we are vectored to 3060 or 3070 via 200E and 2008, respectively. In the former case (3060) 0F is outputted to the LEDs for 5 sec. to signal that we are in the EXTINT routine. We then poll PINT to query whether EXTINT's pending still exists after its ISR was entered. The LEDs will reveal PINT. The EXTINT ISR then ends at HALT (no return). If HSI.0 was the interrupt source, the routine at 3070 outputs F0 to the LEDs for 5 sec. to signal that we are in the HSI.0 routine. We again query PINT to see if HSI.0's pending still exists after its ISR was entered, as revealed at the LEDs. HSI.0's ISR ends at ENUF (no return). The two NOPs at 3042, 3049 will give us the flexibility at run-time to examine the various different possibilities needed to establish the theorem. Again, we use debounced switches at EXTINT and HSI.0 sources.

PROCEDURE

CASE 1: Enter BY 5000 = 00 to select EXTINT rather than ACH.7 as the external source. Enter BY 5001 = 00. This will disable all interrupt lines in the mask register on program execution. Enter BY 3042 = 0FB (global enable), leaving the NOP (0FD) at 3049 as is. Execute (G FR 3020). While the LEDs are all on at P1, and before 5 seconds elapse, create an EXTINT edge transition with a debounced switch. It will not be serviced, as evidenced by the LEDs changing to AA after 5 sec. and remaining that way. Examine BYTE 09 and observe 80 i.e. an EXTINT pending was created, but not serviced because Int. Mask bit #7 was not set by software. Examine PSW. We found PSW.9 = I = 1 and MINT.7 = 0.

CASE 2: ESC and enter BY 5001 = 80H. This will set EXTINT's mask bit in MINT when execution occurs. Leave 0FB and 0FD at 3042 and 3049 from case (1). Execute and create an edge transition at EXTINT, by means of the debounced switch, before 5 secs. are up and while the LEDs still display FF. The LEDs IMMEDIATELY change to 0F for 5 secs. and then change to 00. EXTINT was immediately serviced (0F) because the switch transition created a pending, and PSW.9 (I) and MINT.7 were ALREADY both set to 1 by the software. The fact that the LEDs changed to 00 proves that no pending exists at PINT.7 (the EXTINT ISR at 3060 displays PINT at port P1). Enter PSW. We found PSW.9 was still 1 and MINT.7 was also still 1. ESC and enter BY 5000 = 02 to select ACH.7. Execute and create a 0 to 1 transition at the ACH.7 EXTINT source. Repeat all the above steps and verify all the previous results. Verify that BYTE 09 = 00 after execution, i.e. the pending bit at ACH.7 was cleared.

CASE 3: ESC. Enter BY 5000 = 00 to select EXTINT again. BY 5001 is still 80. Enter BY 3042 = 0FA (DI) and BY 3049 = 0FB (EI). Execute and create an edge transition at EXTINT early on during the 5 secs. that FF shows. FF REMAINS till 5 sec. are over, THEN 0F shows for 5 sec. (EXTINT routine) and then changes to 00 indicating the EXTINT pending, made early, was cleared upon entry into the ISR. A pending was created, but not serviced, till all three conditions were met (MINT bit set, PINT bit set, I bit set). That did not happen till the EI (0FB) was executed at 3049 (actually not till the instruction at 304A was executed - see Expt. 4-4). A query of PSW will reveal that PSW.9 (I) and MINT.7 are still 1. BYTE 09 will indicate the pending bit was cleared (already confirmed at the LEDs).

CASE 4: Repeat case (3), but now create the EXTINT interrupt AFTER 5 sec. of FF i.e. at any time that AA is displayed at the LEDs. Since FB is in force at 3049, you'll observe immediate servicing of the interrupt: AA changes to 0F for 5 sec., then to 00.

CASE 5: Repeat cases (2) and (3) above with BY 5001 = 10, thereby enabling the HSI.0 interrupt source. Thus with FB (EI) at 3042 and FD (NOP) at 3049, execute and this time create an HSI.0 interrupt during the 5 seconds that FF is displayed at the LEDs. FF will immediately change to F0 (HSI.0 ISR) for 5 sec. and then to 00 (the HSI.0 pending was cleared). Enter PSW and confirm that I and MINT.4 (HSI.0 interrupt mask bit) are both still 1. Querying BYTE 09 confirms independently that the HSI.0 pending was removed. If, now, you ESC and change FB at 3042 to FA (DI) and FD at 3049 to FB (EI) and execute again, you'll find that an HSI.0 interrupt, made during the time that P1 shows FF, will not be immediately serviced. It WILL be when 5 seconds are over. Then F0 will be displayed for 5 sec. (HSI.0 ISR) and then change to 00 (pending cleared). PSW will reveal that PSW.0(I) and MINT.4 are both still set.

CASE 6: ESC and enter BY 5001 = 00, BY 3042 = 0FB, BY 3049 = 0FB. Execute. Create an HSI.0 interrupt during the first 5 sec. It will never by serviced. FF changes to AA and stays that way. 00 in 5001 caused all mask bits in MINT to be cleared. The 3 conditions for an interrupt were never met. Examining PSW reveals PSW.9 = 1 and MINT.4 = 0. Entering BYTE 09 should disclose 10 i.e. an HSI.0 pending was created, but since it was never serviced it never cleared.

CASE 7: ESC. Enter BY 5000 = 00, selecting EXTINT; BY 5001 = 80, to set MINT.7 to 1 (enabling EXTINT source), and BY 3042 = 0FA (DI). Starting at 3049, modify the program as follows: enter BY 3049 = 11, 09, 0FB, 11, 0F, 27, FE. 11 09 is machine code for CLRB PINT, FB for EI, 11 0F for CLRB P1, and 27 FE for SJMP THERE. What we are attempting to do here is to show that if a pending interrupt is created (at EXTINT here), and then cleared BEFORE all three conditions for servicing are met, it will not be serviced when the other two conditions are met. This is the corollary to the theorem stated in the opening paragraph to this experiment. To verify it, simply execute this modified program from 3020. Create an EXTINT early during the 5 sec. that FF shows at the LEDs. FF expires at the end of 5 sec., and because the pending created by EXTINT was cleared by CLRB PINT at 3049 BEFORE the EI global enable at 304B, we will not succeed in servicing the EXTINT ISR at 3060. 0F will NOT be displayed. Instead, the main program continues on and, because of CLRB P1 now at 304C, 00 is displayed at the LEDs. If, however, you ESC, enter NOPs (0FD) at 3049, 304A instead of the previous CLRB PINT, and then execute, you'll find that an EXTINT made early during the time that FF is displayed will be serviced after 5 sec. of FF. 0F will come on for 5 sec. followed by 00, indicating servicing at 3060 and automatic clearing of the pending in the ISR. This time EI at 304B causes all 3 conditions to be satisfied and the pending (not cleared at 3049) gets serviced.

CONCLUSION

A 0 to 1 edge triggered interrupt creates a pending interrupt and will be serviced only if and when the global bit I (PSW.9) and its corresponding bit in the interrupt mask register are both 1. It remains pending till those conditions are met. When serviced, the pending is cleared (its bit becomes 0 in the interrupt pending register) but PSW.9 and the mask bit remain set, unless cleared by software. If the pending is created, but then cleared by software (e.g. CLRB PINT) before the mask and global bit conditions are met, it will not be serviced even when the other 2 conditions are eventually met.

IMPORTANT NOTE

The initializations in our main program involved, among other things, the storing of #3060 at the EXTINT vector table location 200E and #3070 at the HSI.0 vector table location 2008. They thus become the addresses of the EXTINT and HSI.0 ISRs. In practise it would not be done that way since the ISR addresses would be programmed into the vector interrupt location table in ROM. To be philosophically consistent, we should have entered WO 200E = 3060 and WO 2008 = 3070 at LOAD TIME, rather than have our program do that. The reason we have done it in the program is to save the reader the steps of having to enter those addresses in the vector table at load time. We have followed the same procedure in all the experiments in the book involving ISR addresses. We repeat: this is not the way it would be done in practise. In fact, the whole RAM area 2000H to 5FFFH on the iSBE-96 is specifically referred to as ROMSIM. That area simulates a ROM.

EXPERIMENT 4-3

THEOREM (C): SOFTWARE INTERRUPTS CAN BE CREATED BY WRITING A 1(S) TO THE RELEVANT BIT(S) IN THE INTERRUPT PENDING REGISTER. THEY ARE SERVICED ONLY IF THE PENDING BIT, THE INTERRUPT MASK BIT, AND THE GLOBAL BIT ARE ALL SET. THE PENDING GETS CLEARED WHEN THE ISR IS ENTERED BUT PSW.9 AND THE INTERRUPT MASK BIT REMAIN SET.

The ability to create software interrupts by WRITING 1s to the pertinent pending bits in the interrupt pending SFR at 09 can be very useful in simulating hardware interrupts. This can allow one to test whether the software and ISRs are acting properly without the necessity of creating the hardware interrupt circuitry until later in the development cycle. These software created interrupts at any of the 8 interrupt sources obey the same rules of Theorem (B) that were demonstrated in Expt. 4-2, as we'll see. Only now the interrupt is not due to a 0 to 1 hardware transition at the source, but rather simply to the existence of a 1 WRITTEN to the relevant bit of SFR 09 by the programmer. The program at 3080 is given below.

```
16 00          IOC1    EQU   16H
09 00          PINT    EQU   09H
08 00          MINT    EQU   08H
0F 00          P1      EQU   0FH              ;LEDs.
0E 20          INVEC1  EQU   200EH
08 20          INVEC2  EQU   2008H
50 00          TEMP    EQU   50H
```

```
3080   A1 C0 00 18                 LD     SP,#00C0H        ;Initialize SP register to 00C0H.
3084   A1 B0 30 50                 LD     TEMP,#30B0H      ;Load interrupt vector table with
3088   C3 01 0E 20 50              ST     TEMP,INVEC1[0]   ;address of EXTINT service routine.
308D   A1 C0 30 50                 LD     TEMP,#30C0H      ;Load interrupt vector table with
3091   C3 01 08 20 50              ST     TEMP,INVEC2[0]   ;address of HSIO service routine.
3096   B1 00 16                    LDB    IOC1,#00         ;Load IOC1 with 00 to select
                                                           ;EXTINT (external interrupt).
3099   11 09                       CLRB   PINT             ;Clear pending interrupt reg. (PINT).
309B   B3 01 01 50 08              LDB    MINT,5001H[0]    ;Load byte at 5001 into interrupt
                                                           ;mask register (MINT).
30A0   FD                          NOP                     ;This will be modified at runtime.
30A1   B3 01 02 50 09              LDB    PINT,5002H[0]    ;Load PINT reg with contents of
                                                           ;memory location 5002H.
30A6   B1 FF 0F                    LDB    P1,#0FFH         ;Output 0FFH to LEDs.
30A9   EF 54 CF                    CALL   TIME             ;Call 5 second time delay routine.
30AC   FD                          NOP                     ;This will be modified at runtime.
30AD   27 FE             NOMOR:    SJMP   NOMOR            ;Loop here.
                         ;
                         ;
                         ;
30B0                               ORG    30B0H
                         ;
                         ; EXTINT SERVICE ROUTINE:
                         ;
30B0   B1 33 0F          EXTINT:   LDB    P1,#33H          ;Output 33H to LEDs.
30B3   EF 4A CF                    CALL   TIME             ;Delay of 5 seconds
30B6   B0 09 0F                    LDB    P1,PINT          ;Output status of pendings to LEDs.
30B9   27 FE             STOP:     SJMP   STOP             ;Loop here.


30C0                               ORG    30C0H
                         ;
                         ; HSI.0 SERVICE ROUTINE:
                         ;
30C0   B1 CC 0F          HSIO:     LDB    P1,#0CCH         ;Output 0CCH to LEDs.
30C3   EF 3A CF                    CALL   TIME             ;Delay 5 seconds.
30C6   B0 09 0F                    LDB    P1,PINT          ;Output status of pendings to LEDs.
30C9   27 FE             FINI:     SJMP   FINI             ;Loop here.
                         ;
30CB                               END
```

In the above program we again work with the EXTINT and HSI.0 interrupts. They'll now be created by writing 1s to bits 7 or 4 in the pending register 09. The first 5 lines of code correspond exactly to their counterparts in Expt. 4-2 except that the EXTINT software - induced ISR is written at 30B0 and the HSI.0 ISR is written at 30C0. These ISRs are exactly the same as their counterparts at 3060 and 3070 in Expt. 4-2, except EXTINT ISR outputs 33 to the LEDs for 5 sec. before changing to 00 (result of outputting PINT to P1) and HSI.0 ISR outputs CC to the LEDs for 5 sec. before changing to 00. Whereas the main program in Expt. 4-2 turned on all LEDs at P1 for 5 sec. and then changed them to AA (unless an ISR was serviced), the main program here simply turns on all LEDs at P1 and keeps them all on (unless an ISR is serviced).

The setting of pending interrupt bits by software is accomplished at address 30A1 where LDB PINT, 5002H[0] loads SFR 09 with the byte entered at 5002 at run-time. Notice, also, that we do not here employ the instruction LDB IOC1, 5000H[0] to choose between EXTINT and ACH.7, but rather LDB IOC1, #00 to select EXTINT. But even this is meaningless and not necessary since we shall be creating an "EXTINT" (or "ACH.7") interrupt, not by hardware, but by software (by writing a 1 to PINT.7) to simulate EITHER EXTINT or ACH.7 hardware interrupts. The time delay (TIME) is the same as in Expt. 4-2 and is still at 3050. SJMP NOMOR represents "other tasks".

PROCEDURE

CASE 1: Enter BY 5001 = 80H (to unmask the EXTINT source line i.e. MINT.7 = 1), BY 5002 = 80 (to create an EXTINT software interrupt by setting PINT.7 = 1), and BY 30A0 = 0FB (EI). Leave the NOP (0FD) at 30AC. Execute from 3080. Since all three conditions (pending, global and interrupt mask bits all set) are met at 30A1, you should observe 33 appear at the LEDs "as soon as" execution starts, remain that way for 5 sec. followed by 00, indicating the pending bit was cleared. FF at the LEDs (instruction at 30A6) never had a chance. Enter PSW. You'll confirm that PSW.9 and MINT.7 are still 1. Enter BY 09 to re-affirm that the pending bit was cleared at PINT.7 when the ISR was entered. Servicing was immediate.

CASE 2: ESC and enter BY 30A0 = 0FA (DI) and BY 30AC = 0FB (EI). Execute and observe FF for 5 sec. at P1s LEDs, then 33 there for 5 sec., and then 00. Servicing was delayed till all three conditions were met at 30AC. Enter PSW and BY 09 to confirm that PSW.9 = MINT.7 = 1 and PINT.7 = 0.

CASE 3: Repeat case (2) with BY 30AC = 0FA (DI). This time FF appears at the LEDs when the program is executed, and does not change. There was no servicing. The 3 conditions were never met. This time PSW will reveal PSW.9 = 0 and MINT.7 = 1 while BY 09 will show that PINT.7 = 1 (the pending is still there since the ISR was not entered).

CASE 4: ESC and enter BY 30A0 = 0FB (EI), BY 30AC = 0FB (EI) and BY 5001 = 00 (all interrupt sources kept masked). Execute. FF comes on at P1 and stays on. There is no interrupt servicing. All three conditions for servicing were not met. PSW shows PSW.9 = 1 and MINT.7 = 0, while BY 09 shows PINT.7 still is 1 (it was not cleared since the EXTINT ISR was not entered).

CASE 5: ESC. This time enter BY 5001 = 10 (to set MINT.4 enabling the HSI.0 interrupt source), BY 5002 = 10 (setting PINT.4 for an HSI.0 interrupt possibility), BY 30A0 = 0FB (EI), BY 30AC = 0FA (DI). Execute and observe CC at P1's LEDs appear immediately. After 5 sec. CC changes to 00 (showing that the pending in PINT was automatically cleared). PSW reveals PSW.9 = 1, MINT.4 = 1, and BY 09 shows PINT.4 = 0. Servicing was immediate because PSW.9 = 1, PINT.4 = 1, MINT.4 = 1 were all satisfied at 30A1 in the program.

CASE 6: ESC. Enter BY 30A0 = 0FA (DI) and BY 30AC = 0FB (EI). Execute and observe FF at P1 appear for 5 sec. (the interrupt has become pending till EI at 30AC is executed), then change to CC for 5 sec (HSI.0 ISR was entered AFTER 30AC when all 3 conditions were met), and then change to 00 (indicating PINT.4 = 0 after servicing of HSI.0). PSW reveals MINT.4 = 1, PSW.9 = 1 while BY 09 shows PINT to be 00.

CASE 7: ESC. Enter BY 30AC = 0FA (DI). Execute and see FF at P1 remain that way. No ISR servicing occurs. PSW shows PSW.9 = 0 and MINT.4 = 1; BY 09 reveals PINT.4 = 1 (pending still there, it was not serviced).

CASE 8: ESC. Enter BY 30A0 = 0FB, BY 30AC = 0FB, BY 5001 = 00 (mask bits all 0). Execution will again result in FF appearing at P1. P1 remains at FF. No ISR service occurred as mask bit 4 in MINT was not set to 1. PSW reveals PSW.9 = 1 and MINT.4 = 0. BY 09 shows 10 (PINT.4 is still 1, as it was not serviced).

CONCLUSION

Software interrupts can be created by writing 1(s) to the appropriate bit(s) in the Pending Interrupt Register (SFR 09). They will be serviced only when and if PSW.9 and the corresponding Int. Mask bit(s) in SFR 08 are all 1. On entering the ISR, the pending bit is automatically reset to 0 but the interrupt mask and PSW.9 bits remain set.

NOTE

In the ISR subroutines of Expts. 4-2 and 4-3 we did not bother to end the ISRs with returns (RET) as is, of course, generally required in any real problem or application. They were ended, instead, on self loops ("halts"), since we were in all cases only interested in: 1. did we get to the ISR for servicing? 2. were the pendings that were created automatically cleared when the ISR was entered? and 3. were the PSW.9(I) and Interrupt Mask Register (08) bits still set after ISR servicing?

In the more realistic interrupt experiments, starting with Expt. 4-5, that is changed. There we ARE interested in the ISR returning to the main program at the point where mainline activity was interrupted, so that it can be resumed from that point after the ISR is serviced. Further interrupts to the same or other ISRs are then possible in the main program, and the ISRs will always return there. Or one ISR can interrupt another ISR and the return will carry us back to the original ISR.

There is still much to investigate concerning 8096 interrupts. Expts. 4-4 through 4-10 continue that study.

EXPERIMENT 4-4

THEOREM (D): THE GLOBAL ENABLE (EI) INSTRUCTION KEEPS ALL INTERRUPTS INHIBITED TILL AFTER THE INSTRUCTION FOLLOWING IT HAS BEEN EXECUTED.

What the above means is simply this: EI does not go into effect till the instruction following it has been executed. This fact can be very important to the success of the interrupt software and must always be taken into account when creating programs dealing with interrupts. The same statement can be made with regard to the DI, POPF, PUSHF, and signed multiply and divide instructions, as well as the TRAP (software trap) instruction (of no concern to us in this book). They all inhibit an interrupt from being executed till after the following instruction has been executed.

One important consequence of this, as we shall see in one of the experiments later on in this chapter, is that a POPF (pops flags and interrupt mask byte back into PSW), follwed by RET (the two instructions that are usually the last ones in an ISR), GUARANTEES that the RET will be executed back to the main program BEFORE further interrupts can occur. If any are pending they will be serviced AFTER the return back to the main program (since the Interrupt Mask Register's unmasked i.e. set bit and I are restored by the POPF). This can be very important in that, if it were not the case, a pending interrupt could be serviced after the POPF instruction, but before the return, and this would leave the return address to the main program still on the stack. This could result in stack overflow if interrupts were occurring at a high rate.

We shall demonstrate the theorem only for the EI instruction and leave it to you to confirm it for the other instructions cited above. The program at 30D0 is presented below.

```
18 00        SP       EQU    18H
0E 00        P0       EQU    0EH
0F 00        P1       EQU    0FH
16 00        IOC1     EQU    16H
08 00        MINT     EQU    08H
09 00        PINT     EQU    09H
0E 20        INVEC1   EQU    200EH
50 00        TEMP     EQU    50H
```

```
30D0                          ORG    30D0H
                        ;
30D0   A1 C0 00 18            LD     SP,#00C0H        ;Initialize SP to 00C0H.
30D4   11 0F                  CLRB   P1               ;Clear LEDs on P1
30D6   FA                     DI                      ;Disable global interrupt bit PSW.9.
30D7   11 09                  CLRB   PINT             ;Clear pending interrupts.
30D9   A1 F6 30 50            LD     TEMP,#30F6H      ;Load TEMP with address of ACH7 intr.
                                                      ;service routine. (30F6H)
30DD   C3 01 0E 20 50         ST     TEMP,INVEC1[0]   ;Store address in VECTOR INT table at
                                                      ;200EH.
30E2   B1 02 16               LDB    IOC1,#02H        ;Load 02 into IOC1 to select ACH7.
30E5   B1 80 08               LDB    MINT,#80H        ;Set bit 7 of Interrupt Mask reg. to
                                                      ;enable ACH7 interrupt.
30E8   30 0E FD         POLL: JBC    P0,0,POLL        ;If P0.0 (switch S0) = 0, then loop
                                                      ;here.
30EB   FD                     NOP                     ;This will be modified at runtime.
30EC   B1 FF 0F               LDB    P1,#0FFH         ;Output 0FFH to LEDs.
30EF   B1 AA 0F               LDB    P1,#0AAH         ;Output 0AAH to LEDs.
30F2   27 FE            HERE: SJMP   HERE             ;Loop here.
                        ;
                        ;
30F6                          ORG    30F6H
                        ;
                        ;
                        ;  ACH.7 SERVICE ROUTINE:
                        ;
30F6   27 FE            STOP: SJMP   STOP             ;Loop here.
                        ;
30F8                          END
```

In the above program we shall select the ACH.7 source of EXTINT, which the instruction LDB IOCI, #02 accomplishes. The ISR service routine is at 30F6. That is specified by the 5th and 6th lines of code (via INVEC1 = 200E in the vector interrupt table). Port 1's LEDs are cleared early on in the program, interrupts are disabled globally in the 3rd line of code, any pendings are cleared in the next line, and MINT.7 is set to 1 in the 8th line to unmask the EXTINT source. The next line polls bit 0 of port P0 where 8 switches are located. As long as switch S0 at that port is low, the JBC loops on itself. When S0 is thrown high program flow falls through to the NOP which in one case we'll leave as is and in another case change to EI. After the

NOP are two instructions: one outputs FF to the LEDs at P1 and the very next one outputs AA to P1. The last instruction in the main program is a "halt", or can represent "other tasks". Finally, the ISR at 30F6 for servicing the ACH.7 interrupt is simply a "halt" (SJMP STOP).

PROCEDURE

1. With the NOP at 30EB as is and switch S0 low, execute (G FR 30D0). Observe LEDs = 00. Create an ACH.7 interrupt from a debounced switch. Then throw S0 from low to high to low. Observe AA at the LEDs. Since the system was globally disabled, the pending ACH.7 never got serviced and FF was output to P1 and immediately followed by AA. AA remains. An EI is needed for servicing.
2. ESC. Replace the NOP with EI by entering BY 30EB = 0FB. Execute. LEDs = 00. Again create an ACH.7 interrupt. Throw S0 from low to high to low. This time you'll observe FF on the LEDs, not AA, nor 00. This proves that the pending got serviced, NOT after EI was executed, but after the NEXT instruction (LDB P1, 0FF) was executed, and that program flow immediately went to the ISR at 30F6, thereby permitting FF to remain on. Had the interrupt been serviced at the conclusion of the EI instruction, 00 would have remained on the display.

CONCLUSION

Execution of EI does not permit ISR servicing, even if a pending bit and the corresponding mask bit are set, until AFTER the instruction following the EI is executed.

PROBLEM

Write programs that will demonstrate the same feature (theorem D) as it applies to the execution of a DI or PUSHF or POPF instruction.

EXPERIMENT 4-5

IMMEDIATE OR PENDING SERVICING OF EXTINT AND HSI.0 INTERRUPTS. SUBROUTINE RETURNS. EITHER SOURCE CAN INTERRUPT THE OTHER. NESTING.

In this experiment the main program at 3100 (below) has pulse generators go on/off/on/off.... at port 1's LEDs with on-time = off-time = 5 sec. The time delay called is the routine TIME (5 sec.) at 3050 of Expt. 4-2. If an EXTINT interrupt is created, the EXTINT ISR outputs 0F at P1 for 5 sec. (either immediately, or EXTINT becomes a pending to be serviced later when 0F will then be output for 5 sec.). A RET at the end of the ISR returns to the main program and the pulse generators resume from exactly where they left off, finishing up the time remaining in the on or off part of the cycle where they were interrupted. The on/off cycles then continue normally. The same behavior will occur if the main program is interrupted by an HSI.0 edge transition, except the HSI.0 ISR outputs F0 (immediately, or later if it becomes a pending) for 5 sec. at port 1's LEDs, replacing the pulse generators there. The return from its ISR will cause the pulse generators to resume from the point at which they were interrupted in the on or off part of their cycle.

The important cases where EXTINT interrupts the HSI.0 ISR before the latter is finished, or vice-versa, are also examined, as is the case where one source interrupts the other a NUMBER OF TIMES before that other's ISR is finished up. Thus, this experiment examines the weaving in and out of the main program to and from the ISRs, and also from ISR to ISR, in an attempt to further solidify your understanding of 8096 interrupts.

Since the ISRs below call TIME, and the main program is also using TIME and will have been interrupted somewhere in TIME, it is important that the ISRs save the time delay registers (TREG1 and TREG2) which are being used by main program, before the ISR calls TIME for itself, and that the TREG1 and TREG2 saved values be restored after the ISR is done with TIME. In that way it can return to the main program and recommence execution of the main program from exactly the point in TIME where it was interrupted, thereby finishing up the remaining on or off-time. In that regard, it is also essential that the status of the LEDs at P1 (i.e. the on or off part of the pulse generator cycle) be saved at the beginning of each ISR routine, and that it be restored to P1 before returning to the main program. In that way the main program can resume with the same LED status it had at the time of interrupt and for the correct amount of remaining on or off-time in the cycle. These points explain the need for the LDB REG1, P1 (or LDB REG2, P1), the LDB P1, REG1 (or LDB P1, REG2), the PUSH TREG2, the LDB REG3, TREG1 (or LDB REG4, TREG1), the LDB TREG1, REG3 (or LDB TREG1, REG4), and the POP TREG2 instructions in the EXTINT and HSI.0 ISRs at 3130 and 3160 below.

As far as the main program (below) is concerned, the EXTINT and HSI.0 ISR addresses are set to 3130 and 3160, respectively, by loading those values into TEMP and then storing them at 200E and 2008 in the interrupt vector table (EXTINT and HSI.0 vector entry addresses). 00 is loaded into IOC1 in order to select EXTINT over ACH.7. 90 is loaded into MINT to set mask bits 7 and 4 (enabling the EXTINT and HSI.0 interrupt sources). CLRB PINT clears any pendings that might be left over from a previous experiment. The NOPs at 311E and 312B (as well as those in the ISRs at 3130 and 3160) will be modified at run-time so that the effects of DI or EI (or neither) there can be studied. (The NOPs at 3147 and 3177 will be modified at run-time as far as Expts. 4-7 and 4-9 are concerned, both of which use the program of this experiment.) We output EE to P1, call 5 sec. time, then output 00 to the LEDs, call the same 5 sec. time again, and then loop back by means of SJMP THERE to initiate another on/off cycle. The program at 3100 is shown below.

```
                        .EXTERNAL TIME
                        .EXTERNAL REG TREG1
                        .EXTERNAL REG TREG2

              ;
              ;
18 00         SP       EQU     18H
16 00         IOC1     EQU     16H
08 00         MINT     EQU     08H
09 00         PINT     EQU     09H
0F 00         P1       EQU     0FH
40 00         TEMP     EQU     40H
50 00         REG1     EQU     50H
60 00         REG2     EQU     60H
70 00         REG3     EQU     70H
80 00         REG4     EQU     80H
0E 20         INVEC1   EQU     200EH
08 20         INVEC2   EQU     2008H
```

```
3100                                ORG     3100H
                          ;
3100  A1 C0 00 18                  LD      SP,#00C0H        ;Initialize SP to 00C0H.
3104  A1 30 31 40                  LD      TEMP,#3130H      ;Load interrupt vector table with
3108  C3 01 0E 20 40               ST      TEMP,INVEC1[0]   ;the address of the EXTINT service
                                                            ;routine. (3130H)
310D  A1 60 31 40                  LD      TEMP,#3160H      ;Load interrupt vector table with
3111  C3 01 08 20 40               ST      TEMP,INVEC2[0]   ;the address of the HSI.0 service
                                                            ;routine. (3160H)
3116  B1 00 16                     LDB     IOC1,#00         ;Select EXTINT interrupt source.
3119  11 09                        CLRB    PINT             ;Clear all pending interrupts.
311B  B1 90 08                     LDB     MINT,#90H        ;Set EXTINT AND HSI.0 Mask bits.
311E  FD                           NOP                      ;This will be modified at runtime.
311F  B1 EE 0F            THERE:   LDB     P1,#0EEH         ;Output 0EEH to LEDs.
3122  EF DB CE                     CALL    TIME             ;Delay for 5 seconds.
3125  B1 00 0F                     LDB     P1,#00H          ;Turn LEDs off.
3128  EF D5 CE                     CALL    TIME             ;Delay for 5 seconds.
312B  FD                           NOP                      ;This will be modified at runtime.
312C  27 F1                        SJMP    THERE            ;Loop back to repeat.


                          ;        EXTINT SERVICE ROUTINE:
                          ;
3130                               ORG     3130H
                          ;
3130  FD                           NOP                      ;This will be modified at runtime.
3131  B0 0F 50                     LDB     REG1,P1          ;Save status of LEDs in REG1.
3134  C8 00                        PUSH    TREG2            ;Save previous value of time delay
                                                            ;WORD register TREG2.
3136  B0 00 70                     LDB     REG3,TREG1       ;Save previous value of time delay
                                                            ;BYTE register TREG1.
3139  B1 0F 0F                     LDB     P1,#0FH          ;Output 0FH to LEDs.
313C  EF C1 CE                     CALL    TIME             ;5 sec. delay.
313F  B0 70 00                     LDB     TREG1,REG3       ;Restore previous value of time delay
                                                            ;BYTE register TREG1.
3142  CC 00                        POP     TREG2            ;Restore previous value of time delay
                                                            ;WORD register TREG2.
3144  B0 50 0F                     LDB     P1,REG1          ;Restore status of LEDs.
3147  FD                           NOP                      ;This will be modified at runtime.
3148  F0                           RET                      ;Return to main routine.
```

```
                    ;       HSI.0 SERVICE ROUTINE:
                    ;
                    ;
3160                        ORG     3160H
                    ;
3160  FD                    NOP                 ;This will be modified at runtime.
3161  B0 0F 60              LDB     REG2,P1     ;Save status of LEDs in REG2.
3164  C8 00                 PUSH    TREG2       ;Save previous time delay WORD
                                                ;register TREG2.
3166  B0 00 80              LDB     REG4,TREG1  ;Save previous time delay BYTE
                                                ;register TREG1.
3169  B1 F0 0F              LDB     P1,#0F0H    ;Output 0F0H to LEDs.
316C  EF 91 CE              CALL    TIME        ;Call 5 second time delay.
316F  B0 80 00              LDB     TREG1,REG4  ;Restore previous value of time delay
                                                ;BYTE register TREG1.
3172  CC 00                 POP     TREG2       ;Restore previous value of time delay
                                                ;WORD register TREG2.
3174  B0 60 0F              LDB     P1,REG2     ;Restore orig. status of LEDs.
3177  FD                    NOP                 ;This will be modified at runtime.
3178  F0                    RET                 ;Return to main routine.
                    ;
                    ;
3179                        END
```

PROCEDURE

CASE 1: Enter BY 311E = 0FB (EI) and leave the NOP at 312B. Execute (G FR 3100) and allow several on/off cycles (EE, 00, EE, 00, etc. at port 1) go by. Create an EXTINT during one of the on-times (say 2 sec. into the on-time). It will be immediately serviced because of the EI at 311E and the 90 in MINT. EE changes to 0F at P1 for 5 sec. Then EE resumes for the remaining 3 sec. of on-time. The off/on/off.... cycles then resume. During one of the off-times create another EXTINT. Again there is immediate servicing with 0F coming on to replace 00 for 5 seconds. 00 then re-appears at P1 for the time remaining in its off part of the cycle (reckoned from the time at which the EXTINT occurred). Then the on/off/on.... cycles resume. Thus PSW.9 and MINT.7 both remained set after the first servicing of EXTINT ISR; the second EXTINT request created another pending, so that the 3 conditions were again satisfied and immediate servicing again took place.

CASE 1(a): Repeat Case (1) with BY 3130 = 0FA (DI). You'll observe that the first EXTINT gets immediate service (observe 0F for 5 seconds, then resumption of the on/off cycles at P1), but another EXTINT request during the on/off cycles is ignored. The DI at 3130 in the ISR disabled the global and the return to the SJMP THERE loop in the main program never re-enables it.

CASE 2: ESC. Put the NOP (0FD) back at 3130. Leave FB at 311E and NOP at 312B. Execute again and repeat case (1) with an HSI.0 interrupt request. HSI.0's ISR at 3160 is immediately entered as evidenced by F0 replacing EE, 00, EE, ... at P1. F0 holds for 5 sec. The EE/00 cycles then resume from the point at which interrupted, with whatever on or off-time remaining from that point being finished up first. Another HSI.0 interrupt will again be immediately serviced because PSW.9 and MINT.4 both remained set after the first HSI.0 ISR servicing.

CASE 2(a): ESC and enter BY 3160 = 0FA (DI). Repeat case (2). Execute. Create an HSI.0 interrupt. Servicing is immediate with F0 replacing the EE/00 ... cycles for 5 sec. The cycles then resume from the point where the interrupt occurred, first finishing up the on or off-time remaining. Another HSI.0 interrupt is not serviced because the DI, now at 3160, leaves PSW.9 = 0 when return to the main program is made.

CASE 3: ESC. Re-enter BY 3130 = 0FD (NOP) and BY 3160 = 0FD. Enter BY 311E = 0FA (DI) and BY 312B = 0FB (EI). Execute and create an EXTINT late during the on-time of the FIRST cycle. It does not get serviced till the off-cycle gets done (when the 3rd necessary condition, EI, comes into effect). At that time we see 0F for 5 sec. at P1, followed by the EE, 00, EE, 00, etc. on/off/on/off... cycles again. Another EXTINT request at any time is IMMEDIATELY serviced with 0F showing for 5 sec. followed by continuation of the on/off cycles FROM WHERE THEY WERE INTERRUPTED. Why? If you ESC and re-run, this time attempting an EXTINT during the SECOND cycle, it will be serviced immediately. Why? When you first ran this program (above) and created EXTINT late during the on-time of the first cycle, you found that it didn't get serviced till the off-cycle got done, and then the on/off cycles resumed after the ISR (0F) was serviced. YOU WERE THUS PROVING THAT THE RETURN FROM ISR IS ALWAYS TO WHERE THE INTERRUPT TOOK EFFECT (GOT SERVICED), NOT TO WHERE IT WAS CREATED (in our case to 311F - remember, the EI takes effect AFTER the instruction at 312C gets executed).

CASE 4: ESC and re-run. Repeat case (3) with HSI.0 being the source of the interrupt. All will repeat in every detail, except that the ISR is now at 3160, so instead of seeing 0F we see F0 at P1 for 5 sec. when the interrupt is serviced. Thus, an HSI.0 request during the on-time of the first cycle does not get serviced till the off-cycle is done. Then we see F0 for 5 sec. followed by EE/00/etc. on-off cycles again. Another HSI.0 at any time will be serviced immediately, followed by resumption of the on/off cycles of EE/00 from the point where the interrupt was made (i.e. finishing up any remaining on or off time first).

CASE 5(a): ESC and enter BY 311E = 0FB (EI), BY 312B = 0FD (NOP), with NOPs still at 3130 and 3160. Execute. After about 3 sec. of on-time (EE at P1), create an EXTINT request. See 0F at P1 immediately. After 3 sec. of 0F create an HSI.0 request. Immediately F0 is displayed at P1. After 5 sec. of F0, observe 0F come back at P1 to finish up its remaining 2 sec. Then EE re-appears at P1 to finish up its 2 sec. of on-time. Off/on/off cycles (00, EE, 00) then resume at P1. THIS NICELY ILLUSTRATES NESTING OF REQUESTS.

CASE 5(b): ESC and re-run. After 3 sec. of EE on-time, create EXTINT. See 0F. After 2 sec. of 0F create HSI.0. See F0. After 5 sec. of F0 see 0F. After 1 sec. of 0F create HSI.0. See F0 for 5 sec., then 0F. After another sec. of 0F create HSI.0 again. See F0. After 5 sec. of F0, see 0F re-appear for 1 sec. Then EE appear for its remaining 2 sec., then off/on/off ... (00, EE, 00, etc.) resume. A perfect example, again, of nesting - this time more complex.

CASE 5(c): After 3 sec. of off-time during the pulse generator's cycles, create an HSI.0 request. F0 immediately appears. After 2 sec. of F0, create an EXTINT request. 0F is immediately displayed. After 5 sec. of 0F note 3 more sec. of F0, then 2 sec. of off-time (00) (finishing up the off-time of the pulse generator's cycle), then a resumption of the EE/00 ... on/off cycles at P1.

CASE 5(d): ESC and re-run. After 3 sec. off-time, create an HSI.0 request. Observe F0. After 2 sec. of F0 create an EXTINT request. See 0F. After 5 sec. of 0F note F0 re-appear. After 1 sec. of F0 create EXTINT again. See 0F. After 5 sec. of 0F, F0 comes on again. After 1 more sec. of F0 create EXTINT. 0F again appears. After 5 sec. of 0F, see F0 come back to finish up the remaining 1 sec. left in its ISR, then note 00 appear at P1 for the 2 sec. re-
maining in its off-time, then the EE/00 on/off cycles resume.

CASE 6: ESC. Re-run. This time we'll try something more ambitious. After 3 sec. of on-time (EE) create an EXTINT request. See 0F. After 3 sec. of 0F, create an HSI.0 request. See F0. After 2 sec. of F0 create EXTINT. See 0F for 5 sec., then F0 for 3 sec., then 0F for 2 sec., then F0 for 2 sec.(!), then 00, EE, 00, EE again at P1. This is not what we'd like to see. We'd like NOT to see the last F0 for 2 sec. but, instead, to observe EE for 2 sec. (finishing up the original remaining on-time when EXTINT first occurred), then 00, EE, 00, etc. In this case REG1 and REG2, which are saving the status of P1 in the EXTINT and HSI.0 ISRs, respectively, get inter-twined after more than 2 nestings: the original EE saved in REG1 at the time of the first EXTINT request gets replaced by saving F0. A careful study of the two ISRs will reveal why this can come about when each source interrupts the other's ISR, and vice-versa, BEFORE either gets done. Now see the problem below.

PROBLEM

Re-write the ISRs so that you can create a number of interrupt nestings, whereby each source interrupts the other's ISR a number of times before the latter gets done, and vice-versa. The aim is that after a number of those interrupts are made back and forth, the history should cleanly unravel in the reverse sense. We want the times of the events remaining at the moments of interrupts to unfold and be realized one after the other till the original pulse generator comes back to finish up its on or off-time remaining before resuming the on/off cycles. Pushing and popping P1 on and off the stack in the ISRs (instead of saving in REG1 and REG2) should do it. Or will it? You can only push a WORD and P1 is at an odd address, 0F. Well, how about a PUSH P0 (P0 is input port 0E)? This will carry both P0 AND P1 on to the stack. Or will it? SFRs 0E and 0F are both BYTE read-able and write-able. You can only push a WORD, so that's out. We, therefore, fall back to loading P1 into an even register, pushing that register (as a word), popping it back later, and then loading the even register back into P1.

EXPERIMENT 4-6

MODIFYING THE STACK TO EFFECT A RETURN TO ANY DESIRED ADDRESS.

There are occasions in applications involving interrupt control where the return from ISR should carry us back to another location in the main program other than to the normal return address where the interrupt was originally acknowledged. An example might be a drilling operation where the drill bit, already embedded in the material, has its associated sensor send out an interrupt signal to indicate the drill bit is approaching a non-reliable state (too thin, weak, etc.) and the operation should halt and the bit be quickly replaced by another one ("automatically"). The interrupt routine would take care of the extraction and replacement, and possibly the discarding of the part in which drilling had already commenced. In that case, we'd want the RET at the end of the ISR to take us back to the main program where drilling a new part starts from the beginning, and not continue from where the old bit was embedded in its drilling cycle. Many other such examples in production-line type of electromechanical operations can be cited where the process has to be interrupted for one reason or another.

The problem can best be handled by loading the desired new return address on top of the stack in the ISR, before the RET, replacing the original return address stored there at the time the interrupt was made. The RET, always popping the top of the stack into the PC, will now guarantee a return to the new desired address in the main program.

The following program at 3190 illustrates the method. HSI.0 is the interrupt source in this experiment.

```
18 00     SP      EQU   18H
0E 00     P0      EQU   0EH
0F 00     P1      EQU   0FH
08 00     MINT    EQU   08H
09 00     PINT    EQU   09H
50 00     REG     EQU   50H
08 20     INVEC2  EQU   2008H
40 00     TEMP    EQU   40H
```

```
3190                              ORG    3190H
                         ;
3190  A1 C0 00 18        BEGIN:  LD     SP,#00C0H        ;Initialize SP to 00C0H.
3194  A1 C0 31 40                LD     TEMP,#31C0H      ;Load address of HSI.0 ISR into TEMP
3198  C3 01 08 20 40              ST     TEMP,INVEC2[0]   ;Store address into INT VECTOR table
                                                          ;at 2008H.
319D  11 09                       CLRB   PINT             ;Clear all pending interrupts.
319F  B1 10 08                    LDB    MINT,#10H        ;Set HSI.0 interrupt mask bit in INT
                                                          ;register.
31A2  FB                          EI                      ;Enable global interrupt PSW.9 bit.
31A3  B1 AA 0F           OLD:     LDB    P1,#0AAH         ;Output 0AAH to LEDs.
31A6  27 FB                       SJMP   OLD              ;Loop back to output to LEDs.
                         ;
                         ;
                         ;
                         ;        NEW  ROUTINE:
                         ;
31B0                              ORG    31B0H
                         ;
31B0  B1 55 0F           NEW:     LDB    P1,#55H          ;Output 55H to LEDs.
31B3  30 0E FA                    JBC    P0,0,NEW         ;If P0.0 = 0 , then continue looping on
                                                          ;output to LEDs.
31B6  27 D8                       SJMP   BEGIN            ;Else goto BEGIN.
                         ;
                         ;
                         ;        HSI.0 INTERRUPT SERVICE ROUTINE:
                         ;
31C0                              ORG    31C0H
                         ;
31C0  B1 FF 0F                    LDB    P1,#0FFH         ;Output 0FFH to LEDs.
31C3  37 0E FD           HERE:    JBC    P0,7,HERE        ;If P0.7 = 0, then continue looping on
                                                          ;output to LEDs.
31C6  A1 B0 31 50                 LD     REG,#31B0H       ;Else load new return address into REG.
31CA  C2 18 50                    ST     REG,[SP]         ;Store new return address onto top of
                                                          ;STACK.
31CD  F0                          RET                     ;Return to address on top of STACK
                                                          ;(31B0H).
                         ;
31CE                              END
```

In the main program above, SP is set to 00C0. The HSI.0 ISR address is placed at 31C0 by having TEMP loaded with 31C0 and then storing it at HSI.0's vector entry address 2008 (INVEC2). MINT.4 is set to 1 to enable the HSI.0 interrupt source;

pendings are cleared; PSW.9(I) is set to 1; and finally AA is output to the LEDs at P1. The SJMP OLD loop really simulates many "other tasks" that the microcontroller is engaged in - we simply represent them by the loop outputting a constant AA.

When an HSI.0 interrupt occurs during looping through "other tasks" at 31A3-31A6, we are vectored to the ISR at 31C0. There the "emergency operation" consists of outputting FF to the LEDs at P1. The "operator" is to throw switch S7 (P0.7) high to signal that the necessary "repairs" have been made (automatically or otherwise) and that the system is functioning. As long as S7 is low, JBC P0,7,HERE causes the ISR to stay "on hold". When S7 is thrown high REG is loaded with 31B0 which represents the new return address (label NEW). There, 55 is output to P1, rather than AA, which would have been the case with the normal return in the ISR (i.e. back to the SJMP OLD loop). To make that happen, we employ ST REG,[SP] which stores 31B0 (in REG) to the address pointed to by SP (indirect addressing). Since SP is pointing to SP-2 i.e. 00BE, at the time we enter ISR (the return address 31A3 or 31A6 was pushed on the stack when the interrupt was made), the ST instruction simply places 31 in 00BF and B0 in 00BE, replacing the old return address (remember, when a word is loaded into a location, low byte goes to lower even address and high byte goes to higher odd address). SP is still at 00BE. The RET pops this word 31B0 from top of the stack, to which SP is pointing, into the PC, effecting a return to 31B0 (NEW) rather than to somewhere in OLD.

At 31B0 55 is output to P1. We keep it that way by the use of the JBC P0,0,NEW instruction which polls switch S0 at P0.0. As long as it is low we loop back to NEW. When S0 is thrown high we fall through to SJMP BEGIN where the jump to BEGIN results in AA being output to P1 again ("other tasks") until another interrupt comes along.

Observe that, had we used NOPs at addresses 31C6 - 31CC in the ISR, the return would have been the normal one to 31A3 - A6 in the main program and AA would have resulted at P1 instead of 55.

All the above are confirmed as we go through the procedure described below.

PROCEDURE

CASE 1: With the switch byte at P0 set to 00, execute (G FR 3190). Observe AA at LEDs. Create an HSI.0 interrupt. Observe FF at P1 replace AA. Throw S7 at P0.7 high/low. FF at the LEDs changes to 55 indicating we returned to NEW instead of OLD. Now throw S0 at P0.0

high/low and observe AA again at the LEDs - we are back into the main program.

CASE 2: ESC and enter BY 31C6 TO 31CC = 0FD, thereby replacing the LD and ST instructions in the ISR with NOPs. Now the top of the stack will retain the original return address (either 31A3 or 31A6). Execute. See AA at P1. Create an HSI.0 interrupt and observe FF there. Throw S7 high at P0.7. This time you'll see AA again at P1. 31B0 (NEW) is bypassed as RET pops either 31A3 or 31A6 back into the PC. 55 is not seen.

NOTE

We could have used the LD REG, 5000H[0] instruction at 31C6 instead of the present one there. Then, before executing, we'd enter WO 5000 = desired return address. This would allow for greater flexibility. The above instruction is 5 bytes long so the ST and RET instructions would now be at 31CB and 31CE, respectively.

EXPERIMENT 4-7

THE ORDER OF SERVICING OF SEVERAL HARDWARE EDGE-TRANSITION CREATED PENDING INTERRUPTS. THE 8096 PRIORITY STRUCTURE.

The program for this experiment is the same one as for Expt. 4-5 at 3100. You are advised to consult that program as we discuss it in what follows.

We wish to examine the order in which pending interrupts get serviced after interrupts have been created (in any order). They will become pending till EI in the program occurs, at which point the 3 necessary conditions for servicing are satisfied. In other words, we wish to confirm the 8096 priority structure: EXTINT (7) highest, down to TIMER OVERFLOW (0) lowest - see Fig. 2-12 p. 2-10 and Fig. 2-10 p. 2-8 Microcontroller Handbook (1985) or ch. 1 section E in this book.

Not only that, but we wish to investigate the important case where the ISR is "unprotected". That is, there is no DI at the beginning of the ISR, so that anothr pending of LOWER priority can interrupt the higher priority's ISR and "seemingly" get serviced "first" before the RET at the end of its ISR allows the higher priority to continue its servicing. This will not contradict or negate the priority structure in the 8096. But it will mean that once your higher priority ISR is entered, it should be protected with a DI at the beginning of the ISR IF YOU WISH THE PRIORITY STRUCTURE TO BE MAINTAINED AGAINST "RAIDING" BY A LOWER ORDER PRIORITY INTERRUPT. You can then re-enable the interrupt system with an EI just before the RET at the end of the higher priority ISR so that, upon return to the main program, the next lower priority pending interrupt can be serviced. The same DI/EI argument holds for that LOWER priority ISR re: "raiding" by a still lower priority interrupt that has been pending. But note, if this method of DI/EI is employed in each ISR, then a higher priority interrupt that attempts later to interrupt an ISR will have to wait till the ISR is finished before it will be serviced. The word "priority" thus has to be treated carefully. Of course, you may want to establish your own TRUE priority structure whereby only certain interrupt sources can immediately interrupt a given ISR, or none can. This is treated in Expts. 4-9, 4-10.

The procedure described below will confirm the points in the above discussion. EXTINT (7) and HSI.0 (4) interrupt sources will be used to demonstrate what we are driving at.

PROCEDURE

CASE 1: Enter BY 311E = 0FA (DI), BY 312B = 0FB (EI), BY 3130 = 0FA (DI), BY 3147 = 0FB (EI), BY 3160 = 0FA (DI), and BY 3177 = 0FB (EI). Refer to the program in Expt. 4-5 which starts at 3100, with the EXTINT ISR at 3130 and HSI.0 ISR at 3160. In this case we are protecting each ISR, once entered, from being interrupted by the other's interrupt source till the end of that ISR when the system is re-enabled with EI. Execute the program (G FR 3100). Create HSI.0 and EXTINT edge triggered requests, IN THAT ORDER, DURING THE ON OR OFF-TIME OF THE FIRST CYCLE OF THE EE, 00 OUTPUT AT P1. They become pending till EI is reached at 312B and SJMP is executed at 312C. Then they'll be serviced i.e. only AFTER the first on/off cycle is finished with its off-time. 311F goes on the stack. At that point you'll observe 0F appear at P1 indicating that EXTINT was serviced first, even though created second. 0F remains for 5 seconds. Then, after its ISR returns to the MAIN PROGRAM with global bit re-enabled, the pending HSI.0 gets serviced immediately and we'll see F0 at P1 for 5 seconds. Its ISR returns to the main program where EE/00/EE.... on/off/on cycles resume. This again demonstrates that the return is to the point in the main program 311F where the interrupts took effect (after EI) and not to the point where they were created (in the on-part, or during the off-part, of the cycle). Query BYTE 09 to confirm that the pendings were cleared after servicing. Priority has been demonstrated. Further interrupts can be created.

CASE 2: ESC and enter BY 3130 = 0FD (NOP), BY 3147 = 0FD (NOP), BY 3160 = 0FD (NOP), BY 3177 = 0FD (NOP). DI and EI are still at 311E, 312B. We are now setting up the case where the ISR, once entered, is not protected from an interrupt by the other interrupt source, even if the latter is of lower priority. Execute. During the on-time of the first EE/00 cycle create EXTINT and HSI.0 interrupts in that order. Nothing happens till the end of the first off-cycle, when EI occurs. At that point F0 appears at P1 (from the HSI.0 ISR) for 5 seconds, THEN 0F from EXTINT ISR for 5 seconds, followed by resumption of the EE/00/EE ... on/off/on ... cycles at P1. It SEEMS that HSI.0 received service before its higher priority cousin EXTINT. That, in fact, is not exactly so. EXTINT got "serviced" first at the end of the off-time of the first cycle. That service took us to 3130 in its ISR where the NOP is GUARANTEED to execute (see section 3.6.4 p. 3-13 Microcontroller Handbook). At that point its pending was CLEARED (see Expts. 4-2, 4-3). However, the HSI.0 interrupt now meets the 3 conditions for servicing: its PENDING is STILL 1, its mask bit MINT.4 is 1 (as is MINT.7), and EI is still in force. Hence, after EXTINT execution of the NOP at 3130, HSI.0 can, and does, interrupt the ISR at 3130, (saving the return address 3131 on the stack) and vectors to its ISR at 3160, where F0 is output for 5 seconds. The RET at 3178 pops the return address 3131 off the stack, taking us to EXTINT's ISR where 0F is output for 5 seconds before its RET carries us back to the main program where the EE/00 ... cycles resume at 311F. (The interrupt call was generated AFTER EI at 312B and SJMP at 312C were executed, leaving return address 311F on the stack.) Query BYTE 09. It should reveal that the HSI.0 and EXTINT pendings were cleared.

MORAL OF THE STORY

Hardware pendings ENTER their ISRs in the order of their 8096 priorities. To ensure that a higher priority ISR FINISHES UP before the next lower priority is serviced, you should include DI at the beginning of each ISR and EI at the end before each RET. IF YOU DON'T DO THAT, THEN, IN FACT, ALL PENDINGS WILL GET SERVICED SEEMINGLY IN REVERSE ORDER! (PUSHF and POPF will accomplish the same as DI/EI - more on that in Expt. 4-10.) This is the result, as we've seen, of an "instantaneous ripple effect" from highest to lowest priority ISR, with the latter's ISR finishing FIRST; then the NEXT higher priority finishes up, etc., as the RET from each of the next lower ISR that just finished up gets us back to the top of the next higher priority ISR to commence its execution. This reverse execution of ISRs ultimately ends up in the main program again. As we've seen, this can be avoided by protecting the ISRs with DI/EI (or PUSHF, POPF).

You can now appreciate how important all the aspects of theorem (B) in Expt. 4-2 are. You must remember that on entering an ISR, the associated interrupt's pending bit is cleared and that particular ISR is an easy target for ANY other interrupt whose pending exists, be it lower OR higher in the priority ordering, unless it is protected with a DI. Also understand that, while the DI/EI solution in each ISR protects that ISR from lower order "raiding", it also protects it from a higher order interrupt being serviced till the ISR finishes up. Thus "priority" has meaning only in the sense that the ISRs are REACHED in the order of "priorities", but once in a given ISR that is protected by DI, another higher order interrupt will not be serviced till that lower order one is finished up. Expts. 4-9 and 4-10 deal with the case where WE CAN ESTABLISH OUR OWN TRUE PRIORITY STRUCTURE so that only certain (or no) interrupt sources can interrupt a given ISR and receive immediate servicing BEFORE that ISR finishes up, regardless of 8096 stated "priorities".

EXPERIMENT 4-8

THE ORDER OF SERVICING OF SOFTWARE CREATED PENDING INTERRUPTS.

In this experiment we are dealing with interrupts whose pendings are created, not by hardware edge transitions as in Expt. 4-7, but rather by the user writing 1s to the relevant bits in the pending interrupt register. This will create one of the three necessary conditions for the pertinent interrupt source to be serviced. The general conclusions will be the same as in Expt. 4-7. The program at 3200 is given below.

```
          18 00           SP      EQU     18H
          0E 00           P0      EQU     0EH
          0F 00           P1      EQU     0FH
          08 00           MINT    EQU     08H
          09 00           PINT    EQU     09H
          0E 20           INVEC1  EQU     200EH
          08 20           INVEC2  EQU     2008H
          40 00           TEMP    EQU     40H
                          ;
                          ;
3200                              ORG     3200H
                          ;
3200      A1 C0 00 18             LD      SP,#00C0H         ;Initialize SP to 00C0H.
3204      A1 30 32 40             LD      TEMP,#3230H       ;Load address of EXTINT ISR into TEMP
                                                            ;(3230H).
3208      C3 01 0E 20 40          ST      TEMP,INVEC1[0]    ;Store address into INT VECTOR table
                                                            ;at 200EH.
320D      A1 40 32 40             LD      TEMP,#3240H       ;Load address of HSI.0 ISR into TEMP
                                                            ;(3240H).
3211      C3 01 08 20 40          ST      TEMP,INVEC2[0]    ;Store address into INT VECTOR table
                                                            ;(2008H).
3216      FA                      DI                        ;Disable global interrupt bit.
3217      11 09                   CLRB    PINT              ;Clear all pending interrupts.
3219      B1 90 08                LDB     MINT,#90H         ;Set HSI.0 and EXTINT intr. mask bits.
                                                            ;in INT register.
321C      B1 10 09                LDB     PINT,#10H         ;Create HSI.0 pending interrupt.
321F      91 80 09                ORB     PINT,#80H         ;Then create EXTINT pending interrupt.
3222      B1 AA 0F        LEDS1:  LDB     P1,#0AAH          ;Output 0AAH to LEDs.
3225      30 0E FA                JBC     P0,0,LEDS1        ;If P0.0 = 0, go back to update LEDs.
3228      FB                      EI                        ;Else enable interrupts.
3229      27 F7                   SJMP    LEDS1             ;Loop back to output to LEDs.
```

```
                    ;       EXTINT INTERRUPT SERVICE ROUTINE:
                    ;
                    ;
3230                        ORG     3230H
                    ;
3230  FA                    DI                      ;Disable global interrupt bit.
3231  B1 0F 0F      LEDS2:  LDB     P1,#0FH         ;Output 0FH to LEDs.
3234  31 0E FA              JBC     P0,1,LEDS2      ;If P0.1 = 0, go back to update LEDs.
3237  FB                    EI                      ;Else enable global interrupt bit.
3238  F0                    RET                     ;Return to main loop.
```

```
                    ;       HSI.0 INTERRUPT SERVICE ROUTINE:
                    ;
3240                        ORG     3240H
                    ;
3240  FA                    DI                      ;Disable global interrupt bit.
3241  B1 F0 0F      LEDS3:  LDB     P1,#0F0H        ;Output 0F0H to LEDs.
3244  37 0E FA              JBC     P0,7,LEDS3      ;If P0.7 = 0, go back to update LEDs.
3247  FB                    EI                      ;Else enable global interrupt bit.
3248  F0                    RET                     ;Return to main program.
                    ;
3249                        END
```

The main program above establishes the EXTINT ISR at 3230 and HSI.0's ISR at 3240. MINT.7 and MINT.4 are set to 1 to enable EXTINT and HSI.0 sources. Any previously established pendings are cleared at 3217. LDB PINT, #10 and ORB PINT, #80 then create, first, a software HSI.0 pending (PINT.4 = 1) and then a software EXTINT pending (PINT.7 = 1), in that order. So far the system is disabled (DI at 3116), so nobody gets service. AA is then output to P1's LEDs and kept that way by the JBC P0, 0, LEDS1 instruction. This instruction loops as long as switch S0 (at P0.0) is maintained low. When it is thrown high, fall-through to EI occurs (system now enabled) and the following SJMP LEDS1 instruction gets executed - but that's all.

Servicing can now occur. The priority structure will have EXTINT serviced first at 3230. In that ISR, DI protects it from any lower order "raiding" and EI re-enables the global upon exiting the ISR. 0F is output to P1 replacing AA. JBC P0, 1, LEDS2 maintains 0F as long as switch S1 (P0.1) is low. When it is thrown high we fall through to EI and RET. The latter takes us back to the JSMP LEDS1 loop at 3222 just for an instant, because the HSI.0 pending can now be serviced in view of the EI at end of EXTINT's ISR. It is. We enter the HSI.0 ISR at 3240 where DI guarantees protection from any other interrupt. F0 is output to P1 replacing the previous 0F. It is maintained by the JBC P0, 7, LEDS3 instruction as long as S7 (P0.7) is kept low. When S7 is thrown high we fall through to EI and RET at 3247, 48. The return is to 3222 in the main program where AA is again output at P1 and the SJMP LEDS1 loop is again entered. The software created interrupts have been serviced in the order of their priority. Their pending bits in SFR 09 are now cleared.

All of the above, and more, will be brought out in the experiment. The procedure is described below.

PROCEDURE

1. With the switches set to 00 at P0, execute and observe AA at the LEDs. HSI.0 and EXTINT software pendings have been created, in that order.
2. Throw S0 (P0.0) hi/lo and see EXTINT get serviced (EI was reached), as evidenced by the appearance of 0F at the LEDs. EXTINT's ISR is protected by DI so HSI.0 can't get serviced till EI is executed. The latter will happen as soon as....
3. you throw S1 (P0.1) hi/lo. Fall-through to EI occurs at 3237 and RET carries us back to the main program. HSI.0's pending can now be serviced (since EI is again in effect). It is, as evidenced by F0 appearing at P1's LEDs.

4. Throwing S7 (P0.7) hi/lo causes fall-through to 3247 where EI occurs. The RET takes us back to the main program's loop where AA is again output to P1. Since the pendings were cleared on entering the ISRs (query BYTE 09 to confirm that), no further (software) interrupts occur, even though mask bits and PSW.9 are 1. HARDWARE INTERRUPTS created subsequently by the SWITCHES at EXTINT and HSI.0 can, however, cause further interrupts which WILL be serviced.
5. ESC. Enter BY 3230 = 0FD, BY 3237 = 0FD, BY 3240 = 0FD, BY 3247 = 0FD (NOPs at those addresses). Execute. See AA. Guess what? HSI.0 is serviced "first" (F0 appears and replaces AA) when S0 is thrown hi/lo. Throw S7 hi/lo. Now see 0F at P1 (EXTINT "appears" to have been serviced next). Throw S1 hi/lo. See AA at P1 again. It's the same story as in Expt. 4-7: EXTINT did get "serviced" first. But as soon as 3230 was entered, without DI protection, HSI.0's existing pending takes over, as EXTINT's has just been cleared and EI is still in effect. So 3231 is placed on the stack and HSI.0's ISR is entered at 3240. HSI.0's ISR is executed (F0 appears) and its RET is to 3231 allowing EXTINT's ISR to "continue". 0F appears. The latter's RET is to the main program where AA is again output. Query BYTE 09 to confirm that pendings no longer exist. Without the DI protection the pendings were serviced in an order apparently reverse to their expected priority ordering.

See end of Expt. 4-7 for "moral of the story" and the related discussion after it. They apply, as well, to the software created interrupts in this experiment.

EXPERIMENT 4-9

ONE WAY TO CREATE OUR OWN LIMITED 8096 INTERRUPT PRIORITIES OR NON-PRIORITIES

The program for this experiment is the same one used in Expt. 4-5 at starting address 3100.

The results of Expts. 4-7, 4-8 have confirmed the following statement made on p. 1-14 of the MCS-96 Macro Assembler User's Guide (ref. 3, Introduction to our Chapter 1).

"WHILE THE 8096 HAS ONLY A SINGLE PRIORITY LEVEL IN THE SENSE THAT ANY INTERRUPT MAY BE ITSELF INTERRUPTIBLE, IT DOES HAVE A PRIORITY STRUCTURE FOR RESOLVING SIMULTANEOUS INTERRUPTS".

The statement about "simultaneous interrupts" refers to the 8096 priorities 7 to 0 i.e. when all or some are simultaneously in contention (as when all or several outstanding PENDINGS can qualify for servicing after the 3 conditions of theorem (B) are met). When in such contention, servicing occurs in the order 7 to 0 (EXTINT down to Timer Overflow). However, once in the ISR, that ISR can be interrupted if it did not receive DI, or other, protection. It can be interrupted by a lower order priority interrupt as well as a higher order one, unless steps are taken to prevent that.

This, and the next experiment, are concerned with several methods that the user can employ to create true, arbitrary priority levels in the sense that any interrupt source can be made highest priority and any other one lowest priority. Meaning that, for example, once in a Timer Overflow ISR (normally lowest priority) no other source would be able to interrupt it for immediate servicing, if that's what we desired. Or, if in an EXTINT ISR (normally highest priority), we might want any other source to be able to interrupt it for immediate servicing. Thus we plan to come to grips with the first half of the statement quoted above. WE WANT TO CREATE OUR OWN PRIORITY LEVELS.

In this experiment we tackle the problem of establishing our own priorities in a limited way i.e. through the employment, or non-employment, of DI/EI in the ISRs (DI at its beginning, EI at its end). This method will work quite well if only two interrupt sources are involved. In the next experiment, 4-10, we indicate a general method of establishing your own priority levels by loading the Interrupt Mask Register at the beginning of an ISR, so as to unmask or mask any interrupt sources you desire. That will allow only those interrupt sources, whose mask bits were set by this procedure, to interrupt the ISR in question. The same procedure will hold true for setting MINT arbitrarily at the beginnings of the other ISRs. But more about that in Expt. 4-10. There PUSHF, POPF, not DI/EI, are used.

In this experiment, employing the DI/EI approach, we'll work with the EXTINT and HSI.0 interrupt sources where, normally, the former is "highest priority" and the latter "lower priority" in the "simultaneous" sense. We'll have the DI/EI procedure allow us to implement the following different priority cases: 1. EXTINT is made highest priority and can immediately interrupt an HSI.0 ISR, but not vice-versa (HSI.0 becomes pending in that case); 2. HSI.0 is made highest priority and can interrupt the EXTINT ISR, but not vice-versa (EXTINT becomes pending in that case); 3. either can immediately interrupt the other (i.e. no priorities at all); 4. neither can interrupt the other (they become pendings - each is "highest priority" when its ISR is executing). The procedure below explains all (refer to the program at 3100 in Expt. 4-5).

PROCEDURE

CASE 1: Enter BY 311E = 0FB and BY 312B = 0FD i.e. EI at 311E and NOP at 312B. Then BY 3130 = 0FA (DI), BY 3147 = 0FB (EI), BY 3160 = 0FD (NOP), BY 3177 = 0FD. These entries will guarantee that the EXTINT ISR can not be interrupted by an HSI.0 interrupt, but that the HSI.0 ISR can be interrupted by an EXTINT interrupt. Thus EXTINT is of higher priority than HSI.0 in the true sense.

a). Execute (G FR 3100). During an EE on-time, throw the EXTINT switch. 0F immediately appears at P1. Before 5 sec. are up, throw the HSI.0 switch. 0F finishes up (EXTINT ISR), then F0 comes on for 5 sec. (HSI.0 ISR), then the EE/00/EE ... cycles are resumed from the point of interruption.

b). Without ESC, create an HSI.0 interrupt during an EE on-time. F0 immediately appears. Before 5 sec., strike the EXTINT switch. F0 immediately changes to 0F which lasts 5 sec. (EXTINT ISR), then F0 finishes up its remaining time. The EE/00 on/off cycles then resume from the point of interruption.

CASE 2: ESC and enter BY 3130 = 0FD (NOP), BY 3147 = 0FD, BY 3160 = 0FA (DI), BY 3177 = 0FB (EI). This will allow HSI.0 to interrupt the EXTINT ISR but not vice-versa. HSI.0 is made to be of higher priority than EXTINT.

a). Execute. During an EE on-time, create EXTINT. Observe 0F immediately appear. Before 5 sec. are up, create an HSI.0 interrupt. Observe F0 appear at once for 5 sec., then 0F come back to finish up its 5 sec., then EE/00 on/off cycles re-appear from where they left off.

b). During another on or off-time create an HSI.0 interrupt. See F0 come on. Before 5 sec., create an EXTINT interrupt. F0 finishes up, then 0F comes on for 5 sec., then the on/off cycles resume at P1 from where they left off. HSI.0 has been made to be of higher priority than EXTINT.

CASE 3: ESC and enter BY 3160 = 0FD (NOP) and BY 3177 = 0FD. Now 3130, 3147, 3160, and 3177 all contain NOPs. This time either interrupt source will be able to interrupt the other's ISR for immediate service i.e. no priorities at all.

a). Execute. During an on or off-time, create an EXTINT interrupt. 0F appears immediately. Before 5 sec., create an HSI.0 interrupt. 0F does not finish up. F0 immediately appears for 5 sec., then 0F finishes up its 5 sec., then the EE/00 cycles resume from the point of interruption.

b). This time create an HSI.0 interrupt. Observe F0. Before 5 sec. create an EXTINT interrupt. Observe 0F immediately replace F0. After 5 sec., F0 comes back to finish up. The EE/00 cycles resume. Thus there are no priorities - either can interrupt the other.

CASE 4: ESC. Enter BY 3130 = 0FA (DI), BY 3147 = 0FB (EI), BY 3160 = 0FA (DI), BY 3177 = 0FB (EI). This time each ISR is protected. Neither interrupt source can interrupt the other's ISR. Each ISR is "highest priority" when its ISR is executing.

a). Execute. During a cycle create an EXTINT interrupt. See 0F. Before 5 sec. create an HSI.0 interrupt. 0F finishes up its 5 sec., then F0 appears for its 5 sec., then on/off cycles resume at P1.

b). During a cycle, create an HSI.0 interrupt. Observe F0 immediately appear. Before 5 sec., create an EXTINT interrupt. F0 finishes up its 5 sec., then 0F comes on for its 5 sec., then the EE/00 on/off cycles resume at P1. Each ISR was of highest priority once entered. The other's interrupt could only become a pending for later servicing after the other's ISR finishes up.

The method illustrated in this experiment works well for any two interrupt sources, but no more. That's because the possibilities are fourfold with the NOP, NOP/DI, EI approach i.e. NOP, NOP in one ISR and DI, EI in the other; DI, EI in the first ISR and NOP, NOP in the other; NOP, NOP in both ISRs; and DI, EI in both ISRs. Thus, relative priorities (or none) are nicely established with this method for two sources.

PROBLEM (not hands-on): extend the method to two GROUPS of interrupts, with one group having equal high priorities, and higher than the second group, but with no priorities WITHIN the second group.

We can deal with all 8 interrupt sources to create any arbitrary priority structure we wish, by software i.e. priority in the true sense. That can be accomplished by setting or clearing any mask bits in SFR 08 at the beginning of each ISR. Only those sources whose mask bits are set to 1 at the beginning of an ISR will be capable of interrupting that ISR (if PSW.9 = 1). That gives us complete flexibility in specifying our own total priority structure for all 8 sources. THE METHOD IS ILLUSTRATED IN EXPT. 4-10. The use of PUSHF and POPF are inherent in the method.

EXPERIMENT 4-10

A MORE GENERAL METHOD OF CREATING EIGHT PRIORITIES BY SOFTWARE. USING PUSHF, POPF IN THE ISRs.

In this method, as explained at the end of Expt. 4-9, we can set priorities among the eight 8096 interrupt sources in any manner we wish, so as to realize priorities on a level basis. As indicated there, the method will depend on the user setting or clearing desired interrupt mask bits (SFR 08) at the beginning of certain (possibly all) ISR routines. Those bits set to 1 represent sources that can interrupt the ISR if PSW.9 = 1. Remember, once in an ISR, the pending for that ISR's interrupt source has automatically been cleared, so that source itself is not a contender till another interrupt is created on that same line. Those mask bits cleared in the ISR will not allow immediate servicing of the associated interrupt sources - they'll become pending till their mask bits are set, at which time they'll get serviced (if PSW.9 = 1). The method is truly simple in its application and illustrates another of the many versatile and powerful features of the 8096.

We'll illustrate the method with the two external interrupts EXTINT and HSI.0, as we've been doing through-out the chapter with respect to other 8096 interrupt features. In demonstrating the method, we will also start using the instructions PUSHF at the beginning of each ISR (it pushes flags (including PSW.9), and the interrupt mask on the stack and replaces them with 00, 00), and POPF at the end of each ISR before RET (it restores flags, PSW.9, and the original interrupt mask to the PSW). This is good interrupt practice technique and should be followed whenever the ISR itself affects the flags and/or the interrupt mask bits (the latter being the case whenever you are setting your own priority levels as we are doing here). We certainly want to get back to the main program with the original flags in-tact and the interrupt mask in-tact (unless there is good reason to want the latter changed on return to the main program - and this we can also do, as explained later).

In the experiment, we'll force the HSI.0 source to be of higher priority than the EXTINT source, so that the former can always interrupt the latter's ISR for immediate servicing, but not the reverse (in that case the EXTINT interrupt becomes a pending). Now this was accomplished with the DI/EI approach in Expt. 4-9 (case (2) there). We are about to accomplish the same thing, but with an approach and method that are much more general and versatile. It is easily extended to control the priorities of all 8 sources, not just the two involved here.

Keep in mind that interrupts are not serviced during POPF/RET instructions. They will be AFTER the return, if there's a pending for the source in question, and its mask bit is set, and if PSW.9 = 1. See Expts. 4-2 and 4-4, theorems (B) and (D).

The program at 3250 for this experiment is shown below.

```
     18 00          SP      EQU     18H
     0E 00          P0      EQU     0EH
     0F 00          P1      EQU     0FH
     16 00          IOC1    EQU     16H
     50 00          REG     EQU     50H
     70 00          REG1    EQU     70H
     80 00          REG2    EQU     80H
     08 00          MINT    EQU     08H
     09 00          PINT    EQU     09H
     0E 20          INVEC1  EQU     200EH
     08 20          INVEC2  EQU     2008H
     40 00          TEMP    EQU     40H
                    ;
                    ;
3250                        ORG     3250H
                    ;
3250 A1 C0 00 18            LD      SP,#00C0H         ;Initialize SP to 00C0H.
3254 A1 80 32 40            LD      TEMP,#3280H       ;Load address of EXTINT ISR into TEMP
                                                      ;(3280H).
3258 C3 01 0E 20 40         ST      TEMP,INVEC1[0]    ;Store address into INT VECTOR table
                                                      ;at 200EH.
325D A1 B0 32 40            LD      TEMP,#32B0H       ;Load address of HSI.0 ISR into TEMP
                                                      ;(32B0H).
3261 C3 01 08 20 40         ST      TEMP,INVEC2[0]    ;Store address into INT VECTOR table
                                                      ;(2008H).
3266 B1 00 16               LDB     IOC1,#00          ;Load 00 into IOC1 to select EXTINT.
3269 11 09                  CLRB    PINT              ;Clear all pending interrupts.
326B B1 90 08               LDB     MINT,#90H         ;Set HSI.0 and EXTINT intr. mask bits.
                                                      ;in INT register.
326E FB                     EI                        ;Enable interrupts.
326F B1 FF 0F       THERE:  LDB     P1,#0FFH          ;Output 0FFH to LEDs.
3272 27 FB                  SJMP    THERE             ;Loop back to output to LEDs.
```

```
                        ;       EXTINT INTERRUPT SERVICE ROUTINE:
                        ;
                        ;
3280                            ORG     3280H
                        ;
3280   F2                       PUSHF                   ;Save PSW (flags and INT mask) and
                                                        ;RESET PSW to 00.
3281   C8 00                    PUSH    TREG2           ;Save previous value of time delay
                                                        ;WORD register TREG2.
3283   B0 00 70                 LDB     REG1,TREG1      ;Save previous value of time delay
                                                        ;BYTE register TREG1.
3286   B1 10 08                 LDB     MINT,#10H       ;Set HSI.0 Mask bit to enable only it.
3289   FB                       EI                      ;Enable global interrupt bit.
328A   B1 0F 0F                 LDB     P1,#0FH         ;Output 0FH to LEDs.
328D   EF 70 CD                 CALL    TIME            ;Delay for 5 seconds.
3290   B0 70 00                 LDB     TREG1,REG1      ;Restore previous value of time delay
                                                        ;BYTE register TREG1.
3293   CC 00                    POP     TREG2           ;Restore previous value of time delay
                                                        ;register TREG2.
3295   F3                       POPF                    ;Restore PSW (flags and INT mask).
3296   F0                       RET                     ;Return to main loop.
                        ;
                        ;
                        ;       HSI.0 INTERRUPT SERVICE ROUTINE:
                        ;
32B0                            ORG     32B0H
                        ;
32B0   F2                       PUSHF                   ;Save PSW (flags and INT mask) and
                                                        ;RESET PSW to 00.
32B1   B0 0F 50                 LDB     REG,P1          ;Save status of LEDs.
32B4   C8 00                    PUSH    TREG2           ;Save previous value of time delay
                                                        ;WORD register TREG2.
32B6   B0 00 80                 LDB     REG2,TREG1      ;Save previous value of time delay
                                                        ;BYTE register TREG1.
32B9   B1 F0 0F                 LDB     P1,#0F0H        ;Output 0F0H to LEDs.
32BC   EF 41 CD                 CALL    TIME            ;Delay for 5 seconds.
32BF   B0 80 00                 LDB     TREG1,REG2      ;Restore previous value of time delay
                                                        ;BYTE register TREG1.
32C2   CC 00                    POP     TREG2           ;Restore previous value of time delay
                                                        ;register TREG2.
32C4   B0 50 0F                 LDB     P1,REG          ;Restore status of LEDs.
32C7   F3                       POPF                    ;Restore PSW (flags and INT mask).
32C8   F0                       RET                     ;Return to main program.
                        ;
32C9                            END
```

Let's analyze it. The main program establishes addresses for EXTINT and HSI.0 ISRs at 3280 and 32B0, respectively. EXTINT is selected over ACH.7 as the source for EXTINT. Previous pendings (if any) are cleared. MINT.7 and MINT.4 are set to 1 for obvious reasons. EI sets I in the PSW to 1 (global enable), necessary for interrupts to be serviced. Finally FF is output to P1's LEDs and a loop (SJMP) representing "busy tasks" is then established.

An EXTINT request in the main program would interrupt this "busy task" loop and vector to its ISR at 3280. Now EACH ISR (EXTINT and HSI.0) is going to be calling TIME (at 3050 in Expt. 4-2), which uses TREG1 and TREG2 as its loop counters. Since we are investigating the possibility that each source can interrupt the other's ISR, it is imperative that TREG1 and TREG2 be saved before that ISR itself calls TIME, and restored after the return from TIME to that ISR occurs. Hence the PUSH TREG2; LDB REG1, TREG1; LDB TREG1, REG1; and POP TREG2 in the EXTINT ISR, and the corresponding instructions in the HSI.0 ISR (at 32B0).

Each ISR starts with a PUSHF instruction to save flags and the interrupt mask on the stack. This is very important, as the general method will involve manipulating the interrupt mask IN THE ISR(s) to establish priorities, and we'd like (in general) to return to the main program with the masks the way they WERE. The POPF instruction at the end of each ISR will guarantee that (see later discussion for the case where we might want to return to the main program with a different interrupt mask). As good practice, flags should be saved - the ISR may well affect those flags. Remember that the PUSHF saves PSW and replaces it with 0000. POPF restores the complete PSW (flags and interrupt mask).

The essence of the method has to do, in our application illustration, with the instruction LDB MINT, #10 in the EXTINT ISR (no corresponding instruction in the HSI.0 ISR is needed for THIS example of the method). That instruction resets MINT.7 to 0 but keeps MINT.4 at 1. The EI, after it, GUARANTEES that an HSI.0 interrupt made any time during the CALL TIME at 328D will get IMMEDIATE service, and that the RET at the end of the latter's ISR will get back to the EXTINT ISR to finish up its activity from the point where it was interrupted by HSI.0. HOWEVER, an EXTINT request while we're in the HSI.0 ISR, can NOT be immediately serviced since the PUSHF at 32B0 left the PSW with 0000 (all mask bits 0 AND PSW.9 = 0). EXTINT will become a pending, which can be serviced only after the POPF instruction at 32C7 restores the original PSW.9 and the original interrupt mask (i.e. 1 and 90 in our example). The EXTINT ISR outputs 0F for 5 sec. (if not interrupted by HSI.0) and HSI.0's ISR outputs F0 for 5 sec. - it can NOT be interrupted.

Finally, we note that HSI.0's ISR saves the status of P1, but EXTINT's doesn't. Suppose EXTINT made a request in the main program. IF it's not interrupted by HSI.0, its ISR will display 0F for 5 sec. and will return to SJMP in the main program where FF is again displayed at P1. If HSI.0 made the request, its ISR can NOT be interrupted by EXTINT. It will display F0 for 5 sec. and will return to main program and display FF again. However, suppose EXTINT made the request and, while we are in its ISR with 0F displayed, an HSI.0 interrupt comes along. We are immediately vectored to 32B0. To guarantee that after HSI.0 ISR's display of F0 for 5 sec. we'll return to the EXTINT ISR with the ability to display 0F (which was in force at P1 at the time HSI.0 interrupted EXTINT), it is necessary to save the status of P1 at the time HSI.0 interrupted EXTINT. This is easily accomplished with LDB REG, P1 and LDB P1, REG instructions in HSI.0's ISR (at 32B1, 32C4). Since EXTINT can not interrupt HSI.0 there's no need for those instructions in the EXTINT ISR.

The result of the above discussion is that HSI.0 will always get immediate attention, whereas EXTINT becomes a pending if it tries to interrupt the HSI.0 service routine. The experimental procedure is described below.

PROCEDURE

CASE 1: Execute from 3250. See FF at P1. Create an EXTINT interrupt. Observe 0F for 5 sec., then FF again. Try it again.

CASE 2: Then create an HSI.0 interrupt. See F0 for 5 sec., then FF again.

CASE 3: On the run, create another HSI.0 interrupt. See F0 again. Before 5 sec. are up, create an EXTINT. F0 remains till its 5 sec. are up. Then we'll see 0F for 5 sec., then FF again upon return to the main program. HSI.0 was top priority, EXTINT became a pending.

CASE 4: On the run, create an EXTINT interrupt. See 0F. Before 5 sec. create an HSI.0 interrupt. F0 immediately appears and remains for 5 sec. Then 0F resumes from the point at which EXTINT was interrupted to complete its remaining time. FF then appears upon return to the main program.

CASE 5: On-the-fly, create another EXTINT. See 0F. After 2 sec. create an HSI.0 interrupt. Observe F0 for 5 sec., then 0F again. After another 2 sec. create another HSI.0. See F0 for 5 sec. again, then 0F re-appear for 1 sec. (to complete its ISR), then FF again as EXTINT's ISR returns to the main program.

CASE 6: On the run, create an HSI.0 interrupt. See F0. Try an EXTINT interrupt TWICE. F0 finishes up its 5 sec., then 0F appears for 5 sec. (once), then FF re-appears.

FINAL NOTE

In using this method, wherein the interrupt mask register is manipulated at the beginning of each (or some) of the ISR(s) to realize priority levels of your own choosing, always use PUSHF and POPF instructions at the beginning and end of each ISR so that you can return with the original mask bits and flags as they were.
SHOULD YOU WISH TO RETURN WITH THE SAME PRIORITIES (OR OTHERS) THAT YOU ESTABLISHED IN MINT AT THE BEGINNING OF THE ISR, RATHER THAN THOSE THAT EXISTED BEFORE ENTERING THE ISR, THAT IS EASILY ACCOMPLISHED BY INSERTING THE FOLLOWING INSTRUCTIONS BETWEEN POPF AND THE RET AT THE END OF THE ISR: DI; LDB MINT, NEW VALUE; EI; RET. THE FLAGS ARE RESTORED, BUT MINT HAS BEEN CHANGED. INTERRUPTS IN THE MAIN PROGRAM OR OTHER ISR WILL HENCEFORTH BE DETERMINED BY THIS NEW MINT BYTE.

This concludes chapter 4. We have explored all the elements of the 8096 interrupt structure using the external interrupt sources EXTINT, HSI.0, and ACH.7 as the vehicles in the experiments. The internal interrupt sources obey all the same theorems and features as do the external sources. We'll be working with those internal interrupt sources extensively in chapters 5 and 6 which follow, and indeed through-out the rest of the book.

CHAPTER 5

WORKING WITH THE 8096'S SPECIAL FUNCTION REGISTERS

INTRODUCTION

8096 on-board I/O devices are controlled as register-mapped I/O (in reality memory-mapped I/O, as the SFR registers are in internal RAM space). This provides fast, efficient, powerful, and convenient software I/O processing. The registers in this register-mapped I/O are called the Special Function Registers, or SFRs. These SFRs form one of the crucial links to the understanding and mastering of the 8096 single-chip 16-bit microcomputer. They provide the means for powerful programmable I/O. The nature and context of the I/O control can be chaned at will, and quickly, by writing to the relevant control SFRs. The status of the I/O control situation can be monitored "on the fly" by reading the relevant status SFRs. Both these features are, in part, responsible for the very fast 8096 through-put and I/O response times. In particular, the High Speed Input/ Output units on the 8096, with their associated SFRs, play a decisive role in implementing the 8096's impressive I/O through-put and control.

Another fact that should be born in mind in this regard is the existence of 232 RAM registers above the SFRs which, in a sense, provide 232 accumulators, in that the RALU (Register/Arithmetic Logic Unit) does not use ONE accumulator. It operates directly on the 256 byte register space (including the SFRs), thereby avoiding the "one-accumulator" bottleneck. You can output from, or input to, any of these registers directly.

The map lay-out of the SFRs, and their meanings, are shown and described in Figs. 2-7, 2-8, pp. 2-6, 2-7 of the Microcontroller Handbook (see also section D, chapter 1 this book). In many of these SFRs, individual bits have very special meanings in controlling various aspects of the I/O one is trying to achieve. In some cases the bits are written to, to implement the desired I/O performance; in other cases they are read to determine the status of various aspect(s) of the I/O hardware situation. In still other cases it's the whole SFR byte or word that has meaning, rather than an individual bit (e.g. Timers 1 and 2). Some SFRs are byte-sized registers, others are word-sized registers (lo byte in even register address, hi byte in higher odd register address). In any event a mastery and understanding of the SFRs and most of their individual bits are absolutely essential.

It is the purpose of this chapter to gain the necessary familiarity and confidence needed to work successfully with the SFRs and their control or status bits. We accomplish this through 25 experiments, many of which will have an applications flavor. Specifically applications-oriented experiments with the SFRs of a more advanced nature will be presented in the 26 experiments of chapter 6.

We remind you that we have already worked with a number of SFRs in chapters 2, 3, and 4. We'll be using them again in this and succeeding chapters. Now, however, we are going to come to grips wth all the other SFRs (except the serial port SFRs which we are saving for chapter 8, where we concentrate exclusively on serial I/O and communications with the 8096). The SFRs that we'll work with in this chapter, besides those already used in chapters 2, 3, and 4, are:

PWM,
The A/D SFRs: AD-RESULT (HI/LO), AD-COMMAND,
and HSO-COMMAND,
Port 2,
Timers 1 and 2,
I/O control Registers: IOC0 and IOC1,
HSIO Status Registers: IOS0 and IOS1,
HSO-COMMAND, HSO-TIME, HSI-MODE, HSI-TIME,
HSI-STATUS.

To keep things in perspective, we list those SFRs that we've already worked with in the previous chapters:

Ports P0 and P1 (0EH, 0FH),
Watchdog Timer (WDT - 0AH),
I/O Control Register IOC1 (16H) (several bits),

ZERO Register R0 (00),
Interrupt Mask Register (08H),
Interrupt Pending Register (09H).

The experiments involving all the SFRs will be realistic and meaningful and should give you the ability to easily work with them. (The applications-oriented experiments with the SFRs in chapter 6 should re-inforce that ability, as well as give you a good idea of the many ways the 8096 can be used in powerful applications). 13 of the 25 experiments in this chapter deal with the SFRs associated with control of the HSO and HSI (High Speed Output/Input) Units. 13 of the 26 applications experiments with the SFRs in chapter 6 are also concerned with the HSO and HSI units. These two chapters thus direct a great deal of emphasis toward the HSIO units. And for good reasons: the HSIO units comprise one of the truly outstanding and unique features of the 8096, responsible for so much of its I/O power.

Care must be exercised in working with the SFRs: 1. Don't attempt to use them as general purpose registers for storage or for purposes OTHER than for which they're intended as SFRs. You have plenty of registers (232) in the register file above the last SFR (17H). 2. Don't attempt to use the registers marked "RESERVED" in the SFR space. Indeterminate results may ensue. They are reserved for future use and new SFR dedication by Intel. 3. Consult the general precautions given in section Q, chapter 1, as they relate to working with the SFRs i.e. which are byte or word-read only, which are byte or word-written only, which are altered on being read, etc.

We repeat again that we will not, in this chapter, treat those SFRs concerned with Serial I/O. They will be examined, fully explained, and used in chapter 8 where Serial I/O applications with the 8096 is dealt with. The pertinent registers are:

SBUF (RX),
SBUF (TX),
BAUD RATE,
SP-STAT,
SP-CON.

EXPERIMENT 5-1

ANOTHER EXAMPLE USING THE WATCHDOG TIMER

We have illustrated how the WDT SFR may be applied in Expt. 2-7 of chapter 2. Refer also to section N of chapter 1. Another example is presented here. We write a "faultless" program and then modify it to simulate a "faulty" program. (You may think of the latter as a program that doesn't progress properly because of either software or hardware induced problems). In the faultless program the WDT never times out (reset will not occur). The program keeps running, monitoring switches at P0 and showing their updated values at P1's LEDs. The program is then modified to simulate a "faulty program", in which the switches are monitored once and the program then "gets lost" (simulated by inserting an endless SJMP loop). In the first case the WDT is periodically cleared before the 16 msec. time-out of the WDT can occur, so that a reset will never happen. In the second case, the jump into the "wild" no longer permits periodic clearing of the WDT. Hence, after 16 msec., the WDT times-out and resets the system, preventing possible undesirable effects at the I/Os in case random code is being executed in "outer space". The program to illustrate this is given below at 2200:

```
      0A 00      WDT     EQU   0AH
      0E 00      P0      EQU   0EH
      0F 00      P1      EQU   0FH
                 ;
                 ;
2200                     ORG   2200H
                 ;
2200  B1 1E 0A   BEGIN:  LDB   WDT,#1EH     ;Load WDT access register (SFR) with
2203  B1 E1 0A           LDB   WDT,#0E1H    ;1EH followed by 0E1H to enable and
                                            ;clear WDT.
2206  B0 0E 0F           LDB   P1,P0        ;Output value of switches to LEDs.
2209  FD         HERE:   NOP                ;NOPs will be modified at runtime.
220A  FD                 NOP                ;
220B  27 F3              SJMP  BEGIN        ;Go back to BEGIN to clear WDT and
                                            ;update LEDs.
```

In the above simple program, the first two instructions enable and clear the WDT (address 0AH). The next instruction reads the switches at P0 out to the LEDs at P1. The two NOPs will be modified later to simulate the "faulty" program. The last instruction is vital: it jumps to BEGIN where the WDT is cleared again before WDT overflow can occur (16 msec). The switches are again read. As we vary their values we'll immediately see their status at P1. If, now, we were to replace the NOPs by 27, FE (i.e. SJMP HERE) and execute again, we'd see the initial switch status once. The SJMP HERE simulates "outer space" (in this case the program loops on itself at HERE) and we never reach SJMP BEGIN to periodically clear the WDT. After 16 msec. WDT times out (overflows) and initiates a hardware reset (pulse on the 8096 RESET pin). The 8096 reset conditions are given in section 0 of chapter 1 (or pp. 2-22, 2-23 Microcontroller Handbook). There we see that port P1, in particular, comes up as FF on reset. Hence the initial switch status observed at P1 should give way to FF after 16 msec. of "random code" execution.

PROCEDURE

1. Execute and vary the switches. Port 1's LEDs mirror the switch status at any given time. The WDT never times out (no reset). Make sure Disable Switch S2 on the iSBE-96 is on.
2. ESC and enter BY 2209 = 27, 0FE to replace the NOPs with SJMP HERE. This now simulates "random code". Set the switches to, say, AA. With the WDT Disable Switch S2 in the on position, execute the modified program. You'll see AA for 16 msec. followed by FF at the LEDs. Turn S2 back off. The WDT timed out in 16 msec. as it was never again cleared. Remember, the WDT is a 16-bit counter that is incremented every state time (1/4 usec. for 12 MHz clock) so that the 64K counts till overflow will take 16K usec. or 16 msec. At that time a pulse is output to the RESET pin.

EXPERIMENT 5-2

THE PWM SFR: PULSE WIDTH MODULATION AND D/A CONVERSION. MOTOR SPEED AND LIGHT INTENSITY CONTROL.

The PWM Special Function Register at 17H allows you to write any value from 00 to FF into it to control the on-time of a pulse train that it outputs at pin P2.5 of port 2. The PERIOD of the pulse train is a FIXED 64 usec. (for 12 MHz clock). Thus duty cycle can be controlled. See pp. 2-16, 2-17 and Fig. 2-23 of Microcontroller Handbook (or section F chapter 1 this book). For example, 80H in the PWM will give an on-time of 50% of the period, FFH will give 99.6%, 40H will give 25%, C0H will give 75%, etc. If, then, an RC filter is employed at the PWM output pin, P2.5, the average output voltage will be directly proportional to the duty cycle i.e. to the fraction of the time the pulse is on, and will vary from 0V (00 in PWM) to close to 5V (FF in PWM) (we'll measure the exact value for our unit soon). Thus a digital byte (the byte loaded into the PWM register) has been converted to a proportional analog voltage - a D to A converter. The R,C values we employed for the output filter at P2.5 were R = 3K, C = .3 uf. (see Fig. 4-11, p. 4-8 Microcontroller Handbook). Don't expect a broadband frequency response with these fixed values.

In this experiment we'll implement a D to A converter using the PWM SFR, first by inputting the digital byte at the switch bank on port 0. Then we'll modify the program slightly so that the external byte will be furnished from the keyboard by entering BY 40 = XY on the fly (XY being any byte from 00 to FF). In both cases we'll use a VTVM to measure the filtered output voltage at P2.5 for various switch or keyboard inputted digital bytes. The program at 2210 for the first part is shown below.

```
        0E 00       P0       EQU    0EH
        0F 00       P1       EQU    0FH
        16 00       IOC1     EQU    16H
        17 00       PWM      EQU    17H
                    ;
                    ;
2210                         ORG    2210H
                    ;
2210    B1 01 16             LDB    IOC1,#01H    ;Load 01H into IOC1 register to select
                                                 ;PWM function of P2.5.
2213    B0 0E 17    THERE:   LDB    PWM,P0       ;Load PWM reg. with data from switches.
2216    27 FB                SJMP   THERE        ;Loop back to pass data from switches
                                                 ;to PWM register.
```

It is simple enough. The first instruction selects the PWM function for pin P2.5 by setting bit 0 of IOC1. The second instruction inputs the switch byte at port P0 directly into the PWM SFR, thereby setting the duty cycle of the 64 usec. period pulses at P2.5's output to a value proportional to the switch byte at P0. The last instruction keeps looping to poll for variations in P0 which would change the output duty cycle, and hence change output (filtered) voltage at P2.5 proportionately.

PROCEDURE

1. Execute the program (G FR 2210). Set the switches to 00, 01, 03, 07, 0F, 1F, 3F, 7F, FF, in turn, measuring the filtered output voltage at P2.5 with a VTVM in each case. We found a range from 0.02V (for byte 00 i.e. an offset) to 4.81V (for byte FF). With switch byte at 80 we measured 2.17V. The non-linearity could be the result of our choice of R,C values (quoted above) for the output filter circuit of Fig. 4-11 p. 4-8 Microcontroller Handbook (or section F chapter 1). If you feed the filtered output voltage to an LED and vary the switch byte you'll observe light intensity control as the byte varies from 00 to FF. If, on the other hand, you tap off the pulse train at P2.5 BEFORE the filter, and apply to the circuit of Fig. 2-3 in chapter 2 to drive the motor shown there, you'll be controlling motor speed as you vary the switch value. This we did and observed the effect with a simple 1-6V DC motor. The motor's inertia and inductance provide the filtering in the collector circuit.
2. ESC and enter BY 2213 = 0B0, 40, 17 which is machine code for LDB PWM, REG where REG = 40H and PWM = 17H. This now replaces LDB PWM, P0 and means that the PWM will be loaded with the contents of 40. Execute the new program and, on the fly, enter BY 40 = 00 from the keyboard, then BY 40 = 10, then BY 40 = 20, ... to BY 40 = 0FF. Measure the corresponding analog filtered output voltages at P2.5. We again found that bytes 00, 80, FF gave, respectively, 0.02V, 2.17V, and 4.81V.
3. ESC, reset, and, without executing any program, enter BY 16 = 01, then BY 17 = 00, then BY 17 = 80, then BY 17 = 0FF. Measure the filtered output voltage at P2.5. What's going on? Explain.

NOTE

We often refer to the voltage measuring instrument through-out this book as a VTVM. Please don't purchase a "Vacuum Tube Voltmeter". A VOM or scope will do perfectly. One of the authors goes back in history. VTVM has become his generic term.

EXPERIMENT 5-3

SIMPLE WAVEFORM GENERATION WITH THE PWM D/A UNIT. A RAMP (SAWTOOTH).

In the last experiment the digital byte to be converted was supplied externally (first from the switch bank at P0, then from the keyboard itself). In a sense, Expt. 5-2 was PWM D to A conversion in STATIC mode: externally inputted bytes were changed slowly over "long" time frames and the output analog voltages responded accordingly. In this experiment, we are in a more DYNAMIC situation where the program will itself INTERNALLY generate the bytes for the PWM SFR and change those bytes at a "fast" rate (relative to the changes made on the external bytes in Expt. 5-2). In that way we will realize rapidly changing duty cycles of the output PWM pulse train at P2.5, so that the filter circuit there will generate voltage waveforms varying with time. In other words instantaneous output voltages will be proportional to the instantaneous varying values of duty cycle being generated by the program. The program to generate a ramp (sawtooth) waveform at 2220 follows. Its slope, and therefore period, will be controllable on-the-fly by entering, at will, different bytes at address 5000 while the program is running. The magnitude of those bytes will control the number of output pulses of given width before a change in their width is permitted.

```
        18 00        SP      EQU    18H
        17 00        PWM     EQU    17H
        16 00        IOC1    EQU    16H
        40 00        REG1    EQU    40H
        90 00        TREG    EQU    90H
                     ;
                     ;
2220                         ORG    2220H
                     ;
2220    A1 C0 00 18          LD     SP,#00C0H     ;Initialize SP to 0C0H.
2224    B1 01 16             LDB    IOC1,#01H     ;Load IOC1 with 01H to select PWM
                                                  ;function of P2.5.
2227    B1 00 40             LDB    REG1,#00      ;Initialize REG1 TO 00H.
222A    B0 40 17     RELOAD: LDB    PWM,REG1      ;Load PWM with contents of REG1.
222D    EF 10 00             CALL   TIME          ;Time Delay of 56usec.
2230    17 40                INCB   REG1          ;Increment byte in REG1 for later
                                                  ;load into PWM register.
2232    27 F6                SJMP   RELOAD        ;Go back to re-load PWM.
```

```
                          ;       TIME DELAY ROUTINE:
                          ;
2240                              ORG     2240H
                          ;
2240  B3 01 00 50 90 TIME:        LDB     TREG,5000H[0]   ;Load TREG with byte from memory
                                                          ;address 5000H.
2245  E0 90 FD         TMORE:     DJNZ    TREG,TMORE      ;Decrement TREG If != 0 continue
                                                          ;to decrement.
2248  F0                          RET                     ;Else return.
```

It is essential to remember that the PWM unit outputs a pulse of a given on-time with a period of 64 usec. i.e. the pulse repeats every 64 usec. Therefore, we have to wait 64 usec. before we can output the same, OR A DIFFERENT, value of on-time for the next pulse. If we want a sawtooth waveform, it is clear that one way of accomplishing that would be to have the on-time of the next pulse incremented (by 1, or some other fixed amount), then have another incrementation take place 64 usec. still later, etc. until the PWM register reaches FF, at which point the PWM will start over from 00, generating the ramp. OR, we can have 2, 3, 4, etc. pulses of the SAME width generated, each every 64 usec., THEN an increment in the width is to occur with ANOTHER 2, 3, 4, etc. pulses generated, each every 64 usec. with THAT same width, etc. In this way, by controlling the number of pulses generated of the same width, each spaced 64 usec. apart before the next increment of the on-time occurs for the next group of pulses, we can control the slope of the ramp, and therefore its period.

The above considerations explain the existence of our time delay TIME at 2240 above. Depending on the byte value loaded into TREG (90H) from address 5000 in memory (at run-time), the time delay program will yield 64 usec. between PWM register increments, or 128 usec. between increments, or 192 usec. between increments, etc. In the first case we have one pulse every 64 usec., with each successive one's on-time having been incremented via the PWM. In that case the period of the ramp should be 64 usec. x 256 or about 16 msec. (about 63 Hz). In the second case, we have 2 pulses of the same width, each 64 usec. apart, followed by two more, each having the same incremented value of PWM on-time and each also 64 usec. apart, etc. In that case, the period will be (2 x 64 usec.) x 256 or about 32 msec. (31 Hz) and the slope of the ramp will be 1/2 that in the first instance. In the third case we'll have 3 pulses of the same width, each 64 usec. apart, followed by three more identical ones of incremented width, each 64 usec. apart, etc. This time the period should be (3 x 64 usec.) x 256 or about

48 msec. (21 Hz) and the slope still smaller (1/3 the original slope). Thus we shall consider incrementations (by 1) of the PWM SFR either every 64, 128, or 192 usec.

We come back to the above TIME considerations after we first analyze the main part of the program at 2220. In it, SP is set to 00C0, IOC1 to 01 (to select the PWM function at P2.5) and REG1 to 00. PWM is then loaded with the value in REG1 (remember PWM is a write-only SFR; incrementing PWM directly would imply the need for the RALU to read it first) and TIME is called. It is during this TIME that 1, 2, 3, etc. pulses of the SAME width at the PWM output are permitted to occur (each 64 usec. apart) before a return from TIME permits execution of the INCB REG1 instruction (after the call). The SJMP RELOAD then causes the incremented REG1 to be loaded into PWM to achieve the incremented on-time for each of the NEXT 1, 2, or 3, ... pulses.

The only thing left in the analysis is the calculation of the byte values needed in TREG at 2240 in TIME to generate the 64 usec. or 128 usec. or 192 usec., etc. time delays before another PWM incrementation is allowed. 64 usec. equates to 256 state times (one state time = 3 oscillator periods = 1/4 usec. for a 12MHz clock). The INCB, SJMP, LDB PWM, REG1, and CALL instructions themselves consume 4 + 8 + 4 + 16 = 32 state times before another increment is permitted. This leaves 256 - 32 = 224 state times to be generated by the T.D. There, the LDB and RET instructions take up 12 + 16 = 28 state times which leaves 224 - 28 = 196 state times to be provided by the DJNZ instruction. The latter takes 9 state times. Thus 196/9 = 22 loops on DJNZ must be executed. This will be the case if we enter BY 5000 = 16 at run time, which then is passed to TREG when the program executes.

In the same way, to produce 128 usec. address 5000 should be loaded with 32H i.e. 128 usec. = 512 state times. 512 - 32 - 28 = 452 and 452/9 = 50 dec = 32H. Finally, for 192 usec., 78 dec = 4EH in 5000 would be required (768 - 60 = 708, 708/9 = 78 dec = 4EH).

PROCEDURE

1. Connect the filtered PWM output at P2.5 to the vertical input of a scope. Enter BY 5000 = 16. Execute. Observe a repetitive ramp (sawtooth) waveform. Measure its period. We found 15.6 msec. (not the 16.38 msec. that exact calculation gives i.e. 64 usec. x 256). Probably our RC filter values are responsible for the slight discrepancy. Here the PWM is incremented for EACH new pulse generated.

2. On-the-fly, enter BY 5000 = 32 observe the waveform's slope on the scope is cut in half immediately. Measure the period. We found 31 msec. vs. the expected 128 usec. x 256 = 32.8 msec. This time PWM is incremented after every TWO pulses of identical width are generated.
3. On-the-fly, enter BY 5000 = 4E and observe a change in the ramp's slope to 1/3 its value in (1) above. We measured the period to be 47 msec. vs. the expected 192 usec. x 256 = 49.14 msec. In this case PWM is incremented after every THREE pulses of identical width are generated.

NOTE

In Expt. 6-19 in chapter 6 we come back to this experiment. There, we implement the sawtooth generator as we did here, except the time delay we employ at 2240 here (based on loops) is no longer used. In 6-19, we engage one of the SOFTWARE TIMERS in the High Speed Output Unit (HSO) to produce the necessary time(s) for us. In that way we can free up the processor for "other tasks" (which we do there) and have the selected Software Timer interrupt "other tasks" whenever its time expires. Incrementation of the PWM can take place in the Software Timer Interrupt Routine. The ISR also asks for another Software Timer interrupt after the same desired time interval in the future before returning to "other tasks". The advantages of that approach are clear.

EXPERIMENT 5-4

THE A TO D SFRs: CONVERSION ON ONE CHANNEL. DISPLAY OF RESULTS.

The 8096 has 8 analog input channels (shared with the 8 pins of input port P0). (See chapter 1, section G or pp. 2-15, 2-16 Microcontroller Handbook). The results of the conversion on each channel are 10 bit values. Each conversion requires 168 state times (42 usec. for 12 MHz clock) The input voltages must be in the range 0 to VREF, the latter being the analog reference and supply voltage (nominally at 5 volts). The pertinent SFRs are AD-COMMAND (02H: write-only), AD-RESULT (LO) (02H: read-only) AD-RESULT (HI) (03H: read only). The two RESULT registers are BYTE-READ only. Sometimes, as in Expt. 5-14, we also employ SFRs HSO-COMMAND (06H: write-only) and HSO-TIME (LO) (04H), HSO-TIME (HI) (05H) to control the FUTURE starting time of the A/D conversion. If conversion is to start NOW, they are not necessary. Working with the AD-COMMAND register is sufficient to accomplish that. (HSO-TIME is a word-write only register).

The simple program below is analyzed to see just how the pertinent A/D SFRs are employed in A/D applications with the 8096. Other experiments in this and the next chapters cover other aspects and features of 8096 A/D conversion (such as the "simultaneous" conversion and display of results of several channels; the starting of A/D conversion, not "now" as in this experiment, but at some time in the future; the use of the A/D Conversion Complete INTERRUPT rather than the POLLING of the status bit S in the AD-RESULT (LO) register to ascertain when the converted byte should be read. The program (at 2260) for this experiment is shown below.

```
        18 00           SP       EQU    18H
        02 00           ADCOM    EQU    02H
        02 00           ADRESLO  EQU    02H
        03 00           ADRESHI  EQU    03H
        0F 00           P1       EQU    0FH
        10 00           P2       EQU    10H

                        ;
                        ;
2260                             ORG    2260H
                        ;
2260    A1 C0 00 18              LD     SP,#00C0H       ;Initialize SP to 00C0H.
```

```
2264  B1 08 02   DOOVER: LDB   ADCOM,#08H       ;Load 08 into A/D Command Reg. which
                                                ;starts A/D conversion on CH. 0.
2267  FD                 NOP                    ;Eight state delay for conversion
2268  FD                 NOP                    ;to start.
2269  3B 02 FD   ADBUSY: JBS   ADRESLO,3,ADBUSY;If Status bit = 1, continue polling.
226C  B0 03 0F           LDB   P1,ADRESHI       ;Else output upper 8 bits of conversion
                                                ;result to LEDs at P1.
226F  B0 02 10           LDB   P2,ADRESLO       ;and output lower 2 bits (D1,D0) to
                                                ;LEDs at P2.7, P2.6.
2272  27 F0              SJMP  DOOVER           ;Loop back to repeat conversion.
```

The first instruction at 2260 initializes the SP. The next instruction is crucial: it loads 08 into the AD-COMMAND SFR. What this does is select channel 0 (the low 3 bits in ADCOM specify one of the 8 channels 0, 1, ...7), and asks for conversion to be initiated "now", at that channel. GO = 1 (bit 3 in ADCOM) requests that conversion start "now", (GO = 0 would ask that conversion should be started by the HSO unit at a FUTURE specified time - see Expt. 5-14). It is very important to bear in mind that every time a conversion is complete and a new one is to be started on any channel, the AD-COMMAND register MUST be written to again. Even though GO = 1 may already have been written to bit 3 of ADCOM, it is necessary to REWRITE a 1 to that bit to start a new conversion "now". It's evidently the 0 to 1 TRANSITION which a "Write 1" at that bit produces that is responsible for the initiation of conversion "now" (we'll prove that in this experiment - see PROCEDURE).

The two NOPs that follow provide the 8 state times necessary before testing whether conversion is complete i.e. 8 state times may be needed before conversion starts. At that point we can safely test the status bit S (bit 3 in the AD-RESULT LO register) to see whether conversion is complete. As long as S is high conversion is in progress and the JBS ADRESLO,3,ADBUSY instruction just loops on itself in a wait mode. When S signals 0, conversion is over (A/D idle) and we fall through JBS to the next instruction at 226C. There we load P1 (LEDs) with the HI byte of the AD-RESULT register and P2.7, P2.6 with the two high bits of AD-RESULT/LO register (LED's were connected to P2.7 and P2.6 of port P2). Thus the hi-byte of the 10-bit result is seen at the 8 LEDs at P1 and the least 2 significant bits of the result are displayed at P2.7, P2.6. The next instruction jumps back to 2264 (DOOVER) to initiate another conversion on channel 0.

We employed a variable 0 to 1K POT, using the 5 volts available on the iSBE-96, to generate the required 0 to 5V analog voltages for channel 0 (ACH.0 at P0.0).

PROCEDURE

1. With the POT connected to channel 0 at P0.0 (ACH.0) execute (G FR 2260) and vary the analog voltage on the POT. Observe the 10-bit result vary accordingly at P1's 8 LEDs and at the 2 LEDs P2.7, P2.6. As the POT output varies from 0 to 5V, you should observe ten 0s at the LEDs vary up to ten 1s there. Measure the voltage across the POT with a VTVM as you vary it and correlate it with the 10-bit digital result. You should, of course, observe 3FF for 5V input. Do you observe 1FF for 2.5V input and 0FF for 1.25V input? How's the linearity?
2. ESC. Enter BY 2265 = 09. This changes the 08 there to 09 and now asks for conversion at channel 1. Connect the POT's output voltage to P0.1 (ACH.1). Execute the modified program and observe the A/D results at (P1, P2.7, P2.6) vary as you vary the input voltage from the POT at ACH.1.
3. ESC. Replace F0 at 2273 with F3 (BY 2273 = 0F3), which means SJMP DOOVER is to loop back to 2267 (NOP) rather than to 2264 (DOOVER). Execute and observe the conversion value at the LEDs corresponding to your POT setting at channel 1. Vary the POT. No changes will be observed at the LEDs. What's your conclusion?

EXPERIMENT 5-5

A/D CONVERSION ON TWO CHANNELS. MULTIPLEXING AND DISPLAYING THE RESULTS

In this experiment, we'll alternately convert channel 0 and channel 1, saving their updated results in REG0 and REG1 (40 and 50). Before jumping back to update the conversions on both channels, switch S7 at port 0 (P0.7) is polled. If it's hi, channel 1's result in REG1 is output to P1's LEDs, if lo channel 0's result in REG0 is displayed at P1. (For simplicity, we are only displaying bits 9-2 of the result i.e. the value in AD-RESULT/HI). After the display of one or the other channel's results, an SJMP back to START initiates a new conversion on first one, then the other channel. Thus as the voltages on either or both channels vary, we can always select one or the other for display of updated results by simply throwing S7 at P0.7 hi or lo. The program at 2280 follows. Two 5V 0 to 1K POTS are used, one at channel 0's input, the other at channel 1's.

```
      18 00         SP       EQU    18H
      02 00         ADCOM    EQU    02H
      02 00         ADRESLO  EQU    02H
      03 00         ADRESHI  EQU    03H
      40 00         REG0     EQU    40H
      50 00         REG1     EQU    50H
      0E 00         P0       EQU    0EH
      0F 00         P1       EQU    0FH
                    ;
                    ;
2280                         ORG    2280H
                    ;
2280  A1 C0 00 18            LD     SP,#00C0H         ;Initialize SP to 00C0H.
2284  B1 08 02      START:   LDB    ADCOM,#08H        ;Load ADCOM with 08H to start
                                                      ;conversion on CH 0.
2287  FD                     NOP                      ;Delay Eight State times for conversion
2288  FD                     NOP                      ;to start.
2289  3B 02 FD      CH0BSY:  JBS    ADRESLO,3,CH0BSY;If A/D busy bit (S) = 1,then continue
                                                      ;to poll busy bit.
228C  B0 03 40               LDB    REG0,ADRESHI      ;Else load upper 8 bits of result into
                                                      ;REG0.
228F  B1 09 02               LDB    ADCOM,#09H        ;Start conversion on CH 1.
2292  FD                     NOP                      ;Delay Eight State times for conversion
2293  FD                     NOP                      ;to start.
```

```
2294  3B 02 FD   CH1BSY: JBS    ADRESLO,3,CH1BSY;If A/D BUSY BIT = 1, then continue
                                                ;to poll busy bit.
2297  B0 03 50           LDB    REG1,ADRESHI    ;ELse load upper 8 bits of result into
                                                ;REG1.
                 ; RESULT DISPLAY
229A  3F 0E 05           JBS    P0,7,CHAN1      ;IF P0.7 = 1, then goto display CH1.
229D  B0 40 0F   CHAN0:  LDB    P1,REG0         ;Else display CH0 result on LEDs.
22A0  27 E2              SJMP   START           ;Go back to repeat conversions.
22A2  B0 50 0F   CHAN1:  LDB    P1,REG1         ;Display CH1 result on LEDs.
22A5  27 DD              SJMP   START           ;Go back to repeat conversions.
```

The analysis of the above program is quite straitforward. LDB ADCOM, #08 selects channel 0 for conversion "now". After waiting 8 state times for conversion to start, the S bit in AD-RESULT (LO) - bit 3 - is tested. When it indicates 0, conversion is over. The high byte of channel 0's conversion result in AD-RESULT (HI) is stored in REG0. Then LDB ADCOM, #09 asks for immediate conversion on channel 1. Again 8 state times pass and the S bit is again tested as to whether conversion is over. When S reports a 0, we fall through and store the high byte of channel 1's conversion result from AD-RESULT (HI) to REG1. We next test bit 7 at P0 (switch S7). If it's low we fall through to CHAN0 where channel 0's result (hi-byte) is output from REG0 to the LEDs at P1. The program then jumps back to START at 2284 where channel 0 and then channel 1 are again converted. The updated results are again saved in REG0 and REG1, respectively. If, however, S7 was high, JBS P0, 7 jumps to CHAN1 where REG1 (hi byte of channel 1's conversion result) is output to P1's LEDs. The program then jumps back to START to initiate new conversions on both channels and store the updated results in REG0 and REG1.

PROCEDURE

Adjust the POTs at channel 0 and channel 1 to different settings. Execute the program from 2280. Throw S7 lo, then hi to see first channel 0's, then channel 1's hi-byte conversion results on the LEDs at P1. For a given setting of S7 (either hi or lo) vary the corresponding channel's voltage from the POT and observe P1's LEDs vary accordingly. Then flip S7 to the other position and vary the other POT's output voltage. Observe that particular channel's hi-byte result on the LEDs. Remember, S7 lo chooses channel 0's conversion result for display at P1, S7 hi chooses channel 1's result for display at P1.

EXPERIMENT 5-6

WORKING WITH PORT P2 (SFR 10) IN ITS "REGULAR FUNCTION" MODE.

Port 2 (P2:SFR 10) operates in a "regular function" mode in which its pins act as ordinary input, output, or quasi-bidirectional pins; or in an "alternate function" mode in which 6 of the pins can have "alternate" roles or functions. These "regular" and "alternate" function pin assignments are summarized below. (see also pp. 2-20, 2-21 Microcontroller Handbook or sections L and M or chapter 1).

P2.0	Regular: output.	Alternate: Serial TXD.	Control bit: IOC1.5
P2.1	Regular: input.	Alternate: Serial RXD.	Control bit: none
P2.2	Regular: input.	Alternate: EXTINT.	Control bit: IOC1.1
P2.3	Regular: input.	Alternate: T2CLK.	Control bit: IOC0.7
P2.4	Regular: input.	Alternate: T2RST.	Control bit: IOC0.5
P2.5	Regular: output.	Alternate: PWM.	Control bit: IOC1.0
P2.6	Always a quasi-bidirectional pin.		
P2.7	Always a quasi-bidirectional pin.		

Thus, setting bit IOC1.1 = 0 selects P2.2 as the input for EXTINT. Setting it to 1 allows P2.2 to be a regular input pin. (We've worked with P2.2 as EXTINT source in chapter 4). Setting IOC1.5 = 1 will allow P2.0 to act as the transmit line (TXD) in serial I/O (we'll use TXD in chapter 8 on Serial I/O). Setting bit IOC0.7 to 0 selects P2.3 for use as the clock source for Timer2 (this we do in Expt. 5-7 and elsewhere). Setting IOC0.5 to 0 selects P2.4 for use as a reset source for Timer2 (this we do in Expt. 5-7 and elsewhere). And, finally, setting IOC1.0 to 1 selects P2.5 as a PWM (pulse train) output pin (we've already employed it in that sense in Expt. 5-2, 5-3 on PWM). Doing the opposite of all the above at IOC0 or IOC1 causes the pins in question to revert to their regular output or input mode functions, as specified in the table above. Pin P2.1 needs no "doing" - it can be a regular input pin in the usual digital sense or it can convey RXD serial I/O input receive pulses (as in chapter 8). The source of its input is immaterial. Pins P2.6 and 2.7 have no alternate functions - they're always quasi-bidirectional pins. For information on quasi-bidirectional pins consult section 2.12.2 p. 2-20 and sections 4.2.1, 4.2.2 pp. 4-5, 4-6 of the Microcontroller Handbook. See also section M, chapter 1 in this book.

The following experiment illustrates the use of P2's pins in their regular, non-alternate function mode i.e. as ordinary input or output pins, as the case may be, conveying "ordinary" digital bits. Note that SFR P0 (0E) is a byte-read (only) SFR (input port) while SFRs 10 (P2) and P1 (0F) can be byte-written or byte-read. (As stated above, we've already worked with pins P2.2 and P2.5 in their alternate modes; we'll be working with pins P2.3, P2.4 in their ALTERNATE modes in Expt. 5-7 and beyond. Pin P2.0 will be used in its alternate mode (TXD serial transmit) in chapter 8 on Serial I/O, and pin P2.1 will be used as the RXD Serial I/O input there as well). The experiment is divided into parts A, B, and C. Their programs are shown below:

```
        0F 00        P1      EQU     0FH
        10 00        P2      EQU     10H
        15 00        IOC0    EQU     15H
        16 00        IOC1    EQU     16H
                     ;
                     ;
                     ;       EXPT. 5-6.
                     ;
                     ;       PART A): Input Function Of P2.1
                     ;
2300                         ORG     2300H
                     ;
2300    31 10 05     HERE1:  JBC     P2,1,THERE1      ;If P2.1 = 0, goto THERE1
2303    B1 AA 0F             LDB     P1,#0AAH         ;Else output 0AAH to LEDs.
2306    27 F8                SJMP    HERE1            ;Go back to continue polling P2.1
2308    B1 55 0F     THERE1: LDB     P1,#55H          ;P2.1 = 0, output 55H to LEDs.
230B    27 F3                SJMP    HERE1            ;Go back to continue polling P2.1
                     ;
                     ;
                     ;       EXPT. 5-6.
                     ;
                     ;       PART B): Input Function Of P2.3 And P2.4
                     ;
2310                         ORG     2310H
                     ;
2310    B1 A0 15             LDB     IOC0,#0A0H       ;Load 0A0H into IOC0 to select
                                                      ;input mode for P2.3 AND P2.4.
2313    3B 10 05     HERE2:  JBS     P2,3,THERE2      ;If P2.3 = 1, goto THERE2.
2316    B1 BB 0F             LDB     P1,#0BBH         ;Else, output 0BBH to LEDs.
2319    27 F8                SJMP    HERE2            ;Go back to poll P2.3.
231B    B1 40 0F     THERE2: LDB     P1,#40H          ;P2.3 = 0, output 40H to LEDs.
231E    27 F3                SJMP    HERE2            ;Go back to poll P2.3.
                     ;
                     ;
                     ;       EXPT. 5-6.
                     ;
                     ;       PART C);  Output Functions Of P2.0 and P2.5
```

```
                                ;
2330                                     ORG     2330H
                                ;
2330    B1 00 16                         LDB     IOC1,#00     ;Load 00 into IOC1 to select P2.0
                                                              ;and P2.5 as outputs.
2333    B1 21 10                         LDB     P2,#21H      ;Output 21H to P2 to make P2.0 and
                                                              ;P2.5 = 1.
2336    27 FE                   STOP:    SJMP    STOP         ;Loop here.
```

In part (A) above (at 2300) we poll input pin P2.1 in its regular function mode (an input pin). As noted before, no control register manipulation is needed to distinguish between P2.1's regular (input) mode or its alternate function (Serial I/O RXD input) mode. With a debounced switch S serving as an input to P2.1, the above program polls S (JBC P2, 1) and, if it's low, jumps to THERE1 where 55 is output to P1's LEDs. An SJMP back to HERE1 then polls P2.1 again. If, and when, P2.1 goes high, a fall-through (JBC) occurs and AA is output to P1 and the ensuing SJMP brings us back to another polling of P2.1. PROCEDURE: Execute (G FR 2300). Throw S hi/lo etc. and observe P1 alternate between AA and 55.

In part (B) we wish to use pins P2.3 and P2.4 as ordinary input pins, rather than in their alternate function roles (T2CLK and T2RST, respectively). To accomplish that requires loading IOC0 with A0. This sets both IOC0.7 and IOC0.5 to 1, thereby NOT selecting P2.3 and P2.4 in their T2CLK, T2RST alternate function roles. This time we'll employ the debounced switch S at P2.3. The program at 2310 in (B) above loads A0 into IOC0, then polls P2.3, jumping to THERE2 if S is high, where 40 is output to P1. If S is low, fall-through to 2316 occurs where BB is output to P1. In either case SJMP HERE2 follows, so that P2.3 can be polled again. PROCEDURE: Execute (G FR 2310). Throw S hi/lo etc. and observe P1 alternate between 40 and BB. Then re-do with S connected to P2.4. The JBS instruction should now be JBS P2, 4, THERE2. You can accomplish this by simply entering BY 2313 = 3C to replace the 3B presently there. Execute and again observe P1 alternate between 40 and BB as S is thrown hi/lo.

In part (C) (program at 2330) we wish to output to pins P2.0 and P2.5 in their "non-alternate" pin modes. To do this requires loading IOC1 with 00 to make IOC1.0 = 0 and IOC1.5 = 0, thus selecting P2.5 and P2.0 in their NON PWM and TXD roles, respectively. The first instruction does that. The LDB P2, #21 instruction outputs 21 to P2 which should turn on LEDs placed at P2.5 and P2.0, respectively. The program then halts. ESC and enter BY 16 = 21 into IOC1, (which places 1s at IOC1.5

and IOC1.0, thereby selecting P2.5 and P2.0 in their alternate function roles of TXD and PWM, respectively). Execute from 2333 (by-passing the LDB of IOC1 with 00 at 2330). We'll not now succeed in turning on the LEDs at P2.5 and P2.0 because those pins are now defined as PWM and TXD pins, rather than as simple output pins. PROCEDURE: Execute from 2330 and observe LEDs at P2.5 and P2.0 go on. ESC. Enter BY 16 = 21. Execute from 2333. The LEDs do not go on.

EXPERIMENT 5-7

EVENT COUNTING WITH TIMER2. USING T2CLK (OR HSI.1) AS TIMER2 CLOCK SOURCE AND T2RST (OR HSI.0) AS TIMER2 RESET SOURCE.

In this experiment we work with SFR 0CH (Timer2). Refer to pp. 2-11, 2-12 Microcontroller Handbook or section I of chapter 1 in this book (in particular Fig. 2-13).

In part (A) of the experiment we connect a debounced switch to the T2CLK pin of the 8096 (pin P2.3 in the alternate mode) and another one to the T2RST pin (P2.4 in the alternate mode). Any 0 to 1 OR 1 to 0 transitions at the T2CLK input increments the value in word SFR 0CH i.e. Timer2. Timer2 thus counts 0 to 1 and 1 to 0 events. Any 0 to 1 transition at the T2RST input will clear (reset) the value in Timer2 to 0. Control register IOC0 plays a vital role [in part (B) below as well as part (A)]. To select T2CLK as T2's event source, IOC0.7 must be set to 0 (a 1 there would select the HSI.1 input pin as T2's event source). To select T2RST as T2's reset source requires that IOC0.5 be set to 0 (a 1 would select the HSI.0 input pin as the reset source for T2). In order that EITHER T2RST or HSI.0 (both EXTERNAL reset sources) be the source for resetting T2, IOC0.3 must be set to 1 (otherwise both those possible external T2 reset sources are disabled). And finally, in order to make sure that T2 is cleared (by software) at the start of the program, one must set IOC0.1 to 1. (EACH time a 1 is WRITTEN to IOC0.1, T2 is cleared; the fact that you wrote out a 1 there previously, cleared it PREVIOUSLY. A NEW write of a 1 there is needed to clear T2 again). Thus the byte 0A loaded into IOC0 will accomplish all of the above. The program (at 2350) is shown below.

```
        18 00           SP      EQU     18H
        15 00           IOCO    EQU     15H
        40 00           REG1    EQU     40H
        0F 00           P1      EQU     0FH
        0C 00           TIMER2  EQU     0CH
                        ;
                        ;
2350                            ORG     2350H
                        ;
2350    A1 C0 00 18             LD      SP,#00C0H       ;Initialize SP to 00C0H.
2354    B1 0A 15                LDB     IOC0,#0AH       ;Load 0AH into IOC0 to select T2CLK
                                                        ;and T2RST functions of P2.3 and P2.4
```

```
                                                  ;respectively; resets T2 to 0.
2357   A0 0C 40      COUNT:  LD      REG1,TIMER2   ;Load REG1 with count in TIMER2.
235A   B0 40 0F              LDB     P1,REG1       ;Output lo-byte of count to LEDs.
235D   27 F8                 SJMP    COUNT         ;Go back to display count.
```

In the program above, SP is set to 00C0 and 0A is loaded into IOC0 for the reasons explained above. The word count in Timer2 is loaded into REG1 so that the low byte (low order count) of REG1 can be output to the LEDs at P1. (Timer2 can not be byte read, only word read, hence the use of REG1 as an intermediary). SJMP loops back to count to continually poll the count in T2.

PROCEDURE (PART A)

Execute (G FR 2350). Create events at T2CLK by throwing and releasing the debounced switch connected there. Observe the count-up at P1's LEDs. Note that each 0 to 1 OR 1 to 0 transition at the switch increments the count in T2. Reset T2 every once in a while by throwing the switch at T2RST high. The count is reset as evidenced by P1 clearing. A new count-up commences there.

In part (B) we wish to use HSI.1 and HSI.0 as sources for T2's events and T2's reset, respectively. This is easily accomplished by changing IOC0.7 to 1 and IOC0.5 to 1. Thus AA is now needed for IOC0. That can most easily be realized by entering BY 2355 = 0AA (replacing 0A there - see the object code in the program print-out). Please NOTE: HSI.1 and HSI.0 can be used as T2's clock and reset sources, respectively, WITHOUT IOC0.0 or IOC0.2 being set to 1. Setting those bits to 1 is NECESSARY when input events at the HSI.0 and HSI.1 input pins are to be recorded in the FIFO of the High Speed Input (HSI) unit (more on that later in this chapter when we treat the HSI unit). Here we are using HSI.1 and HSI.0 in an ALTERNATE role. Note also that HSI.0 need NOT be enabled into the HSI unit (IOC0.0 = 1 not necessary) when using it as a source of external interrupts, as we did in chapter 4.

PROCEDURE (PART B)

Connect debounced switches to input pins HSI.0 and HSI.1. With the program AS IS, execute and attempt inputting events at HSI.1. No count-up takes place at P1. IOC0.7 = 0 has selected T2CLK as T2's count source. ESC. Enter BY 2355 = 0AA. Execute and input events from the switch at HSI.1. The count-up is tracked at P1. Periodically clear the count by throwing HSI.0 high and then starting with new events input from HSI.1. AA at 2355 enables HSI.1 as T2's source of. events and HSI.0 as T2's external reset.

EXPERIMENT 5-8

TIMER2 OVERFLOW. T2CLK DRIVEN BY 6000 Hz CLOCK GENERATED AT P2.7

FORMULATION

1. We shall force event counter T2 (SFR 0CH) into overflow by driving T2CLK (P2.3) with a 6000 Hz square wave generated at P2.7. The period being 1/6 msec., during which 2 counts are registered in T2 (0 to 1 and 1 to 0 transitions), it will take 32,768 periods for T2 to reach overflow from a reset condition, i.e. in 32,768 x 1/6 msec. = about 5.5 sec. The 6000 Hz clock at P2.7 is programmably accomplished by simply turning P2.7 on, calling a 1/12 msec. time delay, turning P2.7 off, calling the 1/12 msec. time delay again, etc.
2. Hi-byte of T2's count-up under the above driving conditions will be viewed at P1's LEDs. It should take about 5.5 sec. for P1 to read out FF before the next P2.7 transition causes T2 to overflow to 00 and P1 to read 00.
3. When T2 does overflow it will generate a Timer Overflow interrupt (we enable bit 0 in the interrupt mask register and set IOC1.3 to 1 and IOC1.2 to 0, thereby unmasking the Timer Overflow interrupt source and selecting T2OV rather than T1OV as the source of such overflow interrupts. Remember, T1 is free-running and will overflow every 65,536 x 2 usec. = 131 msec. We don't want to "hear" any interrupts from it). The Timer Overflow interrupt vectors to our ISR via entry address 2000 in the 8096's interrupt location table. There we "freeze" the count at P1 at 00 (overflow has occurred) as long as switch S0 at P0.0 is maintained low. When S0 is thrown high, we return to the main program from the ISR and count-ups from 00 in T2 proceed again.

The program is presented below and an analysis of it is given at its conclusion. It starts at 2400.

```
18 00        SP      EQU    18H
08 00        MINT    EQU    08H
09 00        PINT    EQU    09H
16 00        IOC1    EQU    16H
15 00        IOCO    EQU    15H
10 00        P2      EQU    10H
0F 00        P1      EQU    0FH
0E 00        P0      EQU    0EH
```

```
        40 00           REG1     EQU     40H
        41 00           REG1HI   EQU     41H
        0C 00           TIMER2   EQU     0CH
        90 00           TREG     EQU     90H
        60 00           TEMP     EQU     60H
        00 20           INVEC    EQU     2000H
                        ;
                        ;
2400                             ORG     2400H
                        ;
2400    A1 C0 00 18              LD      SP,#00C0H          ;Initialize SP to 00C0H.
2404    11 09                    CLRB    PINT               ;Clear all pending interrupts.
2406    B1 01 08                 LDB     MINT,#01H          ;Load 01 into MINT to enable
                                                            ;timer overflow interrupt.
2409    B1 08 16                 LDB     IOC1,#08H          ;Load 08H into IOC1 to enable
                                                            ;TIMER2 overflow interrupt.
240C    A1 50 24 60              LD      TEMP,#2450H        ;Load address of TIMER2 overflow
                                                            ;interrupt service routine.
2410    C3 01 00 20 60           ST      TEMP,INVEC[0]      ;into INT Vector Table.
2415    B1 0A 15                 LDB     IOC0,#0AH          ;Load 0AH into IOC1 to select
                                                            ;T2CLK AND T2RST functions of
                                                            ;P2.3 and P2.4, respectively,
                                                            ;and resets T2 to 0.
2418    FA              THERE:   DI                         ;Disable global interrupt bit.
2419    B1 80 10                 LDB     P2,#80H            ;Set P2.7 equal to 1.
241C    EF 21 00                 CALL    TIME               ;1/12 msec. time delay.
241F    B1 00 10                 LDB     P2,#00             ;Output 0 to P2.7.
2422    EF 1B 00                 CALL    TIME               ;1/12 msec. time delay.
2425    A0 0C 40                 LD      REG1,TIMER2        ;Load REG1 with current count in TIMER2
2428    FB                       EI                         ;Enable global interrupt bit.
2429    B0 41 0F                 LDB     P1,REG1HI          ;Output hi-byte of TIMER2 count to LEDs
242C    27 EA                    SJMP    THERE              ;Go back to generate another clock.
                        ;
                        ;
                        ;        TIME DELAY ROUTINE:

2440                             ORG     2440H
                        ;
2440    B3 01 00 50 90  TIME:    LDB     TREG,5000H[0]      ;Load TREG with byte from memory
                                                            ;location 5000 (LOADED AT RUNTIME).
2445    E0 90 FD        TMORE:   DJNZ    TREG,TMORE         ;Decrement TREG until it = 0.
2448    F0                       RET                        ;Then return.
                        ;
                        .
```

```
                        ;       TIMER2 OVERFLOW INTERRUPT SERVICE ROUTINE:
                        ;
2450                            ORG     2450H
                        ;
2450    30 0E FD        WAIT:   JBC     P0,0,WAIT       ;If P0.0 = 0, loop back to poll.
2453    F0                      RET                     ;Else return.
```

First, let's indicate how the time delay at TIME (2440) can be made to generate 1/12 msec. (used for both on-time and for off-time). One DJNZ loop (on itself) requires 9 state times. The LDB and RET instructions (for external memory fetches) require 28 state times together. A quick calculation will show that 34 DJNZ loops, added to the 28 state times, gives the 334 state times needed for 83.5 usec. or about 1/12 msec. Thus 22H entered at 5000H at run-time will give the required 1/12 msec. from TIME. Of course, you can enter any other value at 5000H at run-time to achieve whatever time you need (up to about 0.5 msec.). Remember, 1 state time = 1/4 usec. at 12 MHz.

Coming back to the main program above, the first 3 lines of code are needed in view of the discussion in (3) of the formulation preceeding the program. Next, 2450 is loaded into 2000H (INVEC) which is the vector entry address for a TOV interrupt. Our TOV (really T2OV) ISR is to commence at 2450. LDB IOC0, #0AH is necessary to 1) reset T2 to 00 (IOC0.1 = 1), 2) select T2CLK and T2RST as the clock and external reset sources for T2 (IOC0.7 = IOC0.5 = 0), 3) enable T2's external reset facility (IOC0.3 = 1). We next disable the interrupt global bit, set P2.7 to 1 for 1/12 msec., then turn it off for 1/12 msec. This will yield the 1/6 msec. period needed for our clock source at P2.7 to drive T2CLK at P2.3. With another period thus realized, we read out T2's count into REG1, enable the global bit, read out the hi-byte of T2's count (from REG1HI) at P1's LEDs and jump back to THERE to generate another P2.7 cycle. (The experiment would probably work as well had we placed EI at 2418 and left a NOP at 2428. Try that later).

When a T2OV interrupt is generated upon T2 overflow (after 5.5 sec.), it will be acknowledged just before the SJMP at 242C is executed. The program then vectors to the Timer2 ISR at 2450. At this point T2 is 00 and P1's LEDs should indicate the same. The JBC instruction at 2450 is simply a wait as long as switch S0 at P0.0 is maintained low. Fall-through to RET will occur when we throw S0 high. The return to the main program at 242C generates P2.7 clocks anew and T2 counts up again from its 00 overflow state. The scenario repeats at the end of another 5.5 sec.

PROCEDURE

1. Connect P2.7's output to P2.3's input (T2CLK in its alternate function). Connect a debounced switch to P2.4 (T2RST in its alternate function). Enter BY 5000 = 22 to set TIME for 1/12 msec. Make sure S0 at P0.0 is low.
2. Execute (G FR 2400). Observe the LEDs at P1 count up the high byte of T2's count. Before P1 reaches FF reset it to 00 every so often by throwing the switch at T2RST high. After each reset of T2, the count-up proceeds anew.
3. Let the count at P1 proceed. You'll see P1 reach FF after 5.5 sec. (verify), then overflow to 00. At this point 00 remains "frozen" on the display (P1s LEDs) proving that we're in the T2OV ISR at 2450 (WAIT) with S0 low.
4. Throw S0 high, then low. You'll immediately see count-up start over from 00 and reach FF (then overflow) after another 5.5 sec. Steps (3) and (4) repeat.
5. ESC and place EI at 2418 and NOP at 2428 i.e. BY 2418 = 0FB, BY 2428 = 0FD. Execute. Do you get the same results as before?

This experiment has dealt with Timer Overflow interrupts generated by Timer2 overflows. The next experiment deals with such interrupts generated by Timer1 overflows. Remember, the IOC1.3 and IOC1.2 bits decide which, if either, of those overflow interrupt sources for Timer Overflow is to be enabled, or whether both are to be enabled (as in Expt. 5-10).

EXPERIMENT 5-9

DEMONSTRATING TIMER1 OVERFLOW

Timer1, unlike T2, is free-running. It is one of the word (read) SFRs (0AH) and is clocked every 8 state times (2 usec. for 12 MHz clock). Hence it overflows every 65,536 x 2 usec. = 131 msec. It can be cleared only by executing a reset.

The program at 2500 below merely initializes the relevant parameters and then loops on itself (SJMP HERE), simulating "busy tasks". Every 131 msec. T1 overflows and, since the T1 overflow interrupt has been enabled, this will cause an interrupt vector to our Timer1 Overflow ISR at 2520. There, REG1 is incremented and its low byte output to the LEDs at P1 before returning to "busy tasks". Thus P1 counts up, in binary fashion, at 131 msec. intervals, the number of T1 overflows (interrupts). It should, therefore, take 131 msec. x 256 = 33.5 sec. for P1 to reach FF before starting over from 00. Further analysis of the program shown below is given at its conclusion.

```
        18 00           SP      EQU     18H
        40 00           REG1    EQU     40H
        08 00           MINT    EQU     08H
        09 00           PINT    EQU     09H
        16 00           IOC1    EQU     16H
        50 00           TEMP    EQU     50H
        00 20           INVEC   EQU     2000H
        0F 00           P1      EQU     0FH
                        ;
                        ;
2500                            ORG     2500H
                        ;
2500    A1 C0 00 18             LD      SP,#00C0H       ;Initialize SP to 00C0H.
2504    01 40                   CLR     REG1            ;Clear word REG1.
2506    FA                      DI                      ;Disable global interrupt bit.
2507    11 09                   CLRB    PINT            ;Clear all pending interrupts.
2509    B1 01 08                LDB     MINT,#01H       ;Load 01H into MINT to enable timer
                                                        ;overflow interrupts.
250C    B1 04 16                LDB     IOC1,#04H       ;Load 04H into IOC1 reg. to enable
                                                        ;TIMER1 Overflow interrupts.
250F    A1 20 25 50             LD      TEMP,#2520H     ;Load address of TIMER1 overflow
                                                        ;Interrupt Service Routine into
2513    C3 01 00 20 50          ST      TEMP,INVEC[0]   ;INT Vector Table.
2518    FB                      EI                      ;Enable global interrupt bit.
2519    27 FE           HERE:   SJMP    HERE            ;Loop here.
```

```
                  ;      TIMER1 OVERFLOW INTERRUPT SERVICE ROUTINE:
                  ;
2520                     ORG     2520H
                  ;
2520   07 40             INC     REG1         ;Increment REG1 on every overflow
                                              ;(0.131 seconds)
2522   B0 40 0F          LDB     P1,REG1      ;Output count of overflows to LEDs.
2525   F0                RET                  ;Return to main routine.
                  ;
2526                     END
```

After SP is set to 00C0 at 2500, REG1 is cleared (it will count the number of T1 overflows). DI and CLRB PINT make sure that no interrupts from T1OV can occur from previous T1 overflows that may have become pendings. LDB MINT sets interrupt mask bit 0 to 1 to enable the Timer Overflow interrupt source. LDB IOC1,#04 sets bit IOC1.2 to 1 to enable the T1OV interrupt source and disable the T2OV interrupt source (IOC1.3 = 0). 2520 (ISR address) is next loaded into INVEC (2000H), which is Timer Overflow's interrupt vector entry location in the interrupt table of the 8096. EI allows T1OV interrupts to now be honored and SJMP HERE loops on itself, simulating "busy tasks". The T1OV ISR at 2520 increments REG1, outputs its count to P1 and returns to "busy loop" at 2519.

PROCEDURE

Execute from 2500 and observe P1 increment at 131 msec. intervals. Record the time for P1 to reach FF before it overflows. It should be about 33.5 sec.

EXPERIMENT 5-10

POLLING SPECIAL FUNCTION REGISTER IOS1 (16H) FOR THE SOURCE (T1 OR T2) OF TIMER OVERFLOW

FORMULATION

1. In this experiment, we are going to allow both T1 and T2 overflows to cause interrupts at the Timer Overflow source. It will then be a question of polling bits 4 and 5 in the SFR Status Register IOS1 (16H) to determine which source, T1OV or T2OV, was responsible for the interrupt to the Timer Overflow ISR. The polling, of course, will be done in the TOV ISR.
2. To generate T2 overflows, we'll generate on/off pulses at P2.7 with on-time of 1 usec. and off-time of 3 usec. (period = 4 usec). P2.7 will drive T2CLK (pin P2.3 in the alternate mode) to cause count-up of events in T2, which will ultimately overflow. One cycle of P2.7 (on/off) generates 2 counts in T2 (0 to 1 and 1 to 0) transitions). Overflow will thus require 32,768 cycles from P2.7 into T2CLK, since 2 counts per cycle are generated. Since the P2.7 oscillation period will be 4 usec. it will require 32,768 x 4 usec. or 131 msec. of time before T2 overflows. How we'll arrange for 1 usec. on and 3 usec. off-times at P2.7 will be explained below.
3. T1 is free-running. It overflows every 131 msec. as we've seen before. Thus we have arranged for T1 and T2 to EACH overflow every 131 msec., but clearly out of phase, as T2 will start from a reset condition when the program executes, and T1 can be anywhere between 0000 and FFFF at that time.
4. The 1 usec. on-time at P2.7 is generated by the instruction ORB P2, #80H, which turns P2.7 on in the program at 256A below. It requires 4 state times (1 usec.) and is immediately followed by ANDB P2, #7FH which turns P2.7 off. The latter also consumes 4 state times (1 usec). The SJMP DRIVE at 2570 in the program takes 8 state times (2 usec.) before ORB P2, #80H again turns P2.7 on. Hence, 1 usec. on and 1 + 2 = 3 usec. off, or a period of 4 usec.
5. Whenever one or the other timer causes an interrupt, due to overflow, the ISR at 2580, to which we're vectored, will immediately poll IOS1 (SFR 16H) to determine the source of the overflow. If it was T1OV then bit 5 in IOS1 would have been set; if it was T2OV then IOSI.4 would be set. If it was a T1OV, we output 01 to the LEDs at P1. If it was a T2OV, we output 02 to the LEDs. That means

we should observe LED bits P1.1 and P1.0 oscillate back and forth at about 0.13 sec. intervals. Depending on the value in T1 when the program is executed, we can have the following three extremes: first T1, then T2 overflow, one behind the other, in which case 01 is seen for a very short time followed by 02 for 0.13 sec., followed by 01 for a very short time etc; or T1 and T2 overflow at more equally spaced intervals, in which case 01 and 02 alternate at roughly equal times. Or, T2, then immediately T1, overflow, in which case 02 is seen for a very short time, then 01 for 0.13 sec.

6. After the polling of IOS1 in TOV's ISR routine, and the taking of appropriate action (01 or 02 output to P1), the ISR returns to the main program to continue driving of P2.7 on/off as the clock source for T2 (through T2CLK).

The program starting at 2550 is given below.

```
        18 00          SP      EQU     18H
        09 00          PINT    EQU     09H
        08 00          MINT    EQU     08H
        15 00          IOC0    EQU     15H
        16 00          IOC1    EQU     16H
        16 00          IOS1    EQU     16H
        40 00          TEMP    EQU     40H
        00 20          INVEC   EQU     2000H
        50 00          REG     EQU     50H
        0F 00          P1      EQU     0FH
        10 00          P2      EQU     10H
                       ;
                       ;
2550                           ORG     2550H
                       ;
2550    A1 C0 00 18            LD      SP,#00C0H        ;Initialize SP to 00C0H.
2554    FA                     DI                       ;Disable global interrupt bit.
2555    11 09                  CLRB    PINT             ;Clear all pending interrupts.
2557    B1 01 08               LDB     MINT,#01H        ;Load 01 into MINT to enable timer
                                                        ;overflow interrupt source.
255A    B1 0C 16               LDB     IOC1,#0CH        ;Load 0CH into IOC1 to enable
                                                        ;TIMER1 and TIMER2 overflow
                                                        ;interrupts.
255D    A1 80 25 40            LD      TEMP,#2580H      ;Load address of timer overflow
                                                        ;Interrupt Service Routine.
2561    C3 01 00 20 40         ST      TEMP,INVEC[0]    ;into INT Vector Table.
2566    B1 0A 15               LDB     IOC0,#0AH        ;Load 0AH into IOC0 to select
                                                        ;T2CLK and T2RST functions of
                                                        ;P2.3 AND P2.4, respectively,
                                                        ;resets T2 to 0.
```

```
2569  FB                      EI                      ;Enable global interrupt bit.
256A  91 80 10      DRIVE:    ORB     P2,#80H         ;Output 1 to P2.7
256D  71 7F 10                ANDB    P2,#7FH         ;Output 0 to P2.7
2570  27 F8                   SJMP    DRIVE           ;Keep looping to generate pulses
                                                      ;with 25% duty cycle and 1 usec.
                                                      ;on-time at P2.7.
                    ;
                    ;
2572
                    ;         TIMER OVERFLOW INTERRUPT SERVICE ROUTINE:
                    ;
2580                          ORG     2580H
                    ;
2580  B0 16 50                LDB     REG,IOS1        ;Copy IOS1 status into REG.

2583  3C 50 05                JBS     REG,4,T2OV      ;If IOS1.4 = 1, goto T2OV
2586  3D 50 07                JBS     REG,5,T1OV      ;If IOS1.5 = 1, goto T1OV
2589  20 08                   SJMP    RETURN          ;Else neither. Goto RETURN.
258B  B1 02 0F      T2OV:     LDB     P1,#02H         ;Output 02 to LEDs.
258E  20 03                   SJMP    RETURN          ;Goto RETURN.
2590  B1 01 0F      T1OV:     LDB     P1,#01H         ;Output 01 to LEDs.
2593  F0            RETURN:   RET                     ;Return.
```

In the above program at 2550, we set the SP, disable the global, clear pendings (no interrupts of any kind are wanted till all initializations are complete), enable the Timer Overflow interrupt bit in the interrupt mask (MINT), and load IOC1 with #0CH. The latter sets both IOC1.2 and IOC1.3, thereby enabling BOTH the T1OV and T2OV interrupt sources to Timer Overflow. 2580 is then loaded into Timer Overflow's vector entry (2000) in the 8096 interrupt location table. LDB IOC0, #0AH loads 0A into IOC0, thereby 1) selecting T2CLK and T2RST as the clock and reset sources for T2, 2) enabling T2's external reset facility (here T2RST), 3) resetting T2 to 0. EI enables the global bit, so that now T1OV and T2OV interrupts can be honored. The next three instructions set P2.7 to 1 (for 1 usec.) and turn P2.7 off (for 3 usec.) i.e. 4, 4, 8 state times for ORB, ANDB, and SJMP, respectively, before P2.7 is turned on again by the SJMP to DRIVE.

The ISR (Timer Overflow) at 2580 reads IOS1 into REG, so that it can be polled twice. If we try to poll IOS1 directly, its contents are lost and, since we need to test it twice for 2 bits, we save it in REG. JBS REG,4,T2OV tests bit 4 of IOS1. If it's set i.e. T2OV was the cause, a jump to T2OV is effected. There 02 is output to P1's LEDs. If bit 4 of IOS1 is 0, fall-through to 2586 occurs where bit 5 is tested (JBS REG,5,T1OV). If that bit is set, a jump to T1OV occurs. There we output 01 to P1s display. T1OV was the source of the TOV interrupt. If, for some reason, we get to the TOV ISR with NEITHER T1OV nor T2OV responsible (??), we fall through to 2589 where SJMP RETURN returns us to the main program's P2.7 oscillator drive loop (256A - 2570). On the other hand, if T1OV or T2OV was responsible for entry into the ISR, the RET or SJMP RETURN, in each respective case, also gets us back to the oscillator drive loop at 256A - 2570. P2.7 increments T2 to overflow again, all the while T1 free-runs.

PROCEDURE

Connect P2.7 to pin P2.3 (in its T2CLK alternate mode). Execute (G FR 2550) and observe the 01, 02 oscillations at P1's 2 least significant LEDs at 0.13 sec. intervals. Note their relative phases. ESC. Execute again. Observe. Are their phases the same as before? ESC and try again. The 0.13 sec. is always an observable quantity but the relative phases will differ depending on where T1's count was relative to T2's 0 value when the program starts execution. Which LED at P1 is on longer depends on the value in T1 relative to T2's 0 value at run-time.

CAUTION

The Microcontroller Handbook (1985, p. 2-11, section 2.6.2) states: "To ensure that all CAM entries are checked each count of Timer 2, the maximum transition speed is limited to once per eight state times". This would indicate that the time between positive and negative transitions at T2 should be NO LESS than 2 usec. In our experiment we drove T2 from pulses generated at P2.7 whose on-times were 1 usec. and off-times 3 usec. This would imply that the 2 counts on the positive and negative transitions at the start and finish of each 1 usec. on-time can not be recorded, but rather only the positive (or negative) transitions separated by 4 usec. That would imply that T2 increments by one every period, rather than by two. Hence overflow of T2 would occur every 262 msec., rather than every 131 msec. as we recorded in section 2 of the FORMULATION. The experiment worked fine, but we may not have noticed that T2 overflows occurred every 262 msec. rather than every 131 msec. as seen at LED P1.1.

EXPERIMENT 5-11

USING TIMER1 AND T1OV INTERRUPTS TO GENERATE TIME DELAY. A PULSE GENERATOR WITH ON-THE -FLY CONTROL OF REP RATE.

In this experiment we come back to SFR 0AH (TIMER1) and use it to generate time delays in arbitrary units of 0.13 sec. based on the overflows that free-running T1 generates every 131 msec. Thus, at run time, we'll enter BY 60 = XY where 60 is REG3's address and XY is an arbitrary byte of our choosing. Decimal value of XY multiplied by 0.13 will specify the desired on or off-time of our pulse generator which will be observed at the LEDs at P1 when the program is executed. XY = 0A will give 1.3 sec., XY = 04 0.5 sec., etc. While the LEDs at P1 are going on/off, one can enter BY 60 = X'Y' (new value) and immediately observe the new on/off times at P1. The program at 2610 is presented below.

```
        18 00           SP      EQU     18H
        00 20           INVEC   EQU     2000H
        16 00           IOC1    EQU     16H
        40 00           REG1    EQU     40H
        50 00           REG2    EQU     50H
        60 00           REG3    EQU     60H
        08 00           MINT    EQU     08H
        09 00           PINT    EQU     09H
        0F 00           P1      EQU     0FH
                        ;
                        ;
2610                            ORG     2610H
                        ;
2610    A1 C0 00 18             LD      SP,#00C0H       ;Initialize SP to 00C0H.
2614    FA                      DI                      ;Disable Global interrupt bit.
2615    11 09                   CLRB    PINT            ;Clear all pending interrupts.
2617    B1 01 08                LDB     MINT,#01H       ;Enable timer overflow interrupt
                                                        ;source.
261A    B1 04 16                LDB     IOC1,#04H       ;Select TIMER1 overflow interrupt
                                                        ;source.
261D    A1 40 26 40             LD      REG1,#2640H     ;Load address of T1 overflow interrupt
2621    C3 01 00 20 40          ST      REG1,INVEC[0]   ;service routine into INT Vector table.
2626    B0 60 50                LDB     REG2,REG3       ;Load REG2 with contents of REG3.
2629    FB                      EI                      ;Enable Global interrupt bit.
```

```
262A  B1 FF 0F            LDB    P1,#0FFH        ;Output OFF to LEDs.
262D  27 FE       HERE:   SJMP   HERE            ;Loop here.
                  ;
                  ;
                  ;       TIMER OVERFLOW INTERRUPT SERVICE ROUTINE
                  ;
2640                      ORG    2640H
                  ;
2640  E0 50 06            DJNZ   REG2,RETURN     ;Decrement REG2. If REG2 != 0
                                                 ;return back to main program
2643  B0 60 50            LDB    REG2,REG3       ;Else reload initial time value,
2646  95 FF 0F            XORB   P1,#0FFH        ;and EXCLUSIVE OR the value
                                                 ;of the LEDs with FF to
                                                 ;to complement P1.
2649  F0          RETURN: RET                    ;Return back to main program.
```

The basic idea is simply this: after the initializations (discussed below) and the turning on of P1 (FF there), the main program loops on SJMP HERE simulating "other tasks". Every 0.13 seconds T1 overflows and, because of the initializations, interrupts "other tasks", vectoring us to the T1 Overflow ISR (see 2640 in program below). There the "magnifying" time delay register REG2 (loaded from REG3 in the main program) is decremented. If REG2 is not 0, the DJNZ jumps to RETURN to return to "other tasks" at SJMP HERE. 131 msec. later it is interrupted again by a T1 Overflow. ISR is entered again. After a number of entries into the ISR, REG2 will have been decremented to 0 and DJNZ falls through to the LDB REG2, REG3 instruction which RELOADS REG2 with the XY byte that was entered into REG3 at run-time. The XORB P1, #0FFH instruction next complements the bit values at P1, so that if the LEDs were on they now go off, and vice-versa. The RET to the main program resumes "other tasks". Further T1OV interrupts repeat the scenario to produce an equal off or on-time, as the case may be.

The main part of the program at 2610 above sets SP, disables the global bit, clears all pendings right away (so that no previous or present T1OV interrupts will be serviced), sets M.0 to 1 in the interrupt mask SFR (MINT) to enable Timer Overflow interrupts, and then enables the T1OV interrupt line (IOC1.2 is set to 1). 2640 is then loaded into the vector interrupt location table at 2000 (the vector entry for Timer Overflow interrupts) to define the address of our T1OV ISR. REG3's value (entered at run-time i.e. BY 60 = XY) is next loaded into REG2, so that REG2 will be decremented in the ISR to achieve the desired time (in multiples of 0.13 sec.), but REG3 will always retain the XY value for further identical on and off-times. The EI instruction will allow T1OV interrupts to be serviced after the next instruction is executed. The latter turns on all bits at P1.

SJMP HERE simulates "other tasks". The ISR at 2640 has already been analyzed.

PROCEDURE

1. Enter BY 60 = 08 to specify about 1 sec. on and off-times for our pulse generators at P1.
2. Execute (G FR 2610). Observe the LEDs toggle on/off/on/off.... with approximately 1 sec. on and 1 sec. off-times.
3. On the fly enter BY 60 = 04 and observe the on and off times change to 0.5 sec., AFTER THE PRESENT ON OR OFF TIME FINISHES UP (why?).
4. Now enter BY 60 = 02 and observe new on/off times of about 0.25 sec. after the present on or off time finishes up.
5. Try other BY 60 entries and observe the results.

The "granularity" of desired times is to within 0.13 sec. with the approach used in this experiment. PROBLEM: After you finish this chapter, re-do this experiment using the HSO High Speed Output unit.

EXPERIMENT 5-12

USING THE "A/D CONVERSION COMPLETE" INTERRUPT LINE AS ALTERNATIVE TO POLLING S BIT TO SIGNAL END OF CONVERSION. MULTITASKING (TWO INTERRUPT SOURCES).

The alternative to polling the S (status) bit (bit 3 in the A/D RESULT (LO) register) to determine when A/D conversion is complete, so that the 10-bit result can be reliably read from the A/D RESULT registers, is the use of the "A/D Conversion Complete" interrupt line. The advantage of having this alternative is again one of through-put: why tie up the processor in a polling mode (even if every-so-often)? It can be doing "other tasks" (background) and handle the foreground task only when the latter requests servicing by means of an interrupt.

In Expts. 5-3 and 5-4 A/D conversion was implemented by initiating conversion and then polling the S bit in A/D RESULT (LO) register for a signal as to when conversion was complete. This wait of 42 usec. (conversion time) is at the expense of other tasks (or part of them) that could be undertaken during that time. S going low was the signal that the 10-bit A/D result was available. Here we shall use the "A/D Conversion Complete" interrupt to signal when conversion is complete. That requires bit 1 in the interrupt mask register be set to 1. The location in the 8096 vector interrupt table where the "A/D Conversion Complete" interrupt vectors to is 2002. There we'll load our address of the "A/D Conversion Complete" ISR. That ISR will simply read bits 9 to 2 of the result from A/D RESULT (HI) register out to P1's LEDs. It then reloads A/D COMMAND register with 08 to start another conversion on channel 0 before returning to the main program ("other tasks"). Thus, perhaps 11 usec. or so (45 state times including the interrupt vectoring) are spent in that ISR, saving 31 usec. of time compared to the S polling approach. This accrues to the benefit of executing "other tasks" (SJMP HERE) in the main program.

To make the experiment even more interesting and powerful, we'll enable the T1OV interrupt line into TOV and write a T1OV ISR (entered every 0.13 sec.) to toggle the LED at P2.7 at 0.13 sec. on and off rates. Thus as P2.7 toggles on/off at 0.13 sec. intervals, the LEDs at P1 will display the hi byte of the A/D result at channel 0, where a 0 to 1K, 5V POT is input. As the POT is varied, the A/D result is immediately seen, all the while that P2.7 toggles on/off, seemingly "unaware" of anything else going on. So we have multitasking at 3 levels: "other tasks" in the main program (SMJP HERE), toggling of P2.7, and A/D conversion of an analog input at channel 0. Two of the 3 tasks are implemented by 8096 INTERNAL INTERRUPTS ("Timer Overflow" and "A/D Conversion Complete").

When you think of the 8 interrupt sources available with the 8096 you can start to appreciate the amount of multitasking and through-put that can be accomplished. We'll slowly come to grips with each of those sources in this chapter. (After working with EXTINT/ACH.7 and HSI.0 in chapter 4, and Timer Overflow and now A/D CONVERSON COMPLETE so far in this chapter, there remain the "Software Timers", "HSO", "HSI", and "Serial Port" interrupt lines. The first three of the latter group will be treated later in this chapter, the last one will be reserved for chapter 8).

The program at 2680 is presented below.

```
        18 00          SP       EQU     18H
        02 00          ADCOM    EQU     02H
        02 00          ADRESLO  EQU     02H
        03 00          ADRESHI  EQU     03H
        16 00          IOC1     EQU     16H
        00 20          INVEC1   EQU     2000H
        02 20          INVEC2   EQU     2002H
        40 00          TEMP     EQU     40H
        08 00          MINT     EQU     08H
        09 00          PINT     EQU     09H
        0F 00          P1       EQU     0FH
        10 00          P2       EQU     10H
                       ;
                       ;
2680                            ORG     2680H
                       ;
2680    A1 C0 00 18             LD      SP,#00C0H         ;Initialize SP to 00C0H.
2684    A1 A4 26 40             LD      TEMP,#T1OV        ;Load address of T1 Overflow
2688    C3 01 00 20 40          ST      TEMP,INVEC1[0]    ;Routine into INT VECT table.
268D    A1 A8 26 40             LD      TEMP,#CMPLT       ;Load address of A/D Conversion
2691    C3 01 02 20 40          ST      TEMP,INVEC2[0]    ;Complete Routine into INT VECT
                                                          ;table.
2696    B1 04 16                LDB     IOC1,#04H         ;Load 04 into IOC1 to enable
                                                          ;timer 1 overflow interrupts.
2699    11 09                   CLRB    PINT              ;Clear all pending interrupts.
269B    B1 03 08                LDB     MINT,#03          ;Load #03 into MINT to enable
                                                          ;Timer Overflow and A/D Complete
                                                          ;interrupts.
269E    FB                      EI                        ;Enable Global Interrupt Bit.
269F    B1 08 02                LDB     ADCOM,#08H        ;Start A/D conversion.
26A2    27 FE          HERE:    SJMP    HERE              ;Loop here.
```

```
                        ;       T1OV INTERRUPT SERVICE ROUTINE
                        ;
26A4   95 80 10         T1OV:   XORB    P2,#80H         ;Complement P2.7 (LED).
26A7   F0                       RET                     ;Return to main routine.
                        ;
                        ;
                        ;       A/D CONV. COMPLETE INTERRUPT SERVICE ROUTINE
                        ;
26A8   B0 03 0F         CMPLT:  LDB     P1,ADRESHI      ;Output HIGH Bits 9-2 of A/D
                                                        ;result to LEDS.
26AB   B1 08 02                 LDB     ADCOM,#08H      ;Start another conversion.
26AE   F0                       RET                     ;Return to main routine.
                        ;
                        ;
26AF                            END
```

The main program above initializes the SP and then loads #T1OV (Timer Overflow ISR address 26A4) into INVEC1 (address 2000 in the vector location table for the Timer Overflow entry). Next #CMPLT (A/D Conversion Complete ISR address 26A8) is loaded into INVEC2 (address 2002 in the vector location table for the A/D Conversion Complete entry). #04 in IOC1 enables Timer1 overflow interrupts into TOV. Any residual pendings are then cleared. 03 in MINT sets the M.0 and M.1 bits in the interrupt mask register to 1 enabling the Timer Overflow (TOV) and A/D Conversion Complete interrupt source lines. EI enables the global bit so that T1OV and A/D conversion interrupts will be accepted AFTER the next instruction. The latter initiates A/D Conversion "now" on channel 0 (08 into A/D - COMMAND register does that). While that conversion is going on (42 usec.) the next instruction (SJMP HERE) is entered. It represents "other tasks".

During "other tasks", T1OV interrupts (every 0.13 sec.) will be made, as will A/D Conv. Complete interrupts (roughly every 42 usec). When the former is made, we are vectored to the T1OV ISR at 26A4, where P2.7 is toggled (the result of the XORB instruction). That ISR then returns to "other tasks" at 26A2. When A/D Conv. Complete interrupts are made, we enter the A/D Conv. Complete ISR at 26A8 where the A/D result at channel 0 is read from the A/D - RESULT (HI) register for display at P1's LEDs (we're neglecting the two LSB bits for simplicity). 08 is then loaded into the A/D - COMMAND register to start another conversion at channel 0, "now". The RET takes us back to "other tasks" at 26A2.

PROCEDURE

1. Execute from 2680 and observe the LED at P2.7 toggle on/off about 4 times a second i.e. 0.13 sec. on-time and 0.13 sec. off-time. Vary the POT setting at the input to channel ACH.0 and notice the hi-byte of the 10-bit conversion result vary accordingly at P1's LEDs, all the while P2.7 continues toggling.
2. ESC and replace B1, 08, 02 at 26AB, AC, AD with NOPs i.e. enter BY 26AB = 0FD, 0FD, 0FD. Execute again. Observe the A/D result at P1 corresponding to the POT setting. Vary the POT. No corresponding variation in the A/D hi-byte result at P1 is observed. P2.7, however, does its toggling. The reload of ADCOM at 26AB needed to start ANOTHER conversion "now" is no longer there - hence no conversions beyond the one ordered at 269F in the main program.

INTRODUCTION TO THE HSO UNIT, ITS SFRs, AND THE HSO EXPERIMENTS 5-13 THROUGH 5-19

The next 8 experiments [counting 5-16(A) and 5-16(B)] are concerned with the High Speed Output Unit's (HSO) SFRs and how they control the HSO unit in I/O outputting. The relevant material on the HSO can be found on pp. 2-13, 2-14, 2-15, 3-14, and 3-15 of the Microcontroller Handbook (1985), or in section K of chapter 1 in this book. The output control that the HSO unit can accomplish is impressive and, at times, awesome. It is based on an understanding of its write control SFRs: HSO-COMMAND 06H (sometimes referred to as the HSO Command Tag) and HSO-TIME (LO, HI) 04H, as well as on a solid comprehension of the block diagram of the HSO unit in Fig. 2-18 of the above references. The latter centers on the HSO-COMMAND and HSO-TIME registers as well as the key (non-SFR) registers: HOLDING REGISTER (H.R.) and CAM FILE [CAM = "Content Addressable Memory". See Expt. 5-16(A).] The MUX, which can choose between T1 and T2 as reference timer or counter, and the COMPARATOR are also extremely important. Status Registers IOS0 and IOS1, and (sometimes) Control Register IOC1 are also needed in working with the HSO unit (see pp. 33, 34 ch. 1 on IOC0, IOC1, IOS0, IOS1).

Very directly stated, the HSO unit accomplishes on its own any one of 14 desired actions (all covered later in chapters 5, 6) at any time of your choosing. It does so if the programmer; 1. loads the HSO Command Tag SFR (06H) with the byte that corresponds to the desired action (actually it's a 7-bit register, bit 8 is undefined), and 2. loads the HSO-TIME (16-bit) SFR (04H) with the time (relative to T1 or T2 as specified in the HSO Command Tag) that the desired action is to take place. Or, as the Intel manuals aptly put it: "what to do" and "when to do it". These two specifications will constitute two instructions in your program. When executed, those instructions (16 bits from HSO-TIME and 7 bits from HSO-COMMAND) enter the Holding Register which is 23 bits wide (actually entry of both into H.R. occurs only AFTER the HSO-TIME instruction is executed). This 23-bit action/time entity in H.R. then enters the 23-bit wide CAM FILE IF there is an empty CAM register available.

The CAM FILE can hold up to 8 of these 23-bit action/time commands. Thus you can write 9 pairs of action/time instructions in your program sequentially, and on execution 8 will enter an empty CAM FILE and the 9th will enter the Holding Register. No more can be entered from the Holding Register until a CAM register becomes available. One will become available if a particular action/time event in the CAM gets done i.e. an entry in the CAM is removed from the CAM when the associated action takes place, at which time an entry in the Holding Register (if there is any) moves up into the CAM FILE. Actions can not take place unless the 23 bit-command for that action has entered the CAM FILE from the Holding Register. The command in the Holding Register will not execute unless it gets into CAM FILE. Entering another action/time command in your program will overwrite the one in the Holding Register, if one is there. Therefore, you must make sure the Holding Register is empty if you want it to receive a new command (its "full" or "empty" status can be ascertained by polling the IOSO Status Register - in particular bit IOSO.7. Our experiments will illustrate this later). WHEN WE SAY THAT A CAM ENTRY GETS REMOVED FROM THE CAM FILE WHEN ITS RELATED ACTION "GETS DONE", WE MEAN WHEN FREE-RUNNING TIMER1 (OR EVENT TIMER2, DEPENDING ON THE REFERENCE CHOSEN IN HSO-COM) MATCHES THE VALUE OF TIME WRITTEN INTO THE HSO-TIME SFR IN YOUR PROGRAM, HENCE THE MUX/COMPARATOR (p. 30).

Further, we can specify in the HSO-COMMAND SFR whether we'd like an interrupt to be generated, or not, when the desired action takes place. This is most important because, after the execution of your program causes entry of one or more action/time commands into the CAM FILE, your program can go on to "other tasks", without disturbance, until said "action interrupt" is generated by the HSO unit. At that point you'd enter the "HSO ISR" service routine where, if desired, you could write another action/time command to be entered into the CAM FILE and then return to your main program's "other tasks". Or, the HSO unit could be made to generate an interrupt only after a GROUP of HSO output events occurred. A significant enhancement in I/O through-put thus becomes possible as the HSO unit takes much I/O responsibility off the "back" of your program. It is an independent I/O sub-entity within the 8096.

The description "High Speed Unit" is apt. If Timer1 is chosen as the reference and you employ the second instruction required for the action/time command e.g. ADD HSO-TIME, T1, #UVWX, where UVWX represents the time count when the action is desired RELATIVE TO THE VALUE IN T1 AT THE TIME THIS INSTRUCTION WAS EXECUTED BY THE 8096 CPU, then the action will occur when free-running T1 matches the value T1 + UVWX entered by the ADD into HSO-TIME. The T1 in "T1 + UVWX" is the value of T1 at the time the ADD instruction was executed by the CPU. Thus, if UVWX is 0001, for example, action is being specified 2 usec. from now since T1 clocks (increments) every 8 state times (2 usec. for 12 MHz clock). That's high speed.

Since it can take up to 8 state times for a command to enter the CAM from the Holding Register (2 usec.), and since the ADD HSO-TIME, T1, #UVWX instruction itself consumes 6 state times (1 1/2 usec.) before the H.R. is loaded with the command, the minimum value to be used for UVWX above should be 0002 (4 usec.) because T1 may already be T1 + 0002 (4 usec.) by the time entry into the CAM is realized. Otherwise, if you chose UVWX = 0000 for action "now," and with T1 already at T1 + 4 usec. by the time the command entered the CAM, you'd have to wait a full 131 msec. (FFFF x 2 usec.) before T1 overflowed to reach T1 + 0000 for the action "now" to occur. And that wouldn't be action "now". Hence action "now" is associated with UVWX = 0002. In that case we are asking for action "now", "now" being the value of T1 when the command gets into the CAM. If UVWX were 0003 then we'd have the action occur 2 usec. from "now". To play it extra safe, we have chosen T1 + 0003 for action "now" in many of our experiments.

PLEASE ALSO NOTE THAT IF IT CAN TAKE UP TO 8 STATE TIMES FOR A COMMAND TO ENTER CAM FROM HOLDING REGISTER, THEN TWO SUCCESSIVE ACTION/TIME COMMAND PAIRS SHOULD BE SEPARATED BY 8 STATE TIMES IN YOUR PROGRAM, OTHERWISE THE SECOND COMMAND MIGHT OVER-WRITE THE FIRST COMMAND STILL IN H.R. THUS, IF YOU ARE NOT POLLING IOS0.7 TO TELL WHEN THE HSO's H.R. IS EMPTY AND AVAILABLE FOR A NEW COMMAND, THEN MAKE SURE YOUR INSTRUCTIONS BETWEEN TWO SUCCESSIVE CAM LOAD COMMANDS EXPEND AT LEAST 8 STATE TIMES. IF YOU HAVE NO INSTRUCTIONS BETWEEN SUCCESSIVE LOADS, THEN INSERT TWO NOPs - THEY TAKE 4 STATE TIMES EACH. WHEN MORE THAN 8 CAM LOAD COMMANDS ARE BEING ATTEMPTED, THEN YOU HAVE NO CHOICE BUT TO POLL IOS0.7 FOR H.R. BEING AVAILABLE BEFORE THE NEXT LOAD IS ATTEMPTED, OTHERWISE H.R. WILL BE OVERWRITTEN. IT WILL BECOME AVAILABLE WHEN ONE OF THE COMMANDS IN A FULL CAM IS EXECUTED AND THE COMMAND IN THE H.R. ENTERS THE CAM. REMEMBER, THE CAM CAN HOLD 8 COMMANDS AND THE H.R. ONE. IN THIS CONNECTION, SEE EXPTS. 5-18 AND 5-19.

Thus the two instructions the CPU must execute to have an "action/time" specification enter the H.R. are: LDB HSO-COM, #B1 and ADD HSO-TIME, T1, #B2B3 (if T1 is selected), where #B1 specifies the DESIRED ACTION and #B2B3 specifies WHEN the action is to occur i.e. (B2B3) from "now", where "now" is the T1 value in 2 usec. interval timer T1 AT THE TIME THE ADD INSTRUCTION IS EXECUTED BY THE CPU. The latter is a 3-operand ADD, i.e. T1 + #B2B3 is placed into HSO-TIME for entry (with HSO-COM) into the H.R. When T1 INCREASES to T1 + #B2B3, the "action/time" will be implemented and that CAM entry will be removed from the FILE.

The best way to understand the HSO unit is through experiments which illustrate all the above discussion AND MUCH MORE. This we do in the next 8 experiments and in a host of others in the applications of the SFRs in chapter 6 and beyond. We re-iterate that the experiments in this chapter with the SFRs are also applications-oriented. A different aspect and feature of the HSO unit will be separately illustrated in each of the following 8 experiments.

EXPERIMENT 5-13

USING A SOFTWARE TIMER IN THE HSO UNIT TO IMPLEMENT A PULSE GENERATOR. ON/OFF TIMES CONTROLLED ON-THE-FLY.

As stated in the previous introduction, working with the HSO-COMMAND and HSO-TIME SFRs is key to achieving HSO output control. In this experiment we are asking that port P1 exhibit 8 pulse generators with on or off-times that are multiples of 65 msec. The 65 msec. time units will be generated by one of the "Software Timers" in the HSO unit (we'll work with Software Timer 0). The multiple desired will be entered at run-time (into REG2, address 60H). Every time ST0 (Software Timer 0) expires (65 msec. from "now") we'll ensure that it generates an interrupt. That will vector us to ST0's ISR, via 200AH, where a re-load of the CAM FILE is made asking for another 65 msec./interrupt combination from ST0. REG1 (loaded from REG2) is decremented and if not 0, the ISR returns to "other tasks" in the main program. Another ST0 interrupt occurs 65 msec. hence and the ISR scenario repeats. Eventually REG1 (the multiple count) is decremented to 0, it is reloaded from REG2 and P1 is complemented (XORB) to the on or off-state, as the case may be. The ISR returns to "other tasks" where all repeats for another on (or off)-time.

The key instructions to accomplish the basic 65 msec. time interval from ST0 are simply LDB HSO-COM, #38H followed by ADD HSO-TIME, T1, #8000H. Why? A study of the HSO Command Tag register SFR (06H) shows that the ACTION we desire is accomplished by loading 00111000 = 38H into it. 1000 in the lower nibble ("channel") of HSO-COM selects Software Timer 0 (ST0). Bit 4 = 1 asks for an interrupt to be generated by the Software Timer section of the HSO unit at the time ST0 expires. Bit 5 = 1 is not necessary (SET/CLEAR bit) - 0 would work just as well. (SET/CLEAR is most important for setting or clearing HSO output pins - more on that in subsequent experiments). Bit 6 = 0 ensures that free-running Timer1 is the reference for ST0 in the comparator in determining when "time is up". It increments at 2 usec. intervals.

The instruction ADD HSO-TIME, T1, #8000H adds 8000H to the "current value" of T1 (i.e. T1 at the time the instruction is executed) and places it into HSO-TIME for entry into the HSO Holding Register (along with the HSO Command Tag byte just discussed) when the instruction is executed. 8000H = 32,768 dec. Thus when T1 free-runs from T1 (present value) up to

T1 + 32,768, ST0 will expire and kick out a Software Timer interrupt. This clearly will happen 32,768 x 2 usec. or 65 msec. from "now" ("now" being the time of execution of the ADD instruction). Software Timer interrupts vector through 200A in the vector interrupt location table. There, we specify the address of our Software Timer 0 ISR (in our case, 26E4).

Let us present the program at 26C0 now and continue our discussion of it after.

```
        18 00          SP       EQU     18H
        04 00          HSOTIME  EQU     04H
        06 00          HSOCOM   EQU     06H
        0A 20          INVEC    EQU     200AH
        40 00          TEMP     EQU     40H
        08 00          MINT     EQU     08H
        09 00          PINT     EQU     09H
        0A 00          T1       EQU     0AH
        0F 00          P1       EQU     0FH
        50 00          REG1     EQU     50H
        60 00          REG2     EQU     60H
                       ;
                       ;
26C0                            ORG     26C0H
                       ;
26C0    A1 C0 00 18             LD      SP,#00C0H        ;Initialize SP to 00C0H.
26C4    FA                      DI                       ;Disable globle interrupt bit.
26C5    B1 20 08                LDB     MINT,#20H        ;Load MINT to enable software
                                                         ;timer interrupt source.
26C8    A1 E4 26 40             LD      TEMP,#SOFTIME    ;Load address of software timer
26CC    C3 01 0A 20 40          ST      TEMP,INVEC[0]    ;interrupt service routine into
                                                         ;INT VECT table.
26D1    B0 60 50                LDB     REG1,REG2        ;Load REG2 (total on or off times)
                                                         ;into REG1.
26D4    B1 38 06                LDB     HSOCOM,#38H      ;Load HSOCOM to select software
                                                         ;timer0 with T1 as reference and
                                                         ;generation of a software timer
                                                         ;interrupt.
26D7    45 00 80 0A 04          ADD     HSOTIME,T1,#8000H; Load HSOTIME with delay time
                                                         ;value of 8000H (65msec.) plus T1.
26DC    B1 FF 0F                LDB     P1,#0FFH         ;Output FF to LEDs.
26DF    11 09                   CLRB    PINT             ;Clear all pending interrupts.
26E1    FB                      EI                       ;Enable global interrupt bit.
26E2    27 FE          HERE:    SJMP    HERE             ;Loop here.
```

```
                          ;       SOFTWARE TIMER INTERRUPT SERVICE ROUTINE
                          ;
26E4    B1 38 06          SOFTIME:LDB   HSOCOM,#38H        ;Reload HSO CAM file with command 38.
26E7    45 00 80 0A 04          ADD     HSOTIME,T1,#8000H;Reload HSOTIME with value of
                                                          ;8000H (65msec.) plus T1.
26EC    E0 50 06                DJNZ    REG1,RETURN       ;Decrement REG1 and if REG1 != 0
                                                          ;then return.
26EF    B0 60 50                LDB     REG1,REG2         ;Else reload REG1 with off or on time.
26F2    95 FF 0F                XORB    P1,#0FFH          ;Complement LEDs.
26F5    F0                RETURN: RET                     ;Return to main routine.
```

In the main program above, SP is initialized, the global bit is disabled, 20 is loaded into MINT to enable the Software Timer interrupt source. ISR address # SOFTIME (26E4) is then entered at INVEC (200A) in the interrupt vector location table (Software Timer interrupt entry point). REG1 is loaded from REG2 with the time multiple desired (the latter being specified at run-time). Then come the Command Tag and HSO-TIME instructions explained before. Again, they are specifying that the action be an STO time delay of amount specified in the HSO-TIME instruction, with T1 being used as the reference for that time delay, and that an interrupt should be generated when STO expires. The interrupt is to be generated at T1 + 8000H i.e. 65 msec. from "now" (any other value could have been chosen instead of 8000). FF is next output to the LEDs at P1, pendings, if any, are cleared, and the global bit is enabled so that STO interrupts will be acknowledged after the next instruction SJMP HERE is executed. It simulates "other tasks".

When STO interrupts are generated, we are carried to SOFTIME's ISR at 26E4 where a RELOAD of the CAM FILE with the same action/time request is made. Remember, the previous HSO Command from the main program has been removed from the CAM FILE because it has just been executed, as evidenced by the fact that an STO interrupt was generated after 65 msec. We want another 65 msec. of time from STO. REG1 (multiples) is decremented and, if it's not 0, DJNZ jumps to RETURN and we are back doing "other tasks" in the main program. Further STO interrupts at 65 msec. intervals are thus guaranteed, each action/time command being removed from the FILE and replaced by an identical one in the ISR. DJNZ in the ISR will ultimately produce 0 in REG1. Fall-through to LDB REG1, REG2 then reloads REG1 with the desired multiple. XORB complements the LED status at P1 to effect the pulse generator operation there. RET takes us back to "other tasks" and all repeats for possibly a new on-time or off-time multiple (if we entered a new byte into REG2 (60H) on-the-fly. Otherwise, the existing byte in REG2 will continue to give the same on/off times).

PROCEDURE

1. Reset the unit and enter BY 09 = 00 to make sure the HSO CAM FILE is empty and that no pendings exist. Enter BY 60 = 10 (into REG2) to give 16 multiples of 65 msec., or about 1 sec. on and off-times.
2. Execute (G FR 26C0). Observe the LEDs at P1 go on/off/on... with about 1 sec. on and off-times.
3. On-the-fly enter BY 60 = 20. Observe 32 x 65 msec. or 2 sec. on and off-times.
4. Enter BY 60 = 08 and note the on and off-times change to about 0.5 sec.
5. Enter BY 60 = 02 and observe the on/off-times change to about 1/8 sec.
6. ESC. Reset and change the byte at 26D5 from 38 to 28 i.e. enter BY 26D5 = 28. This specifies to the HSO Command Tag register that we do NOT want an STO interrupt when it expires. Execute. Observe FF at P1 go on and remain on. Interrupts into the ISR were not generated and XORB there was never executed.

EXPERIMENT 5-14

USING THE HSO UNIT TO SPECIFY WHEN A TO D CONVERSION IS TO START.

In this experiment we demonstrate the use of the HSO Command Tag and HSO-TIME SFRs to start an A/D conversion at a specific time. This time is programmed to be relative to T1's value at the time the ADD.... instruction is executed. Additionally, the program disables generation of interrupts from the HSO unit or Software Timer at the start of conversion. However, we will ask for an interrupt to be generated at the END of conversion ("A/D Conv. Complete" interrupt) just as we did in Expt. 5-12.

To make things happen at times that the human eye can follow, we'll have the action (start of A/D conversion) occur .131 sec. from "now". When we execute the program we'll see LED P2.7 turn on and P1's LEDs clear. That will establish time = 0 ("now"). Then 0.173 sec. later we'll see the digital result of the A/D conversion of channel ACH.0 appear at P1's LEDs (as a result of the "A/D Conversion Complete" ISR). Remember A/D conversion takes 42 usec. = 0.042 msec. Thus 0.131 + 0.042 = 0.173 sec.

A glance at the HSO Command Tag format shows that we should load SFR 06H with 00101111 = 2FH. The low nibble (channel) is F which defines the "action" to be: "start A/D conversion". Bit 4 = 0 specifies that no interrupt is to be generated when A/D conversion STARTS. Such an interrupt, if generated, would vector to 200AH. Bit 6 = 0 selects Timer 1 as the reference. Bit 5 = 1 chooses SET (immaterial here). Bit 7 = 0 is immaterial. The HSO-TIME register is loaded from the instruction ADD HSO-TIME, T1, #0FFFFH to specify that A/D conversion is to start 131 msec. from "now" ("now" being the current value of T1 when the ADD is executed). We must not forget that the A/D COMMAND register is also involved. It should be loaded with 00 to specify that conversion on channel 0 is wanted and that its conversion is to start, NOT "NOW", but at the time specified by us in HSO-TIME (131 msec. from now).

The program at 2700 is presented below.

```
18 00        SP       EQU    18H
02 00        ADCOM    EQU    02H
02 00        ADRESLO  EQU    02H
03 00        ADRESHI  EQU    03H
02 20        INVEC    EQU    2002H
```

```
        40 00          TEMP    EQU    40H
        08 00          MINT    EQU    08H
        09 00          PINT    EQU    09H
        06 00          HSOCOM  EQU    06H
        04 00          HSOTIME EQU    04H
        0A 00          T1      EQU    0AH
        0F 00          P1      EQU    0FH
        10 00          P2      EQU    10H
                       ;
                       ;
2700                           ORG    2700H
                       ;
2700    A1 C0 00 18            LD     SP,#00C0H       ;Initialize SP to 00C0H.
2704    FA                     DI                     ;Disable global interrupts
2705    B1 02 08               LDB    MINT,#02H       ;Load MINT with 02 to enable A/D
                                                      ;conv. complete interrupt source.
2708    A1 26 27 40            LD     TEMP,#CMPLT     ;Load address of "A/D Conversion
270C    C3 01 02 20 40         ST     TEMP,INVEC[0]   ;Complete" service routine into INT
                                                      ;VECT table.
2711    11 0F                  CLRB   P1              ;Output 00 to LEDs.
2713    91 80 10               ORB    P2,#80H         ;Turn P2.7 ON.
2716    B1 2F 06               LDB    HSOCOM,#2FH     ;Load HSOCOM with 2FH to select T1
                                                      ;as ref. and trigger start of A/D
                                                      ;without generation of a software timer
                                                      ;interrupt.
2719    45 FF FF 0A 04         ADD    HSOTIME,T1,#0FFFFH;Load HSOTIME with .131 sec.
                                                      ;(start time).
271E    B1 00 02               LDB    ADCOM,#00       ;Load 00 into ADCOM to specify start
                                                      ;of A/D Conversion on Channel 0
                                                      ;initiated by HSO at a future time.
2721    11 09                  CLRB   PINT            ;Clear all pending interrupts.
2723    FB                     EI                     ;Enable global interrupt bit.
2724    27 FE          HERE:   SJMP   HERE            ;Loop here.
                       ;
                       ;
                       ;       A/D CONVERSION COMPLETE INTERRUPT SERVICE ROUTINE
                       ;
2726    B0 03 0F       CMPLT:  LDB    P1,ADRESHI      ;A/D conversion complete output result
                                                      ;to LEDs.
2729    F0                     RET                    ;Return to main routine.
```

In the main part of the above program the various steps are 1. loading 02 into MINT to enable the "A/D Conv. Complete" interrupt source line, 2. the loading of #CMPLT (2726) into address 2002 (INVEC) in the vector interrupt location table (point of entry for the "A/D Complete" interrupt vector), 3. clearing of P1 and any pendings, 4. the turning on of P2.7

by the ORB P2, #80H instruction, 5. the selection of the desired action (start A/D conversion by the LDB HSOCOM, #2FH instruction previously analyzed), 6. the specification of the time the A/D conversion is to start by the ADD HSOTIME, T1, #0FFFFH instruction i.e. 131 msec. from "now", 7. the loading of 00 into ADCOM to select channel ACH.0 for conversion at the time specified above BY THE HSO UNIT, 8. The SJMP HERE loop which simulates "other tasks".

As for the "A/D Conversion Complete" ISR at 2726 (CMPLT), it simply reads out the A/D result (high byte) from A/D RESULT (HI) register to port 1's LEDs and then returns to "other tasks" in the main program.

PROCEDURE

1. Reset the unit and enter BY 09 = 00 to clear the HSO CAM FILE and to make sure no pendings exist. A LED should be used at P2.7. Make sure the 1K POT (5V) is connected as the analog source for ACH.0. Set it to some intermediate value.
2. Execute (G FR 2700). Immediately see LED P2.7 go on and P1's LEDs clear. About 0.17 sec. after P2.7 went on you should see the hi-byte of the A/D result appear at P1's LEDs.
3. Set the POT to a new value. Nothing should change at P1 since we are back in the SJMP loop and have not reloaded the CAM FILE with another identical action/time request (the last one was executed and, therefore, taken out of the FILE). Nor have we re-initiated ADCOM with 00.
4. ESC. Reset. Execute again. You'll see the new A/D result corresponding to the new POT setting appear at P1 0.17 sec. after P1 went off and P2.7 went on.

EXPERIMENT 5-15

USING THE HSO UNIT TO RESET TIMER2 WHEN IT HAS COUNTED A SPECIFIED NUMBER OF EVENTS

A glance at the HSO Command Tag register shows that one of the 14 actions the HSO unit is capable of implementing is the resetting of the count in T2 to 0. To ask for this action requires loading HSOCOM with #6E = 01101110. The low nibble (E) in the "channel" specifies that a reset of T2 is wanted. Bit 4 = 0 specifies that no interrupt is to be generated when T2 is reset. (Such an interrupt, if generated, would vector to 200AH). Bit 5 = 1 chooses SET (immaterial here). Bit 6 = 1 chooses the event counter T2 as our reference. Bit 7 is immaterial.

To cause the reset to happen when T2 reaches a specified count we will have to write the instruction ADD HSO-TIME, T2, #0000 as the "when to do it" companion to the loading of HSOCOM with 6E (above), where T2 is the specified count. In this form we are asking that reset occur when T2 reaches the value T2 + 0000 that the above instruction places in HSO-TIME. This simply means that it is to be reset at the CURRENT value of T2, not one count later. We'll insure that the T2 in T2 + 0000 is the specified count limit.

The program at 2750 is shown below.

```
        18 00           SP      EQU     18H
        40 00           REG1    EQU     40H
        15 00           IOCO    EQU     15H
        06 00           HSOCOM  EQU     06H
        04 00           HSOTIME EQU     04H
        0C 00           T2      EQU     0CH
        0F 00           P1      EQU     0FH
                        ;
                        ;
2750                            ORG     2750H
                        ;
2750    A1 C0 00 18             LD      SP,#00C0H       ;Initialize SP to 00C0H.
2754    11 0F                   CLRB    P1              ;Initialize LEDs (for Expt. 6-18).
2756    B1 02 15                LDB     IOCO,#02H       ;Load 02 into IOCO to select T2CLK,
                                                        ;disable T2RST pin, and reset T2 to 0.
2759    A0 0C 40        EVENTS: LD      REG1,T2         ;Load REG1 with count of events in T2.
275C    B0 40 0F                LDB     P1,REG1         ;Output count of events to LEDs
                                                        ;(lo byte).
```

```
275F   9B 01 00 50 40   CMPB  REG1,5000H[0]   ;Compare count of events with value in
                                              ;memory location 5000H.
2764   D7 F3            JNE   EVENTS          ;If count != value in 5000H, jump
                                              ;back to EVENTS.
2766   B1 6E 06         LDB   HSOCOM,#6EH     ;Else load HSOCOM with 6EH to select
                                              ;T2 as reference and to reset T2
                                              ;without generation of an interrupt.
2769   45 00 00 0C 04   ADD   HSOTIME,T2,#0000H;T2 should be reset 0 counts of T2
                                              ;later.
276E   FD               NOP                   ;Two NOPs needed for Expt. 6-18.
276F   FD               NOP                   ;
2770   27 E7            SJMP  EVENTS          ;Loop back to display new events.
```

In the above program after SP is set, P1 is cleared (needed in Expt. 6-18), and 02 is loaded into IOC0. This selects T2CLK as the source for T2 events, DISBLES the EXTERNAL T2 reset facility, and resets T2 to 0 in case it is not already 0 for some reason. The next two instructions read T2's count into REG1 and outputs its low byte count value from there to P1's LEDs. The CMPB REG1, 5000H[0] instruction compares that count (lo-byte) with the DESIRED LIMIT at which T2 is to be reset. That limit will be specified at run-time in address 5000. If the present count is not equal to that desired limit, the JNE loops back to EVENTS to continue to read future counts out to P1 and to continue to make the comparison. If, however, T2 reaches the specified value, fall-through occurs to the action/time requested of the HSO i.e. to choose T2 as reference, to reset T2 without interrupt, and to do it NOW at the PRESENT value in T2 (T2 + 0000) which, because of the fall-through, is indeed the specified count limit.

The two NOPs are reserved for Expt. 6-18 in chapter 6, which comes back to use this program to implement a pre-scalar. The last instruction jumps back to EVENTS to start all over with a reset T2 and, if desired, new value of the count limit entered at 5000.

PROCEDURE

1. Reset the unit and enter BY 09 = 00 to make sure the HSO CAM FILE is empty and that no pendings exist. Connect a debounced switch to the T2CLK pin (P2.3). Enter BY 5000 = 08 specifying a count limit of 8 at which time reset of T2 is to occur.
2. Execute (G FR 2750). Observe 00 at P1.
3. Create events at T2CLK. Read out their number at P1.

4. Observe P1 clear when the number of events reaches 8. T2 has been reset to 0.
5. Continue creating T2CLK events. P1 counts to 8 again and then clears.
6. On-the-fly enter BY 5000 = 0A specifying the count limit is to reach 10 before resetting to 0.
7. Create T2CLK events till 0A (10) is reached on the LEDs. They clear when 0A is reached.
8. Create more events. P1 reaches 0A and then clears.
9. Enter BY 5000 = 0C. Counts at P1 are now observed till dec. 12 is reached at which point P1 clears.
10. Finally, enter BY 5000 = 06. P1 counts T2CLK events up to 6 and then clears.

NOTE TO READER

It is suggested you go on to Expt. 6-18 which is based on the program in Expt. 5-15 here. Expt. 6-18 modifies the above program to implement a pre-scalar using the HSO unit. After doing Expt. 6-18, continue on to Expt. 5-16(A).

EXPERIMENT 5-16(A)

COMMANDS IN THE HSO CAM FILE ARE EXECUTED ON A TIME ORDERING BASIS. THE CAM FILE IS NOT A FIFO FILE.

The HSO's comparator checks ALL eight CAM 23-bit "action/time" registers in 8 state times. The one whose T1 + t value in the HSO-TIME field matches the CURRENT value of T1 in Timer1 is selected for action NOW. (In T1 + t, T1 is the value of Timer1 AT TIME OF EXECUTION OF THE INSTRUCTION "ADD HSO-TIME, T1, #t" and t = time RELATIVE to THAT T1 when the action is desired). The "action" is the one defined by the instruction that was written into the HSO Command Tag. Hence, no matter in what ORDER the CAM is loaded, actions go into effect on a monatonic time basis. The ones demanding action first get done first, those asking for action at a later time get done later, regardless of their position (order of entry) in the CAM FILE. The comparator does not look at the Holding Register, so any action/time commands in the latter are not executed. The command has to get into the CAM first. The following simple program at 2780, when executed, proves this.

```
      06 00          HSOCOM  EQU   06H
      04 00          HSOTIME EQU   04H
      0A 00          T1      EQU   0AH
      18 00          SP      EQU   18H
                     ;
                     ;
2780                         ORG   2780H
                     ;
2780  A1 C0 00 18            LD    SP,#00C0H        ;Initialize SP to 00C0H.
2784  B1 20 06               LDB   HSOCOM,#20H      ;Load command to turn ON
                                                    ;HSO.0
2787  45 FF FF 0A 04         ADD   HSOTIME,T1,#0FFFFH;It is to go on .131 sec.
                                                    ;from now with no interrupt.
278C  FD                     NOP                    ;Delay 4 state times
278D  FD                     NOP                    ;Delay 4 state times.
278E  B1 21 06               LDB   HSOCOM,#21H      ;Load command to turn on HSO.1
                                                    ;without interrupt.
2791  45 03 00 0A 04         ADD   HSOTIME,T1,#0003H;HSO.1 is to go on 6 usec. from
                                                    ;now.
2796  27 FE          HERE:   SJMP  HERE             ;Loop here.
```

In the above program, the first entry into the CAM FILE demands that HSO.0 is to be set, without generation of any HSO interrupt, at the time FFFF relative to the value in Timer1 at the time of execution of the ADD HSOTIME instruction i.e. at 131 msec. from "now". 20 into HSOCOM specifies channel 0 (i.e. action at the HSO.0 pin) and that HSO.0 is to be set to 1 without the generation of an HSO interrupt. Two NOPs are then executed to allow 8 state times to pass, to make sure the command just described gets into the CAM FILE from the Holding Register, leaving the latter free to accept the next command (at 278E, 91 in the program). The latter command asks that pin HSO.1 is to be set to 1 without generation of interrupt (21 into HSOCOM specifies channel 1: pin HSO.1) at the time 0003 relative to the value in T1 at the time of execution of the second "ADD HSOTIME" instruction. (The values of T1 at 2787 and at 2791 will only differ by about 18 state times or no more than 5 usec). The program ends with a "halt".

Thus we are loading the CAM FILE with the first entry demanding action at HSO.0 0.131 sec. from "now" and with the second entry demanding action at HSO.1 practically "right now". Yet, as we'll see, when the program executes it's the second entry that gets taken care of first, and the first entry second. We'll observe HSO.1 go on immediately and HSO.0 go on 0.131 sec. later.

PROCEDURE

1. Reset the unit and enter BY 09 = 00 to clear out the CAM FILE and eliminate any pending interrupts. Connect LEDs to the HSO.0 and HSO.1 pins.
2. Execute (G FR 2780). Observe HSO.1 go on at once and HSO.0 go on about 0.13 sec. later.

NOTE

The term CAM (Content Addressable Memory) is an apt one, as this experiment confirms. We see that the "address" of an entry into the HSO's CAM file is not based on its physical position (sequential address) in the file, but rather on the CONTENT of that entry i.e. the first entry executed out of the CAM is the one with the lowest (specified time value) content, the next one out is the one with the next higher (time value) content, etc. This is quite different from a FIFO (first in, first out) file where addresses of entries are in sequentially increasing ordering with lowest address out first, then next higher address out next, etc. The HSI unit's FIFO will be studied later. It is the COMPARATOR in the HSO unit that is responsible for "CAM" type action (addressing).

EXPERIMENT 5-16(B)

HAVING THE HSO UNIT GENERATE A CONTINUOUS PULSE TRAIN OF ARBITRATY DUTY CYCLE AND PERIOD.

We shall have the HSO unit generate a continuous pulse train at HSO.0 of arbitrary duty cycle and of any period up to 131 msec. While the program below generates a fixed 131 msec. period, we could easily arrange for it to be anything less by simply changing the value FFFF appearing in the "ADD HSOTIME, T, #0FFFFH" instruction. The duty cycle can be changed on-the-fly simply by entering any arbitrary word value (less than the period value), into address 5000, which is then added to T1 and placed in the HSOTIME register by the LDCAM routine. The experiment requires a LED at HSO.0, where the pulse train is output, and a scope to see the pulse waveform so that the resulting on-time and period can be measured for comparison with the expected values. Values larger than 131 msec. can be achieved with "magnifying" registers.

We present the program at 27A0 below and analyze it afterward. Pulse generation with the HSO unit is certainly one of the important HSO applications, so the analysis of the program below is crucial to understanding manipulation of the HSO unit through its SFRs.

```
        18 00          SP       EQU    18H
        06 20          INVEC    EQU    2006H

        06 00          HSOCOM   EQU    06H
        04 00          HSOTIME  EQU    04H
        50 00          REG1     EQU    50H
        60 00          REG2     EQU    60H
        40 00          TEMP     EQU    40H
        08 00          MINT     EQU    08H
        09 00          PINT     EQU    09H
        0F 00          P1       EQU    0FH
        0A 00          T1       EQU    0AH
                       ;
                       ;
27A0                            ORG    27A0H
                       ;
27A0    A1 C0 00 18             LD     SP,#00C0H        ;Initialize SP to 00C0H.
27A4    FA                      DI                      ;Disable global interrupts.
27A5    B1 08 08                LDB    MINT,#08H        ;Load MINT with 08 to enable
                                                        ;HSO interrupt.
```

```
27A8   A1 D9 27 40                  LD     TEMP,#HSOINT     ;Load address of HSO interrupt service
27AC   C3 01 06 20 40               ST     TEMP,INVEC[0]    ;routine into INT VECT table.
27B1   11 09                        CLRB   PINT             ;Clear all pending interrupts.
27B3   EF 4A D8                     CALL   LDCAM            ;Call CAM load routine.
27B6   FB                           EI                      ;Enable global interrupt bit.
27B7   27 FE              HERE:     SJMP   HERE             ;Loop here.
                          ;
                          ;
                          ;         HSO EXECUTION INTERRUPT SERVICE ROUTINE
                          ;
27D9                                ORG    27D9H
                          ;
27D9   EF 24 D8           HSOINT:   CALL   LDCAM            ;All HSO commands were executed.
                                                            ;Call reload of CAM.
27DC   F0                           RET                     ;Return to main routine.



       06 00              HSOCOM    EQU    06H
       04 00              HSOTIME   EQU    04H
       0A 00              T1        EQU    0AH
                          ;
                          ;
27B9                                ORG    27B9H
                          ;
                          ;
                          ;         LOAD CAM ROUTINE
                          ;
27B9   B1 20 06           LDCAM:    LDB    HSOCOM,#20H      ;Load CAM with command to turn HSO.0
                                                            ;ON without generating an interrupt.
27BC   45 03 00 0A 04               ADD    HSOTIME,T1,#0003H;Program command to execute
                                                            ;now
27C1   FD                           NOP                     ;Delay 4 state times.
27C2   FD                           NOP                     ;Delay 4 state times.
27C3   B1 00 06                     LDB    HSOCOM,#00H      ;Load CAM with command to turn HSO.0
                                                            ;OFF (without interrupt).
27C6   47 01 00 50 0A               ADD    HSOTIME,T1,5000H[0];Program command to execute at
       04
                                                            ;time loaded in 5000H memory location.
27CC   FD                           NOP                     ;Delay 4 state times.
27CD   FD                           NOP                     ;Delay 4 state times.
27CE   B1 30 06                     LDB    HSOCOM,#30H      ;Load CAM with command to turn HSO.0
                                                            ;ON and generate interrupt.
27D1   45 FF FF 0A 04               ADD    HSOTIME,T1,#0FFFFH;Program command to execute .131
                                                            ;seconds from now.
27D6   FD                           NOP                     ;Delay 4 state times.
27D7   FD                           NOP                     ;Delay 4 state times.
27D8   F0                           RET                     ;Return to main routine.
```

The main part of the program above is straightforward: SP is set, the global bit is disabled to protect against any interrupts, MINT is loaded with 08 to enable the HSO interrupt source (M.3 = 1), #HSOINT (27D9) is stored at 2006 (INVEC) in the vector interrupt location table (2006 being the entry address for an HSO interrupt), pendings (if any) are cleared, the LDCAM routine is called at 27B9 (where the action/time commands to HSOCOM and HSOTIME to generate the pulse train are written), and the global bit is then enabled to accept HSO interrupts. The main program then ends on SJMP HERE which simulates "other tasks". The pulse train will appear at HSO.0 all the while "other tasks" are executing. The HSO unit takes care of that multitasking.

The LDCAM (CAM LOAD routine) is crucial and needs careful analysis. The first two instructions at 27B9, BC enter 20 into HSOCOM in order to set HSO.0 to 1 (without the generation of any HSO interrupt) and load T1 + 0003 into HSOTIME so that HSO.0 will go on essentially "now" i.e. when T1 = T1 + 0003. Two NOPs are written to allow the above command to enter the CAM from the Holding Register (8 state times needed) before the next action/time pair at 27C3, C6 is written. In these next two commands 00 is written into HSOCOM asking that HSO.0 be turned off (no HSO interrupt to be generated) and T1 + (5000) is placed in HSOTIME. The latter is asking that HSO.0 be turned off at a time given by the word contents of address 5000 relative to "now" i.e. when Timer1's value equals the present T1 value + (5000). Thus (5000) defines the ON-TIME of the pulse. The value in 5000 will be entered at run-time and can subsequently be changed as the program is running, so as to control on-time (duty cycle) on-the-fly.

The next two NOPs need no explanation. The two action/time commands at 27CE and 27D1 turns HSO.0 back on, WITH A REQUEST FOR AN HSO INTERRUPT WHEN IT HAPPENS (30 into HSOCOM accomplishes this), and asks that this happen at a time FFFF (131 msec.) from "now" i.e. when Timer1 = the T1 + FFFF value in HSOTIME (the ADD instruction at 27D1 does that). (Should we want a VARIABLE PERIOD) instead of the fixed 131 msec. as here, we could write the ADD instruction at 27D1 in the 6 byte form ADD HSOTIME, T1, 5002H[0] and then enter a word in 5002 at run-time and subsequently change it on the fly). The next two NOPs are not necessary (the RET consumes 16 state times) but we inserted them anyway. The RET takes us back to "other tasks" at 27B7 after EI at 27B6 is executed. It is important to mention here that, in general, one should poll IOS0.7 to make sure that the Holding Register is empty before each new load of HSOCOM and HSO-TIME into the Holding Register is attempted, otherwise we may over-write a previous command there that hasn't yet entered the CAM. It doesn't matter here since the LDCAM routine attempts three entries into CAM with 8 state time spacings. See Expt. 5-19 where this matter is treated and discussed. IT CAN BE IMPORTANT.

While "other tasks" are proceeding, the HSO unit is removing the commands just entered into the CAM FILE, as one after the other gets executed by the HSO unit in time order (as Expt. 5-16 (A) demonstrated). By the time the third command in LDCAM gets executed HSO.0 has gone hi, then lo, then back hi (i.e. one pulse period) and at this last hi the HSO generates an interrupt as requested. The interrupt causes a vectoring out of "other tasks" to the HSO ISR at 27D9.

Our aim now is to produce another identical pulse. (If we wanted another pulse of DIFFERENT on-time (duty cycle) we'd have to change (5000). This would give us PWM and hence the possibility of D/A conversion by means of the HSO unit, as well as the PWM unit. This we do in Expt. 6-25). To produce another identical pulse means calling LDCAM and this is exactly what we do at 27D9, - the first instruction in the HSO ISR. LDCAM then enters into the CAM FILE three commands identical to the ones previously executed out of the CAM FILE. THIS TIME the T1 appearing in the ADD HSOTIME commands in LDCAM are the NEW PRESENT VALUES in Timer1 at the time LDCAM is executed when the CALL occurs in the HSO ISR. So everything will be repeated RELATIVE to these present T1 values i.e. ANOTHER IDENTICAL PULSE WILL BE GENERATED. The RET at the end of the LDCAM routine (27D8) returns us to 27DC in the HSO ISR and the RET there sends us back to "other tasks" at 27B7 in the main program. This second identical pulse is generated by the HSO unit and then interrupts "other tasks" again, so that still another identical pulse can be generated by the HSO ISR, etc., etc.

PROCEDURE

1. Reset the unit and enter BY 09 = 00 to clear out CAM FILE and clear any possible pendings.
2. Enter WO 5000 = 4000. Execute (G FR 27A0) and observe HSO.0 blink on/off/on/off etc.
3. Connect HSO.0 to the input of your scope. Observe the pulse train. Measure the on-time. We found 33 msec. Measure the period. It should be 131 msec. The 25% duty cycle is in keeping with 4000 in address 5000 relative to FFFF (see the second and third pair of HSO commands in the LOADCAM routine).

4. On-the-fly enter WO 5000 = 8000H and immediately see the pulse train on-time change on the scope. The on-time should now be about 65 msec. and the period should not have changed. This we verified. 8000 relative to FFFF gives a 50% duty cycle.
5. On-the-fly enter WO 5000 = 0C000 and observe the duty cycle change to 75% with the on-time measuring about 99 msec. and the period still 131 msec. (ratio 75%).
6. On-the-fly enter WO 5000 = 1000 and measure the new on-time. It should be a little over 8 msec. (1/4 the on-time in step 2 above).

PROBLEM

Modify the program so that you can enter any period up to 131 msec. from the keyboard. Also try to achieve periods and on-times greater than 131 msec. by use of "magnifying" registers and the DJNZ instruction operating on those registers.

EXPERIMENT 5-17

HAVING THE HSO UNIT CREATE A FINITE NUMBER OF PULSES OF ARBITRARY DUTY CYCLE AND PERIOD.

This experiment is a take-off on Expt. 5-16(B). We shall now have the HSO unit produce a FINITE number of puses of arbitrary duty cycle and period. Again, we work with a fixed period of 131 msec., but it can easily be made to be a variable parameter. To accomplish this, we need a different HSO ISR routine. It should be entered every time ANOTHER pulse has been generated until the DESIRED number of them (written into REG1 at run-time) have been generated. No further entries into the ISR are then to take place.

The HSO ISR will now be written at 27E0 (see below). Hence we must change the vector address from 27D9 (at 27A8 in 5-16(B)'s program) to 27E0. This is easily realized by entering BY 27A9 = 0E0. This establishes #HSOINT at 27A8 in that program as 27E0 instead of 27D9.

The new HSO ISR routine at 27E0 will be entered at the end of each new generated pulse, as in Expt. 5-16(B). The first instruction at 27E0 below is now DJNZ REG1, ANOTHER. This decrements REG1 (address 50H), whose contents were specified at run-time and represent the desired number of pulses. If REG1 has not been decremented to 0 by DJNZ, then the latter jumps to ANOTHER where a call to LDCAM occurs, just as in Expt. 5-16(B). This results in the reloading of the CAM FILE with the same action/time commands to implement another pulse. A return to "other tasks" is then made. If, however, REG1 has been decremented to 0 because of execution of the desired number of pulses, fall-through to 27E3 in the ISR occurs. There, we ask to turn HSO.0 off "now" WITHOUT THE GENERATION OF AN HSO INTERRUPT. 00 into HSOCOM requests the turn-off without interrupt, and ADD HSOTIME, T1, #0003 asks that it be done "now" i.e. when Timer 1's value equals T1 + 0003, where T1 is the present value of Timer 1. SJMP RETURN then gets us back to "other tasks" in the main program. Since no further interrupts can occur from the HSO, we never get back to the ISR where more pulses would be created. HSO.0 has been turned off permanently.

The modified HSO ISR at 27E0 is presented below. No further discussion of it is necessary in view of its explanation above.

```
      0A 00          T1       EQU     0AH
      50 00          REG1     EQU     50H
      04 00          HSOTIME  EQU     04H
      06 00          HSOCOM   EQU     06H

                     ;
27E0                          ORG     27E0H
                     ;
27E0  E0 50 0A       HSOINT:  DJNZ    REG1,ANOTHER     ;If REG1 != 0 then more pulses.
27E3  B1 00 06                LDB     HSOCOM,#00H      ;Else load command to turn HSO.0
                                                       ;OFF (without interrupt).
27E6  45 03 00 0A 04          ADD     HSOTIME,T1,#0003H;Program command to execute now.
27EB  20 03                   SJMP    RETURN           ;Jump to return to main routine.
27ED  EF 10 D8       ANOTHER:CALL     LDCAM            ;Load CAM with commands for
                                                       ;another pulse.
27F0  F0             RETURN:  RET                      ;Return to main routine.
                     ;
27F1                          END
```

PROCEDURE

1. Reset the unit and enter BY 09 = 00 to clear the CAM FILE and any pendings that may exist.
2. Enter BY 27A9 = 0E0 to change #HSOINT in Expt. 5-16(B) from 27D9 to 27E0, as the new HSO ISR address here.
3. Enter WO 5000 = 8000 asking for an on-time of 65 msec. (period 131 msec.) i.e. a square wave of 50% duty cycle.
4. Enter BY 50 = 08, (REG1 is address 50), asking for 8 pulses.
5. Execute from 27A0. Observe exactly 8 pulses.
6. ESC. Reset. Enter BY 50 = 01 for one pulse. Execute and observe just one pulse.
7. ESC. Reset and enter BY 50 = 0F. Execute and observe 15 pulses.

PROBLEM

Employ more registers to have the on, off-times greater than 0.131 sec., e.g. 1 sec. on, 2 sec. off.

NOTE

It is suggested that you now do Expt. 6-20 before going on to Expt. 5-18. Expt. 6-20 is concerned with subharmonic generation and is based on a modification of the program in Expt. 5-16(B).

EXPERIMENT 5-18

INDEPENDENT PULSE GENERATORS ON TWO HSO PINS. POLLING IOS0 AS ALTERNATIVE TO HSO INTERRUPTS. USING "ACTION/TIME" TABLES TO LOAD CAM.

In this experiment we shall have two independent pulse trains generated at HSO.0 and HSO.1, respectively. They shall be independent as to their on and off-times. They'll both have the same periods, although we could easily arrange for the periods to be independent as well.

We'll be referring to the following figure from time to time.

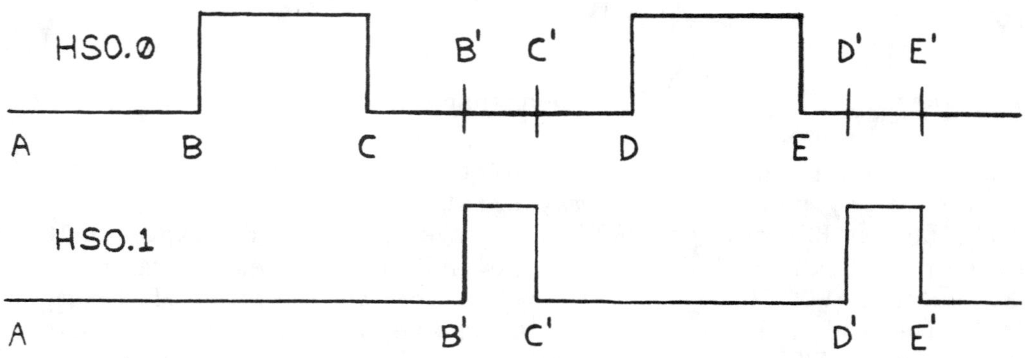

FIGURE 5-1. HSO.0 and HSO.1 independent pulse generator waveforms. Reference points.

As stated, we are treating the case of equal periods (BD = B'D'), but that poses no restrictions as to the general method involved. They could be made different.

The salient points of the method we shall employ follow. Read them carefully.

FORMULATION

1. Four action/time commands will be entered into the CAM FILE for HSO execution: the action/time at B, the action/time at C, the action/time at B', and the action/time at C'. The CAM FILE will be reloaded with these commands every time they have been executed to guarantee continuous pulse trains.

2. These four action/time commands will be written into HSO-COM/HSOTIME, respectively, from a TABLE of "actions" and a TABLE of "times", entered at run time. We call those tables CMDTBL and TMTBL, respectively. One is a byte table (the actions), the other is a word table (the times). Indexed mode addressing into the tables will be used to fetch the byte actions and word times for the HSOCOM and HSOTIME SFRs.
3. The LOAD CAM routine (which we now label as NLDCAM since it is a new routine, different than LDCAM used in Expts. 5-16(B) and 5-17) has just ONE action/time pair of instructions. It is called as many times as there are action byte entries in CMDTBL (or time word entries in TMTBL). In that way we can conveniently load the CAM FILE with, in this case, the four entries corresponding to the action/times desired at B, C, B', C' in Fig. 5-1.
4. We must make very sure in the general case, where more than 8 entries into the CAMFILE might be desired for subsequent additional action/time commands, that the Holding Register is empty, otherwise the 10th and subsequent command entries will overwrite the 9th one in the Holding Register if it did not yet enter the CAM FILE (see Expt. 5-19). Remember, a command can only enter the CAM FILE from the Holding Register if there is room for it there. If the CAM FILE is loaded with 8 entries, the only way the 9th in the Holding Register can enter the CAM and leave the Holding Register empty, is if one entry in a possibly loaded CAM FILE has been executed. To make sure the Holding Register is empty before entering another command into it requres the polling of status bit 7 in Status Register IOS0 ("HSO Holding Register is Full"). This we do the very first thing in the NLDCAM routine with a JBS IOS0, 7, NLDCAM loop i.e. a blocking action until bit 7 of IOS0 goes low indicating Holding Register is empty. Only then do we fall through to load another action/time into the Holding Register for subsequent entry into the CAM FILE. (See Expt. 5-19 for the possible consequences if we didn't poll IOS0.7).
5. After the number of desired action/time entries are made into the CAM FILE (and possibly Holding Register) no further call of NLDCAM is made until all the basic action/times are executed (here B, C, B', C' in Fig. 5-1). At that time we'll enter the same action/times into the CAM FILE by calling NLDCAM the same number of times again.
6. How will we know when the basic number of action/time commands have been executed so that we can repeat the process to generate continuous pulse trains? We could do it by having the HSO unit produce an interrupt only when the action/time C' in Fig. 5-1 has been executed, as a signal

to us that the basic B, C, B', C' chain of events has completed and another is desired. Instead, we'll do it by polling the "HSO.1 current state" - bit 1 in status register IOS0. We'll do that by remaining in a blocking action while HSO.1 is clear (interval AB' in Fig. 5-1), then remaining in another blocking action while HSO.1 is high (interval B'C' in Fig. 5-1), then falling through when HSO.1 goes low again (C' in Fig. 5-1). This will land us on a jump back to a reload of the CAM FILE for a repeat of the B, C, B', C' scenario at D, E, D', E' in Fig. 5-1, etc.

7. At run-time the following kinds of entries will have to be made: a). The number of table (byte or word) entries for the particular application - in our case four. This will be done by entering BY 40 = 04 (REG1 = 40H). b). The kinds of actions desired in CMDTBL at 5000 by entering BY 5000 = X1Y1, X2Y2, X3Y3, X4Y4 - the four desired action bytes to be loaded into HSOCOM in our application. c). The relative time values of the desired actions in TMTBL at 5100, by entering WO 5100 = T1U1V1W1, T2U2V2W2, T3U3V3W3, T4U4V4W4 - the four desired relative times to be loaded into HSOTIME in our application.
8. You can appreciate the power of this general approach in which "action/time" tables are employed. It simplifies the LOADCAM routines significantly. Only one general pair of action/time (HSOCOM, HSOTIME) instructions are needed in that routine. Table look-up and repeated use of that routine do the rest to load the CAM FILE with the desired number of commands, always separated by a poll of IOS0.7.
9. As for our specific application described in Fig. 5-1, B should be associated with a load of 20 into the HSOCOM SFR (20 will set HSO.0 without an HSO generated interrupt), C with 00 for HSOCOM (00 will clear HSO.0 with no interrupt), B' with 21 (21 will set HSO.1 with no HSO interrupt), and C' with 01 (01 will clear HSO.1 with no HSO interrupt). As for the relative times associated with these actions, let us ask them to be 4000 for B, 8000 for C, A000 for B', and C000 for C'. These values will define a 33 msec. HSO.0 pulse-width BC [8000 - 4000 = 4000 = 1/4 (FFFF), with FFFF = 131 msec.] and a 16 msec. HSO.1 pulse-width B'C' [C000 - A000 = 2000 = 1/8 (FFFF)]. The off-time for HSO.0 between C and D in Fig. 5-1 will be (C' - C) + (D - C') = (C000 - 8000) + 4000, since D will occur 4000 after C' (the CAM is reloaded at C'). Thus the off-time will be 4000 + 4000 = 8000 = 65 msec. The period of HSO.0 will thus be 33 + 65 = 98 msec. A similar consideration holds for HSO.1's off-time [D'C' = A000 = 5/8 (FFFF) = 82 msec.] and period (16 msec. + 82 msec. = 98 msec).

10. The values chosen in (9) above are entered at run-time as follows: BY 5000 = 20, 00, 21, 01 and WO 5100 = 4000, 8000, 0A000, 0C000. Additionally BY 40 = 04 is required to stipulate four entries in the table.
11. A last point before presenting the program is this: the offset into CMDTBL and TMTBL starts out at 0. Since the CMDTBL table is a byte table and TMTBL is a word table, we must multiply the offset by 2 after accessing CMDTBL before accessing the NEXT entry in TMTBL, and then restore it by dividing it by 2 before again accessing the CMDTBL next time NLDCAM is called. The NLDCAM in the program below does that with a SHL OFFSET, #1 instruction after CMDTBL was accessed to load HSOCOM, and then restores OFFSET with a SHR OFFSET, #1 instruction after TMTBL was accessed to load HSOTIME (one multiplies by 2, the other divides by 2). Naturally, the main program increments the offset (INC OFFSET) before NLDCAM is called again so that we can access the next CMDTBL byte entry properly.

The program at 2800 is presented below. The extended discussion above should make it unnecessary to analyze it any further. Just remember: 1). the JBS instruction at 2819 waits till we're sure the Holding Register is empty before loading in another command, 2). the JBC, JBS instructions at 2811, 2814 wait until all four commands (in our case) were executed so that B, C, B', C' are implemented and another load of the CAM is to be initiated by the SJMP AGAIN to 2804, 3). that the NEXT reload of the (in this case) 4 CAM commands means that the time words in TMTBL (4000, 8000, A000, C000 in our case) ARE NOW TIMES RELATIVE TO THE POINT IN TIME AT WHICH HSO.1 WENT LOW (C' IN FIG. 5-1). This is a very important point. This is what will cause the period of each pulse train to be 98 msec. and not the 131 msec. that we've generally adopted. 4). that CMDTBL [OFFSET] or TMTBL [OFFSET] in indexed addressing means accessing memory address CMDTBL + OFFSET or TMTBL + OFFSET for the byte or word stored there.

```
06 00        HSOCOM  EQU    06H
04 00        HSOTIME EQU    04H
00 50        CMDTBL  EQU    5000H
00 51        TMTBL   EQU    5100H
0A 00        T1      EQU    0AH
18 00        SP      EQU    18H
15 00        IOS0    EQU    15H
40 00        REG1    EQU    40H
50 00        REG2    EQU    50H
60 00        OFFSET  EQU    60H
```

```
2800                          ORG     2800H
                      ;
2800   A1 C0 00 18            LD      SP,#00C0H          ;Initialize SP to 00C0H.
2804   B0 40 50       AGAIN:  LDB     REG2,REG1          ;Load number of CAM loads into
                                                         ;counter.
2807   01 60                  CLR     OFFSET             ;Initialize OFFSET
2809   EF 0D 00       LOAD:   CALL    NLDCAM             ;Call routine to load CAM.
280C   07 60                  INC     OFFSET             ;Adjust OFFSET parameter
280E   E0 50 F8               DJNZ    REG2,LOAD          ;If REG2 != 0 goto load CAM.
2811   31 15 FD       HSO1LO: JBC     IOS0,1,HSO1LO      ;If HSO.1 is low loop here.
2814   39 15 FD       HSO1HI: JBS     IOS0,1,HSO1HI      ;If HSO.1 is high loop here.
2817   27 EB                  SJMP    AGAIN              ;Loop back to create another
                                                         ;pulse pair.
                      ;
                      ;
                      ;
                      ;       LOAD CAM ROUTINE
                      ;
2819   3F 15 FD       NLDCAM: JBS     IOS0,7,NLDCAM                ;Loop until HSO Holding Reg.
                                                                   ;can accept a new command.
281C   B3 61 00 50 06         LDB     HSOCOM,CMDTBL[OFFSET]        ;Load HSOCOM with command
                                                                   ;from Command Table.
2821   09 01 60               SHL     OFFSET,#1                    ;Multiply OFFSET by two since
                                                                   ;TIME is a WORD variable.
2824   47 61 00 51 0A         ADD     HSOTIME,T1,TMTBL[OFFSET];Load HSOTIME from TIME Table.
       04
282A   08 01 60               SHR     OFFSET,#1                    ;Divide to correct for WORD
                                                                   ;access.
282D   F0                     RET                                  ;Return to main routine.
                      ;
                      ;
282E                          END
```

PROCEDURE

1. Reset the unit and enter BY 09 = 00. Connect the HSO.0 and HSO.1 pins to a dual trace scope. LEDs at those pins would also be useful.
2. Enter BY 40 = 04 = number of CAM entries desired.
3. Enter BY 5000 = 20, 00, 21, 01 to establish a CMDTBL of bytes for HSOCOM.
4. Enter WO 5100 = 4000, 8000, 0A000, 0C000 to establish a TMTBL of word values for HSOTIME.
5. Execute from 2800 and observe the blinking LEDs at HSO.1 and HSO.0 and the waveforms on the scope. We measured the on-time of HSO.0 to be 33 msec. and its off-time to be 65 msec. (period = 98 msec). HSO.1's on-time was measured

to be 16 msec. and its off-time 82 msec. (period = 98 msec). These are exactly in accordance with the predicted values that our previous discussion indicated (see section 9 of the Formulation earlier).

6. ESC, reset, enter BY 09 = 00, and repeat after first setting up a new table of time values. Measure the new on/off times and see if they agree with what you'd expect.

PROBLEMS

1. Extend the program to allow for 4 independent pulse generators at HSO.0, HSO.1, HSO.2, and HSO.3 (8 entries in CAM FILE, 8-byte and 8-word tables). Modify it to have a 4-bit sequencer at those pins.

2. Redo the program of the 2 pulse generators here to employ an HSO interrupt after C' in Fig. 5-1 rather than the polling technique we used in conjunction with IOSO. This will allow "other tasks" to be accomplished in the main program while the HSO unit takes care of the pulse generation.

3. Redo the program of the 2 pulse generators here so that the periods of each are different.

The above problems are applications-oriented. Chapter 6 pursues experiments of that nature in greater depth in its 26 experiments.

EXPERIMENT 5-19

ATTEMPTING TO LOAD MORE THAN 9 ENTRIES INTO THE HSO CAM FILE/HOLDING REGISTER. THE NEED TO POLL IOS0.7.

We have already indicated in Expt. 5-18 the need to poll bit IOS0.7 ("HSO Holding Register is Full") before attempting to load entries into the HSO CAM and Holding Register. This was done there. Should the CAM FILE have 8 entries and the Holding Register be loaded with a 9th entry, then any attempt to load more entries will write over the 9th one in the Holding Register and lead to other than expected I/O results. We must make sure the Holding Register is empty i.e. that it has loaded the CAM FILE with its contents when space in the file is available (which it will be when one of the 8 entries in it has been executed or if less than 8 entries were originally loaded into it).

This experiment is intended to give vivid proof of the above need by demonstrating what can happen if you don't poll IOS0.7 for the existence of an empty Holding Register before attempting to enter another command in the CAM. We can best describe what we have in mind by presenting the following formulation.

FORMULATION

1. We shall load the CAM with 8 identical entries each asking for the SAME action/time i.e. HSO.0 is to go on at a specific time e.g. at about 0.5 msec. from "now". A 9th entry will also be made (into the Holding Register) asking that HSO.0 go off 65 msec. from "now". Generation of HSO interrupts will not be requested.
2. We shall attempt to enter a 10th entry into the Holding Register under two different conditions:
   a. without asking whether the Holding Register is empty, in which case the 10th entry will over-write the 9th one if none of the 8 CAM entries was executed.
   b. only after asking whether, and ascertaining that, the Holding Register is empty, in which case the 9th entry will enter the CAM FILE when one of the 8 entries in it is executed and the 10th can then enter the then empty Holding Register.
3. The 10th entry alluded to above asks that HSO.1 is to go on 131 msec. from "now".

In case 2(a) above we should observe HSO.0 go on 0.5 msec. from "now", stay on forever, while HSO.1 should go on 131 msec. from "now" and also stay on forever. In case 2(b) above HSO.0 should go on 0.5 msec. from now, then go off 65 msec. from now and stay off, while HSO.1 should go on 131 msec. from "now" and stay on. The two results are clearly significantly different.

The program at 2A00 is given below. Note how 20 is loaded into HSOCOM and 0100 into HSOTIME 8 times, each time requesting that HSO.0 go on 0.5 msec. from "now" without an HSO interrupt being generated. Notice the 8 state times that the NOPs provide between successive entries. REG (40H) is employed as the counter to signify when 8 entries into the CAM FILE are made. The DJNZ falls-through after the 8th entry is made, instead of going back to LOAD for another entry. The fall-through loads the 9th entry into the H.R. requesting that HSO.0 go off 65 msec. from "now" (00 into HSOCOM and 8000 into HSOTIME are the relevant numbers), again without HSO interrupt generation.

After that, 5 NOPs are provided. The first two will provide the 8 state times needed before another entry into the Holding Register is attempted [really not necessary in view of the next 3 NOPs which will become a JBS instruction (9 state times)]. The 3rd, 4th, and 5th NOPs will allow us to implement cases 2(a) and 2(b) in the above formulation. In the first case, 2(a), we'll leave in the three NOPs at 2A1E, 1F, 20. This means that we sail through to the 10th entry attempt at 2A21 which will overwrite the 9th one in the Holding Register, with the anticipated results as already explained. In the 2nd case, 2(b), we'll replace the NOPs at 2A1E, 1F, 20 with a JBS IOS0, 7, FULL instruction (machine code: 3F, 15, 0FD i.e. a jump on itself) which blocks the fall-through as long as the Holding Register is full (IOS0.7 = 1). When one of the 8 CAM entries is executed, the Holding Register empties the 9th entry into the CAM and it is now empty. JBS falls through as IOS0.7 is now 0. The 10th entry (at 2A21, 24) can now safely get into the Holding Register. The results to be expected for this case were already explained. The program ends on a "halt".

```
06 00          HSOCOM  EQU     06H
04 00          HSOTIME EQU     04H
40 00          REG     EQU     40H
0A 00          T1      EQU     0AH
18 00          SP      EQU     18H
```

```
2A00                              ORG    2A00H
                        ;
2A00   A1 C0 00 18                LD     SP,#00C0H        ;Initialize SP to 00C0H.
2A04   B1 08 40                   LDB    REG,#08H         ;Number of CAM loads in REG.
2A07   B1 20 06         LOAD:     LDB    HSOCOM,#20H      ;Load command to turn ON
                                                          ;HSO.0 (no interrupt).
2A0A   45 00 01 0A 04             ADD    HSOTIME,T1,#0100H;Program to execute .5 msec. from now.
2A0F   FD                         NOP                     ;Delay 4 state times
2A10   FD                         NOP                     ;Delay 4 state times.
2A11   E0 40 F3                   DJNZ   REG,LOAD         ;If REG != 0, then go back and
                                                          ;load another command.
2A14   B1 00 06                   LDB    HSOCOM,#00H      ;Eight entries have been loaded
                                                          ;now try to load the 9th (HSO.0 to
                                                          ;go off without HSO interrupt).
2A17   45 00 80 0A 04             ADD    HSOTIME,T1,#8000H;Program to execute 65 msec.
                                                          ;from now.
2A1C   FD                         NOP                     ;Delay 4 state times
2A1D   FD                         NOP                     ;Delay 4 state times
2A1E   FD                         NOP                     ;This will be modified at runtime.
2A1F   FD                         NOP                     ;
2A20   FD                         NOP                     ;
2A21   B1 21 06                   LDB    HSOCOM,#21H      ;Nine entries have been loaded
                                                          ;now try to load the 10th (HSO.1 to
                                                          ;go on     without HSO interrupt).
2A24   45 FF FF 0A 04             ADD    HSOTIME,T1,#0FFFFH;Program to execute .131 sec. from
                                                          ;now.
2A29   27 FE            HERE:     SJMP   HERE             ;Loop here.
```

PROCEDURE

1. Reset the unit. Enter BY 09 = 00. With NOPs at 2A1E, 1F, 20, execute from 2A00 and observe HSO.0 go on and stay on, and HSO.1 go on 131 msec. after HSO.0 went on, and stay on. Use LEDs at HSO.0, HSO.1.
2. ESC. Reset. Enter BY 09 = 00. Enter BY 2A1E = 3F, 15, 0FD i.e. JBS IOS0, 7, FULL for a polling of IOS0.7. Execute and observe HSO.0 go on, then go off 65 msec. later, and HSO.1 go on 131 msec. after HSO.0 went on.

INTRODUCTION TO THE HSI UNIT, ITS SFRs, AND THE HSI EXPERIMENTS 5-20 THROUGH 5-24.

The last 5 experiments in this chapter are concerned with the High Speed Input Unit's SFRs and how they control the HSI unit I/O inputting. The relevant reference material on the HSI unit can be found on pp. 2-12, 2-13, 3-14, 3-15 of the Microcontroller Handbook (1985), or in section J of chapter 1 in this book. The workings of the powerful and fast HSI unit are based on an understanding of its three associated SFRs: the HSI-STATUS (06H) and HSI-TIME (04H) read-only registers, and the write-only HSI-MODE (03H) register. Other SFRs that are frequently involved with HSI control are control registers IOC0 (15H), IOC1 (16H), and Status Register IOS1 (16H).

An understanding of the HSI unit block diagram in Fig. 2-14 of the above references is essential. The crucial elements of that diagram are the Change Detector, reference Timer 1, (clocked every 8 state times to record times of an input event occurance on any of the 4 HSI input pins - hence 2 usec. resolution with a 12 MHz clock), the HSI-MODE, HSI-TIME, and HSI-STATUS SFRs, the FIFO (20 bits side, 7 registers deep, which can hold a record of which HSI pin(s) had a past transition occurrence, and when) and the Holding Register. The HSI FIFO, being 20 bits wide, holds 4 bits which tell which of the four HSI pins recorded an incoming "event" ("event" meaning a 0 to 1 or 1 to 0 CHANGE occurred at an HSI pin), with the other 16 bits telling us the time at which the event occurred. Every time such "event/time" happening occurs, it enters the FIFO through both the HSI pin Change Detector and Timer 1. From there it seeps down into the Holding Register - if the latter is empty. It will be empty if it has been read into 4 bits of the HSI-STATUS register and into the 16-bit HSI-TIME register. If the Holding Register is not empty, the FIFO itself starts to fill up and can ultimately hold up to 7 event/time entries. FIFO here implies that the first event/time entry accepted by it is the first to enter the Holding Register, when empty, AND SO ON FOR SUCCEEDING ENTRIES IN ORDER OF ACCEPTANCE.

If FIFO and Holding Register are full, additional event/times are lost - they will not be recorded. Each reading of the H.R. (Holding Register) allows an entry in the FIFO (if any) to drop down into the H.R. for future reading. It can take up to 8 state times (2 usec.) for the FIFO entry to get into the H.R. Hence, attempting to read out successive event/times from the FIFO through the H.R., will require 8 state times between successive reads to make sure the next event/time from FIFO got into the H.R. after the first was read out of the H.R.

A reading of the Holding Register to gain information on what type of transition (0 to 1 or 1 to 0) occurred at which pin, and when, is done as follows: a read of HSI-STATUS is made (e.g. LDB REG, HSI-STATUS) followed by a read of HSI-TIME (e.g. LD REG1, HSI-TIME). It is the second read (of HSI-TIME) which empties out the Holding Register and allows another FIFO event/time occurrence (if any) to enter H.R. Clearly then, reading HSI-TIME BEFORE reading HSI-STATUS will give us the correct time of the event occurrence that's in H.R., but, since a new FIFO entry will now replace the previous one in H.R., a subsequent read of HSI-STATUS will give us the status (event) information of an event other than the one we're interested in.

Further, one should make sure that, when a read of the HSI-STATUS and TIME registers is made, the H.R. has valid data available (it may still be seeping down from the FIFO, as it can take 8 state times to do so). This can be assured by first polling bit IOS1.7 ("HSI Holding Register Data Available") and falling through to make the H.R. read ONLY when that bit is a 1. If this is not done, the STATUS and TIME values read will be indeterminate as H.R. may not yet have the valid event/time data we're interested in. If, alternatively, you employ an "HSI interrupt when H.R. is loaded" to let you know when H.R. is loaded with event data, there'll be no need to poll IOS1.7. That will be explained more fully later in this section (consult IOC1.7).

While the reading of HSI-TIME tells the exact time (referenced to Timer 1) when a 0 to 1 or 1 to 0 triggered event occurred, the reading of HSI-STATUS gives us four 2-bit pieces of information about the nature of the event that occurred. Each of the four HSI input pins is associated with 2 bits in the HSI-STATUS register. The LOWER of the two bits tells us if an "event" has occurred on that pin i.e. a 1 would be telling us that a 0 to 1 or 1 to 0 triggered event occurred on that pin at the time given in the HSI-TIME register. A 0 would indicate that no event occurred on THAT pin - that the time in HSI-TIME is the time corresponding to an event that occurred on ANOTHER pin (the one for which the lower bit is a 1). The UPPER of the two bits tells us the CURRENT state of the pin. Thus, a 0,0 combination says that no triggered (0 to 1, 1 to 0) event occurred on that pin at the time given in HSI-TIME and that its state is now a 0. A 0,1 would tell us that a triggered event occurred on the pin at HSITIME and that the current state of the pin is 0 (so it must have been a 1 to 0 transition). A 1,0 would tell us no triggered event occured on the pin at HSITIME and that its state was and still is 1. A 1,1 would indicate that a triggered event occurred on the pin at the time given in HSI-TIME and that the current state of the pin is 1 (so it must have been a 0 to 1 transition).

That certainly is a lot of information to be had from the HSI unit about the nature and time of input events.

What's more, with the HSI-MODE SFR we can arrange to have the HSI unit record only SELECTED types of events on the various HSI pins (and programmably change that selection as execution proceeds, if that's needed in the particular application). Thus, we may want the FIFO to record only 0 to 1 transitions on a given pin and ignore other types; or we may want it to record only 1 to 0 transitions on a pin; or to record either kind; or, finally, only to record every eighth positive transition. INDEPENDENT mode selection for each of the four HSI input pins HSI.0, .1, .2, .3 can thus be made. This is easily implemented by writing into HSI-MODE (SFR 03). The bits in HSI-MODE occur in 4 pairs corresponding to each of the four pins HSI.0, HSI.1, HSI.2, HSI.3. For each pair you can write a 0,0; 0,1; 1,0; or 1,1 combination. 0,0 stipulates that the FIFO is to record only the 8th of 8 positive transitions on that pin; 0,1 would stipulate that only 0 to 1 transitions are to be recorded; 1,0 that only 1 to 0 transitions are to be recorded; and 1,1 that both 0 to 1 and 1 to 0 transitions are to be recorded in the FIFO. Each HSI pin can be assigned its own mode.

Mode selection is most useful, as the remaining experiments in this chapter will indicate, and as the applications experiments with the HSI in chapter 6 will confirm. For example, if you'd want to measure periods or time between 0 to 1 events, the 0,1 mode would be useful. For measuring pulse-widths, the 1,1 mode would be employed. For determining the end of switch bounce, for example, or the times between 1 to 0 transitions, the 1,0 mode would be chosen. An example of the 0,0 mode would be the implementation of a pre-scalar. These cases, and other examples, will be covered in the HSI experiments in this and the next chapters.

As with the HSO unit, a powerful feature is the ability to program the HSI unit to generate an HSI interrupt when either a NEW event/time occurrence has ENTERED the H.R. from the FIFO, OR when the FIFO ITSELF GOES FROM A 5 (OR LESS) LEVEL OF ENTRIES TO 6 OR MORE. (THUS "FIFO FULL" REALLY MEANS THE SITUATION WHERE THE FIFO THRESHOLDS FROM 5 OR LESS ENTRIES TO 6 OR MORE - IMPORTANT!). (Don't confuse these possible interrupts from the HSI unit with the HSI.0 EXTERNAL interrupt source which can be enabled. The latter use of HSI.0 has nothing to do with its possible use as an input pin to the FIFO, if enabled for that purpose - see below). Don't be led into the trap of thinking that HSI interrupts can be generated AS LONG AS the H.R. is loaded or AS LONG AS the FIFO is "full". They can be generated ONLY in going from an UNLOADED H.R. or NON-FULL (5 or less) FIFO to a LOADED H.R. or FULL (6 or more) FIFO. The experiments will prove that.

These interrupts can be generated by setting bit 7 in the IOC1 control register to either 0 or 1, respectively; unmasking the "HSI Data Available" interrupt source; and enabling the global bit. The beauty of this, of course, is the ability gained thereby of having the program execute "other tasks" while the HSI unit worries about incoming events to be monitored and recorded. The HSI can interrupt "other tasks" only when it has new input information in its H.R. or when it has a full file of such new events in its FIFO. This is another example of increasing through-put, this time by having the HSI monitor the high-speed (2 usec. resolution) input I/O while the 8096 CPU is engaged in "other tasks". The HSI interrupt routine can then concern itself with processing the input information just made available in the H.R. or FIFO.

If one chooses not to enable the "HSI Data Available" interrupt source, then a polling of either bit 6 in Status Register IOS1 ("HSI FIFO IS FULL") or bit 7 in IOS1 ("HSI HOLDING REGISTER DATA AVAILABLE") would be necessary as the alternative to using HSI interrupts to let one know of the existence of input information. Only after a 1 is indicated for the relevant bit in IOS1, could you proceed to read the H.R. for a single entry, or to read it repeatedly for the various entries in a full FIFO. Caution: polling or reading IOS1 clears it. So if you are concerned with the status of more than one bit in IOS1, it should be read into a register BEFORE testing the relevant bits in the register. In a number of cases we don't do that since we're interested, in that application or experiment, in only one bit (IOS1.7 or IOS1.6, for example). In others, we are concerned with various bits in IOS1. In that case we copy it into a register for subsequent testing.

Finally the HSI pins that are to record events and times into the FIFO must be enabled for that purpose. That's easily done by writing 1s into the relevant HSI enable bits in IOC0. IOC0.0, .2, .4, and .6 control the enabling or disabling of HSI.0, HSI.1, HSI.2, and HSI.3 into the FIFO, respectively. HSI.1 can be used, as we've seen in Expt. 5-7, as a source for clock events into Timer 2. In that case IOC0.2 need not be set to 1, but IOC0.7 does. Likewise, HSI.0 can be used as an external interrupt source even if IOC0.0 is set to 0. Interrupt Mask bit 4 and global bit PSW.9 should be set to 1 in that case. Also note that HSI.2, and HSI.3 share common pins with HSO.4 and HSO.5. Bits 4 and 6 of IOC0 and IOC1 will enable one or the other.

This, then, is a summary of the significant points needed to understand 8096 HSI operation. The remaining 5 experiments in this chapter stress HSI fundamentals, the HSI SFRs, and all the points of the above discussion. They will put us in a good position to understand the applications experiments with HSI in chapter 6 and beyond.

NOTE

Please note the distinction already made between the HSO's CAM FILE and the HSI's FIFO, but repeated here for emphasis. The CAM FILE is based on a Content Addressable Memory scheme where the order of execution of entries in that file occurs on the basis of the CONTENT (specified time value) of each entry. The lower content (time value) entries are addressed (executed) first, the higher content ones later. This is implemented by the COMPARATOR section of the HSO. The HSI's FIFO, on the other hand, accepts entries one after the other and deposits them one after the other in the Holding Register (if empty) in the same order they were accepted. Thus, each entry's physical address is one higher than the preceding entry, with the lower physical addresses being emptied into the H.R. first.

EXPERIMENT 5-20

USING THE HSI UNIT AND ITS HSI MODE, STATUS, AND TIME SFRs. PART I: POLLING IOS1.7 AS TO AVAILABILITY OF DATA IN THE HOLDING REGISTER.

FORMULATION

1. A debounced switch will be used to input 0 to 1 or 1 to 0 transitions through HSI.0 into the FIFO and Holding Register. A debounced switch (normally low) will be used at input pin P0.0 for other purposes described below. Working with HSI.0 requires that we write a 1 out to IOC0.0 to enable it into the FIFO.
2. The program will allow HSI-MODE to be loaded with the byte (entered at run-time) at address 5000. Four different cases will be tried: BY 5000 = 00 (FIFO will record every 8th positive transition on HSI.0); BY 5000 = 01 (FIFO will record only positive transitions on HSI.0); BY 5000 = 02 (FIFO will record only negative transitions on HSI.0); and BY 5000 = 03 (FIFO will record either positive or negative transitions on HSI.0).
3. We shall poll IOS1.7 to ascertain when Holding Register data is available for read-out. It will be loaded with data after an event at HSI.0, corresponding to the mode selected, is triggered. IOS1.7 = 1 signals that there is data in the H.R.
4. When IOS1.7 is 1 (Holding Register data is available), fall-through the polling instruction will occur and we'll read HSI-STATUS out to the LEDs at P1 in order to see a) if bit 0 of P1 is a 1 (corresponding to the fact that an event (0 to 1 or 1 to 0) at HSI.0 occurred); and b) what the current status of HSI.0 is, as revealed by bit 1 of P1 (it should be 1 if the event was a 0 to 1 transition, and 0 if it was a 1 to 0 transition).
5. After throwing the switch at P0.0 high/low the program will read out the low byte of the time of the event's occurrence (from HSI-TIME) to P1's LEDs.
6. The above will be repeated (for the same HSI-MODE) just to record a new event time at P1.
7. All the above will be done for each of the four possible trigger/event modes, in turn.

The program at 2850 below will be analyzed after it is presented.

```
          18 00          SP       EQU    18H
          15 00          IOCO     EQU    15H
          16 00          IOS1     EQU    16H
          03 00          HSIMODE  EQU    03H
          06 00          HSISTAT  EQU    06H
          04 00          HSITIME  EQU    04H
          40 00          REG      EQU    40H
          0E 00          PO       EQU    0EH
          0F 00          P1       EQU    0FH
                         ;
                         ;
2850                              ORG    2850H
                         ;
2850      A1 C0 00 18             LD     SP,#00C0H         ;Initialize SP to 00C0H.
2854      B1 01 15                LDB    IOC0,#01H         ;Enable recording of HSI.0 in FIFO.
2857      B3 01 00 50 03          LDB    HSIMODE,5000H[0]  ;Load HSIMODE with mode byte
                                                           ;from address 5000H.
285C      11 0F          CLEAR:   CLRB   P1                ;Initialize LEDs.
285E      37 16 FB                JBC    IOS1,7,CLEAR      ;If IOS1.7 = 0, then loop back to
                                                           ;CLEAR.
2861      B0 06 0F                LDB    P1,HSISTAT        ;Else output HSI status to LEDs.
2864      30 0E FD       STOP:    JBC    P0,0,STOP         ;If P0.0 = 0, then loop on STOP.
2867      A0 04 40                LD     REG,HSITIME       ;Else load HSITIME into REG.
286A      B0 40 0F                LDB    P1,REG            ;Output low byte of HSITIME to LEDs.
286D      38 0E FD       WAIT:    JBS    P0,0,WAIT         ;If P0.0 = 1, then loop on WAIT.
2870      27 EA                   SJMP   CLEAR             ;Else jump back to wait for new entry
                                                           ;into HSI FIFO.
```

The first line of code sets SP, as usual. The second instruction enables HSI.0 for inputting transitions/times to the FIFO. The next instruction loads HSI-MODE with the byte entered at 5000 at run-time to select the transition mode desired. The LEDs at P1 are then cleared and a polling of IOS1.7 is undertaken by means of the JBC IOS1, 7, CLEAR instruction, which keeps P1 at 00 as long as no data is available in the H.R.

When data is available in H.R. (at the time we throw HSI.0 high and/or low, as the case may be, through the debounced switch there) a fall-through JBC will occur. Our next instruction is to read out the HSI-STATUS byte to the LEDs at P1. Matters remain that way as long as P0.0 is low. When we throw the switch at P0.0 high, fall-through the JBC P0, 0, STOP instruction will allow us to read out HSI-TIME to REG. Then the low byte of the time of occurrence of the event is outputted to P1's LEDs (THIS EMPTIES THE H.R.). The next instruction (JBS) waits as long as S0 at P0.0 is high. Only when S0 is released do we fall through to SJMP back to CLEAR, where the LEDs are cleared and a polling of IOS1.7 is again undertaken. The scenario repeats when another HSI.0 event is entered and the H.R. is again available for reading.

PROCEDURE

1. Reset the unit to clear the FIFO. Clear any pendings (BY 09 = 00) in case they exist. Use debounced switches at HSI.0 and P0.0 inputs.
2. Enter BY 5000 = 00 to specify that an event will enter the FIFO only after the 8th 0 to 1 transition on HSI.0 occurs. Execute from 2850. Throw HSI.0 lo/hi/lo eight times. On the 8th positive throw observe the HSI-STATUS at P1. It's 03 indicating an event occurred on HSI.0 (P1.0 = 1) and the current status at HSI.0 is 1 (P1.1 = 1), in keeping with expectations. Throw S0 (P0.0) hi, and keep hi. We read the low byte of HSI-TIME at P1's LEDs to be F4 (which was the time the 8th positive transition occurred). Release S0. The LEDs clear. Try 8 more throws of HSI.0 and again observe 03 appear at P1 on the 8th throw high. Throw S0 high and read the new lo-byte of time. We found 9E this time. Release S0. The LEDs at P1 clear. Etc.
3. ESC. Enter BY 5000 = 01 to specify that only positive edge transitions on HSI.0 will be recorded in the FIFO. The FIFO and H.R. are clear because we read out the single event in H.R. in part (2) above. Execute. Throw HSI.0 hi and keep it hi. Read the HSI-STATUS on the LEDs. You'll find 03 there. It appears the moment HSI.0 goes hi. 03 was input to the H.R. via the FIFO at that moment. 03 indicates an event occurred at HSI.0 and that the pin is PRESENTLY high. Throw S0 high and read the low-byte of time on the LEDs. We found BF. Release S0. LEDs clear. NOW release HSI.0 to 0. No effect is observed on the LEDs (why?). Throw HSI.0 hi/lo. Read the status. It's again 03 (when HSI.0 went hi). Throw S0 hi. Read the new event time. We found 1C for its low byte. Release S0. LEDs clear. Etc. H.R. and FIFO are now empty. Why?
4. ESC. Enter BY 5000 = 02 to specify that only negative edge transitions on HSI.0 are to be accepted into the FIFO. Execute. Throw HSI.0 high. No effect at the LEDs. Release HSI.0. Observe HSI-STATUS = 01 at the LEDs. This says an event occurred at HSI.0 and that its current status is 0, in keeping with a 1 to 0 transition. Throw S0 hi. Read low-byte of the event's time occurrence. We read CB. Release S0. LEDs clear. Repeat. Status = 01 is again observed when HSI.0 goes 1 to 0 and a new time (14) was read on the LEDs. The LEDs again clear on release of S0 to 0. H.R. and FIFO are now both empty.
5. ESC. Enter BY 5000 = 03 specifying that HSI.0 entries into

the FIFO will be accepted when a positive or negative transition on that pin occurs. Execute and throw HSI.0 hi. Keep it high. Read the status at P1. It should be 03 (a 0 to 1 event at HSI.0 occurred and its current state is 1). Throw S0 high and read the low-byte of the time of the event (we read F4). Release S0. LEDs at P1 clear. Release HSI.0 to 0. Read the new status at P1. It should be 01 (an event at HSI.0 occurred and its current state is 0 in keeping with the 1 to 0 transition just created there). Throw S0 high. Read the low byte of the 1 to 0 event's time occurrence at P1. We found FF. Release S0. LEDs clear. Etc.

EXPERIMENT 5-21

THE HSI UNIT. PART II: POLLING IOS1.6 AS TO WHEN FIFO IS FULL.

FORMULATION

1. We shall, as before, enable HSI.0 into the FIFO and have HSI-MODE loaded from address 5000. Address 5000, in turn, is loaded at run-time with the byte establishing one of the four possible modes or conditions under which the FIFO will accept specific HSI.0 events. Each mode will be investigated in turn. A full FIFO will be signaled when bit IOS1.6 becomes 1.
2. Two debounced switches will be used, one for inputting events through HSI.0, the other (S0) for control at P0.0.
3. After initializations of SP, IOC0 (to enable HSI.0), HSI-MODE, and the clearing of P1, the program polls bit 6 of Status Register IOS1 ("HSI FIFO IS FULL"). Events will be input at HSI.0 and when the FIFO is full (IOS1.6 = 1) the program will fall through the JBC polling of IOS1.6 and output FF to the LEDs. The appearance of FF will signify that the FIFO is full. We want to observe how many transitions (events) at HSI.0 are necessary before FF appears (FIFO becomes full). FF remains as long as P0.0 is low. Remember, "FIFO full" means the FIFO has gone from 5 or less entries to 6 or more entries. If FIFO is full AT LEAST 7 events must have occurred with one of them now in H.R.
4. When S0 at P0.0 is thrown high another fall-through occurs. The program reads out HSITIME into a "dummy" register (REG) FOR THE PURPOSE OF EMPTYING THE HOLDING REGISTER, thereby causing one of the FIFO entries to seep down to the H.R. THE FIFO WILL NOW BE 1 LESS THAN FULL. The next instruction jumps back to the clearing of P1 and the polling of IOS1.6 again (with the FIFO one less than full).
5. This time only ONE further event at HSI.0 should be necessary to make the FIFO full (as revealed by the presence of FF at P1 again). This is so because we sucked out ONE FIFO entry via the H.R. when we loaded HSI-TIME into the dummy register.

The program at 2880 below needs no further analysis.

```
        18 00           SP       EQU    18H
        15 00           IOCO     EQU    15H
        16 00           IOS1     EQU    16H
        03 00           HSIMODE  EQU    03H
        04 00           HSITIME  EQU    04H
        40 00           REG      EQU    40H
        0E 00           PO       EQU    0EH
        0F 00           P1       EQU    0FH
                        ;
                        ;
2880                             ORG    2880H
                        ;
2880    A1 C0 00 18              LD     SP,#00C0H          ;Initialize SP to 00C0H.
2884    B1 01 15                 LDB    IOCO,#01H          ;Enable recording of HSI.0.
2887    B3 01 00 50 03           LDB    HSIMODE,5000H[0]   ;Load HSIMODE with mode byte
                                                           ;from address 5000H.
288C    11 0F           CLEAR:   CLRB   P1                 ;Initialize LEDs.
288E    36 16 FB                 JBC    IOS1,6,CLEAR       ;If IOS1.6 = 0, then loop back to
                                                           ;CLEAR.
2891    B1 FF 0F                 LDB    P1,#0FFH           ;Else output 0FF to LEDs.
2894    30 0E FD        HERE:    JBC    PO,0,HERE          ;If PO.0 = 0, then loop on HERE.
2897    A0 04 40                 LD     REG,HSITIME        ;Else load HSITIME into REG.
289A    27 F0                    SJMP   CLEAR              ;Jump back to wait for new entry
                                                           ;into the FIFO.
```

PROCEDURE

1. Reset the unit to clear the FIFO and enter BY 09 = 00. Enter BY 5000 = 01 so that the mode will be set specifying entry of events/times into the FIFO only on 0 to 1 transitions at HSI.0. Execute the program from 2880. Throw HSI.0. lo to hi a number of times. You'll observe FF appear at P1 on the 7th 0 to 1 transition at HSI.0. The FIFO filled up with 6 entries, and one (7th) resides in the H.R. as expected. Clear P1 by throwing S0 at P0.0 hi/lo. This time only one 0 to 1 transition at HSI.0 is needed to cause FF to appear again at P1. We had created one vacancy in the FIFO when we read HSI-TIME into REG. Reading HSI-TIME emptied the H.R., and one FIFO entry then seeped down to H.R. FIFO then had 5 entries. Thus only one more entry from HSI.0 was needed to fill the FIFO again (to 6). Throw S0 hi/lo again. P1 clears. Again, only one more HSI.0 positive transition is needed to see FF again.
2. ESC. Reset the unit to clear the FIFO. Enter BY 5000 = 02 to establish the mode in which only 1 to 0 transitions at HSI.0 will enter as events into the FIFO. Execute the program. This time you'll see FF appear at P after the 7th negative (1 to 0) transition of the switch at HSI.0.

Clear P1 and remove one entry in the FIFO by throwing S0 hi/lo. Throw HSI.0 hi/lo and note FF appear at P1 after the FIRST negative transition at HSI.0. Clear P1. FF appears again when HSI.0 is again made to go hi to lo. This is all in keeping with expectations. The FIFO fills with 6 entries, with the 7th in the H.R. Reading H.R. causes one of the 6 FIFO entries to enter the H.R. Only one more event is needed to fill FIFO again.

3. ESC and reset to clear out the FIFO. Enter BY 5000 = 03. This time the mode will be such that the FIFO will accept 0 to 1 AND 1 to 0 transitions at HSI.0. Execute. Throw HSI.0 hi/lo a number of times. Note that FF appears on the fourth throw of HSI.0 hi (a total of 7 0 to 1 and 1 to 0 transitions were made and the FIFO is full). Release HSI.0 to low. That's another event but can't get into the full FIFO. Clear P1 and remove one entry in the FIFO by throwing S0 hi/lo. This time FF will re-appear on the first throw of HSI.0 hi (0 to 1), filling the FIFO again. Release HSI.0. Another event (1 to 0) has just been created but it won't get into the FIFO as the latter is full again. Clear P1 by throwing S0 hi/lo. This also empties one entry from the FIFO. Throw HSI.0 high again. FF re-appears (full FIFO). MAINTAIN HSI.0 high and throw S0 hi/lo to clear P1 and empty one FIFO entry. Release HSI.0 from high to low. FF re-appears (full FIFO) because the 1 to 0 transition found room in the FIFO and filled it again.
4. ESC and reset. Enter BY 5000 = 00 to set the mode for a FIFO entry only on every 8th positive transition at HSI.0. Execute. Throw HSI.0 hi/lo a number of times. To be exact, throw it high 8 times, 7 times over i.e. 7 times in groups of 8. On the 56th throw high you'll see FF at P1. The FIFO filled with 7 EVENTS, one event being defined as the 8th positive transition on HSI.0. Throw S0 hi/lo to clear P1 and EMPTY ONE EVENT from FIFO into H.R. (due to the reading of HSI-TIME in the program). Throw HSI.0 high a number of times again. FF will re-appear on the 8th throw high i.e. another EVENT has been made and fills the FIFO again from 5 to 6 entries.

EXPERIMENT 5-22

THE HSI UNIT. PART III: HSI IS MADE TO INTERRUPT WHENEVER AN EVENT ENTERS THE HOLDING REGISTER. READ-OUT OF STATUS/TIME IN THE ISR.

The key word in the above title is ENTERS. The formulation, method, and procedure are exactly as in Expt. 5-20 except that, instead of polling IOS1.7 as to when the Holding Register is full with data to be read, we shall now have the HSI unit generate an interrupt to indicate that the H.R. BECAME full. In that way our program can be engaged in "other tasks". It will be interrupted only when the HSI has data available in the H.R. from a new event. At that time a vector to the "HSI Data Available" ISR is made to read out the status and time in the H.R. associated with the event that entered the FIFO and then seeped into the H.R. Our ISR in this case will do EXACTLY what the program of Expt. 5-20 did after the fall-through of the polling of IOS1.7 there. The ISR then returns to "other tasks".

Generation of an interrupt from the HSI unit when the H.R. has been loaded with an event can be arranged by doing the following: 1. set bit 2 in the Interrupt Mask Register ("HSI Data Available" mask bit); 2. set the global bit (PSW.9) to 1 with an EI instruction; 3. set IOC1.7 to 0 to ask for an HSI interrupt based on the Holding Register having been loaded (rather than on the FIFO having been filled, as in Expt. 5-23). Also remember that the address in the interrupt location table for an HSI interrupt is 2004. That location must be loaded with the address of the HSI ISR (28C3 in our program below).

The program at 28A0 is presented below. No need to analyze the ISR at 28C3 as it is the same set of steps as in Expt. 5-20 after the JBC IOS1, 7, CLEAR there i.e. reading out HSI's status at P1, then the time of the event at P1, then back to the main program clearing P1 (and in this case doing "other tasks"). The main program enables HSI.0 transitions into the FIFO (IOC0.0 = 1), asks for an HSI interrupt when the H.R. has been loaded (IOC1.7 = 0), sets the HSI mode from the byte written to 5000 at run-time, sets M.2 = 1 to enable the HSI interrupt source, loads address of HSIINT (28C3) into address 2004 (INVEC), enables the global bit after pendings are cleared, clears the LEDs at P1, and engages in "other tasks" at SJMP CLEAR.

```
      18 00            SP       EQU      18H
      15 00            IOC0     EQU      15H
      16 00            IOC1     EQU      16H
      03 00            HSIMODE  EQU      03H
      06 00            HSISTAT  EQU      06H
      04 00            HSITIME  EQU      04H
      50 00            TEMP     EQU      50H
      04 20            INVEC    EQU      2004H
      08 00            MINT     EQU      08H
      09 00            PINT     EQU      09H
      40 00            REG      EQU      40H
      0E 00            P0       EQU      0EH
      0F 00            P1       EQU      0FH
                       ;
                       ;
28A0                            ORG      28A0H
                       ;
28A0  A1 C0 00 18               LD       SP,#00C0H        ;Initialize SP to 00C0H.
28A4  FA                        DI                        ;Disable global interrupt bit.
28A5  B1 01 15                  LDB      IOC0,#01H        ;Enable recording of HSI.0.
28A8  B1 00 16                  LDB      IOC1,#00         ;Select the generation of interrupt
                                                          ;on a loading of the HSI Holding
                                                          ;Register.
28AB  B3 01 00 50 03            LDB      HSIMODE,5000H[0];Load HSIMODE with mode byte
                                                          ;from address 5000H.
28B0  B1 04 08                  LDB      MINT,#04H        ;Load MINT to enable "HSI Data Avail."
                                                          ;Interrupt.
28B3  11 09                     CLRB     PINT             ;Clear all pending interrupts.
28B5  A1 C3 28 50               LD       TEMP,#HSIINT     ;Load the address of the HSIINT
28B9  C3 01 04 20 50            ST       TEMP,INVEC[0]    ;Interrupt Service Routine into INT
                                                          ;VECTOR table.
28BE  FB                        EI                        ;Enable global interrupt bit.
28BF  11 0F            CLEAR:   CLRB     P1               ;Clear LEDs.
28C1  27 FC                     SJMP     CLEAR            ;Jump back to wait for new entry
                                                          ;(interrupt).
                       ;
                       ;
                       ;
                       ;        HSI INTERRUPT SERVICE ROUTINE
                       ;
28C3  B0 06 0F         HSIINT:  LDB      P1,HSISTAT       ;Output HSI status to LEDs.
28C6  30 0E FD         STOP:    JBC      P0,0,STOP        ;If P0.0 = 0, then loop on STOP.
28C9  A0 04 40                  LD       REG,HSITIME      ;Else load HSI time word into REG.
28CC  B0 40 0F                  LDB      P1,REG           ;Output low byte of time word to

                                                          ;LEDs.
28CF  38 0E FD         WAIT:    JBS      P0,0,WAIT        ;If P0.0 = 1, then loop on WAIT.
28D2  F0                        RET                       ;Else return to main routine.
```

PROCEDURE

1. Reset to clear out the FIFO. Enter BY 09 = 00 to clear any pendings. Enter BY 5000 = 01 for the FIFO to accept only 0 to 1 transitions at HSI.0. Execute from 28A0. Throw HSI.0 high. Observe 03 at P1. An HSI interrupt was generated because H.R. was loaded with an event. HSI-STATUS was read out to P1 in the ISR. 03 indicates an event (0 to 1) occurred at HSI.0 and that its current status is 1. Throw S0 at P0.0 high. HSI-TIME is then read out at P1 (lo-byte). We found 1D. Throw S0 low and see P1 clear. Throw HSI.0 high again and observe 03 on P1. S0 high produced 7B at P1 (event time, lo-byte). S0 low cleared P1 again.
2. ESC and reset. Enter BY 09 = 00. Enter BY 5000 = 02 to have the FIFO accept only 1 to 0 transitions on HSI.0. Execute the program. Throw HSI.0 high then low. 01 appeared at P1 only when HSI.0 went from 1 to 0. Throw S0 high. HSI-TIME (lo-byte at P1) was 3A in our case. Throw S0 low. P1 clears. The status 01 at P1 indicated an event occurred at HSI.0 and that its current state is 0, as expected. Repeat and observe the status (always 01 when HSI.0 goes 1 to 0) and then the lo-byte of time at P1.
3. ESC and reset. Enter BY 09 = 00. Enter BY 5000 = 03 for the FIFO to accept 0 to 1 and 1 to 0 transitions. Execute the program. Throw HSI.0 high and keep high. Observe status 03 at P1, as expected for a 0 to 1 transition. Throw S0 high and read time at P1 (we read 8B for its low byte). Throw S0 low. P1 clears. Release HSI.0 (1 to 0 transition). Observe 01 at P1 for the status of HSI.0 i.e. an event (1 to 0) occurred at HSI.0 and its current state is 0. Throw S0 high and read time at P1 (we found 5A). Throw S0 low. P1 clears. Repeat, keeping HSI.0 high after the 0 to 1 transition. 03 appears at P1 again. Read out low byte of time by throwing S0 high. Clear P1 by throwing S0 low. Release HSI.0 (1 to 0) and see status 01 at P1 again. Read the time and then clear P1.
4. ESC. Reset. Enter BY 09 = 00. Enter BY 5000 = 00 so that the FIFO will only accept an event on the 8th positive transition at HSI.0. Execute the program. Throw HSI.0 0 to 1 eight times. On the 8th throw 03 appears at P1 showing the expected status. Throw S0 high to read lo-byte of the time of occurrence. We read 31 at P1. Throw S0 low to clear P1. Repeat. After 8 throws of HSI.0 hi/lo, 03 is again observed at P1. Throwing S0 high, then low, produced 6B (time) at P1 followed by a clear of P1.

EXPERIMENT 5-23

THE HSI UNIT. PART IV: HSI IS MADE TO INTERRUPT WHENEVER THE HSI FIFO GOES TO A FULL STATE.

The key word in the above title is GOES. This experiment uses a modified form of the program of Expt. 5-22 just done. To have the HSI unit create HSI interrupts when the HSI FIFO BECOMES full requires only that IOC1.7 be set to 1. All we need do is change LDB IOC1, #00 to LDB IOC1, #80 i.e. enter BY 28A9 = 80 at address 28A9 in the program of Expt. 5-22. The ISR (new) for this experiment will now be located at 28D5. This requires only that we change C3 at 28B6 to D5 i.e. enter BY 28B6 = 0D5 so that #HSIINT (address of ISR) is now 28D5. The ISR program itself is shown below at 28D5. It is entered only when the FIFO BECOMES full (6 or more entries). When entered, the global bit is disabled so that no further HSI interrupts will occur. FF is output to P1 and remains there until S0 at P0.0 is thrown high, at which point the ISR returns to main program. P1 then clears. The FIFO is still full because nothing has been read out of H.R. No more interrupts would be produced when transitions at HSI.0 are made as a result of DI. However, even WITHOUT DI at 28D5, no further FIFO interrupts would be generated on HSI.0 transitions BECAUSE, BEING STILL FULL, FIFO CAN NOT GO FROM THE NECESSARY LESS THAN FULL STATE TO A FULL STATE. We'll verify this later.

```
        0E 00       P0       EQU    0EH
        0F 00       P1       EQU    0FH
                    ;
                    ;
28D5                         ORG    28D5H
                    ;
                    ;        HSI INTERRUPT SERVICE ROUTINE
                    ;
28D5    FA          HSIINT:  DI                   ;Disable global interrupt bit.
28D6    B1 FF 0F             LDB    P1,#0FFH      ;Output 0FF to LEDs.
28D9    30 0E FD    STOP:    JBC    P0,0,STOP     ;If P0.0 = 0, then loop on STOP.
28DC    F0                   RET                  ;Else return to main routine.
```

PROCEDURE

1. Reset. Enter BY 09 = 00. Enter BY 28A9 = 80, then BY 28B6 = 0D5, and BY 5000 = 01 (for HSI.0 0 to 1 transitions only). Execute from 28A0 (same as for Expt. 5-22). Throw

HSI.0 hi/lo a number of times. FF appears at the LEDs after 7 throws of HSI.0 i.e. only after the FIFO itself is full with 6 entries (one is in H.R.). Throw S0 hi/lo. LEDs clear. Throw HSI.0 hi/lo. FF does NOT appear again because of the DI instruction. Redo the above (after a reset) with DI at 28D5 replaced by NOP i.e. enter BY 28D5 = 0FD. You'll find even then that when FF appears at P1 (after 7 throws of HSI.0) and is then cleared by S0, further throws of HSI.0 will not cause FF to reappear. The FIFO became "full" after 7 throws and remained full. It can only generate an interrupt when it goes from a LESS THAN FULL TO FULL STATE. Remember our ISR does not read out an entry in the H.R. so FIFO remains at 6.

2. Reset. Enter BY 09 = 00 and BY 5000 = 00 for the eight 0 to 1 transitions mode. Leave the NOP at 28D5. Execute from 28A0. Throw HSI.0 0 to 1 56 times (one "event" per 8 transitions, 7 events required to fill FIFO). FF appears at P1 after the 56th throw is completed. Throw S0 hi/lo to clear P1. No further FIFO interrupt occurs whether or not you throw HSI.0 hi again many or a few times. A FULL FIFO BY ITSELF DOES NOT GENERATE THE INTERRUPT. IT MUST GO FROM A LESS THAN FULL TO FULL STATE.

EXPERIMENT 5-24

USING THE HSI UNIT TO GENERATE A) A DIVIDE-BY-8 PRESCALAR, B) A DIVIDE-BY-56 PRESCALAR.

PART (A). DIVIDE-BY-8 PRESCALAR

This experiment is based on the program in Expt. 5-22 with 00 back at 28A9 and 0C3 at 28B6, so that HSI interrupts to the ISR at 28C3 will be generated each time the Holding Register is loaded with a new event/time. To realize a divide-by-8 prescalar only requires that the ISR increment the LEDs at P1 every time it is entered, and that it should be entered once every 8 (0 to 1) transitions on HSI.0. The latter is easily provided for by entering BY 5000 = 00 at run-time, which is passed to HSIMODE by the program. It is also necessary, before the ISR returns to the main program after the INCB P1 we propose, that the H.R. be "sucked out" artificially by a read of HSI-TIME into a "dummy" register. This will ensure that, after the return, the now empty H.R. can generate another HSI interrupt when another event/time enters it (after another 8 (0 to 1) transitions at HSI.0). Finally, the SJMP CLEAR at 28C1 in Expt. 5-22 should be changed so that the LEDs are NOT continually cleared by "other tasks" in the main program. This is easily realized by replacing FC at 28C2 with FE. A debounced switch is used at HSI.0.

PROCEDURE

1. Reset and enter BY 09 = 00. Enter BY 28A9 = 00 and BY 28B6 = 0C3, their original values in Expt. 5-22. Enter BY 28C2 = 0FE. Establish the ISR program by entering BY 28C3 = 17, 0F, 0A0, 04, 40, 0F0. This is code for INCB P1 (17, 0F) followed by LD REG, HSITIME (where A0 is code for LD, REG is 40, and HSITIME is 04), and then RET (F0). Finally, enter BY 5000 = 00 to select the 8 transition mode.
2. Execute the program from 28A0. Throw the switch at HSI.0 high 8 times and see P1 = 01 appear on the 8th throw. Another 8 throws creates P1 = 02, then 03, etc. i.e. a divide-by-8 prescalar.
3. Reset. Replace A0, 04, 40 by NOPs i.e. enter BY 28C5 = 0FD, 0FD, 0FD. Enter BY 09 = 00 and BY 5000 = 00. Execute from 28A0 again. Throw HSI.0 high 8 times. See P1 = 01 on the 8th throw. Try another 8, then another 8, etc. P1 remains "stuck" at 01. Reason: H.R. was not now emptied out in the ISR. Hence it could not go from an empty to loaded

state, the requirement needed to produce the associated HSI interrupt. Thus we never enter ISR again to increment P1. This is a very important point.

PART (B). DIVIDE-BY-56 PRESCALAR

To accomplish a divide-by-56 prescalar, we should use the "FIFO Full" HSI interrupt in conjunction with mode 00. Then eight 0 to 1 transitions on the HSI pin (here HSI.0) will cause one "event/time" to enter the FIFO, and 7 such groups of 8 will be necessary before the FIFO fills (one in H.R. and six in FIFO) and an HSI interrupt is generated. The interrupt to the ISR will then result in an increment of P1 by 1. We will then have our ISR read out H.R. and all 6 entries in the FIFO, thereby making FIFO and H.R. TOTALLY EMPTY before returning to the main program of Expt. 5-22. In that way we can assure ourselves that another 56 0 to 1 transitions on HSI.0 will fill up H.R. AND FIFO (to 6), thereby causing HSI to generate another "FIFO Full" interrupt to ISR where P1 is incremented once again, etc.

The best way to accomplish the emptying of H.R. and the FIFO in the ISR is to empty the Holding Register by a read of HSI-TIME into REG (40H in Expt. 5-22) as many times as necessary until bit IOS1.7 ("HSI Holding Register Data Available") is 0. This will indicate ALL FIFO entries have successively entered the H.R. and ALL were read out (no more data is available in the H.R.). Thus our ISR is now to read: INCB P1; LD REG, HSI-TIME; NOP; NOP; JBS IOS1, 7, READ; RET; where READ is the label to be associated with the LD instruction. As long as IOS1.7 is 1, a loop back to another READ (of the H.R.) is done until IOS1.7 is finally 0, indicating an empty FIFO AND H.R. The two NOPs are inserted to guarantee the 8 state times needed between successive reads of the H.R. They're really not needed here since the JBS instruction consumes 9 state times if obeyed. The machine code to be entered for this ISR at 28C3 is accomplished by entering BY 28C3 = 17, 0F, 0A0, 04, 40, 0FD, 0FD, 3F, 16, 0F8, 0F0 (check that this is so). In addition, we now need to enter BY 28A9 = 80 in Expt. 5-22 (to ensure HSI interrupt generation when FIFO becomes full) and BY 28C2 = 0FE (to replace FC there).

PROCEDURE

1. With the changes indicated in the last paragraph made, reset and enter BY 09 = 00. Execute from 28A0. Observe P1 increment once for every 56 throws of HSI.0 (0 to 1) verifying a divide-by-56 prescalar.

2. Reset and replace JBS IOS1, 7, READ with JBS IOS1, 6, READ-easily realized by merely entering BY 28CA = 3E (replacing 3F there). This means we'll now be testing IOS1.6 ("HSI FIFO IS FULL"). Fall-through this JBS instruction means IOS1.6 = 0 which signifies the FIFO is NO LONGER FULL i.e. it has less than 6 entries (5). If you execute from 28A0 you'll find P1 will read 01 after 56 transitions on HSI.0. But P1 will increment to 02 after only another 8 throws of HSI.0, and to 03 after only another 8 throws of HSI.0, etc. Easy to explain: upon RET from ISR, FIFO now had 5 entries (it's not full). One more entry will make it full and kick off a FIFO FULL interrupt to ISR again. 8 throws will produce that next event to fill the FIFO. The story repeats in the ISR. A very important point.

CHAPTER 6

APPLICATIONS WITH THE 8096 USING ITS SPECIAL FUNCTION REGISTERS AND HIGH SPEED I/O UNITS. CLASSIC APPROACH VS. THE HIGH SPEED WAY.

INTRODUCTION

In this chapter we shall apply the understanding and mastery of the 8096's SFRs gained in chapter 5 to problems of an applications nature specifically centered around the use of those SFRs. Some 26 applications experiments are presented which will illustrate the power that can be achieved in I/O control through the SFRs. While many of the experiments in chapter 5 already had an applications orientation, the ones here go farther. 13 of the 26 experiments are specifically concerned with the HSO and HSI units. Thus we'll be able to appreciate the many advantages which the High Speed Units offer in I/O control versus the more classic SFR approach expressly used in other applications experiments in this chapter for purposes of comparison. Where the latter approach was adopted, the experiment usually ends with a problem suggesting that the reader try to implement the same application the "High Speed way". In some cases we do that ourselves later in the chapter. The table of contents for chapter 6 indicates the scope of applications we'll cover in this chapter.

Chapter 5 did not concern itself with the Serial I/O port's related SFRs, nor will this chapter. We leave that for chapter 8 where Serial I/O is treated exclusively.

EXPERIMENT 6-1

USING PWM TO REALIZE A VOLTAGE SYNTHESIZER. LIGHT INTENSITY OR MOTOR SPEED CONTROL.

In this experiment we wish to have the PWM unit produce an output voltage at P2.5 that numerically equals the value entered on-the-fly at the keyboard. Thus entering 11 should produce 1.1V, 05 should produce 0.5V, etc. The PWM pulses output at P2.5 are converted to smooth D.C. voltage levels proportional to pulse duty cycle by the RC filter circuit added at P2.5 (see Fig. 4-11 p. 4-8 Microcontroller Handbook).

FORMULATION

1. When the program is executed, we would like to enter e.g. WO 40 = 00 and measure 0 volts at the filtered PWM output at P2.5, then enter WO 40 = 05 and measure 0.5 volts, then enter WO 40 = 11 and observe 1.1, volts, ... up to WO 48 to produce 4.8 volts. Assuming FF in the PWM register (100%) duty cycle) produces 4.8V at the filtered output at P2.5 (which was true in our unit), and assuming linearity between % duty cycle and voltage output at P2.5, then the following table is to govern the implementation of our voltage synthesizer:

BYTE at 40	DESIRED OUTPUT	REQUIRED BYTE FOR PWM REG.
00H	0.0V	00H
05	0.5V	1B
11	1.1V	3A
16	1.6V	55
22	2.2V	75
35	3.5V	BA
41	4.1V	D9
48	4.8V	FF

2. From the above table, we are led to the following relationship that will be stored as a table starting at address 2100:

2100	00
2105	1B
2111	3A
2116	55
2122	75

2135	BA
2141	D9
2148	FF

The above table, when properly accessed by the program, will assure that WO 40 = 16 will produce 1.6 V, WO 40 = 35 will produce 3.5V, etc.

3. The program must be such that when executing, entering e.g. WO 40 = 16 will access address 2116 in the table and read the byte 55 there into the PWM (17H) to produce the 1.6V at P2.5. Likewise, entering WO 40 = 35 on-the-fly will access address 2135 in the table and read the byte BA there into PWM to produce 3.5 V at P2.5. (40 here is the address of what we call REG1 in the internal RAM register file. Remember from chapter 2 that entering e.g. WO 40 = 16 places the word 0016 into REG1 i.e. 16 goes to 40 and 00 to 41 - important in what follows in the program).

The program itself starts at 2160, the table above, entered by user, starts at 2100. We present the program at 2160 below.

```
        18 00          SP      EQU    18H
        17 00          PWM     EQU    17H
        16 00          IOC1    EQU    16H
        40 00          REG1    EQU    40H
        50 00          REG2    EQU    50H
                       ;
                       ;
2160                           ORG    2160H
                       ;
2160    A1 C0 00 18            LD     SP,#00C0H        ;Initialize SP to 00C0H.
2164    B1 01 16               LDB    IOC1,#01H        ;Load IOC1 to select PWM function.
2167    45 00 21 40 50 RDREG1: ADD    REG2,REG1,#2100H;Add 2100H to contents of REG1,
                                                       ;store result in REG2.
216C    B2 50 17               LDB    PWM,[REG2]       ;Load PWM reg. with contents of
                                                       ;memory location pointed to by REG2.
216F    27 F6                  SJMP   RDREG1           ;Loop back to continue polling.
```

The second line of code selects the PWM function for pin P2.5. The next line is our way of accessing the table at 2100. The base address 2100 is added to the word value in REG1 (which is entered and altered at will as the program is running: i.e. WO 40 = XY, where XY = 00, 05, 11, 16, 22, 35, 41, or 48). The word sum is stored in word REG2 (at 50H) - a three operand ADD. REG2 is now pointing to 2100, or 2105, or 2111, ... or 2148 depending on the value XY entered for WO 40 on-the-fly. Next, the PWM register is loaded with the byte stored at the address in the table to which REG2 is pointing. This drives pin P2.5.

There we measure the (filtered) output voltage with a VTVM. Finally the SJMP to RDREG1 polls REG1 for any update in the value at 40, should we wish to produce another (synthesized) output voltage.

PROCEDURE

1. Enter the table at 2100, 2105, 11, 16, 22, 35, 41, 2148 with the bytes listed in (2) of the formulation section. Enter WO 40 = 0000 (or simply WO 40 = 00) to produce an initial voltage of 0.
2. Execute from 2160. Measure the voltage at P2.5 with a VTVM. Do you find any offset from the expected 0 volts? We found 0.02V.
3. On-the-fly, enter WO 40 = 05. We found .51 volts at P2.5. Enter WO 40 = 11. We measured 1.1 volts output. Enter WO 40 = 16. We observed 1.63 volts on the VTVM. Enter WO 40 = 22. We read 2.22 volts. With WO 40 = 48 we found 4.79 volts. Try other entries corresponding to the table at 2100.
4. Connect the P2.5 pin's filtered output to any LED on your board making sure that the LED is disconnected from its other input source. As you vary WO 40 note how the light intensity produced at the LED varies accordingly.
5. ESC. This time connect the unfiltered output at P2.5 to a 1-6V d.c. motor (see Fig. 2-3, chapter 2). Execute and enter the various values at WO 40, as before. Notice the speed vary as the output voltage (pulses) drive the base of the transistor in the motor circuit of Fig. 2-3. The pulses are integrated out to a smooth motor response by the circuit inductance and motor inertia.

EXPERIMENT 6-2

WAVEFORM GENERATION USING THE PWM UNIT: SAWTEETH AND TRIANGLES OF VARIABLE SLOPE.

In this application, the PWM unit will be used to generate sawtooth and triangular waveforms of arbitrary slope. The program will increment (or increment and decrement) the byte to be loaded into the PWM SFR, thereby continually varying the pulse width of one or more groups of pulses at P2.5. With our RC filter there, this will lead to the expected waveforms.

FORMULATION

1. Triangular waveforms will ge generated and observed on a scope by periodically incrementing the byte in the PWM register by a given amount (equal to the byte stored at address 5000 at run-time) until FF (divisible by that byte) is reached, and then periodically decrementing the byte in the PWM by a given amount (equal to the byte stored at address 5001 at run-time). When 00 in the PWM is reached on the way down, the incrementations shall start over again, etc. It is clear that if the incrementations are in steps of 1, the PWM - outputted pulse width keeps incrementing the least possible amount and the slope of the integrated voltage output will be small. If the incrementations are in steps of, say, 3 or 5, the pulse widths increment by those step amounts and the slope will be correspondingly larger (ditto for the decrementations; note the stored bytes at 5000 and 5001 can be different, if you wish, to produce asymmetric triangles).
2. To produce a sawtooth waveform, it will only be necessary to replace the test as to when the PWM reaches FF with NOPs, so that the jump to the decrementations of the PWM bytes is not achieved. Instead FF will overflow to 00 and the incrementations will continue.
3. We shall incorporate a time delay in the program that will allow any desired number of pulses of the SAME width to be generated before a change in their width is permitted. Recall that the period of the PWM pulse output at P2.5 is a fixed 64 usec. so that we must wait AT LEAST that amount of time before the PWM is incremented to produce the next pulse width at P2.5. Or we can wait a MULTIPLE of 64 usec. to allow several pulses of identical width to be outputted before the NEXT group of identical pulses, but of incremented width, is generated. The byte stored at address 5002

will determine the time delay between pulse width incrementations or decrementations i.e. the number of pulses generated of given width before any change in their width is permitted. This will allow for a second parameter controlling the slope of the triangle or sawtooth, inasmuch as a large time delay will allow a larger number of pulses of identical width to be generated before incrementations of width occur - hence a smaller slope.

4. In the program, we shall test the state of switch S0 at P0.0 (which we'll keep in the low state in this experiment). When FF in the PWM on the way up, or 00 in the PWM on the way down, is reached, the state of S0 is tested. If it's 0 (as in this experiment), fall-through occurs and decrementations (or incrementations) of the PWM are immediately realized, thus effecting the triangle waveform. If, however, S0 is kept high (as in Expt. 6-3), the test prevents fall-through and the PWM is maintained at FF or 00, as the case may be UNTIL S0 is thrown low, when fall-through occurs. In that way the triangular waveform becomes trapezoidal. The latter is extensively used in the area of efficient motor speed control. We treat that application in Expt. 6-3. Here we keep S0 low so that triangular waveforms are output for observation on a scope.

The program starts at 2220 and is reproduced below.

```
      18 00          SP       EQU    18H
      17 00          PWM      EQU    17H
      16 00          IOC1     EQU    16H
      40 00          REG1     EQU    40H
      50 00          REG2     EQU    50H
      0E 00          P0       EQU    0EH
                     ;
                     ;
2220                          ORG    2220H
                     ;
2220  A1 C0 00 18             LD     SP,#00C0H        ;Initialize SP to 00C0H.
2224  B1 01 16                LDB    IOC1,#01H        ;Load IOC1 to select PWM function.
2227  B1 00 40                LDB    REG1,#00         ;Load REG1 with 00H.
222A  B0 40 17       THERE0:  LDB    PWM,REG1         ;Load PWM reg. with contents of REG1.
222D  EF 30 00                CALL   TIME             ;Call TIME to allow N pulses of
                                                      ;equal widths.
2230  99 FF 40                CMPB   REG1,#0FFH       ;Test value of REG1.
2233  DF 07                   JE     THERE2           ;If REG1 = 0FFH then jmp to THERE2.
2235  77 01 00 50 40 THERE1:  ADDB   REG1,5000H[0]    ;Else add contents of 5000H to REG1.
223A  27 EE                   SJMP   THERE0           ;Loop back to repeat.
223C  38 0E FD       THERE2:  JBS    P0,0,THERE2      ;Poll switch S0. If = 1 jmp to THERE2.
```

```
223F  7B 01 01 50 40 THERE3: SUBB   REG1,5001H      ;Else subtract contents of memory loc
                                                    ;5001H from REG1. Store result in REG1.
2244  B0 40 17               LDB    PWM,REG1        ;Load PWM reg. with contents of REG1.
2247  EF 16 00               CALL   TIME            ;Call TIME to allow N pulses of
                                                    ;equal widths.
224A  99 00 40               CMPB   REG1,#00        ;Test value of REG1.
224D  D7 F0                  JNE    THERE3          ;If REG1 != 00, then goto THERE3.
224F  38 0E FD      THERE4:  JBS    P0,0,THERE4     ;Else poll switch S0; if = 1 jmp
                                                    ;THERE4.
2252  27 E1                  SJMP   THERE1          ;Else loop back to THERE1 to repeat.
                    ;
                    ;
                    ;
                    ;        Time Delay Routine
                    ;
2260                         ORG    2260H
                    ;
2260  A3 01 02 50 50 TIME:   LD     REG2,5002H[0]   ;Load REG2 with contents of memory
                                                    ;location 5002H.
2265  05 50         AGAIN:   DEC    REG2            ;Decrement REG2.
2267  D7 FC                  JNE    AGAIN           ;If REG2 != 0, goto AGAIN.
2269  F0                     RET                    ;Else return to main program.
```

In the main part of the above program, REG1 is initialized to 00 and then loaded into the PWM. TIME is called and a comparison of REG1 with FF is then made to see if we've reached the apex of the triangle. If yes, then a jump to THERE2 will start to decrement REG1 (and hence the PWM) if S0 is 0. If not, REG1 is incremented by the amount stored in 5000 and its value is then transferred to PWM as a result of SJMP to THERE0. This continues until FF in REG1 is reached (with TIME deciding how many pulses of that incremented width are to be produced before we go on to the next incrementation of the PWM). When FF is reached JE THERE2 lands us on the test of S0. If S0 is low, we fall through to SUBB which starts decrementations of REG1 (and hence of PWM). TIME is again called between decrementations of the pulse width to control the number of pulses of given width that are output at P2.5 before the next decrement of pulse width for the next group of outputted pulses is permitted. Finally, REG1 is compared to 00 (trough of the triangle). If 00 is reached, fall-through to THERE4 occurs where S0 is tested. If S0 is low, fall-through to SMJP THERE1 starts incrementing PWM again. If 00 is not reached JNE THERE3 continues the decrementations of REG1 (and PWM). In this manner we achieve a triangular waveform. It should be apparent that if we place NOPs (0FD) at addresses 2230-2234 inclusive, we eliminate the test as to whether the upper limit FF in PWM is achieved. In that case, there'll never be a JE THERE2 to the decrementations of REG1 and PWM (assuming S0 is low). There will only be incrementations of REG1 with the attendant SJMP to THERE0 where REG1 is transferred to PWM. Hence a ramp is produced till FF overflows to 00 and another ramp commences. This, then, will produce a sawtooth waveform.

The time delay routine at 2260 (TIME) needs analysis. The LD, DEC, JNE, and RET take up 12, 4, 8 and 16 state times, respectively. With one state time equal to 3 oscillator periods, each state time is equivalent to 1/4 usec. for a 12 MHz clock. Allowing 54 states = 14 usec. for the CALL, CMPB, ADDB (or SUBB), SJMP, LDB, JE (or JNE) instructions in the main program in between successive calls to TIME, leaves about 50 usec. of TIME needed to produce the 64 usec. minimum delay before the PWM may be incremented to produce a different pulse width. 50 usec. of TIME requires 200 state times. 28 of them are accounted for by LD and RET in TIME, leaving 172 to be accounted for by DEC and JNE. The latter consume together 12 state times. Hence 172/12 = 14 loops of DEC/JNE are needed. This requires that 000EH be loaded into REG2. This we do by means of the LD REG2, 5002H[0] instruction at the start of TIME at 2260. Address 5002 is loaded at run-time with word 000E (or other word values as now discussed). With 000E in 5002, we conclude that 64 usec. TIME is produced so that ONE pulse, and ONLY one pulse, is generated of a specific width by PWM, BEFORE the NEXT incremented or decremented width is generated. To produce 2 such identical pulses before a change in width is permitted would require (128 - 14) usec. = 114 usec. = 456 state times = (456-28) DEC/JNE states = 428/12 = 35 (DEC/JNE) loops = 0023H. i.e. 0023H must now be loaded into REG2 from the word 0023 stored at 5002 at run-time. In the same way 0039H stored in 5002 will produce sufficient TIME for 3 PWM pulses of identical width to be produced before the next incrementation or decrementation. 004E in 5002 will allow TIME to generate 4 pulses of identical width before any increment or decrement of the pulse width occurs (verify these conclusions with your own calculations).

For this experiment you'll need to connect the output of the PWM unit at P2.5 (after it's been filtered with the RC integrator circuit of Fig. 4-11, p. 4-8 of the Microcontroller Handbook) to the vertical input of an internally swept oscilloscope.

PROCEDURE

CASE 1. Connect the filtered PWM output at P2.5 to the vertical of your scope. Enter BY 5000 = 01, BY 5001 = 01, WO 5002 = 000E. This will assure increments and decrements of the PWM by one, and allow only one pulse of given width to be produced before another increment or decrement of the width is to take place. Hence the time to reach FF (max. width) from 00 (min. width) should be 64 usec. x 256 increments = 16.38 msec. Keep switch S0 at P0.0 low. Execute the program from 2220. Triangular waveforms will be seen. We measured the rise from zero to apex of the triangle to be 15.6 msec.

CASE 2. ESC and enter BY 5000 = 03, BY 5001 = 03, and leave WO 5002 at 000E as before. This time one pulse is again produced between increments or decrements, but the latter are now to be in steps of 3. Hence 85 such 3-step increments will bring us to FF. The rise time, therefore, should now be 64 usec. x 85 = 5.45 msec. Execute the program. Triangles again appear on the scope. We found the rise time now to be 5.4 msec.

CASE 3. ESC and enter BY 5000 = 05, BY 5001 = 05, but leave WO 5002 at 000E. Again one pulse between increments or decrements is to be produced, but this time the latter are to be in steps of 5. 51 such 5-step increments will be needed to reach FF. The rise time, therefore, should now be 64 usec. x 51 = 3.28 msec. Execute and measure the rise time of the triangles. We found approximately 3 msec.

CASE 4. Leave BY 5000 and BY 5001 at 05 but on-the-fly change WO 5002 to 0023. The latter will guarantee that 2 pulses of identical width will be produced before incrementations in steps of 5 occur. Since the time between pulses is 64 usec. and 51 5-step increments are needed to reach FF, the rise time should be 2 x 64 usec. x 51 or 6.56 msec. The triangle slope changes. We found about 6 msec. for the new rise time.

CASE 5. Enter WO 5002 = 0039H with the same byte values at 5000 and 5001 (i.e. 05). This will assure that 3 pulses of identical width are produced before the next 5-step increment on pulse width is allowed. Hence the rise time should now be 3 x 64 usec. x 51 = 9.84 msec. We observed triangles of about 10 msec. rise time when WO 5002 = 0039 was entered.

CASE 6. Enter WO 5002 = 004E, leaving 05 at 5000 and 5001. This will allow the production of 4 pulses of identical width before another 5-step increment or decrement is allowed. Hence the rise time now should be 4 x 64 usec. x 51 or 13.12 msec. We observed about 13 msec. for the rise time as soon as we entered WO 5002 = 004E.

CASE 7. ESC and place NOPs at 2230 - 2234 i.e. BY 2230 TO 2234 = 0FD. Enter BY 5000 = 01 and WO 5002 = 000E. This should produce ramps (sawteeth) from 00 to FF, then over again and again. One pulse between increments of 1 will occur leading to a sawtooth rise time of 64 usec. x 256 = 16.4 msec. Executing from 2220 did indeed produce ramps. We measured the rise time to be about 16 msec. If you change BY 5000 to 03, then to 05, etc. (on-the-fly), you should observe 5.4 and 3.26 msec. rise times. Why? This we verified.

CONCLUSION

Most, if not all, of the essential points concerning pulse-width-modulation generation and D to A conversion with the 8096's PWM SFR were covered and verified in this experiment. Our roughly measured rise-times (observed on the scope) were in good agreement with all expected theoretical values. It is essential that you keep in mind that the PWM function produces one pulse of whatever width every 64 usec. Multiples of that time must be allowed before trying to change the width by loading in a new value into PWM. To this end we used our time delay routine at 2260, based on loops, to allow for the required time. In Expt. 6-19 we re-do this waveform generation experiment, but in that case we employ one of the four Software Timers internal to the 8096 and part of the HSO unit. We'll have it generate an INTERRUPT at some multiple of 64 usec. The Interrupt Service Routine will then increment the PWM the desired number of times. In this way we free up the 8096 for "other tasks" instead of keeping it pinned down in time delay loops, as we've done here.

EXPERIMENT 6-3

TRAPEZOIDAL PROFILE MOTOR SPEED CONTROL IMPLEMENTED WITH THE PWM UNIT.

The program for this experiment is exactly the same as the one in Expt. 6-2 just concluded (make sure you enter BY 2230 = 99, 0FF, 40, 0DF, 07 to replace the NOPs that we inserted at addresses 2230 - 2334 in case 7 of Expt. 6-2. That will restore the CMPB and JE instructions that were previously there). Trapezoidal motor speed control is desirable for efficient motor operation. Final motor speed is attained with a gradual ramp-up, and halting of the motor is achieved gradually from its maximum speed. That is desirable from the standpoint of power consumption and wear and tear.

FORMULATION

1. To achieve a trapezoidal profile at P2.5's PWM output now requires that S0 at P0.0 be kept high, so that the test of S0 at 223C maintains PWM at FF as long as S0 stays high. When S0 is then thrown lo/hi, fall-through to THERE3 at 223F will occur to start the ramp-down to 00. When 00 is reached, fall-through JNE at 224D will occur and, since S0 is now high again, the PWM will be maintained at 00 till S0 is again thrown lo/hi. That will cause fall-through at 224F to SJMP THERE1, starting a ramp back up till FF is again reached. Since S0 is back high, FF is maintained in the PWM till S0 is again thrown lo/hi, etc. etc. In this way, we have S0 control the production of a trapezoidal profile, as contrasted to the triangular waveforms produced in Expt. 6-2 when S0 was always kept lo.
2. P2.5's PWM pulses will be fed directly to the base of the transistor drive circuit of Fig. 2-3 in unfiltered form. The motor does its own integrating as a result of its inertia and circuit inductance.
3. As an example, let's have the PWM's rise-time from 00 to FF, or its fall-time from FF to 00, be 3 seconds, so that the d.c. motor's speed will proceed from rest to its maximum value in 3 sec., then remain at that maximum speed as long as S0 is high, start back down to 0 in 3 sec. when So is thrown lo/hi, remain at rest as long as S0 is high, start back up when S0 is again thrown lo/hi, etc. etc. In that way we should be able to observe the trapezoidal motor speed profile.
4. To achieve 3 sec., we'll work with BY 5000 = 01 and BY 5001 = 01 i.e. increases or decreases in the pulse width will be in steps of 1. Let n be the number of pulses

generated of identical width before the next increment or decrement of their width is permitted. Then the time for the PWM to reach FF will be n x 64 x 256 usec. We want this to equal 3 seconds. This leads to n = 183 as the required number of identical pulses before any increment or decrement is allowed. Since the time that elapses between identical pulses is 64 usec., the required time delay for the n = 183 identical pulses to be produced must be 64 x 183 = 11,712 usec. This translates to 46,848 state times that our time delay program at 2260 in Expt. 6-2 must produce. Since the LD and RET instructions in the T.D. account for 28 states, and the CALL, CMPB, ADDB, etc. instructions in the main program between the time delay entries themselves require 48 state times, we are left with 46,772 state times that the DEC/JNE instructions in the T.D. must provide. DEC/JNE provide 12 states, so 46,772/12 = 3898 loops are needed. This means loading REG2 at 2260 in the T.D. program with the word 0F3A (which we'll enter at address 5002 at run-time).

PROCEDURE

1. Connect the unfiltered PWM output at P2.5 to the base of the transistor whose collector circuit contains the d.c. motor (see Fig. 2-3). Enter BY 5000 = 01, BY 5001 = 01, and WO 5002 = 0F3A. Keep switch S0 high. Execute the program of Expt. 6-2 from 2220. Note the motor speed increase from 0 to a max. in about 3 sec., which WO 5002 = 0F3A assures. The speed remains constant as long as S0 is high. Throw S0 lo/hi and note the decrease in speed to 0, also in 3 sec. The motor remains at rest till S0 is again thrown lo/hi, when its speed again increases to a max. in 3 sec., etc. etc.
2. ESC and enter WO 5002 = 1F3A. Execute the program and observe the motor speed increase to a max. or decrease to a min. in about 6 sec. time intervals, with constant max. or min. speeds maintained for as long as S0 is maintained high. (1F3A is a little more than double 0F3A).
3. ESC and enter WO 5002 = 3F3A. Execute and observe the motor speed ramp up or down in about 18 sec. time intervals (3F3A is about 3 times the value of 1F3A).
4. ESC. At address 224B in the program, where CMPB REG1, #00 is present, enter BY 224B = 0B0 so that the comparison on the way down will now be with B0, not 00. In other words, the limits on speed will be a max. (FF) and a min. B0 (not 0). Leave WO 5002 at 3F3A. Execute and note the motor speed ramp up from 0 to a max., remain at max. as long as S0 is high, ramp down to some smaller speed when S0 is thrown lo/hi, stay at that smaller speed as long as

S0 is high, ramp back up to the max. speed when S0 is again thrown lo/hi, etc. etc. The ramp-up and ramp-down times between max. and min. speed limits is now less than the 18 sec. observed in case 3 above. FF - B0 = 79 dec. so the new ramp speeds should be about (79/255) x 18 sec., or something less than 6 sec. Verify that.

5. ESC. Enter By 17 = XY, where XY is any value you like between 00 and FF. Keep changing it. What's hapening to the motor speed and why?

EXPERIMENT 6-4

A TO D CONVERSION OF ALL EIGHT ANALOG CHANNELS. STORING THE RESULTS AND MULTIPLEXING THEM FOR DISPLAY.

The method can be applied to any number of channels less than or equal to eight. We illustrate it for all eight channels.

FORMULATION

1. Each analog input channel will be converted, one after the other, and the 10-bit results will be stored in memory at word addresses 5000, 5002, 5004, etc. Thus converted byte ACH.0 (lo) will be stored at 5000 and ACH.0 (hi) will be stored at 5001; ACH.1 (lo) will be stored at 5002 and ACH.1 (hi) will be stored at 5003; .... ACH.7 (lo) will be stored at 500E and ACH.7 (hi) will be stored at 500F.
2. At run-time we'll enter WO 70 = 0000 to select channel 0's digital results for initial display at P1s LEDs (bits 9-2) and at P2.7, P2.6 (bits 1,0). Here REG4 will be RAM location 70.
3. Upon execution of the program at 22B0 (see below) each channel's analog input is converted, one after the other, and the results stored at the mentioned eight word addresses in memory. The LEDs at P1 and P2 will immediately display bits 9-2 and 1,0 (at P2.7, 2.6), respectively, of channel 0's conversion results.
4. As we then enter WO 70 = 0001, or 0002, or 0003, ... or 0007 (in turn, or in any order) we'll see channel 1's, or 2's, or 3's, ... or 7's 10-bit conversion results at port P1's and P2's LEDs (P1.7 .... P1.0; P2.7, P2.6).
5. If we change the POT settings at the ACH input channels, and then enter WO 70 = 0008, conversions of all the NEW ACH analog inputs will start and the new results will be stored in the same 8 memory word locations 5000 - 500E.
6. Entering WO 70 = 00, then 01, then 02, ... then 07, in any order, will result in the display of each channel's conversion results at the P1, P2 LEDs.
7. Changing POT settings at the ACH channels and entering WO 70 = 0008 from the keyboard will result in conversions of all the new analog inputs and the storage of the respective digital results in the aforementioned memory locations. Selection of various channels for display then proceeds as in (6) above.

The program to accomplish the above is shown below, starting at 22B0. We analyze it at its conclusion.

```
                        ;  EXPERIMENT 6-4:  MULTI-CHANNEL A/D CONVERSION.
                        ;
                        ;
       18 00            SP       EQU    18H
       02 00            ADCOM    EQU    02H
       02 00            ADRESLO  EQU    02H
       03 00            ADRESHI  EQU    03H
       0F 00            P1       EQU    0FH
       10 00            P2       EQU    10H
       40 00            REG1     EQU    40H
       50 00            REG2     EQU    50H
       60 00            REG3     EQU    60H
       60 00            REG3LO   EQU    60H
       61 00            REG3HI   EQU    61H
       70 00            REG4     EQU    70H
       80 00            REG5     EQU    80H
       90 00            REG6     EQU    90H
                        ;
                        ;
22B0                             ORG    22B0H
                        ;
22B0   A1 C0 00 18               LD     SP,#00C0H         ;Initialize SP to 00C0H.
22B4   A1 00 50 40      BEGIN:   LD     REG1,#5000H       ;Load REG1 with base of result
                                                          ;table.
22B8   B1 08 50                  LDB    REG2,#08H         ;Load REG2 with start command
                                                          ;for A/D conversion on channel 0 now.
22BB   B0 50 02         THERE:   LDB    ADCOM,REG2        ;Load ADCOM to start A/D conversion.
                                                          ;Channel number is 3 LSBs of REG2.
22BE   FD                        NOP                      ;Allow eight state times before
22BF   FD                        NOP                      ;polling conversion done bit.
22C0   3B 02 FD         BUSY:    JBS    ADRESLO,3,BUSY    ;If BUSY BIT = 1, then loop and test.
22C3   B0 02 60                  LDB    REG3LO,ADRESLO    ;Else conversion is over,store results
22C6   B0 03 61                  LDB    REG3HI,ADRESHI    ;in REG3.
22C9   C2 41 60                  ST     REG3,[REG1]+      ;Store 10 bit result as TWO bytes
                                                          ;in table.
22CC   17 50                     INCB   REG2              ;Increment REG2 to next A/D channel.
22CE   99 10 50                  CMPB   REG2,#10H         ;Test if last channel done.
22D1   D7 E8                     JNE    THERE             ;If CHANNEL != LAST, then go to THERE.
                        ;
                        ;        DISPLAY RESULTS
                        ;
22D3   A0 70 90         RDREG4:  LD     REG6,REG4         ;Else load REG6 with channel/command
                                                          ;from input variable location.
22D6   99 08 90                  CMPB   REG6,#08H         ;Test for start new convert command.
22D9   DF D9                     JE     BEGIN             ;If REG6 = new convert command,then
                                                          ;go back to begin.
22DB   09 01 90                  SHL    REG6,#01H         ;Else logical shift left to multiply
                                                          ;input data by 2.
```

```
22DE    45 00 50 90 80      ADD     REG5,REG6,#5000H;Add modified input data
                                                    ;with table base and store into pointer.
22E3    B2 81 10            LDB     P2,[REG5]+      ;Output channel conversion value to
22E6    B2 80 0F            LDB     P1,[REG5]       ;LEDs at P2 and P1.
22E9    27 E8               SJMP    RDREG4          ;Go back to poll for input data.
```

The main program from 22B0 through 22D2 accomplishes the following: REG1 is loaded with the base address of 5000 of the table in which the 10-bit converted results of each of the 8 channels are to be stored. 08 is loaded into REG2, and from there into ADCOM to start immediate A/D conversion on channel 0 (ADCOM is a write-only SFR and therefore can not be incremented directly to proceed from channel to channel. We increment it through REG2). The two NOPs are needed to provide the eight state times necessary before conversion starts. ADRESLO, bit 3, (the status bit S) is then polled to ascertain whether conversion is over. When S = 0 conversion is over and fall-through to 22C3 then loads ADRESLO into REG3LO (with bits 1,0 of the A/D result going into bits 7,6 of REG3LO), followed by a loading of bits 9-2 of the A/D result from ADRESHI to REG3HI. The ST instruction then stores REG3's A/D word result into the table at the address pointed to by REG1, with the latter then being double-incremented so that REG1 is now ready to point to the next WORD ADDRESS in the table for storing the next channel's A/D result. REG 2 is then incremented in preparation for its loading into ADCOM to start a conversion on the next channel. Before that is done, the incremented value of REG2 is compared with the byte 10H. If all 8 channels have been converted REG2 would have gone from 08 to 0F, then to 10 after the last increment. If the comparison indicates that REG2 has not yet been incremented to 10, then another channel needs to be converted. The JNE THERE accomplishes that, since the incremented value of REG2 is loaded into ADCOM at THERE to start conversion on the next channel. When REG2 equals 10, fall-through 22D1 occurs to "DISPLAY RESULTS". All 8 channels have been converted and the results stored as words in the table starting at 5000 (and ending at 500E).

At 22D3 we start the "DISPLAY RESULTS" routine. REG4 (entered at-run-time, and changed on-the-fly from the keyboard i.e. WO 70 = 000n where n will be 0, 1, 2, ... 7, or 8 and REG4 = 70H) is loaded into REG6. A comparison of REG6 with 08 is made. An entry WO 70 = 0008, as the program is executing, will be our way of initiating another conversion of all 8 channels. In that case the JE BEGIN is taken and 8 new conversions, with storage of new results in the same table, will take place. If, however, WO 70 = 000n was entered on-the-fly, with n = 0, 1, 2, ... 7 (but not 8) then fall-through to 22D9 occurs. SHL then multiplies 000n by 2. Thus, for example, if n were 3, asking to display channel 3's results, SHL would produce 0006 in REG6 and, in that case, the 3-operand ADD instruction that follows would leave e.g. 5006 in REG5. The LDB at 22E3 would then go to address 5006 and load the byte found there (holding the 2 low bits of the A/D conversion result of channel 3) out to port P2 (where the LEDs at P2.7 and P2.6 would display those 2 low bits). REG5 would then be auto-incremented by 1 to 5007 so that the next LDB instruction at 22E6 would fetch the byte at 5007 and output it to the 8 LEDs at port P1. That byte at 5007 contains the hi bits (9-2) of the A/D conversion result of channel 3, in this case. The SJMP RDREG4 goes back to 22D3 to poll for another WO 70 entry either asking for the same, or another, channel's results to be displayed, or for the start of 8 new conversions for subsequent display. The SHL instruction is clearly needed to access even word boundaries in the table.

PROCEDURE

1. We used two 5V POTS at channels 6 and 7 to supply variable analog input signals there, and simple digital switches at channels 0 - 5 (so that conversion results at channels 0 - 5 would be either 00 or FF depending on the switch setting). This was done for the sake of simplicity. The method will be perfectly well demonstrated with this simple set-up.
2. Enter WO 70 = 0000, asking for the display of channel 0's results. Adjust the POTs to definite analog settings at channels 6, 7 and set channels 5 - 0 to e.g. 5V, 0V, 5V, 0V, 5V, 0V, respectively, by setting the switches there to 1, 0, 1, 0, 1, 0.
3. Execute the program from 22B0. Observe channel 0's 10-bit results at the LEDs at P1 and P2 (P2.7, P2.6). In this case the result is 000 - all LEDs are out. Enter, in turn, WO 70 = 01, 02, ... 07 and read the 10-bit results for the requested respective channels 1, 2, ... 7 at the 10 LEDs. In this case the results will be 3FF for channel 1, 000 for channel 2, 3FF for channel 3, 000 for channel 4, 3FF for channel 5, and the relevant values for channels 6 and 7 corresponding to the POT settings there.
4. Change the POT settings at channels 6 and 7 and this time set the switches at channels 5 - 0 so that the input voltages on channels 5 - 0 are now 0V, 5V, 0V, 5V, 0V, 5V, respectively. No change will appear on the LEDs. The latter are still displaying the results of the old POT setting at channel 7. Enter WO 70 = 08. This requests 8 new, updated conversions and storage. Then enter WO 70 = 0, 1, 2, ... 7 and observe the new conversion results at the respective channels 0, 1, 2, ... 7. Are they consistent with your settings?

EXPERIMENT 6-5

EVENT COUNTING FROM TWO DIFFERENT SOURCES (T2CLK and HSI.1) WITH DIFFERENT MAXIMUM EVENT REQUIREMENTS.

We will here demonstrate the use of two possible event sources for Timer 2. These are the T2CLK pin (P2.3) and the HSI.1 pin (53). Events (0 to 1 or 1 to 0 transitions) on those two pins will be counted by Timer 2 when the appropriate T2 source is selected by the programming of IOC0 bit 7. We will also demonstrate use of one of the two possible external hardware inputs for the resetting of T2. They are the T2RST (P2.4) or HSI.0 (54) pins. Programming bit 5 in IOC0 selects which of these two pins is to reset T2. A 0 to 1 transition on the selected pin will cause T2 to be cleared to 0. Bit 3 in IOC0 must be set to 1 for either of these two external hardware T2 reset sources to be enabled. Finally, we'll demonstrate use of one of the two possible software T2 reset sources, namely either bit 1 of IOC0 or channel 14 (E) of the HSO Command Tag. We'll work with the T2RST pin as our hardware T2 reset source and IOC0.1 as our software T2 reset source. See Expt. 6-6 and 5-7, where channel E in HSOCOM is used to reset T2 by software and HSI.0 is used to reset T2 by hardware, respectively.

In the experiment, we'll use three debounced switches connected to T2CLK, HSI.1, and T2RST. When the program described below is executed, we are to allow the T2CLK source to input no more than 6 events - they'll be recorded at P1's LEDs. Further T2CLK events will not be recorded. Events are now to come only from HSI.1 to the extent that no more than 4 from HSI.1 will be recorded (as add-ons to the 6 recorded at P1 from T2CLK). When P1 shows 10, no further events at HSI.1 will be recorded. Instead the count at the LEDs clears and only new events at T2CLK will be recorded. The scenario repeats - 6 from T2CLK, then 4 from HSI.1, then 6 from T2CLK, etc. Further, during the T2CLK inputs, T2 (and P1) can be cleared by throwing the switch at T2RST; you can then input 6 more T2CLK clocks again, before HSI.1 takes over for its 4 events.

The program starting at 2370 is given below.

```
18 00        SP      EQU     18H
15 00        IOC0    EQU     15H
40 00        REG1    EQU     40H
0F 00        P1      EQU     0FH
0C 00        T2      EQU     0CH
```

```
2370                           ORG     2370H
                         ;
2370    A1 C0 00 18              LD      SP,#00C0H         ;Initialize SP to 00C0H.
2374    B1 0A 15         LOAD15H:LDB     IOC0,#0AH         ;Load IOC0 to select T2CLK and
                                                           ;T2RST, and reset T2.
2377    A0 0C 40         RDT2CLK:LD      REG1,T2           ;Load value of T2 into REG1
237A    B0 40 0F                 LDB     P1,REG1           ;Output low byte of T2 value to LEDs.
237D    99 06 40                 CMPB    REG1,#06H         ;Test if value of T2 = 6.
2380    D7 F5                    JNE     RDT2CLK           ;If T2 != 6,then go back to read it.
2382    B1 88 15                 LDB     IOC0,#88H         ;Else load IOC0 to select HSI.1 as
                                                           ;T2 input clock (T2 not reset).
2385    A0 0C 40         RDHSI1: LD      REG1,T2           ;Load value of T2 into REG1.
2388    B0 40 0F                 LDB     P1,REG1           ;Output low byte of T2 value to LEDs.
238B    99 0A 40                 CMPB    REG1,#0AH         ;Test if value of T2 = 10.
238E    D7 F5                    JNE     RDHSI1            ;If T2 != 10,then go back to read it.
2390    27 E2                    SJMP    LOAD15H           ;Else jump back to repeat.
```

The LDB at 2374 programs T2CLK as the source for T2 events and T2RST as the external source for a T2 reset (note that this also enables the external reset for T2). The LDB also clears T2 because it sets bit IOC0.1 to 1. T2 is then polled and its value loaded into word REG1. The low byte (lo count) of REG1 is then output to the LEDs at P1 (T2 can not be byte-read). The CMPB instruction tests whether REG1 has reached 6 (from events at T2CLK recorded by T2). If not, a jump back to a reading of T2 occurs. When the CMPB indicates that 6 events have indeed been input from T2CLK, fall-through occurs to 2382. There IOC0 is loaded with 88. This selects HSI.1 as the source for T2 events and keeps T2RST as the external source for hardware resets of T2. Importantly, it does not software reset T2 (bit IOC0.1 is now 0). Hence TOTAL counts will be displayed (6 plus any additional ones now to come from HSI.1). Again T2 is loaded into REG1 and then output to P1 (lo-byte of count). This time another CMPB tests whether the total count in T2 has reached 0A (10 dec.) i.e. whether 4 counts from HSI.1 have been recorded. If not, then the JNE instruction will send the program to another reading of T2. (The source of T2 events is still HSI.1, so the jump goes back to RDHSI.1, not to RDT2CLK.) If 10 counts total have been reached, fall-through to 2390 occurs where SJMP to LOAD15H again selects T2CLK as the source for T2 events and resets T2 to 0 (by software). The sequence of happenings repeats all over.

PROCEDURE

1. Execute the program from 2370. Remember to connect debounced switches to the T2CLK, HSI.1, and T2RST input pins.
2. Create more than 6 events at the T2CLK switch. Only 6 will show at P1's LEDs. Now create more than 4 events at the HSI.1 switch. The count at the LEDs increases to 10, but no more. The LEDs at P1 clear just after the count there reaches 10. Create events again at T2CLK. The features of the results just observed repeat.
3. During the time T2CLK is inputting its events you can throw the switch at T2RST to effect a reset of T2. The LEDs at P1 will clear and you can then start over with new counts from T2CLK till 6 are reached, as previously. What happens if 6 are reached, you input 2 more from HSI.1, so that the LEDs indicate 8 total counts, and you THEN throw the switch at T2RST? You'll clear T2 and the LEDs at P1, but now 10 events from HSI.1 will be required before the LEDs clear and the process starts all over, normally again. Why?

PROBLEM

Modify the program so that the maximum event limits on T2CLK and HSI.1 can be changed on-the-fly as the program is running. Think up other practical variations of the problem whereby alarms are set off when certain critical numbers of events from either source, or the total number of events, are reached. Having two independent sources of events for T2, which can be programmably controlled to flexibly operate in conjunction with one another, can be very useful in real applications.

EXPERIMENT 6-6

COUNTING SPECIFIED NUMBERS OF EVENTS IN T2, STARTING OVER, TRACKING TOTALS. TWO SOFTWARE WAYS TO RESET T2.

In this experiment, we again demonstrate the use of T2 to record events at the T2CLK input. The objective is both to keep a running total of events while providing intermediate count limits to trigger a simulated event whenever the count reaches these limits.

FORMULATION

1. A debounced switch is used at T2CLK (P2.3) to input events to T2. Another debounced switch S0 is used at input bit P0.0. S0 is initially kept low.
2. Address 5000 contains the desired number of events to be counted (entered at run-time) before T2 is to be cleared. The counts will be observed at P1's LEDs. The latter also clear when the specified number of events is reached. Further events are recorded in T2 (and at P1) until the specified number is again input, at which time T2 and P1 again clear.
3. REG2 will keep track of the total number of counts as multiples of the desired limit. Thus, for example, if 5000 contains the number 6 as the limit of input events at which time T2 is to be cleared, then inputting 30 events will cause T2 and P1 to each count to 6 and then clear before another 6 events are input. In this case they'll clear 5 times over, but REG2 will store the number 30 up to that point.
4. If, in the numberical example presented in (3) above, 4 more events are input, REG2 will still hold 30 BUT REG3 WILL STORE THE TOTAL RUNNING COUNT i.e. 34 in this case.
5. Displaying the total number of events that were input at any point in time can be achieved by throwing switch S0 high. The total number of events to that point will be displayed at the LEDs at P1. Throwing S0 back low will allow port P1 to resume showing the count WITHIN THE LIMIT (6 IN THIS EXAMPLE) THAT WAS LAST REACHED and to increment from that point, clearing only when the desired limit is again reached. Thus S0 low allows P1 to show the event count-up in groups of the desired limit, in which P1 clears every time the limit is reached, while S0 high asks for the total count-up to that point in time to be displayed at P1. S0 going low again resumes the event count,

within the limit, at P1.

The program at 23A0 is shown below.

```
         18 00         SP       EQU    18H
         0E 00         P0       EQU    0EH
         0F 00         P1       EQU    0FH
         15 00         IOC0     EQU    15H
         40 00         REG1     EQU    40H
         50 00         REG2     EQU    50H
         60 00         REG3     EQU    60H
         0C 00         T2       EQU    0CH
                       ;
                       ;
23A0                            ORG    23A0H
                       ;
23A0     A1 C0 00 18            LD     SP,#00C0H          ;Initialize SP to 00C0H.
23A4     11 50                  CLRB   REG2               ;Initialize BYTE register REG2.
23A6     B1 0A 15               LDB    IOC0,#0AH          ;Load 0AH into IOC0 to select
                                                          ;T2CLK and T2RST and reset T2.
23A9     30 0E 03      POLLS0:  JBC    P0,0,RDT2          ;If P0.0 = 0,then jump to continue
                                                          ;loading REG1.
23AC     EF 20 00               CALL   TOTAL              ;Else Call DISPLAY TOTAL routine.
23AF     A0 0C 40      RDT2:    LD     REG1,T2            ;Continue loading REG1 with
                                                          ;count.
23B2     B0 40 0F               LDB    P1,REG1            ;Output interim count to LEDs
                                                          ;(low byte).
23B5     54 40 50 60            ADDB   REG3,REG2,REG1     ;Update total counts in REG3.
23B9     9B 01 00 50 40         CMPB   REG1,5000H[0]      ;Test if present count is equal
                                                          ;to limit.
23BE     D7 E9                  JNE    POLLS0             ;IF limit not reached, then go
                                                          ;back to poll P0.0 and record cnts.
23C0     77 01 00 50 50         ADDB   REG2,5000H[0]      ;Else add the limit to previous
                                                          ;limit.
23C5     B1 0A 15               LDB    IOC0,#0AH          ;Reload IOC0 to reset T2 and
                                                          ;start a new count.
23C8     FD                     NOP                       ;These NOPs will be modified
23C9     FD                     NOP                       ;at runtime.
23CA     FD                     NOP                       ;
23CB     FD                     NOP                       ;
23CC     FD                     NOP                       ;
23CD     27 DA                  SJMP   POLLS0             ;Jump back to poll P0.0 and repeat.
23CF     B0 60 0F      TOTAL:   LDB    P1,REG3            ;Output total events to LEDs.
23D2     38 0E FD      HERE:    JBS    P0,0,HERE          ;If P0.0 = 1 loop here.
23D5     F0                     RET                       ;Else return to main program.
```

Let us analyze the program. SP initialized to 00C0 and REG2, which will hold the total count-up in MULTIPLES of the desired basic event limit, is cleared. 0A loaded into IOC0 selects T2CLK and T2RST as the event and external reset sources for T2, enables the external T2 reset facility, and clears T2 (IOC0.1 = 1 clears T2). S0 at P0.0 is next polled. If S0 is low (which it initially is), the JBC at POLLS0 jumps to RDT2 which reads the event count in T2 into REG1. The low byte of REG1 (lo count of T2) is then output to the LEDs at P1. Next the total count to this point is stored in REG3 by adding the present count in REG1 (which is less than or equal to the specified limit of event counts desired) to the total count in REG2 (which is a multiple of the limit count to this point). The ADDB instruction is of the 3-operand type so that the result of REG1 + REG2 is stored in REG3. The CMPB instruction compares the present count in REG1 (a count which is, so far, less than or equal to the desired limit) with the desired limit which has been stored in address 5000 at run-time. If that limit is not reached, the following JNE causes a jump back to POLLS0 and the whole description repeats, as long as S0 is low.

If, and when, the desired limit is reached, fall-through to ADDB REG2,5000H[0] results in the limit stored at 5000 being added to the previous value (multiples of the limit) stored in REG2, with that updated multiple replacing the previous multiple in REG2. Since the limit has been reached, we should now reset T2 and clear P1. The LDB IOC0, #0AH clears T2 (IOC0.1 = 1). Five NOPs follow to leave room for a modification to be made later after we perform the basic part of the experiment - of no concern to us now. The SJMP POLLS0 causes a jump back to the JBC test. If S0 is still low, the jump taken by JBC to RDT2 outputs the cleared value of T2 to the LEDs at P1, and all starts over again - BUT with REG2 containing the updated value of the MULTIPLES of the LIMIT input so far at T2CLK, and with REG3 containing the actual TOTAL number of events input to this point at T2CLK.

What happens when S0 is thrown high? The JBC at POLLS0 falls through to "CALL TOTAL". TOTAL is located at 23CF. There the total count in REG3 is output to the LEDs at P1. This display is maintained as long as S0 is high. When S0 is thrown low fall-through to RET takes us back to RDT2 at 23AF where the LAST attained count in T2 (somewhere between 0 and the desired limit) is restored to P1 and all proceeds as before.

NOTE

We could have eliminated the LDB IOC0, #0AH instruction at 23C5 and replaced it, instead, with an SJMP back to 23A6 where we already have that instruction. Recall that this latter instruction resets T2, among other things. Our purpose of inserting it at 23C5, with the 5 NOPs that follow, has to do with a program modification we'll be making after the basic experiment is done. That modification will allow us to examine another method of resetting T2 - one which will involve the HSO unit. (See the latter parts of the Procedure below).

PROCEDURE

1. Connect two debounced switches to T2CLK (P2.3) and P0.0 (S0). Keep S0 low. Enter BY 5000 = 06 i.e. we are to allow 6 input events at T2CLK before T2 and P1 clear. Further input events will cause T2 and P1 to count up from 0 again to a max. of 6, etc.
2. Execute from 23A0 and input events from the switch at T2CLK. Observe the count-up at P1's LEDs. The count at P1 is cleared when 6 is reached. Do it three times over so that P1 will clear 3 times and 18 events will have been input thus far. Key in 2 more events. P1 now shows 2. Throw S0 high and keep it high. Observe the total events input thus far at P1. P1 reads 14H = 20 dec., as expected. Release S0. See P1 = 2 again. Key in 4 more events from T2CLK. P1 clears. Throw S0 high. See P1 = 18H = 24 dec., as expected. Release S0. P1 reverts to 0. Key in another 4 events at T2CLK. See P1 = 4. Throw S0 high. Observe P1 = 1C = 28 dec., again as expected. Release S0 and observe P1 = 4 again. Key in an additional 2 events and see P1 clear, etc.
3. ESC and enter BY 5000 = 08 as the desired limit when T2 and P1 are to clear. Execute and repeat the steps in 2. All repeats, except that the limit when T2 and P1 clear is now 8.
4. We can have the HSO unit reset T2 as follows: LDB HSOCOM, #4EH followed by ADD HSOTIME, T2, #0000 are the two instructions needed by the HSO unit to reset T2. This is so for the following reasons: 4E loaded into the HSO Command Tag (HSOCOM:SFR 06H) selects T2 as the reference timer and channel 14, the "Reset T2" channel (in the lower nibble of HSOCOM). Thus we are programming the action to be a RESET of T2 when T2 reaches a certain value. That value is to be T2 + 0000 as dictated by the next instruction ADD HSOTIME (where HSOTIME is SFR 04H). T2 + 0000 means "now" i.e. the reset is to occur for the present value of T2 and NOT after T2 is incremented any further. Hence, if these two instructions can be inserted at 23C5 - 23CC in the program, then a reset of T2 will be accomplished, just as the LDB IOC0, #0AH instruction at 23C5 presently accomplishes it. The code for these two instructions is B1, 4E, 06

followed by 45, 00, 00, 0C, 04. Hence all we need do to modify our program is to enter BY 23C6 = 4E, 06, 45, 00, 00, 0C, 04 (the B1 is already present at 23C5 from the previous LDB). With these changes made, enter BY 5000 = 06 again and execute from 23A0. Enter events at T2CLK and see all the results that were observed in step 2 above.

EXPERIMENT 6-7

A PRESCALAR WITH T2 AS THE EVENT COUNTER.

In this experiment timer T2 is used to count events occurring at T2CLK's input. A register is used, in conjunction with the DIVB instruction, to scale the counts by a factor loaded into memory prior to execution of the program. The scaled count is displayed at P1's LEDs.

FORMULATION

1. T2CLK is connected to a debounced switch which, when pressed or released, will simulate an event. For every such y events, we wish to have the LEDs at P1 increment by 1. The desired prescale number y will be entered in address 5000 at run-time. y is the prescale factor. A debounced switch S0 at P0.0 is maintained lo.
2. When S0 at P0.0 is thrown high the remainder will be displayed i.e. the number of additional events that occurred since the last increment of the prescale value at P1.
3. At any time, we can throw a switch (not necessarily debounced) at T2RST to start all counts over again from 0.

The program at 2400 is presented below.

```
        18 00         SP      EQU     18H
        15 00         IOCO    EQU     15H
        40 00         REG1    EQU     40H
        41 00         REG1HI  EQU     41H
        0E 00         P0      EQU     0EH
        0F 00         P1      EQU     0FH
        0C 00         T2      EQU     0CH
                      ;
                      ;
2400                          ORG     2400H
                      ;
2400    A1 C0 00 18           LD      SP,#00C0H       ;Initialize SP to 00C0H.
2404    B1 0A 15              LDB     IOC0,#0AH       ;Load 0AH into IOC0 to select
                                                      ;T2CLK and T2RST,and reset T2.
2407    A0 0C 40      COUNT:  LD      REG1,T2         ;Load REG1 with number of events
                                                      ;from T2.
240A    FE 9F 01 00 50        DIVB    REG1,5000H[0]   ;Divide count by prescaler in
        40
                                                      ;memory location 5000.
```

```
2410   B0 40 0F             LDB    P1,REG1         ;Output quotient to LEDs.
2413   30 0E F1             JBC    P0,0,COUNT      ;IF P0.0 = 0, then continue event
                                                   ;counting.
2416   B0 41 0F             LDB    P1,REG1HI       ;Else display remainder on the LEDs.
2419   38 0E FD    HERE:    JBS    P0,0,HERE       ;IF P0.0 = 1, then loop here.
241C   27 E9                SJMP   COUNT           ;Else jump back to repeat.
```

The instruction at 2404 resets T2 to 0, selects T2CLK as the event source for T2 and T2RST as the reset source for T2. It also enables T2's external reset facility. The event count in T2 is then read into REG1. Remember that Timer 2 can only be word-read, and this has bearing on why we load REG1 with the value in T2 as far as the DIVB instruction is concerned. DIVB divides the count in REG1 by the prescale value y stored in 5000 at run-time. The quotient is written into REG1(LO) while the remainder is placed in REG1(HI). This ensures that for every y events, REG1(LO) will increment by 1. The LDB P1, REG1 instruction, then, in fact, outputs that incremented (scaled) REG1(LO) value to the LEDs at P1. The JBC instruction at 2413 polls S0 at P0.0. If it's low, a jump to COUNT keeps counting events into T2 and outputting scaled-down values to P1. If, however, S0 is thrown high, fall-through to 2416 takes the count remainder from REG1(HI) and displays it at P1 as long as S0 remains high. When S0 is thrown back low, fall-through to SJMP COUNT results in a continuation of the recording of scaled-down events at P1's LEDs.

NOTE

A prescalar based on HSO Unit control is implemented in Expt. 6-18.

PROCEDURE

1. With debounced switches connected to T2CLK and P0.0 and any switch connected to T2RST, enter BY 5000 = 06 (prescale factor). Make sure S0 at P0.0 is in the low position and that the switch at T2RST is low.
2. Execute the program from 2400 and create a group of 6 events, 5 times over, then 4 more at T2CLK. You should observe 0, 1, 2, 3, 4, 5, appear at P1's LEDs.
3. Throw and maintain S0 high. You'll see 04 at P1 (the remainder after 5 prescales).
4. Release S0. You'll observe 05 at P1 again.
5. Create 2 more events at T2CLK. You'll now see 06 appear at P1. Create another 2 events at T2CLK. Throw S0 high and maintain it high. 02 appears at P1 (the remainder). Release S0. 06 re-appears at P1. Etc.

6. Keep creating T2CLK events. Then throw T2RST from low to high at any stage in the event process. T2, REG1, and the LEDs all revert to 0 (reset).
7. On-the-fly, enter BY 5000 = 0A (for a new prescale value of 10), but only after you've cleared the count in T2 by throwing T2RST lo/hi. Create 24 events at T2CLK. Observe 02 at P1, as you'd expect. Throw and maintain S0 high. Observe 04 (remainder) at P1's LEDs. Release S0. Observe 02 at P1 again.

EXPERIMENT 6-8

EVENT COUNTING WITH T2 DURING A REPETITIVE MANUFACTURING OPERATION. APPLICATION TO QUALITY CONTROL.

FORMULATION

1. In this experiment we simulate a widgit manufacturing process. n widgits are to be produced and, if the number of defectives is less than the tolerable limit d when n are produced, the batch of n is to go through and another batch of n is to be produced. If, however, the number of defectives in any batch reaches d before the number of widgits produced reaches n, then production of widgits is to halt and an alarm is to go on. The operator comes on to reject that batch and to re-tool. When he/she throws a switch, the alarm goes off and production of new batches is to commence. This is the general desription of the problem. Further details now follow.
2. The production quota n will be stored at run-time at address 5000 and the tolerable limit on defectives, d, will be stored at address 5001 at run-time.
3. Production of one widgit will consist of P2.6 going on for 1 sec. (the "drill"), then going off, and P2.7 coming on for 1 sec. (the "rivet" or "bolt" machine), then going off. That cycle of on/off for P2.6 and on/off for P2.7 repeats for each new widgit that is to be produced.
4. The number of widgits produced up to any given time (within a batch of n that is to be produced) is stored in REG1 and can be displayed at any time by simply entering BY 40 on-the-fly, where REG1 will be address 40 in RAM file.
5. As production of widgits is observed (LEDs are to be connected to pins P2.6 and P2.7), defectives will be simulated by periodically throwing a debounced switch connected to T2CLOCK. Timer T2 records a new event for each positive or negative transition at T2CLK, but our program will count ONE event as the positive, negative transition PAIR at the lever microswitch we employed for T2CLK's input. The LEDs at P1 will count up the number of defectives as they are produced, and REG4 will store that updated number, as will, of course, T2. You can think of a defective widgit as one that is outside some required critical dimension which will cause a limit switch (connected to T2CLK) to trip as that widgit moves on down the assembly line.
6. As stated in (1) above, if the number of defectives is less than d when n widgits are produced, that batch is to go

through. T2, P1, and REG1 are to be cleared and a new batch production of widgits is to start from a 0 defective count. This should happen automatically.

7. If, however, the number of defectives reaches d before n widgits have been produced, the count of defectives at P1 is to "freeze", production is to halt (i.e. P2.6 = P2.7 = 0) and an alarm is to go on (P1.7 = 1). The operator then rejects the batch and possibly re-tools. He/she can read the number of units produced in that batch to that point by entering BY 40. This gives the operator an idea of how bad the problem really is e.g. a low number produced with a relatively large number of defectives turned out would be quite serious. The operator can, if desired, enter a new production quota (BY 5000 = n') and/or a new value for the tolerable number of defectives (BY 5001 = d'). When the operator throws a switch S0 (at P0.0) high, the alarm goes off, P1 and T2 clear (previous defective count), and a new production run starts with a new count-up of defectives from a 0 value.
8. At any time during a production run, we can throw another switch S7 (at P0.7) high to freeze the count of defectives at P1 (even though less than d), clear P2.6, P2.7 (stopping production), and put on the alarm at P1.7. This might be desirable so that the operator can have the opportunity to enter new n, d values at 500, 5001, respectively, if he/she realizes the previous values entered there were wrong, or suddenly new requirements on n, d are needed. BY 40 again tells us the number produced. The operator can then throw S0 high to clear P1 and T2, shut the alarm and start production all over again from scratch. Thus we can abort and reject the latest run even though neither n nor d were reached during that run.

The program at 2490 is presented below. A detailed analysis is made at its conclusion.

```
18 00        SP      EQU     18H
15 00        IOC0    EQU     15H
40 00        REG1    EQU     40H
50 00        REG2    EQU     50H
60 00        REG3    EQU     60H
70 00        REG4    EQU     70H
0E 00        P0      EQU     0EH
0F 00        P1      EQU     0FH
10 00        P2      EQU     10H
0C 00        T2      EQU     0CH
```

```
2490                        ORG     2490H
                        ;
2490  A1 C0 00 18     BEGIN:  LD      SP,#00C0H       ;Initialize SP to 00C0H.
2494  11 0F                   CLRB    P1              ;Initialize LEDs to 00.
2496  01 40                   CLR     REG1            ;Initialize REG1 to 00.
2498  B1 0A 15                LDB     IOC0,#0AH       ;Load IOC0 with 0AH to select
                                                      ;T2CLK and T2RST and reset T2.
249B  71 3F 10        CYCLE:  ANDB    P2,#3FH         ;Initialize LEDs on P2.6,P2.7
                                                      ;to 0.
249E  91 40 10                ORB     P2,#40H         ;Set P2.6 to 1 (turn on "drill").
24A1  EF 32 00                CALL    TIME            ;Call time delay of approx. 1 sec.
24A4  71 BF 10                ANDB    P2,#0BFH        ;Set P2.7 to 1 and P2.6 to 0.
24A7  91 80 10                ORB     P2,#80H
24AA  EF 29 00                CALL    TIME            ;Call time delay of approx. 1 sec.
24AD  07 40                   INC     REG1            ;Increment COUNT of produced "parts".
24AF  3F 0E 19                JBS     P0,7,FREEZE     ;If P0.7 = 1,then jump to FREEZE
24B2  9B 01 00 50 40          CMPB    REG1,5000H[0]   ;Else test number produced.
24B7  D7 09                   JNE     AHEAD           ;If prod. number != limit (5000H),
                                                      ;jump to AHEAD.
24B9  9B 01 01 50 70          CMPB    REG4,5001H[0]   ;Else test number of defectives
24BE  D7 D0                   JNE     BEGIN           ;If number defectives != limit,then
                                                      ;production complete, jump to BEGIN.
24C0  20 09                   SJMP    FREEZE          ;Else go poll switch P0.0.
24C2  9B 01 01 50 70 AHEAD:   CMPB    REG4,5001H[0]   ;Production less then limit.
24C7  DF 02                   JE      FREEZE          ;If defectives = limit,then goto poll
                                                      ;switch.
24C9  27 D0                   SJMP    CYCLE           ;Else continue cycle.

24CB  71 3F 10        FREEZE: ANDB    P2,#3FH         ;P2.7 and P2.6 are cleared
                                                      ;("stop production").
24CE  91 80 0F                ORB     P1,#80H         ;Turn "alarm" on leaving display
                                                      ;of defective count on LEDs.

24D1  30 0E FD        HERE:   JBC     P0,0,HERE       ;If P0.0 = 0,then loop here.
24D4  27 BA                   SJMP    BEGIN           ;Else go back to BEGIN.
                        ;
                        ;       TIME DELAY ROUTINE
                        ;
24D6  B1 02 50        TIME:   LDB     REG2,#02H       ;Load REG2 with major loop count.
24D9  A1 FF FF 60     LOAD:   LD      REG3,#0FFFFH    ;Load REG3 with minor loop count.
24DD  A0 0C 70        READT2: LD      REG4,T2         ;Load REG4 with defective count in T2.
24E0  08 01 70                SHR     REG4,#01H       ;Logical shift right once to divide
                                                      ;number by 2.
24E3  B0 70 0F                LDB     P1,REG4         ;Output number of defectives to LEDs.
24E6  05 60                   DEC     REG3            ;Decrement minor loop.
```

```
24E8   D7 F3          JNE    READT2        ;If minor loop != 0,then go poll def.
                                           ;count.
24EA   E0 50 EC       DJNZ   REG2,LOAD     ;Else decr. major loop. If major
                                           ;count != 0 go back to reload minor
                                           ;loop count.
24ED   F0             RET                  ;Else return to main routine.
```

The main program above starts by clearing P1, which will display number of defectives, and REG1, which will keep track of the number of widgits produced. IOC0 is then loaded with 0A in order to select T2CLK as the event source for T2 and reset T2 to 0. 02 would do as well since we are not using the external hardware reset facility here. The ANDB and ORB instructions turn P2.6 (drill) on and P2.7 (rivet or bolt machine) off to start production. TIME is then called to keep P2.6 on for about 1 sec. Returning from TIME finds the ANDB and ORB instructions this time turning P2.6 off and P2.7 on. TIME is again called to keep the rivet or bolt machine on for 1 sec. One widgit has been produced and so we increment REG1, the production count register. A test is then made of switch S7 at P0.7. If it's high, we jump to FREEZE where, as we'll see, production stops, alarm goes on, and new numbers n and d of production quota and tolerable defectives can be entered at 5000 and 5001. If S7 is not high fall-through to the CMPB instruction occurs. There we test if the number produced has reached the value n stored in 5000. If not, a jump is taken to AHEAD where a test is made as to whether the number of defectives (stored in REG4 in the TIME routine to be analyzed shortly) has reached the tolerable limit d stored in 5001. If it has, then we have produced less than n and reached the tolerable limit d. The JE instruction at 24C7 jumps to FREEZE where production stops and the alarm goes on. If not, we should produce another widgit - all is O.K. so far. In that case fall-through the JE instruction to SJMP CYCLE starts production of another widgit (P2.6 = 1, P2.7 = 0).

On the other hand, back at 24B2 where we tested if the number produced reached n (we assumed it did not in the above), if the number produced did, in fact, reach n then fall-through the JNE occurs and a test is made at 24B9 as to whether the number of defectives (stored in REG4) reached the tolerable limit d stored in 5001. If it did not, then a batch n has been produced with defectives less than the critical value d and the JNE at 24BE takes us back to BEGIN where a whole new batch is started from scratch with everything cleared - the whole process and above descriptions repeat. If, however, the number of defectives did reach d, then fall-through JNE at 24BE occurs to SJMP FREEZE. The latter jumps us to FREEZE where production stops and the alarm goes on. We have achieved the production quota, n, at the SAME TIME that the tolerable number of defectives, d, has been reached (a sort of singular, but possible, case).

Note that the FREEZE routine at 24CB turns P2.6 and P2.7 off (production stops), the alarm goes on at P1.7, and the production count at P1 is frozen at the value attained for the last widgit produced. The FREEZE routine, as indicated above, is reached if EITHER S7 is thrown high at ANY time OR if d is reached before n is reached, OR if n is reached at the same time d is reached. S0 is polled at 24D1 in FREEZE. If it's low, we stall in a wait loop. This can allow us to enter new n, d values at 5000, 5001 if we wish. When S0 is thrown high at P0.0, fall-through to SJMP BEGIN occurs. Alarm is shut, P1 is cleared, REG1 is cleared, and T2 is cleared. Production starts over from scratch with these new (or same) values of n, d as the pertinent parameters.

An analysis of TIME at 24D6 follows. TIME not only provides the 1 sec. delays for the P2.6 and P2.7 on-times, but also has embedded in it the polling of Timer T2 for defectives entered in it via the debounced ("limit") switch at T2CLK which is "tripped" by defective widgits. (Of course, T2CLK doesn't have to be driven by a limit switch. Defectives could block light from reaching a photodetector circuit, so that the latter's output goes from 0 to 1 to 0, with that output being input to T2CLK to record another event (defective) in T2). The loading of 02 in REG2 and FFFF in REG3 will provide the 1 sec. delay when account is taken of the state times of ALL the instructions in the loops of the TIME routine. T2 is then read into REG4 (number of defectives so far). That number is divided by 2 (SHR instruction) to correct for the fact that T2 increases by two when our lever switch goes 0 to 1 and then 1 to 0 (on release) to simulate ONE defective. The number of defectives (lo-byte from REG4) is then output to P1 and displayed on the LEDs there. Only then do we commence the usual decrements on REG3 and REG2 to achieve delay. Note that if REG2 is not 0 after the DJNZ on it, the jump is taken, as always, to LOAD where FFFF is again loaded into REG3, and that is immediately followed by another polling of T2 and updating of the defective count at P1. If REG3 is not 0 after DEC we jump back to READT2 to poll T2 again before another DEC. Thus we are polling for defectives on a very "tight" basis, all the while delay is being generated by the loops. The RET from TIME takes us back to either 24A4 or 24AD in the main program.

PROCEDURE

1. Provide LEDs at P2.6 and P2.7. Use a debounced switch at

P2.3 for T2CLK event inputs to T2. S0 and S7 will be used from the switch bank at port P0. Keep S0 and S7 low. Remember, each thrown and release of T2CLK represents ONE more defective in our program.

2. Enter BY 5000 = 0A and BY 50001 = 04 specifying that the number to be produced in a batch is n = 10 and the tolerable number of defectives is to be d = 4.
3. Execute from 2490. Observe P2.6 and P2.7 oscillate, in turn, with one second on-times for each. One additional widgit is produced every time P2.7 goes on/off AFTER P2.6 goes on/off. Make a mental count of the number being produced as they oscillate (simply count up the number of times P2.6 goes on).
4. Before 10 widgits are produced, throw the T2CLK switch 4 times. P1 counts up the defectives and FREEZE occurs. Production stops (P2.7 = P2.6 = 0) and the alarm goes on (P1.7 = 1). P1 shows 84 (P1 is serving as the source for the alarm (P1.7) AND as the display for the number of defectives). Enter BY 40 to read the number of widgits produced. Does it agree with your count-up at P2.6?
5. Throw S0 hi/lo. Production at P2.6, P2.7 starts all over with P1 cleared and the alarm off. Previous batch was "discarded".
6. Thrown T2CLK 2 times. P1 shows 02. Let 10 widgits be produced. P1 clears and a new batch starts. The previous one was let through as 10 was reached before 4 defectives were turned out.
7. Throw T2CLK 2 times. P1 shows 02. Before 10 widgits are produced throw S7 hi/lo. Alarm goes on (P1 shows 82) and P2.7 = P2.6 = 0. Production stops and FREEZE occurs. Read out BY 40 for the number that were produced. It should agree with the count you made at P2.6. Now enter BY 5000 = 06 and BY 5001 = 02. We are now specifying new production parameters: the batch is to consist of n = 6 widgits and the number of tolerables is to be d = 2. Throw S0 hi/lo. P1 is cleared (alarm goes off) and a new production run starts from 0 with T2 = P1 = REG1 = 0.
8. Throw T2CLK 2 times before 6 widgits are produced. Alarm goes on and P1 shows 82. P2.6, P2.7 are both 0. FREEZE again occurs. Throw S0 hi/lo. A new production batch starts from scratch, the previous one being "discarded".
9. Throw T2CLK once. P1 shows 01. Let 6 widgits be produced. P1 clears to 00 as a new batch is started. 1 in 6 is a tolerable result.
10. After 4 or 5 widgits are produced (no defectives), throw S7 hi/lo. FREEZE occurs. Alarm goes on. P1 shows 80 (no defectives). Read BY 40 for the number produced in this new batch. It should be 4 or 5 as the case may be. Enter BY 5000 = 10 and BY 5001 = 06. Throw S0 hi/lo. Production

starts up again. Repeat various cases and situations.

PROBLEM

Come back to this problem after you've concluded this chapter and try to re-do Expt. 6-8 employing the HSO unit. To simplify matters for yourself, take the on-times at P2.6 and P2.7 to be e.g. 131 msec. i.e. T1 + #0FFFF in HSOTIME (a high speed cutting/spraying operation). Take n to be a large number in that case e.g. enter FF in address 5000 so that you'll have about 64 seconds to input defectives at T2CLK before the batch clears.

EXPERIMENT 6-9

MEASURING SWITCH CONTACT TIME (OR PULSE WIDTH) USING TIMER T1.

In this experiment we shall demonstrate the use of timer T1 to measure the pulse width of a switch contact.

FORMULATION

1. We shall throw a debounced lever switch S0 at P0.0 from low to high and quickly release it to its low position. We wish to measure the time it remained in the high state. The method will be equally applicable to measuring pulse width i.e. the time a pulse remains in its high state after transitioning from 0 to 1 and before dropping back to 0. Timer T1, which is free-running, will be read into REG1 at the moment S0 goes high, and then again into REG2 the moment it is released to the 0 state.
2. During the contact time, T1 may well overflow. Certainly, if the contact time is long, T1 will overflow a NUMBER of times. Hence the contact time is not simply (REG2 - REG1) x 2 usec., but rather (REG2 - REG1) x 2 usec. + (REG3 x 65,536) x 2 usec., where REG3 will contain the number of T1 overflows. Remember that T1 will overflow each time it counts from 0000 to FFFF at 2 usec. intervals, i.e. every 131 msec., but that the FIRST overflow, if one occurs, will be offset from the value of T1 read into REG1. Hence the formula for contact time is:

   t = [(REG2 - REG1) + REG3 x 65,536] x 2 usec.

   However, the formula should be re-written to apply to two cases, since the first T1 overflow is offset from the value of T1 in REG1:

   a). If REG3 = 0 (no T1 overflows):
   t = (REG2 - REG1) x 2 usec.

   b). If REG3 is greater than or equal to 1 (one or more overflows of T1 during contact time):
   t = [(65,536 - REG1) + REG2 +
   (REG3 - 1) x 65,536] x 2 usec.

3. The number of T1 overflows will be stored in REG3 by having our program do the following: the Timer Overflow interrupt source will be enabled by setting MINT.0 = 1 in the interrupt mask register; IOC1.2 will be set to 1, thereby enabling the T1 overflow interrupt source to TOV, rather than

the T2 overflow interrupt source; the T1OV ISR's service address will be established by loading it into the Vector Interrupt Location 2000H that is appropriate to TOV interrupts; the T1OV ISR will consist simply of incrementing REG3 (which is initialized to 0 in the main program) and returning to the main program where contact is possibly still being made by S0.

4. After S0 is thrown high and released, we simply read out the REG1, REG2, REG3 values for insertion into the formulas in (2) above. This is accomplished by entering WO 50, WO 60, and WO 70, where 50, 60, and 70 are the RAM file addresses that we've assigned to REG1, REG2, and REG3.

The program to accomplish the above is presented below, starting at 2500. Our analysis then follows.

```
        18 00           SP      EQU     18H
        16 00           IOC1    EQU     16H
        50 00           REG1    EQU     50H
        60 00           REG2    EQU     60H
        70 00           REG3    EQU     70H
        0A 00           T1      EQU     0AH
        09 00           PINT    EQU     09H
        08 00           MINT    EQU     08H
        00 20           INVEC   EQU     2000H
        80 00           TEMP    EQU     80H
        0E 00           P0      EQU     0EH
                        ;
                        ;
2500                            ORG     2500H
                        ;
2500    FA                      DI                      ;Disable global interrupt bit.
2501    A1 C0 00 18             LD      SP,#00C0H       ;Initialize SP to 00C0H.
2505    B1 01 08                LDB     MINT,#01H       ;Load MINT with 01H to enable
                                                        ;timer overflow interrupt.
2508    A1 2B 25 80             LD      TEMP,#252BH     ;Load address of T1OV Interrupt
250C    C3 01 00 20 80          ST      TEMP,INVEC[0]   ;Handler Routine into INT VECT
                                                        ;Table.
2511    30 0E FD        S0LO:   JBC     P0,0,S0LO       ;If P0.0 = 0,then loop here.
2514    A0 0A 50                LD      REG1,T1         ;Else load value of T1 into REG1.
2517    01 70                   CLR     REG3            ;Clear REG3.
2519    B1 04 16                LDB     IOC1,#04H       ;Load IOC1 with 04H to enable
                                                        ;T1 overflow interrupt source.
251C    11 09                   CLRB    PINT            ;Clear all pending interrupts.
251E    FB                      EI                      ;Enable global interrupt bit.
251F    38 0E FD        S0HI:   JBS     P0,0,S0HI       ;If P0.0 = 1,then loop here.
2522    A0 0A 60                LD      REG2,T1         ;Else read T1 into REG2.
2525    FA                      DI                      ;Disable global interrupt bit.
```

```
2526   27 E9            SJMP    SOLO          ;Jump back to test P0.0.
                  ;
                  ;
                  ;     T1 Overflow Interrupt Service Routine
                  ;
252B                    ORG     252BH
                  ;
252B   07 70            INC     REG3          ;Increment REG3.
252D   F0               RET                   ;Return to main routine.
```

The above program implements the details set forth in the FORMULATION as follows: DI, the first instruction will prevent any free-running T1 overflows from being serviced until switch contact is made - otherwise invalid incremented values of REG3 in the ISR will occur. The SP is then initialized and the TOV interrupt source unmasked by loading MINT with 01. 252B is then stored in INVEC i.e. at TOV's vector entry address 2000, establishing T1OV's ISR address as 252B. We now poll switch S0 for contact. The JBC instruction at 2511 waits until S0 is first thrown high. Fall-through then occurs and the value of T1 at initial contact time is read into REG1. Next REG3 is cleared (REG3 will hold the number of T1 overflows made during contact time). 04 into IOC1 selects the T1 overflow interrupt source for TOV interrupts, rather than the T2OV source. CLRB PINT clears all pendings, so that any PREVIOUS T1 overflow pendings (made even though DI disabled the global interrupt bit) will not be serviced after the EI instruction is next executed. We are only interested in T1 overflows that occurred since FIRST SWITCH CONTACT was made. The JBS instruction at 251F establishes another wait loop as long as S0 remains high (contact).

It is during this wait loop that relevant T1 overflows (if any) might occur, in which case there will be vectoring to the ISR at 252B (T1OV ISR), where REG3 is incremented each time such overflow occurs. The ISR ends on RET to 251F and the wait loop. As long as S0 is high we remain in the wait loop with T1OV interrupts to 252B occurring every 131 msec. (after the first overflow happened). Finally, when S0 is released, fall-through to 2522 occurs. There T1 is read into REG2. DI then prevents any further T1 overflow from being serviced (which would increment REG3 and give a false value of contact time if such overflows were serviced). SJMP SOLO jumps back to the wait loop at 2511. We remain there until another throw of S0 is made should we wish to measure another pulse width or contact time.

PROCEDURE

1. With a debounced switch S0 connected to P0.0, execute the program from 2500. Throw S0 high and QUICKLY release it. Enter WO 50, WO 60, and WO 70 to access the values in REG1, REG2, and REG3, respectively. We found REG1 = 54F9, REG2 = BC0C, and REG3 = 0000. Using formula (a) in section (2) of the formulation, with all REG values converted to decimal, gives t = 26,387 x 2 usec. = 53 msec. (approx), which seemed perfectly consistent with our quick release of S0.
2. Repeat, throwing S0 high and quickly releasing it. This time we read WO 50 as 8869, WO 60 as DB06, and WO 70 as 0000 again. Using formula (a) in section (2) of the formulation gives t = 21,149 x 2 usec. = 42 msec. (approx), again in keeping with our quick release of S0.
3. This time throw S0 high and keep it high for 2 or 3 seconds before releasing it. Read out the word values in 50, 60, and 70. We found REG1 = 5E5A, REG2 = D061, and REG3 = 0014. Now we must use formula (b) in section (2) of the formulation. Doing so gives us t = [(65,563 - 24,154) + 53,345 + 19 x 65,536] x 2 usec. or t = 2678 msec. (approx) = 2.68 sec. (approx), totally in keeping with the stopwatch we used to track the time from initial S0 contact to its release.

NOTE

We come back to measuring pulse widths with the HSI High Speed Unit in Expt. 6-21.

EXPERIMENT 6-10

USING T2 AND T1 TO MEASURE THE NUMBER OF SWITCH BOUNCES AND THE TIME FROM FIRST CONTACT TO LAST BOUNCE.

FORMULATION

1. In this experiment REG1 will store the value of T1 when the bouncing switch FIRST went high. The switch to be tested is a bouncing switch connected to T2CLK at P2.3, so that Timer T2 will record the number of bounces.
2. REG2 will contain the value of T1 just after the last bounce was made i.e. when the switch finally went low and stayed low.
3. REG4 will contain the number of T1 overflows (passed to it from REG3) made during the time interval between the first contact high and the last bounce to low. We again employ a T1OV interrupt routine where REG3 counts up the number of T1 overflows as in Expt. 6-9.
4. As in Expt. 6-9, the formula to be used to determine the time t between first contact high and last bounce to low is either t = (REG2 - REG1) x 2 usec. or t = [(65,536 - REG1) + REG2 + (REG4 - 1) x 65,536] x 2 usec. The first one holds if REG4 = 0 (no overflows), the second if REG4 is greater than or equal to 1. The reasoning is the same as given in the formulation to Expt. 6-9.
5. REG5 will contain the true number of switch bounces. This is accomplished by loading T2 into REG5, incrementing it and then shifting REG5 right 1 bit to divide by 2. We do this because T2 records not merely 1 bounce, but rather increments by 2 for every bounce (it records every transition positive or negative). Thus, for example, if a third bounce were just made, T2 would contain 5, the increment of REG5 would give 6, and the SHR right 1 bit would leave 3 in REG5 - correct. Only then is REG5 output to the LEDs at P1 to display the number of true bounces. P1 will thus display the number of bounces, as they occur, from first to last, until there are no further bounces.

A detailed analysis of the program at 2700 is given after the latter is presented below. Elements of it are similar to the one in Expt. 6-9.

```
        18 00          SP       EQU     18H
        16 00          IOC1     EQU     16H
        15 00          IOCO     EQU     15H
        40 00          REG1     EQU     40H
        50 00          REG2     EQU     50H
        60 00          REG3     EQU     60H
        70 00          REG4     EQU     70H
        80 00          REG5     EQU     80H
        90 00          TEMP     EQU     90H
        0A 00          T1       EQU     0AH
        0C 00          T2       EQU     0CH
        09 00          PINT     EQU     09H
        08 00          MINT     EQU     08H
        00 20          INVEC    EQU     2000H
        0F 00          P1       EQU     0FH
        10 00          P2       EQU     10H
                       ;
                       ;
2700                            ORG     2700H
                       ;
2700    FA                      DI                        ;Disable global interrupt bit.
2701    A1 C0 00 18             LD      SP,#00C0H         ;Initialize SP to 00C0H.
2705    B1 01 08                LDB     MINT,#01H         ;Load 01 into MINT to enable
                                                          ;timer overflow interrupts.
2708    A1 40 27 90             LD      TEMP,#T1OV        ;Load address of T1OV routine into
270C    C3 01 00 20 90          ST      TEMP,INVEC[0]     ;INT VECTOR table.
2711    B1 0A 15                LDB     IOC0,#0AH         ;Load 0A into IOC0 to select T2CLK
                                                          ;and T2RST, also resets T2 to 0.
2714    3B 10 02       LOW:     JBS     P2,3,FIRSTHI      ;IF P2.3 = 1,then go to FIRSTHI.
2717    27 FB                   SJMP    LOW               ;Else continue polling switch.
2719    A0 0A 40       FIRSTHI:LD       REG1,T1           ;Load value of T1 into REG1 to
                                                          ;record T1 value at time of first
                                                          ;contact.
271C    01 60                   CLR     REG3              ;Initialize REG3 TO 0.
271E    B1 04 16                LDB     IOC1,#04H         ;Load 04H into IOC1. Enables overflow
                                                          ;interrupt from T1.
2721    11 09                   CLRB    PINT              ;Clear all pending interrupts.
2723    FB                      EI                        ;Enable global interrupt bit.
2724    33 10 FD       LOAGAIN:JBC      P2,3,LOAGAIN      ;If P2.3 = 0 then continue looping
                                                          ;here.
2727    A0 60 70                LD      REG4,REG3         ;Else load REG4 with contents of REG3.
272A    A0 0A 50                LD      REG2,T1           ;Update REG2 with T1 value.
272D    A0 0C 80                LD      REG5,T2           ;Update REG5 with T2 count.
2730    07 80                   INC     REG5              ;Increment T2 count.
2732    08 01 80                SHR     REG5,#01H         ;Shift right 1 bit to give number
                                                          ;of bounces.
2735    B0 80 0F                LDB     P1,REG5           ;Output number of bounces to LEDs.
2738    27 EA                   SJMP    LOAGAIN           ;Loop back to check switch.
```

```
                    ;       T1OV Interrupt Service Routine
                    ;
2740                        ORG     2740H
                    ;
2740    07 60       T1OV:   INC     REG3            ;Increment REG3 for time record.
2742    F0                  RET                     ;Return to main program.
                    ;
                    ;
2743                        END
```

The first 5 lines of code are exactly the same as the first 5 lines in Expt. 6-9 and need no comment here. Except that the T1OV Overflow ISR's address is now programmed to be 2740. Loading 0A into IOC0 selects T2CLK as T2's event source and resets T2 to 0 (02 will also do). The JBS instruction at 2714 tests the status of the switch at T2CLK (pin P2.3). If it's low (no contact yet) fall-through occurs to SJMP LOW and we are back at 2714 to keep testing T2CLK. When the switch at T2CLK is finally thrown high, JBS jumps to FIRSTHI at 2719 where the value of T1 is loaded into REG1. This is the reference time at which FIRST contact was just made. REG3, which will hold the number of free-running T1 overflows, if any occur, is next cleared to 0. Loading 04 into IOC1 selects the T1OV source for TOV (Timer Overflow) interrupts. Then all pendings are cleared, so no past pending T1 overflows can be serviced to haunt us, and the global interrupt bit is enabled. T1OV interrupts from this point on will be serviced. At this point T2 = 1.

The crucial part then follows. T2CLK (P2.3) is again tested, this time with a JBC instruction at 2724. If T2CLK is STILL high, as it is, fall-through to 2727 occurs where REG4 is loaded with REG3's value, the latter containing the NUMBER of T1 overflows to the ISR that occurred so far (if any). We'll understand later why we drag in REG4 for that purpose. Next T1 is loaded into REG2. Remember, T2CLK is still high and T1 is free-running, so "time marches on" AND WE WANT TO KNOW THE LATEST VALUE OF T1 FOR WHICH T2CLK IS STILL HIGH. The number of true bounces (1) made so far is output to the LEDs at P1 by means of the instructions at 272D, 2730, 2732, and 2735 in keeping with our discussion in section 5 of the formulation. P1 WILL SHOW 01 TO THIS POINT - ONE BOUNCE SO FAR. SJMP LOAGAIN then jumps us back to 2724 where T2CLK is again tested. As long as it's high, we fall-through and the loop between 2724 and 2738 repeats. REG2 keeps increasing, as does REG4 (from possible T1OV interrupts) since T1 is free-running. Finally, the switch goes back low (T2 = 2) and the JBC at 2724 goes into a wait loop. T1 keeps increasing and T1 overflow interrupts to the ISR probably continue to be made. On the next bounce, T2CLK goes high again (T2 = 3) and fall-through to 2727 occurs. The number of overflows made so far (stored in REG3) is passed to REG4, the value of the number of BOUNCES made is (3 + 1)/2 = 2. So 02 shows at P1's LEDs, and the on-going T1 value is placed in REG2. Everything has been updated. T1OV interrupts continue. We're again in the JBC, SJMP LOAGAIN loop as long as T2CLK remains high on this second contact. Again, when T2CLK goes low (T2 = 4), we're caught in the wait at 2724's JBC instruction, but T1 keeps increasing, as does REG3 from continuing T1OV overflows. The next high causes T2 = 5 and P1 will show (5 + 1)/2 = 3.

It is not hard to see that when the LAST bounce is made and T2CLK goes, and stays, low, we'll remain locked at 2724. REG4 will now contain the number of T1OV overflows made from first to last bounce (REG4 will NOT change any more even though REG3 keeps on incrementing due to FURTHER T1 overflows. That's because we're locked in at 2724. Any T1 overflows vector from there to the ISR and RETURN to 2724 in the LOAGAIN loop. Now you see why we passed REG3 to REG4.) REG2 will contain the value of T1 when T2CLK was LAST high i.e. the value of T1 JUST BEFORE T2CLK went low - essentially the value of T1 when the switch went low for the FINAL time. P1 will show the total number of bounces and, of course, REG1 holds the value of T1 when the first contact was made. Application of the formulas in section 4 of the formulation can then be made to find total elapsed bounce time. (We have assigned RAM addresses 40, 50, 60, 70, 80 to REG1, REG2, REG3, REG4, and REG5). The T1OV ISR at 2740 is exactly as in Expt. 6-9: REG3 is incremented every time the ISR is entered due to another T1 overflow. Thus, AFTER the first overflow, REG3 measures time in units of 131 msec.

PROCEDURE

1. First connect a debounced switch to T2CLK at P2.3. Execute the program from 2700. Throw the switch 5 times at one second intervals between throws. See P1 increment up to 5. We should have a total time between first contact hi and last contact low of ABOUT 4.5 sec. Why? 1 sec. from first high to second high + 1 sec. from second high to third high + 1 sec. from third high to fourth high + 1 sec. from fourth high to fifth high + ABOUT 0.5 sec. from fifth high to ensuing and final LOW. We found the following values in REG1, REG2 and REG4: WO 40 = 934F, WO 50 = 16BC, and WO 70 = 0022H. Using the appropriate formula in section (4) of the formulation gives:
   t = [(65,536 - 37,701) + 5820 + 33 x 65,536 x 2 usec.
   t = 67.3 msec. + 4325 msec. = 4.39 sec. (approx).

This is in excellent agreement with what we expected, given also the fact that we threw the switch 5 times at APPROXIMATELY 1 sec. intervals - estimated times. ESC.

2. Next connect a bouncing switch to T2CLK at P2.3. This can easily be realized from a debounced switch if you are using the debounced switch circuit shown in Fig. 2-2 of chapter 2. Simply take the switch output at pin 1 of the 7400 IC instead of at pin 6. The switch output then will certainly bounce. Execute from 2700. Throw and quickly release the switch. P1 read 16 bounces. Query REG1, REG2, and REG4. We found WO 40 = 9B4E, WO 50 = 0CE3, WO 70 = 0001. Using the second of the two formulas in section (4) of the formulation gives 58.14 msec. from time of first contact till last bounce. ESC, re-run and throw the switch again. P1 read 17 bounces. This time we found 77FD, EF0E, and 0000 in 40 (REG1), 50 (REG2), and 70 (REG4), respectively. The first formula with this data gives 60.96 msec. ESC once more and execute again. Throw and very quickly release the switch. P1 displayed 15 bounces and REG1, REG2, REG4 contained 3E68, 87AE, and 0000, respectively. Using the first of the two formulas in section (4) of the formulation now gives 37.52 msec. These various bounce transient times are totally in keeping with expected values for typical bouncing switches. The lever microswitch we employed was a particularly highly bouncing switch. The various values reflect different switch contact times that we permitted before release.

NOTE

Expt. 6-23 employs the High Speed Input Unit to solve this same switch bouncing problem. It will be instructive to compare the "HSI way" with the classic approach taken here. In Expt. 6-23 we also construct a table that records the precise time of EVERY bounce.

EXPERIMENT 6-11

TIMER T1 IS USED TO PRODUCE DELAYS FOR A PULSE GENERATOR WHILE TIMER T2 INDEPENDENTLY COUNTS EVENTS.

FORMULATION AND APPROACH

1. A debounced switch will be used to create events at the T2CLK source for T2. When the program is executed, an LED placed at P2.7 will oscillate on/off/on/off ... at about 1 second on and off-times. All the time the oscillations at P2.7 are taking place, and transparent to them, the number of events input from the debounced switch at T2CLK will be recorded at the LEDs at port P1.
2. The 1 sec. time delays alluded to above will be produced by having timer T1 produce 8 overflow interrupts (.131 sec. x 8 = 1.05 sec.) before P2.7 is complemented with an XORB instruction in the T1OV ISR. Of course, the number 8 can be made a parameter whereby any multiple of .131 sec. delay can be achieved. That number is loaded into REG2 in the main part of the program and each time the T1OV ISR is reached, REG2 is decremented until it reaches 0. Then P2.7 is complemented. The return from the T1OV ISR is to the main program where the event count in T2 is being polled and output to P1. When REG2 reaches 0, it is reloaded in the ISR (with 8, for example) just before P2.7 is complemented. This time we'll let T2 record "events" on each positive and negative transition.

The program at 2550 is shown below.

```
18 00        SP      EQU     18H
16 00        IOC1    EQU     16H
15 00        IOCO    EQU     15H
50 00        REG1    EQU     50H
60 00        REG2    EQU     60H
70 00        REG3    EQU     70H
0A 00        T1      EQU     0AH
0C 00        T2      EQU     0CH
09 00        PINT    EQU     09H
08 00        MINT    EQU     08H
00 20        INVEC   EQU     2000H
0F 00        P1      EQU     0FH
10 00        P2      EQU     10H
```

```
2550                         ORG    2550H
                     ;
2550  A1 C0 00 18            LD     SP,#00C0H      ;Initialize SP to 00C0H.
2554  FA                     DI                    ;Disable global interrupt bit.
2555  B1 01 08               LDB    MINT,#01H      ;Load 01 into MINT to enable timer
                                                   ;overflow interrupts.
2558  B1 04 16               LDB    IOC1,#04H      ;Load 04H into IOC1 to select
                                                   ;T1 overflow interrupt.
255B  A1 90 25 50            LD     REG1,#T1OV     ;Load address of T1OV routine into
255F  C3 01 00 20 50         ST     REG1,INVEC[0]  ;INT VECTOR table.
2564  B1 08 60               LDB    REG2,#08H      ;Load REG2 with 08 for 1 sec. delay.
2567  B1 0A 15               LDB    IOC0,#0AH      ;Load 0A into IOC0 to select T2CLK
                                                   ;and reset T2.
256A  11 09                  CLRB   PINT           ;Clear all pending interrupts.
256C  FB                     EI                    ;Enable global interrupt bit.
256D  71 7F 10               ANDB   P2,#7FH        ;Clear P2.7.
2570  A0 0C 70       READT2: LD     REG3,T2        ;Load REG3 with event count in T2.
2573  B0 70 0F               LDB    P1,REG3        ;Output event count to LEDs.
2576  27 F8                  SJMP   READT2         ;Go back to update event count display.
                     ;
                     ;
                     ;       T1OV Interrupt Service Routine.
                     ;
2590                         ORG    2590H
                     ;
2590  E0 60 06       T1OV:   DJNZ   REG2,RETURN    ;Decrement REG2 and test if zero.
                                                   ;If REG2 != 0,then jump to RETURN.
2593  B1 08 60               LDB    REG2,#08H      ;Else reload time delay reg.
2596  95 80 10               XORB   P2,#80H        ;Complement P2.7 (toggle)
2599  F0             RETURN: RET                   ;Return to main program.
```

Analysis of the above program is straight-forward. SP is initialized, MINT.0 is set to 1 to unmask the TOV interrupt line, IOC1.2 is set to 1 to select T1OV as the source of TOV interrupts, 2590 is loaded into VECTOR TABLE address 2000 (TOV interrupt entry address) to establish our T1OV ISR at 2590, REG2 is loaded with 08 to ensure 8 T1OV overflow interrupts (each separated in time by .131 sec.), and T2CLK is established as the source of T2 event counts (at the same time T2 is reset to 0). Pending interrupts are then cleared (so that any PREVIOUS T1OV overflow pending interrupts will "disappear") and the system is enabled to honor FUTURE T1OV interrupts.

With the above initializations out of the way, P2.7 is cleared by the ANDB instruction. Finally, T2's event count is read into REG3 and its low byte output to the LEDs at P1. The SJMP READT2 keeps polling T2 for additional events. It is in this READT2 loop that T1OV overflow interrupts to T1OV's ISR at 2590 will occur every 0.131 sec. (after the first overflow). A complement of P2.7 will be made only after 8 entries into that ISR; otherwise, a return to the polling of T2 in the main program (READT2 loop) will take place. Thus P2.7 will toggle at about 1 sec. intervals.

The T1OV ISR at 2590, each time that it is entered, decrements the contents of REG2 (initially 08 in our case). If REG2 is still not 0, a jump to RETURN is asked for, and we're back into the main program polling events in T2 for display at P1. Time goes on. After (in our case) 8 entries into the T1OV ISR, REG2 will have been decremented to 0, and fall-through from 2590 to 2593 will take place. There REG2 is reloaded with (in our case) 08 in order that another 1 sec. delay be guaranteed AFTER P2.7 is complemented by the XORB instruction at 2596. The following RET takes us back to the main program where updated events in T2 are polled for display at port P1.

PROCEDURE

1. Connect a debounced switch to T2CLK at P2.3 and execute the program from 2550. Nothing happens at P2.7 (it's off) for a time less than or equal to about 1 sec. P2.7 then goes on for about 1 sec., then off for 1 sec., etc. as we enter the T1OV ISR every 131 msec. (after the first entry).
2. During the on/off cycles at P2.7, create asynchronous events with the debounced switch at T2's T2CLK input. Observe the count-up of events at P1 (one for switch contact, another for switch release), all the while the pulse generator at P2.7 continues its on/off cycles (multitasking).
3. ESC and replace 08 at 2565 and at 2594 with 10 by entering BY 2565 = 10 and BY 2594 = 10. Then execute from 2550 again. Observe the oscillations at P2.7 with 2 sec. on and 2 sec. off-times. Create events at T2CLK and observe the count-up of events at P1's LEDs while P2.7 toggles.

EXPERIMENT 6-12

PULSE GENERATOR WITH REP. RATE CONTROLLED FROM KEYBOARD ON-THE-FLY.

In this application, time delay is implemented with classical software loops. You should compare the classical approach we take here with the method used when the HSO unit is employed to implement pulse generators in Expt. 5-16 (B) and later in Expt. 6-16. In both the latter cases the on-times are also controlled from the keyboard on-the-fly. The differences in approaches are instructive, and will show the advantages the HSO unit provides in substantially increasing through-put (multi-tasking).

FORMULATION

1. REG1 and REG3 will contain values for the outer and inner loops of the software time delay program at 2616. Those values will determine the time delay itself. While REG1 will contain a fixed value 14H, REG3 will contain the value passed to it from REG2 where REG2, in turn, can be loaded from the keyboard at run-time or on-the-fly. With REG1 = 14H and REG3 = FFFFH, 4 sec. time delay results. The value of time delay will be directly proportional to the size of the word passed into REG3 so that, e.g. for REG3 = 8000, 2 sec. time results. The word in REG2 is passed to it on-the-fly by simply entering WO 60 = UVWX, where we've assigned RAM location 60 to REG2 and UVWX is any word value from 0001 to FFFF.
2. The pulse generator will be implemented at P2.7 where we connect an LED. The on and off-times will be controllable by the word value passed to REG2.
3. The number of cycles gone through at P2.7 is constantly updated and displayed at P1's LEDs.

The program is shown at 2600 below. It is quite simple. After setting SP, P1 is cleared and P2.7 is turned on. TIME is called and the subsequent return to 260C causes P2.7 to be turned off. TIME is again called and, when the return to 2612 is made, another cycle has been done. We increment P1 to display that fact and then jump back to CYCLE to start another on/off cycle at P2.7. The time delay at 2616 loads 14H into REG1 and the value in REG2 into REG3. REG3 is then decremented till it's 0, at which point REG1 is decremented. If REG1 is not 0, then a jump back to RELOAD starts the inner loop of decrements all over with REG3 reloaded with REG2's value again. This continues till the outer loop forces REG1 to 0. Time is up and we return to the main program.

```
        18 00          SP       EQU     18H
        50 00          REG1     EQU     50H
        60 00          REG2     EQU     60H
        70 00          REG3     EQU     70H
        0F 00          P1       EQU     0FH
        10 00          P2       EQU     10H
                       ;
                       ;
2600                            ORG     2600H
                       ;
2600    A1 C0 00 18             LD      SP,#00C0H       ;Initialize SP to 00C0H.
2604    11 0F                   CLRB    P1              ;Initialize LEDs to 00.
2606    91 80 10       CYCLE:   ORB     P2,#80H         ;Set P2.7 to 1.
2609    EF 0A 00                CALL    TIME            ;Call Time Delay
260C    71 7F 10                ANDB    P2,#7FH         ;Reset P2.7 to 0.
260F    EF 04 00                CALL    TIME            ;Call Time Delay.
2612    17 0F                   INCB    P1              ;Increment and display cycle cnt.
2614    27 F0                   SJMP    CYCLE           ;Repeat cycle.
                       ;
                       ;
                       ;        TIME DELAY ROUTINE:
                       ;
2616    B1 14 50       TIME:    LDB     REG1,#14H       ;Load major loop counter.
2619    A0 60 70       RELOAD:  LD      REG3,REG2       ;Load minor loop counter from
                                                        ;data from "keyboard" entry.
261C    05 70          MORE:    DEC     REG3            ;Decrement minor loop counter.
261E    D7 FC                   JNE     MORE            ;If REG3 != 0,then loop back to MORE.
2620    E0 50 F6                DJNZ    REG1,RELOAD     ;Else go back to reload minor loop
                                                        ;counter if REG1 != 0.
2623    F0                      RET                     ;Else return to main program.
                       ;
                       ;
2624                            END
```

PROCEDURE

1. With an LED connected to P2.7, enter W0 60 = 0FFFF so that the initial on and off-times will be 4 sec.
2. Execute from 2600 and observe P2.7 toggle with 4 sec. on and off-times. Note the cycle count-up at P1's LEDs.
3. On-the-fly enter W0 60 = 8000 and observe the on, off-times change to 2 sec.
4. On-the-fly enter W0 60 = 2000 and observe the on, off-times change to 1/2 sec.
5. Enter W0 60 = 1000 and observe the on, off-times change to 1/4 sec.

6. Enter WO 60 = 4000 and observe the on, off-times change to 1 sec.
7. All the while you're doing the above, the number of cycles traversed keeps incrementing at P1.

PROBLEMS

In the above, the response time to the newly entered word values in REG2 (at 60) will be NO MORE than 0.2 sec. Why? Modify the program so that the response to the new keyboard entry will be "instantaneous". (You'll have to poll a keyboard entry in the tight inner loop.) As another problem, try to implement this experiment with the HSO unit (without consulting Expts. 5-16 (B) or 6-16).

EXPERIMENT 6-13

A COMPUTER CONTROLLED "DRILL PRESS" (PUMP, VALVE, ETC).

In this application we again implement time delay in the classical manner (software loops). We suggest a problem at the end of the experiment for you to modify the program we present here so that the application can be realized by employing the HSO unit (à la Expts. 5-13 or 5-16 (B) or 6-16, etc.)

FORMULATION

1. Two switches (not necessarily debounced) are employed: S0 at P0.0 and S7 at P0.7. LEDs are used at P2.7 and P2.6. P2.7's LED will act as a prompt for us to enter the parameters of the problem (desired on-time, desired off-time, and desired number of cycles), while the LED at P2.6 will represent the drill, pump, valve etc. going on/off/on/off ....
2. With S0 low, you'll observe the P2.7 LED go on when the program is executed. This is the prompt for us to enter 3 parameters: on-time, off-time, and # of cycles. We do so by entering BY 50 = XY, BY 60 = X'Y', and BY 0A0 = X''Y'', where REG1, REG2, and REG6 have been assigned RAM addresses 50, 60, 0A0 respectively, and XY, X'Y', X''Y'' are the values of desired on-time (in REG1), desired off-time (in REG2), and desired # of cycles (in REG6).
3. After the three parameters are entered, S0 will be thrown high to initiate the physical activity at P2.6 and to turn the prompt LED, P2.7, off. P2.6 goes on for the time XY, then off for the time X'Y', and this is repeated for X''Y'' cycles. Meanwhile, P1 counts up the number of cycles as they unfold. When the cycles are complete P2.6 stays off, P1 clears, and P2.7 goes on again, prompting us for entry of new XY, X'Y', and X''Y'' parameters (or we may leave the old parameters in REG1, REG2, and REG6, if desired). This is again done by entering the desired values in BY 50, BY 60, and BY 0A0. Throwing S0 high initiates new cycles.
4. At any time during the EXECUTION of the cycles you can abort by throwing switch S7 high, in which case P2.6 immediately goes off, P2.7 goes on, P1 clears and we can enter new parameters (or leave the old ones) before S0 is thrown high to initate new cycles.

The program at 2650 is shown below. It is analyzed at its conclusion.

```
      18 00        SP      EQU    18H
      40 00        REG     EQU    40H
      50 00        REG1    EQU    50H
      60 00        REG2    EQU    60H
      70 00        REG3    EQU    70H
      80 00        REG4    EQU    80H
      90 00        REG5    EQU    90H
      A0 00        REG6    EQU    0A0H
      0E 00        P0      EQU    0EH
      0F 00        P1      EQU    0FH
      10 00        P2      EQU    10H
                   ;
                   ;
2650                       ORG    2650H
                   ;
2650  A1 C0 00 18  BEGIN:  LD     SP,#00C0H       ;Initialize SP to 00C0H.
2654  11 0F                CLRB   P1              ;Initialize LEDs to 00.
2656  71 BF 10             ANDB   P2,#0BFH        ;Turn P2.6 OFF.
2659  91 80 10             ORB    P2,#80H         ;Set P2.7 to 1.
265C  30 0E FD     HERE:   JBC    P0,0,HERE       ;Poll P0.0 (S0).If P0.0 = 0
                                                  ;data has not been loaded yet.
265F  B0 A0 70             LDB    REG3,REG6       ;Data input complete. Load REG3
                                                  ;from REG6 with number of cycles.
2662  17 0F        NEWCYC: INCB   P1              ;Data has been loaded, start
                                                  ;new cycle count.
2664  71 7F 10             ANDB   P2,#07FH        ;Turn P2.7 OFF and P2.6 ON.
2667  91 40 10             ORB    P2,#40H         ;
266A  B0 50 40             LDB    REG,REG1        ;Retrieve ON time.
266D  EF 0E 00             CALL   TIME            ;Call Time delay
2670  71 BF 10             ANDB   P2,#0BFH        ;Turn P2.6 OFF.
2673  B0 60 40             LDB    REG,REG2        ;Retrieve OFF time.
2676  EF 05 00             CALL   TIME            ;Call Time Delay.
2679  E0 70 E6             DJNZ   REG3,NEWCYC     ;Decrement cycle counter.If REG3!=0
                                                  ;then go back and do another cycle.
267C  27 D2                SJMP   BEGIN           ;Else jump to BEGIN and wait for
                                                  ;new data entry.
                   ;
                   ;
                   ;       TIME DELAY ROUTINE:
                   ;
267E  A1 FF FF 80  TIME:   LD     REG4,#0FFFFH    ;Initialize minor loop counter.
2682  3F 0E 09     AGAIN:  JBS    P0,7,STKTOP     ;IF P0.7 = 1,then update stack
                                                  ;and return.
2685  05 80                DEC    REG4            ;Else decrement minor loop counter.
2687  D7 F9                JNE    AGAIN           ;If minor loop != 0,keep decr.
```

```
2689   E0 40 F2                DJNZ    REG,TIME       ;Else decr. major loop. If major
                                                      ;loop != 0 keep decr.
268C   20 07                   SJMP    RETURN         ;Else return. Do normal return.
268E   A1 50 26 90   STKTOP:   LD      REG5,#BEGIN    ;Load BEGIN address into REG5 to
2692   C2 18 90                ST      REG5,[SP]      ;modify STACK for return to BEGIN.
2695   F0            RETURN:   RET                    ;Return to main routine.
```

The first 5 lines of code initialize SP, clear P1, turn P2.6 off and P2.7 on, and sets up a wait loop (JBC) as long as S0 is low. This gives the operator a chance to enter the desired parameters in REG1 (on-time), REG2 (off-time), and REG6 (# cycles). When he/she has done so and is ready for the activity to unfold, switch S0 is thrown high. Fall-through to 265F occurs where the # cycles is retrieved from REG6 and loaded into REG3. Since the first cycle is about to start P1 is incremented to show 01 at its LEDs. ANDB turns the prompt, P2.7, off and ORB turns P2.6 (drill, pump, etc.) on. The on-time is next retrieved from REG1 and loaded into REG (REG will be decremented in the outer software loop of the time delay at 267E and is thus instrumental in generating time delay along with REG4 for the inner loop). At 266D TIME is now called. We'll analyse TIME shortly. Upon return from TIME, P2.6 is turned off by the ANDB instruction at 2670. This time the off-time is retrieved from REG2 and placed in REG prior to calling TIME again. (Again REG is decremented in the outer software loop of TIME, only now it will generate the correct off-time, whereas before it generated the correct on-time.) Returning from TIME to 2679 finds a DJNZ on REG3. One more cycle has been done and we want to know if all the cycles have finished. Remember, REG3 was originally loaded with the # of cycles from REG6. If REG3 is not 0 after DJNZ, a jump to NEWCYC at 2662 increments P1 for the next cycle and all repeats. Finally, REG3 is 0 when the desired number of cycles have been executed. Fall-through DJNZ to SJMP BEGIN clears P1, turns P2.7 on, keeps P2.6 off, and allows the operator to enter new on/off time parameters and # cycles before throwing S0 high to initiate a new run.

The time delay program at 267E starts off by loading inner loop register REG4 with FFFF. Before decrementing REG4, a polling of switch S7 takes place. As long as S7 is low, fall-through to 2685 occurs where REG4 is decremented and, if not 0, a jump back to 2682 is made to poll S7 again. Delay is unfolding with a tight polling of S7. If, at any time, S7 is thrown high, the JBS at 2682 jumps to STKTOP at 268E where we load REG5 with the address (2650) of BEGIN and then store it on the top of the stack i.e. at the address pointed to by SP, namely at 00BE, BF (remember, SP is at 00BE after the CALL TIME in the main program, with the return address 2670 or 2679 stored in 00BF, 00BE.

We are simply replacing 2670 or 2679 there by 2650). The RET instruction will then pop 2650 into the PC from the top of the stack, forcing a return to BEGIN where P1 is cleared, P2.6 is turned off, the prompt P2.7 is turned on and new parameters can be entered as long as S0 is low. In that way we can abort the execution of cycles at any time, should we so desire, for whatever reason.

If, however, S7 is not thrown high, the inner and outer loops (REG4, REG registers) of the time delay finish up and fall-through DJNZ to SJMP RETURN takes us to 2695 where now the RET pops the normal contents of the top of the stack (2670 or 2679) into the PC. A normal return to the main program occurs. The cycles continue on.

PROCEDURE

1. With S0 and S7 low, execute from 2650. The LED at P2.7 goes on, the one at P2.6 goes or stays off. Enter the following parameters: BY 50 = 04, BY 60 = 08, and BY 0A0 = 06. This is asking for 1 sec. on-times, 2 sec. off-times (approx.) and 6 cycles at P2.6. (Remember, our time delay now consists of 17 state times in the inner loop and 65,536 such loops will be made, so that the inner loop gives about 0.26 sec. delay).
2. Throw S0 high/low. Observe the on/off cycles at P2.6's LED unfold. Count-up 1, 2, ... 6 at P1's LEDs is displayed. When the last cycle has been done, P1 clears and P2.7 goes on prompting for new parameters. P2.6 remains off.
3. Enter new parameters as follows: BY 50 = 02, BY 60 = 04, BY 0A0 = 0A asking for 1/2 sec. on-time, 1 sec. off-time, and for 10 cycles. Throw S0 hi/lo and observe the new cycles commence at P2.6. During one of the on cycles throw S7 hi/lo and observe the process abort: P1 clears, P2.6 stays off, and P2.7 goes on. Enter new parameters, or simply throw S0 high/low with the same parameters in place. In the latter case, observe P2.6 do its 10 cycles of 1/2 sec. on and 1 sec. off-times, after which P1 clears, P2.6 stays off, and P2.7 goes on.

PROBLEM

Re-do the experiment using the HSO unit and several of its HSO output pins. You may want to come back to this problem after you finish the chapter.

EXPERIMENT 6-14

AN EXAMPLE OF SIGNAL PROCESSING USING A/D INPUT AND PWM (D/A) OUTPUT: VOLTAGE CLAMPING WITH AN HSO BACKGROUND TASK.

FORMULATION

1. In this experiment we shall employ a POT connected between 5V and ground at analog A/D input channel ACH.0. The A/D converted byte will be used in modified (processed) form as input to the PMW unit. We'll observe the latter's filtered analog output voltage at pin P2.5 in its PWM alternate function. A LED will be connected to pin HSO.0 where we'll have the HSO unit generate pulses with on/off times of 65 msec. The latter will constitute a "background activity". The main signal processing activity will center around varying the potentiometer at ACH.0 through its 0 to 5V range and outputting an analog (integrated) voltage at the PWM output pin P2.5. The PWM output voltage is to be constant at some lower limit value as the POT input varies from 0 to a certain lower value; the output is then to increase linearly as the POT input varies from the lower value to some upper value; and finally the output at P2.5 is to be constant at some upper limit value as the POT input varies beyond the upper limit value to 5V. This would represent achievment of software generation of a clamping circuit by signal processing the input voltage and outputting the desired analog voltage to P2.5 in its PWM function role.
2. Symbols used in this experiment and their meanings are as follows: vin refers to the analog input voltage to ACH.0 from the POT. vout refers to the analog (filtered) output voltage at pin P2.5 generated by the PWM unit. XY refers to the 9, 8, 7, ...2 bits (byte) that results from the conversion of the input voltage vin at channel ACH.0. We shall use the notation vin(XY) to denote the analog input voltage and its converted byte. WE ARE NEGLECTING THE 1,0 BITS OF THE CONVERSION RESULT. ERROR IS LESS THAN 0.4%.
3. The specifications defining the problem are the following: a) for vin(XY) between 0(00) volts and vin1(X1Y1) volts, the output at P2.5 is to be a constant value vout1; b) for vin(XY) between vin1(X1Y1) and vin2(X2Y2), vout at P2.5 is to vary linearly from vout1 to some value vout2; c) for vin(XY) between vin2(X2Y2) volts and 5(FF) volts, the output at P2.5 is to be the constant value vout2. This defines clamping action.

4. The input limits vin1(X1Y1) and vin2(X2Y2) will be specified at run-time by simply entering the desired values BY 5000 = X1Y1 and BY 5001 = X2Y2, where X1Y1 is less than X2Y2, and each can be anywhere from 00 to FF. These limits can be changed at will on-the-fly as the program is executing.
5. As stated before, background activity will consist in toggling at pin HSO.0 with approximately 65 msec. on and off-times, transparent to the main problem.
6. As the input potentiometer at ACH.0 is varied, the converted byte XY will be displayed at the LEDs at port P1 (i.e. the upper bits 9-2). In that way we can verify if linear rise in vout does indeed commence at the value X1Y1 we entered into 5000 and whether the linear rise does indeed end at the value X2Y2 we entered into 5001.
7. A VTVM or oscilloscope with probe will be needed to measure the output (filtered) analog voltages, vout, produced by the PWM at P2.5 to confirm clamping at the X1Y1, X2Y2 limits.

The program starts at 2697 and is presented below.

```
        06 00           HSOCOM  EQU     06H
        04 00           HSOTIME EQU     04H
        09 00           PINT    EQU     09H
        08 00           MINT    EQU     08H
        06 20           INVEC   EQU     2006H
        40 00           TEMP    EQU     40H
        16 00           IOC1    EQU     16H
        02 00           ADRESLO EQU     02H
        03 00           ADRESHI EQU     03H
        02 00           ADCOM   EQU     02H
        17 00           PWM     EQU     17H
        0A 00           T1      EQU     0AH
        18 00           SP      EQU     18H
        0F 00           P1      EQU     0FH
                        ;
                        ;
2697                            ORG     2697H
                        ;
2697    A1 C0 00 18             LD      SP,#00C0H        ;Initialize SP to 00C0H.
269B    B1 01 16                LDB     IOC1,#01H        ;Select PWM function.
269E    FA                      DI                       ;Disable global interrupt.
269F    B1 08 08                LDB     MINT,#08H        ;Enable HSO interrupt source.
26A2    A1 FA 26 40             LD      TEMP,#HSOINT     ;Load address of HSO interrupt
26A6    C3 01 06 20 40          ST      TEMP,INVEC[0]    ;service routine into INT VECT
                                                         ;table.
26AB    EF 52 D9                CALL    LDCAM            ;Call CAM load routine.
```

```
26AE   11 09                      CLRB    PINT              ;Clear all pending interrupts.
26B0   FB                         EI                        ;Enable global interrupt bit.
26B1   B1 08 02          CONVERT:LDB      ADCOM,#08H        ;Start Conversion on ch. 0.
26B4   FD                         NOP                       ;Wait 4 state times
26B5   FD                         NOP                       ;Wait 4 state times
26B6   3B 02 FD          BUSY:    JBS     ADRESLO,3,BUSY    ;If status = 1,keep polling.
26B9   B0 03 0F                   LDB     P1,ADRESHI        ;Else output upper 8 bits of result.
26BC   9B 01 00 50 03             CMPB    ADRESHI,5000H[0]  ;Compare result with lower limit
26C1   D1 0C                      JNH     LOWLIM            ;If result <= low limt, goto LOWLIM
26C3   9B 01 01 50 03             CMPB    ADRESHI,5001H[0]  ;Else compare with upper limit
26C8   D9 0C                      JH      HILIM             ;If result > high limit, goto HILIM
26CA   B0 03 17                   LDB     PWM,ADRESHI       ;Else load input A/D result into
                                                            ;PWM reg. In between limits.
26CD   27 E2                      SJMP    CONVERT           ;Go back to do another A/D conversion.
26CF   B3 01 00 50 17 LOWLIM:     LDB     PWM,5000H[0]      ;A/D result was <= low limit. Load
                                                            ;PWM reg. with low limit.
26D4   27 DB                      SJMP    CONVERT           ;Go back to do another convert.
26D6   B3 01 01 50 17 HILIM:      LDB     PWM,5001H[0]      ;A/D/ result was > high limit. Load
                                                            ;PWM reg. with high limit.
26DB   27 D4                      SJMP    CONVERT           ;Go back to do another conversion.


                         ;
                         ;
26FA                              ORG     26FAH
                         ;
                         ;        HSO INTERRUPT SERVICE ROUTINE
                         ;
26FA   EF 03 D9          HSOINT: CALL     LDCAM             ;Call CAM load routine to generate
                                                            ;another pulse.
26FD   F0                         RET                       ;Return to main program.
                                  .GLOBAL LDCAM
                         ;
                         ;
       06 00             HSOCOM   EQU     06H
       04 00             HSOTIME  EQU     04H
       0A 00             T1       EQU     0AH
                         ;
                         ;
26DD                              ORG     26DDH
                         ;
                         ;
                         ;
                         ;        LOAD CAM ROUTINE
                         ;
26DD   B1 20 06          LDCAM:   LDB     HSOCOM,#20H       ;Load HSOCOM with command to turn
                                                            ;HSO.0 ON and not to generate
                                                            ;HSO interrupt.
26E0   45 03 00 0A 04             ADD     HSOTIME,T1,#0003H ;Program command to execute now.
```

```
26E5   FD               NOP                          ;Delay 8 state times before next entry.
26E6   FD               NOP                          ;
26E7   B1 00 06         LDB   HSOCOM,#00H            ;Load CAM with command to turn HSO.0
                                                     ;OFF (no interrupt).
26EA   45 00 80 0A 04   ADD   HSOTIME,T1,#8000H      ;Program command to execute
                                                     ;.065 seconds from now.
26EF   FD               NOP                          ;Delay 8 state times.
26F0   FD               NOP                          ;
26F1   B1 30 06         LDB   HSOCOM,#30H            ;Load CAM with command to turn HSO.0
                                                     ;ON and generate HSO interrupt.
26F4   45 FF FF 0A 04   ADD   HSOTIME,T1,#0FFFFH     ;Program command to execute
                                                     ;.131 seconds from now.
26F9   F0               RET                          ;Return to main routine.
```

The first 6 lines of code sets the SP, selects the PWM function at pin P2.5, disables the interrupt system, sets bit 3 in the interrupt mask register so that the HSO interrupt source is unmasked, and loads #HSOINT (26FA) into INVEC (2006), thereby establishing the address of our HSO ISR at 26FA (via HSO's vector entry address 2006). We next call the LDCAM routine at 26DD. That routine loads the HSOCAM with the three necessary commands to produce one pulse of 65 msec. on-time and 65 msec. off-time at pin HSO.0. We'll analyze it after first going through the rest of the main program.

The return from LDCAM to 26AE results in the clearing of any previous pendings of whatever kind in PINT, followed by the enabling of the interrupt system. (We shall be using the HSO interrupt source to help in producing the pulses at HSO.0.) The program between 26B1 (CONVERT) and 26DB tackles the main task: the implementation of a clamping type voltage at the PWM output in relation to a linear increase in input voltage at A/D channel 0. LDB at 26B1 starts A/D conversion at ACH.0 NOW. The two NOPs provide the 8 state times that may be needed till conversion starts. Bit 3 (S bit) in the A/D RESULT (LO) register is then tested. As long as S is high conversion is in progress. When it's over, S drops to 0 and fall-through to 26B9 occurs. There we output the digital result in A/D RESULT (HI) register (bits 9-2) to the LEDs at P1. We are now at the heart of the matter. We want to know in which region the converted digital byte, XY, finds itself: region (1) where XY is between 00 and X1Y1, region (2) where XY is between X1Y1 and X2Y2, or region (3) where XY is between X2Y2 and FF. The two CMPB instructions at 26BC and 26C3 will decide for us. The CMPB at 26BC compares the result XY in the A/D RESULT (HI) register with X1Y1 that has been stored in address 5000 at run-time. The JNH instruction at 26C1 (Jump if Not Higher - unsigned) jumps to 26CF (LOWLIM) if XY is less than or equal to X1Y1. At 26CF the byte X1Y1 is retrieved from 5000 and loaded into the PWM to produce the CONSTANT lower limit voltage vout1 (as long as vin(XY) lies between 0(00) and vin1(X1Y1)]. That is followed by SJMP CONVERT to start another conversion.

If, however, the test at 26C1 shows that XY in ADRESHI register is greater than X1Y1 in 5000, then fall-through to the next CMPB instruction takes place. There we compare the result XY in ADRESHI with the byte X2Y2 that was stored in address 5001 at run time. If XY is higher than X2Y2, the JH (Jump if Higher - unsigned) instruction jumps us to 26D6 (HILIM) where the byte X2Y2 is retrieved from 5001 and loaded into the PWM to produce the CONSTANT upper limit voltage vout2 [as long as vin(XY) lies between vin2(X2Y2) and 5(FF)]. The next instruction jumps back to CONVERT to start another conversion.

If the test at 26C8 proves that XY in ADRESHI is less than or equal to X2Y2 in 5001, fall-through to 26CA occurs. There we simply take XY from ADRESHI, as is, and load it into the PWM to produce an output voltage vout proportional to the XY byte that drives the PWM [which in turn was proportional to the vin voltage at ACH.0, so that vout is proportional to vin in the region vin1(X1Y1) to vin2(X2Y2)]. The next instruction at 26CD jumps back to CONVERT to accomplish another A/D conversion.

The above constitutes the signal processing of the A/D input to produce the clamped signal at the PWM output. All the while the program to produce this clamping is running, the HSO unit is producing background pulses at HSO.0. Let's now analyze how this comes about. Back at 26AB we called LDCAM at 26DD. As we see, LDCAM first loads 20 into the HSO Command Tag register (HSOCOM) specifying that HSO.0 be turned on without generation of an HSO interrupt and that T1 be used as the reference timer. The next instruction loads T1 + 0003 into HSOTIME which specifies that HSO.0 be turned on essentially NOW. 8 state times are provided by the 2 NOPs to allow for the command just described to enter the CAM file from the Holding Register before the next one is written into the H.R. (otherwise over-write of the H.R. would occur). The next command places 00 into HSOCOM and T1 + 8000H into HSOTIME. This specifies that HSO.0 be turned off 65 msec. from now without any interrupt being generated by the HSO unit. Again 2 NOPs are needed for 8 state times. The final command at 26F1 places 30 into HSOCOM and T1 + FFFFH into HSOTIME. This specifies that HSO.0 go back on 131 msec. from now and that the HSO unit create an interrupt. The RET returns us to 26AE in the main program. Those three commands will guarantee the generation of one pulse of 65 msec. on-time and 65 msec. off-time with HSO interrupt then generated.

Now that we're back in the main program implementing the solution to the clamping problem, the HSO unit on its own is removing the 3 commands that we've just entered into the CAM file and executes them. When the pulse has been generated and HSO.0 goes high again after 131 msec. from "now", the HSO unit generates an HSO interrupt, as our third command requested. Wherever we are in the main program, that interrupt will vector us to our HSO ISR at 26FA. The HSO ISR there simply calls LDCAM to reload the CAM file with the same 3 commands analyzed above specifying that another identical pulse be produced at HSO.0. The RET returns us to the main program where the HSO interrupt occurred and A/D conversion and PWM output continue to be implemented. And so it goes!

PROCEDURE

1. Reset the unit and enter BY 09 = 00 to clear out the HSO CAM and clear any pendings. Enter BY 5000 = 50 and BY 5001 = 90H. This establishes X1Y1 = 50H and X2Y2 = 90H as limits.
2. Execute from 2697. Observe the pulse generator at HSO.0 with 65 msec. on/off times. Vary the POT at ACH.0 from 0 to 5 volts and note the A/D conversion byte displayed at P1's LEDs. P1 will vary from 00 to FF as the POT is varied from 0 to 5 volts. Measure the filtered output voltage vout at P2.5. We found that as vin varied from 0 to vin1 (50), vout remained constant at vout1 = 1.44 volts. P1's LEDs show the conversion bytes and they varied from 00 to X1Y1 = 50. As we increased vin further, we noted that the byte at P1 increased from 50, but now, for the first time, the output voltage vout at P2.5 started to increase. It kept increasing as vin continued to increase until the byte 90 = X2Y2 at P1 was reached, corresponding to vin2(90). At that point we measured vout to be 2.63 volts. As vin was inreased further to the 5 volt limit, P1 increased from 90 up to FF but vout remained constant at the value vout2 = 2.63 volts. The results are consistent in that vout is constant until 50 is reached at P1 (X1Y1 = 50 was specified for the upper limit on the low region); vout rises linearly in the middle region till 90 is reached at P1 (X2Y2 = 90 was specified as the upper limit on the middle region); and vout is again constant as P1 increases from 90 to FF in the high region. Notice that the voltage swing 2.63V - 1.44V = 1.19V corresponds nicely to what we'd expect i.e. (90H - 50H) x 5V/FFH, which works out to be 1.25V.
3. On-the-fly, enter BY 5000 = 60 and BY 5001 = 80. X1Y1 and X2Y2 limits are thus changed to 60 and 80, respectively. Again vary the POT at ACH.0 from 0 to 5 volts and measure vout at P2.5. This time we found vout = vout1 = 1.73 volts

as vin increased from 0 volts till P1 showed the byte 60 at its LEDs. Further increase in vin caused P1's byte to increase from 60 and vout started to increase linearly from 1.73V until P1 showed 80 and vout measured 2.32 volts. At that point further increase in vin gave no further increase in vout. vout remained constant at vout2 = 2.32 volts and P1 increased from 80 to FF. Again the results are totally consistent. And HSO.0 keeps toggling. Again notice the swing 2.32V - 1.73V = 0.59V corresponds to what we'd expect: (80H - 60H) x 5V/FFH = 0.625V.

EXPERIMENT 6-15

CONCURRENT USE OF TWO HSO SOFTWARE TIMERS TO IMPLEMENT TWO INDEPENDENT PULSE GENERATORS.

This experiment will demonstrate the use of the HSO Software Timers. The application provides two independent pulse generators. WE EMPHASIZE THE NEED TO POLL THE IOS1 STATUS REGISTER WHENEVER A SOFTWARE TIMER INTERRUPT OCCURS. That need arises because all four HSO Software Timers share a common interrupt vector location. By polling IOS1, the programmer can determine which timer caused the interrupt.

FORMULATION

1. Software Timer 0 (STIMER0) and Software Timer 2 (STIMER2) will control the independent on/off times of LEDs at P1.0 and P1.1, respectively. Those timers can be brought into action by loading channels 8 and A, respectively, into the low nibble of the HSO Command Tag register (06H). In order to realize on and off times larger than 131 msec. we'll use other registers to effect loops whereby independent multiples of the times produced by STIMER0 and STIMER2 can be realized. By themselves the Software Timers can only produce times up to 131 msec. in accordance with the loading of HSOTIME. Thus we'll associate REG1 with the on/off times of P1.0 i.e. with STIMER0, and REG3 with the on/off times of P1.1 i.e. with STIMER2. Further, REG1 and REG3 will be loaded with the "magnification" bytes entered in REG2 and REG4, respectively, at run-time. For simplicity we'll have the on and off-times equal for each oscillator, but different for one oscillator vs. the other.
2. Each software timer will be programmed to generate an interrupt when the requested time (loaded into HSOTIME) expires. Recall that Software Timer interrupts are associated with bit 5 in the interrupt mask register and with the vector entry address 200A in the vector interrupt location table. The purpose of these interrupts is to vector to the Software Timer ("Time Up") Interrupt Routine. In that routine we shall want to decrement either REG1 or REG3 (depending upon which timer's interrupt was generated) in order to start building up multiples of the basic on or off-time that that timer was programmed to generate via the HSOTIME register. In order to know which Software Timer expired, so that we can decrement the appropriate register, REG1 or REG3, before reloading the HSO Command Tag for

another Software Timer delay and another interrupt, it will be necessary to poll IOS1 (16H), in particular its bits 0 and 2 ("Software Timer 0 Expired" or "Software Timer 2 Expired"). Whichever bit is 1 indicates which Software Timer was responsible for the interrupt. Appropriate jumps within the ISR to STIMER0 or STIMER2 routines can then effect the time build-up through decrements on REG1 or REG3, as the case may be. Of course, we'll have to reload REG1 and REG3 with the values in REG2 and REG4, respectively, whenever either has reached 0 as a result of the decrements of either after STIMER0 or STIMER2 has "expired" and generated an interrupt.

3. The independence of the pulse generators stems from the fact that we can program any basic expiration time for STIMER0 and STIMER2 by simply loading HSOCOM and HSOTIME twice with the desired expiration times i.e. ADD HSOTIME, T1, #UVWX where UVWX can be anything from 1 to FFFF (131 msec. from "now"). Further, the program can address itself to "other tasks" in between the Software Timer generated interrupts which take us to the ISR where two pulse generators are implemented. Thus through-put is enhanced while the Software Timers are counting down 10 or 20 or ... 130 msec. of time.

The program at 2760 is presented below.

```
        06 00          HSOCOM  EQU     06H
        04 00          HSOTIME EQU     04H
        09 00          PINT    EQU     09H
        08 00          MINT    EQU     08H
        0A 20          INVEC   EQU     200AH
        40 00          TEMP    EQU     40H
        16 00          IOS1    EQU     16H
        0A 00          T1      EQU     0AH
        18 00          SP      EQU     18H
        0F 00          P1      EQU     0FH
        50 00          REG1    EQU     50H
        60 00          REG2    EQU     60H
        70 00          REG3    EQU     70H
        80 00          REG4    EQU     80H
        90 00          REG5    EQU     90H
                       ;
                       ;
2760                           ORG     2760H
                       ;
2760    A1 C0 00 18            LD      SP,#00C0H       ;Initialize SP to 00C0H.
2764    FA                     DI                      ;Disable global interrupt.
2765    B1 20 08               LDB     MINT,#20H       ;Enable Software timer intr. source.
```

```
2768   A1 91 27 40              LD     TEMP,#SOFTINT    ;Load address of HSO interrupt
276C   C3 01 0A 20 40           ST     TEMP,INVEC[0]    ;service routine into INT VECT
                                                        ;table.
2771   B0 60 50                 LDB    REG1,REG2        ;Load REG1 with ON/OFF time variable.
                                                        ;for P1.0
2774   B0 80 70                 LDB    REG3,REG4        ;Load REG3 with ON/OFF time variable
                                                        ;for P1.1
2777   B1 38 06                 LDB    HSOCOM,#38H      ;Enable software timer0 interrupt.
277A   45 08 70 0A 04           ADD    HSOTIME,T1,#7008H ;STimer0 is to expire in 57 msec.
277F   FD                       NOP                     ;Delay 4 state times.
2780   FD                       NOP                     ;Delay 4 state times.
2781   B1 3A 06                 LDB    HSOCOM,#3AH      ;Enable software Timer2 interrupt.
2784   45 FF FF 0A 04           ADD    HSOTIME,T1,#0FFFFH ;STimer2 is to expire in 131 msec.
2789   11 09                    CLRB   PINT             ;Clear pending interrupts.
278B   FB                       EI                      ;Enable global interrupt bit.
278C   B1 03 0F                 LDB    P1,#03H          ;Output 03H to LEDs to turn P1.0 ,P1.1
                                                        ;on.
278F   27 FE           HERE:    SJMP   HERE             ;Loop here.

                       ;        SOFTWARE TIMER INTERRUPT SERVICE ROUTINE
                       ;
                       ;
2791   B0 16 90        SOFTINT:LDB     REG5,IOS1        ;Load status reg into REG5.
2794   38 90 05                 JBS    REG5,0,STIMER0   ;If IOS1.0 = 1 Timer1 caused intr.
2797   3A 90 16                 JBS    REG5,2,STIMER2   ;Else if ISO1.2 = 1 Timer2 caused
                                                        ;interrupt.
279A   20 27                    SJMP   RETURN           ;Jump to RETURN. (neither).
279C   FA              STIMER0:DI                       ;Disable global interrupt bit.
279D   B1 38 06                 LDB    HSOCOM,#38H      ;Enable software timer0 interrupt.
27A0   45 08 70 0A 04           ADD    HSOTIME,T1,#7008H STimer0 is to expire in 57 msec.
27A5   E0 50 1A                 DJNZ   REG1,ENAB        ;Decrement and test. If REG1 != 0,
                                                        ;jump to enable intr. and return.
27A8   B0 60 50                 LDB    REG1,REG2        ;Else reload ON/OFF time.
27AB   95 01 0F                 XORB   P1,#01H          ;Toggle status of P1.0.
27AE   20 12                    SJMP   ENAB             ;Now jump to enable intr. and return.
27B0   FA              STIMER2:DI                       ;Disable global interrupt.
27B1   B1 3A 06                 LDB    HSOCOM,#3AH      ;Enable software Timer2 interrupt.
27B4   45 FF FF 0A 04           ADD    HSOTIME,T1,#0FFFFH STimer2 is to expire in 131 msec.
27B9   E0 70 06                 DJNZ   REG3,ENAB        ;Decrement and test. If REG3 != 0,
                                                        ;jump to enable intr. and return.
27BC   B0 80 70                 LDB    REG3,REG4        ;Else reload ON/OFF time.
27BF   95 02 0F                 XORB   P1,#02H          ;Toggle status of P1.1.
27C2   FB              ENAB:    EI                      ;Enable global interrupt bit.
27C3   F0              RETURN: RET                      ;Return to main routine.
```

The first 7 lines of code initialize SP, disable the interrupt system, set bit 5 in the interrupt mask to 1 enabling the Software Timer Interrupt source, load #HSOINT (2791) into INVEC

(200A: the vector interrupt entry for Software Timer interrupts), and load REG1 and REG3 with the on/off time "magnifications" for P1.0 and P1.1 from REG2 and REG4 (entered at run-time), respectively. Our Software Timer ISR is thus to be written at 2791. Next we load 38 into HSOCOM. This asks that STIMER0 (channel 8) count down and generate an interrupt at its expiration. T1 is to be the reference timer. The amount of time programmed is 57 msec. from "now", as we see from the next instruction which loads T1 + #7008H into HSOTIME. Two NOPs are required (8 state times) before the next HSO Command can be loaded into the Holding Register on its way to CAM file. This new command addresses itself to STIMER2 (channel A in HSOCOM) and specifies that it also count down (INDEPENDENTLY of STIMER0!) and generate an interrupt at its expiration. 3A into HSOCOM will accomplish that. T1 is again the reference. The amount of time programmed is 131 msec. from "now", as the next instruction shows, in which T1 + #FFFF is loaded into HSOTIME. Pendings are then cleared so no unwanted interrupts can be serviced from any prior pendings. The global bit is enabled, the oscillators at P1.0 and P1.1 are turned on simultaneously (we could have done otherwise, but no loss in generality results), and we end the main program on SJMP HERE which simulates the processor executing "other tasks". Thus independent STIMER times can be generated.

So far so good. When one of the timers expires (in our case it will be STIMER0 first, but no matter) the associated interrupt carries us to the Software Timer ISR at 2791. There we read IOS1 into REG5 (because we intend to poll IOS1 twice and the first read would clear IOS1, leaving it invalid for the second poll). Bit 0 in REG5 (IOS1.0) is tested. If it's 1 it was STIMER0's interrupt that was received and we jump to the label STIMER0. If not, we fall-through to a test of bit 2 in REG5 (IOS1.2). If the latter is 1 we jump to label STIMER2. If it was neither (hard to envisage, but perhaps a fault) we fall-through and return to the main program to await an STIMER0 or 2 interrupt.

Suppose it was an STIMER0 interrupt (IOS1.0 = 1). We are now at 279C (STIMER0's subroutine). The interrupt system is disabled - other interrupts (from e.g. STIMER2) will become pending. First thing we then do is reload 38 and T1 + #7008H into HSOCOM and HSOTIME, respectively, to have STIMER0 count down another 57 msec. and generate an interrupt. Remember, the previous such command at 2777, 277A has been REMOVED FROM THE CAM FILE by the very fact that we're in the ISR at 279C i.e. T1 MATCHED T1 + #7008H and count-down with interrupt were performed as requested. So we reload the CAM with the VERY SAME COMMAND (since it's no longer there). The STIMER2 command (3A, FFFFH) is still in the CAM. We next decrement the "multiples" register REG1 to build up P1.0 time. If REG1 is not yet 0, the DJNZ at 27A5 jumps to ENAB where the interrupt system is re-enabled and a return to the main program is made. When another STIMER0 interrupt occurs (either after or before an STIMER2 interrupt, or whatever) the same picture unfolds. We always reload the CAM file with the STIMER0 (38, #7008) command to replace the one removed. Eventually, this will lead to REG1 being 0 and we fall-through the DJNZ at 27A5 to 27A8 where REG1 is reloaded with the multiples byte still in REG2. The toggle at P1.0 is now effected since on (or off) time for P1.0 is over. XORB P1, #01 at 27AB does that. SJMP ENAB jumps to 27C2 where the interrupt system is re-enabled and we return to the main program.

The exact same analysis holds if STIMER2 caused the interrupt (IOS1.2 = 1). This will bring us to STIMER2's subroutine at 27B0. After the DI at 27B0, we reload HSOCOM and HSOTIME with 3A and T1 + #0FFFF, respectively, to replace the identical command that had to have been removed from the CAM by virtue of the fact that we are in the ISR at 27B0. This places the STIMER2 command in the CAM behind the STIMER0 command that was previously re-loaded into the CAM in the STIMER0 routine. Remember [Expt. 5-16(A)] that CAM commands are executed on a time ordering basis so it doesn't matter who's behind whom in the CAM. The main thing is that the command that was executed out of the CAM be replaced so as to generate another count-down and interrupt. From that point on at 27B9 the analysis is identical, except that the DJNZ is on REG3 (P1.1 on or off-time "multiple"). After a number of STIMER2 interrupt entries to the ISR, REG3 will be 0, we fall-through the DJNZ at 27B9 and reload REG3 with its multiples byte (still in REG4). The on or off-time for P1.1 is over and we toggle it with the XORB P1, #02 instruction at 27BF. EI and RET follow.

PROCEDURE

1. Reset the unit and enter BY 09 = 00 to clear the CAM and all pendings. Enter BY 60 = 04 and BY 80 = 08 where REG2 and REG4 are addresses 60 and 80, respectively. These should give 4 x .057 sec. and 8 x .131 sec. for the on/off times of P1.0 and P1.1, respectively (about 1/4 sec. and 1 sec., respectively). Execute from 2760 and observe the LEDs at P1.0 and P1.1. We found good agreement with the expected on/off times at each oscillator. Note the independence of the two oscillators.
2. ESC and enter BY 60 = 13 and BY 80 = 02. This should produce 19 x .057 and 2 x .131 sec., respectively, i.e. about 1 sec. for P1.0 and 1/4 sec. for P1.1 on or off-times. Execute from 2760. We observed excellent agreement with the expected on/off times at P1.0 and P1.1.

3. ESC and enter BY 60 = 09 and BY 80 = 04. This should give 9 x .057 and 4 x .131 sec., respectively i.e. about 1/2 sec. for P1.0's on/off times and the same for P1.1.

PROBLEM

Try four independent pulse generators with their own individual on/off times generated by the four HSO Software Timers. Then try making the on and off times unequal.

EXPERIMENT 6-16

CREATING SEVERAL IDENTICAL PULSE GENERATORS AT HSO OUTPUT PINS USING THE HSO UNIT.

FORMULATION

In Expt. 6-15 we used the HSO unit to generate independent pulse generators in the sense that we used two of the four Software Timers in the HSO unit and its software interrupts to control time. We had to address the HSOCOM and HSOTIME registers, as is to be expected whenever the HSO unit is used. However, we did not produce the pulses at any of the HSO output pins but rather, by choice, at P1.0 and P1.1. We could have produced the pulses at HSO output pins by using ADDITIONAL appropriate HSO commands in the Software Timer ISR (try it as a PROBLEM). In this experiment we'll implement identical pulse generators at the HSO.0 and HSO.1 pins to which we connect LEDs. The Software Timers will not be explicitly used to generate time. HSOTIME and T1 will do that directly for us. This time HSO pin interrupts will be used. We'll again use "magnification" registers to build up on/off times to exceed .131 sec., if so desired. The on and off-times will now be independent of each other. REG1 and REG2 will be associated with off-times at each pin and REG3, REG4 with the on-times. REG2 and REG4 will be specified at run-time by entering values at 60 (REG2) and at 80 (REG4). They will be passed to REG1 and REG2 in the program at execution time. Compare our approach here with those in Expts. 5-16(B) and 6-12. Again the processor can speed most of its time in "other tasks".

The program at 2800 follows.

```
06 00          HSOCOM  EQU     06H
04 00          HSOTIME EQU     04H
09 00          PINT    EQU     09H
08 00          MINT    EQU     08H
06 20          INVEC   EQU     2006H
40 00          TEMP    EQU     40H
0A 00          T1      EQU     0AH
18 00          SP      EQU     18H
15 00          IOS0    EQU     15H
50 00          REG1    EQU     50H
60 00          REG2    EQU     60H
70 00          REG3    EQU     70H
80 00          REG4    EQU     80H
```

```
2800                            ORG     2800H
                        ;
2800   A1 C0 00 18              LD      SP,#00C0H          ;Initialize SP to 00C0H.
2804   FA                       DI                         ;Disable global interrupt.
2805   B1 08 08                 LDB     MINT,#08H          ;Enable HSO intr. source.
2808   A1 24 28 40              LD      TEMP,#HSOINT       ;Load address of HSO interrupt
280C   C3 01 06 20 40           ST      TEMP,INVEC[0]      ;service routine into INT VECT
                                                           ;table.
2811   B0 60 50                 LDB     REG1,REG2          ;Load REG1 with OFF time variable.
2814   B0 80 70                 LDB     REG3,REG4          ;Load REG3 with ON time variable
2817   B1 36 06                 LDB     HSOCOM,#36H        ;Command to set HSO.0 and HSO.1 on
                                                           ;with interrupt.
281A   45 FF FF 0A 04           ADD     HSOTIME,T1,#0FFFFH ;Command is to execute in 131 msec.
281F   11 09                    CLRB    PINT               ;Clear all pending interrupts.
2821   FB                       EI                         ;Enable global interrupt bit.
2822   27 FE            HERE:   SJMP    HERE               ;Loop here.
                        ;
                        ;
                        ;       HSO INTERRUPT SERVICE ROUTINE
                        ;
                        ;
2824   30 15 06         HSOINT: JBC     IOSO,0,LOW         ;If IOSO.0 = 0, then jump to LOW.
2827   E0 70 09         HIGH:   DJNZ    REG3,KEEPHI        ;Else decrement REG3. If REG3 != 0
                                                           ;then jump to KEEPHI.
282A   B0 80 70                 LDB     REG3,REG4          ;Else reload ON time.
282D   E0 50 0D         LOW:    DJNZ    REG1,KEEPLO        ;Decrement REG1, If REG1 != 0, then
                                                           ;jump to KEEPLO.
2830   B0 60 50                 LDB     REG1,REG2          ;Else reload OFF time.
2833   B1 36 06         KEEPHI: LDB     HSOCOM,#36H        ;Command to set HSO.0 and HSO.1 on
                                                           ;with interrupt.
2836   45 FF FF 0A 04           ADD     HSOTIME,T1,#0FFFFH ;Command is to execute in 131 msec.
283B   20 08                    SJMP    RETURN             ;Jump to RETURN.
283D   B1 16 06         KEEPLO: LDB     HSOCOM,#16H        ;Command to set HSO.0 and HSO.1 off
                                                           ;with interrupt.
2840   45 08 70 0A 04           ADD     HSOTIME,T1,#7008H  ;Command is to execute in 57 msec.
2845   F0               RETURN: RET                        ;Return to main program.
```

The main part of the program disables the global bit, sets MINT.3 = 1 to enable the HSO interrupt source, loads INVEC (2006: vector entry address for an HSO interrupt) with #HSOINT (2824 in our case i.e. the address of our HSO ISR), passes the off-time multiplier from REG2 to REG1, then the on-time variable from REG4 to REG3 (where REG2 and REG4 are loaded at run-time), loads 36 into HSOCOM and T1 + #FFFF into HSOTIME, clears all pendings, enables the global bit and goes on to "other tasks" at SJMP HERE. Loading 36 into HSOCOM specifies that pins HSO.0 and HSO.1 be set to 1 (channel 6 in lower nibble of HSOCOM) and that an interrupt be generated when they are set to 1. It also specifies that T1 be the reference timer. Those pins are to be set to 1 at the time specified in the ADD HSOTIME instruction i.e. at a time 131 msec. from "now", that is, from whatever time value exists in T1 when the command pair is executed by the CPU. Hence 131 msec. from "now", while the CPU is executing "other tasks" at 2822, HSO.0 and HSO.1 will go on and an interrupt to 2824 will be generated.

Let us now analyze that HSOINT ISR. The pins are high. We want to keep them high till the desired on-time is over. To that end we poll bit IOS0.0 ("HSO.0 current state"). As long as it's high, we fall-through the JBC instruction at 2824 and decrement the REG3 on-time multiplier at 2827. If REG3 is not 0 after the decrement, we jump to KEEPHI at 2833. There we reload the CAM with 36 and T1 + 0FFFF, so that HSO.0, HSO.1 will go (remain) high 131 msec. from NOW (NOW being the time in T1 when the instruction at 2836 is executed by the CPU), with generation of HSO interrupt. We then SJMP to RETURN where we return to "other tasks" in the main program. 131 msec. later HSO.0 and HSO.1 go (remain) on and another HSO interrupt is generated. The whole scenario and above explanation repeat. Eventually, the DJNZ at 2827 decrements REG3 (on-time multiplier) to 0 and we fall-through to 282A where REG3 is re-loaded with the on-time multiplier from REG4. The next instruction at 282D "ANTICIPATES" HSO.0, HSO.1 going low by FORCING THE ISSUE and "losing" one of the multiplier counts in REG1, the off-time multiplier register. We DJNZ REG1. If not 0, we jump to KEEPLO. There, we load the CAM with the command that will turn HSO.0, HSO.1 off 57 msec. from "now" (7008 + T1 is loaded into HSOTIME) and generate an HSO interrupt at that time (16 loaded into HSOCOM asks for that action). That is followed by a return to "other tasks" in the main program. After 57 msec. HSO.0 and HSO.1 will indeed go low and generate another interrupt to the ISR at 2824.

This time the JBC instruction at 2824 finds IOS0.0 (state of HSO.0 pin) low, and thus the jump to LOW at 282D is taken. There REG1 (off-time multiplier) is again decremented. If REG1 is not 0, DJNZ at 282D jumps to KEEPLO at 283D where we again load 16 into HSOCOM and 7008 + T1 into HSOTIME, ensuring that HSO.0 and HSO.1 will go (remain) off 57 msec. from now with generation of another HSO interrupt. The following instruction returns us to "other tasks" in the main program. 57 msec. later HSO.0 and HSO.1 are still low and another interrupt to the ISR is generated. The events repeat. Eventually, REG1 will be decremented to 0 and we fall-through the DJNZ at 282D.

REG1 is re-loaded with the off-time multiplier from REG2 and the CAM is asked to turn HSO.0 and HSO.1 on again 131 msec. from now with generation of an HSO interrupt. Return is then made to "other tasks". Remember, REG3 has been re-loaded previously (at the expiration of the first on-time) with the on-time multiplier from REG4. 131 msec. from now HSO.0 and HSO.1 go back on with an HSO interrupt generated to the ISR. The JBC at 2824 finds IOSO.0 high and fall-through to HIGH at 2827 occurs. Everything repeats. We are LOCKED in to pulse generation at HSO.0 and HSO.1 in which the on-times are controlled, in this case, by the value loaded into REG4 at run-time multiplied by the basic HSO on-time we've specified (131 msec.); and the off-times are controlled, in this case, by the value loaded into REG2 at run-time multiplied by the basic HSO off-time fo which we've programmed (57 msec).

PROCEDURE

1. Reset the unit to clear out the CAM file and enter BY 09 = 00 to remove pendings.
2. Enter BY 60 = 13 (for REG2 off-time multiplier) and BY 80 = 04 (for REG4 on-time multiplier). These values should lead to 19 x .057 = about 1 sec. off-time and 4 x .131 = about 1/2 sec. on-time. Execute from 2800 and observe identical pulse generators at HSO.0 and HSO.1's LEDs with on-times of about 1/2 sec. and off-times about 1 sec.
3. On-the-fly, enter BY 60 = 09 and BY 80 = 08. These should give 9 x .057 = about 1/2 sec. off-time, and 8 x .131 = about 1 sec. on-time. We observed the immediate change to those new on/off times at the LEDs at HSO.0, HSO.1.
4. On-the-fly enter BY 80 = 04H. The off-time should remain at 1/2 sec., but the on-time should change to 1/2 sec. This we observed at both pulse generators.
5. On-the-fly enter BY 60 = 13 and BY 80 = 08. This should produce 19 x .057 = about 1 sec. off-times and 8 x .131 = about 1 sec. on-times. We observed the change to these new off/on time values at HSO.0, HSO.1 as soon as the entries were made.

PROBLEMS

1. Redo for the HSO.4 pin (consult IOC1 control register).
2. How would you make the SUB-UNIT TIME DIVISIONS at addresses 281B, 281C, 2837, 2838, 2841, and 2842 readily controlled on-the-fly, so that we are freed from the FFFF, 7008 basic values we've employed? Modify the program to do that (only 3 extra bytes will be needed). This will give a much finer tuning of the on/off times than will REG2 and REG4 alone. Word (time) parameters will now be entered at 5000, 5002 at run-time.

EXPERIMENT 6-17

USING THE HSO UNIT TO GENERATE A SEQUENCER AT FOUR HSO OUTPUT PINS. SPEED CONTROLLABLE ON-THE-FLY.

FORMULATION

1. Four LEDs will be connected to HSO.3, HSO.2, HSO.1, HSO.0 and the following sequencing patter is to be implemented (bit 3 on left, bit 0 on right):

```
0 0 0 0
0 0 0 1
0 0 1 1
0 1 1 1
1 1 1 1
0 0 0 0
0 0 0 1
0 0 1 1
0 1 1 1
1 1 1 1
0 0 0 0
  etc.
```

2. The time interval between one bit pattern to the next in the above sequencer table will be determined by the word entered at address 5000 at run-time. Thereafter, it can be varied on-the-fly by simply entering another word value in the range 0001 to FFFF into address 5000 as the program is executing. The value of the word in 5000 is added to T1 and the result placed in HSOTIME. The HSO unit then takes care of generating the requested action (turning on of another pin in the sequence, or turning them all off) at the time (5000) from "now" i.e. at time T1 + (5000), where T1 is the value in Timer 1 when the ADD HSOTIME, T1, 5000H[0] is executed.
3. Essential to the method will be a polling of IOS0.3 ("HSO.3 current state"). When it is found to be high, a jump in the program will be made to turn off all the LEDs (they're all on if HSO.3 is high) at a time (5000) from "now". Sequencing will recommance thereafter.

The program at 2870 is shown below.

```
     06 00        HSOCOM  EQU    06H       40 00        TEMP   EQU   40H
     04 00        HSOTIME EQU    04H       0A 00        T1     EQU   0AH
     09 00        PINT    EQU    09H       18 00        SP     EQU   18H
     08 00        MINT    EQU    08H       15 00        IOSO   EQU   15H
     06 20        INVEC   EQU    2006H     50 00        REG1   EQU   50H
2870                      ORG    2870H
                  ;
2870  A1 C0 00 18         LD     SP,#00C0H        ;Initialize SP to 00C0H.
2874  FA                  DI                      ;Disable global interrupt.
2875  B1 08 08            LDB    MINT,#08H        ;Enable HSO intr. source.
2878  A1 92 28 40         LD     TEMP,#HSOINT     ;Load address of HSO interrupt
287C  C3 01 06 20 40      ST     TEMP,INVEC[0]    ;service routine into INT VECT
                                                  ;table.
2881  B1 30 50            LDB    REG1,#30H        ;Load REG1 with HSO command.
2884  B0 50 06            LDB    HSOCOM,REG1      ;Command to set HSO.0 on (with
                                                  ;HSO interrupt generated).
2887  47 01 00 50 0A      ADD    HSOTIME,T1,5000H[0] ;Command is to execute at
      04
                                                  ;time stored in location 5000H.
288D  11 09               CLRB   PINT             ;Clear all pending interrupt.
288F  FB                  EI                      ;Enable global interrupt bit.
2890  27 FE       HERE:   SJMP   HERE             ;Loop here.
                  ;
                  ;
                  ;       HSO INTERRUPT SERVICE ROUTINE
                  ;
                  ;
2892  FA          HSOINT: DI                      ;Disable global interrupt bit.
2893  3B 15 0D            JBS    IOSO,3,REPEAT    ;If IOSO.3 = 1, then goto REPEAT
2896  17 50               INCB   REG1             ;Else increment REG1.
2898  B0 50 06            LDB    HSOCOM,REG1      ;Load HSO command from REG1.
289B  47 01 00 50 0A      ADD    HSOTIME,T1,5000H[0] ;Set time of execution to value
      04
                                                  ;in location 5000H with HSO interrupt.
28A1  20 17               SJMP   RETURN           ;Goto RETURN.
28A3  B1 2F 50    REPEAT: LDB    REG1,#2FH        ;Load REG1 with #2F to start over.
                                                  ;All pins (0 to 3) have gone on.
28A6  B1 06 06            LDB    HSOCOM,#06H      ;Load HSO command to clear HSO.0 and 1.
28A9  47 01 00 50 0A      ADD    HSOTIME,T1,5000H[0] ;Set time of execution to value
      04
                                                  ;in location 5000H without HSO
                                                  ;interrupt.
28AF  FD                  NOP                     ;Delay 4 state times.
28B0  FD                  NOP                     ;Delay 4 state times.
28B1  B1 17 06            LDB    HSOCOM,#17H      ;Load HSO command to clear HSO.2 and 3.
28B4  47 01 00 50 0A      ADD    HSOTIME,T1,5000H[0] ;Set time of execution to value
      04
                                                  ;in location 5000H with HSO interrupt.
28BA  FB          RETURN: EI                      ;Enable global interrupt bit.
28BB  F0                  RET                     ;Return to main routine.
```

The first 5 lines of code initializes the SP, disables the interrupt system, unmasks bit 3 in MINT (the HSO interrupt source), and loads #HSOINT (2892) into the HSO vector interrupt entry location INVEC (2006). We then load REG1 with #30H. Since HSOCOM can not be read, we can not directly increment it (in order to sequence from one HSO pin to the next in the turn-on process). So we'll be incrementing REG1 and then loading HSOCOM from REG1 to get to the next pin. Thus at 2884, HSOCOM is loaded with the present 30 in REG1. This specifies that HSO.0 be turned on at the time specified in HSOTIME in the ADD instruction at 2887 i.e. at the time T1 + (5000), where T1 is the present time in Timer 1 and (5000) are the word contents found in address 5000 (entered at run-time or changed on-the-fly). Further, the loading of 30 in HSOCOM specifies that an HSO interrupt to the HSO ISR at 2892 be generated when HSO.0 is turned on at the programmed time. Before the interrupt system is enabled at 288F all pendings are cleared at 288D. Finally, "other tasks" get executed at 2890, simulated by the SJMP loop.

At the above specified time HSO.0 goes on and the HSO interrupt vectors us to the ISR at 2892. There we disable the system and then poll IOS0.3 (state of HSO.3). Since it's not yet high, we fall-through the JBC and increment REG1 (to 31 on the first ISR entry) and load it into HSOCOM. The effect of this is to specify that the HSO.1 pin be turned on and to generate an interrupt at that time. The instruction at 289B specifies that HSO.1 be turned on (5000) from "now". We then SJMP to RETURN at 28BA where the interrupt system is re-enabled and a return is then made to "other tasks" at HERE in the main program.

(5000) later in time another interrupt is generated as HSO.1 is turned on. The events repeat in the ISR. HSO.3 is still not high so we fall-through JBS and increment REG1 again (to 32). It is loaded into HSOCOM asking that HSO.2 be turned on, also (5000) from "now" as specified in the instruction at 289B. Again an HSO interrupt is wanted. We again return to "other tasks". (5000) from "now" another interrupt to the ISR is made when HSO.2 is turned on. Eventually, REG1 gets incremented to 33 which is passed to HSOCOM specifying that HSO.3 be turned on (5000) from "now" with HSO interrupt generated. Back we go to "other tasks". Finally HSO.3 is turned on with interrupt generated. We again vector to the ISR. This time JBS finds IOS0.3 high and the jump is taken to REPEAT. To get prepared for another sequencing, we load #2F into REG1 (the next time REG1 is incremented it will be 30, the right value to turn HSO.0 on again, with interrupt). But first we must turn all four pins OFF for the same period of time, (5000). This is accomplished by loading 06 into HSOCOM, which specifies that HSO.0 and HSO.1

both be turned off WITHOUT the generation of an HSO interrupt. The instruction at 28A9 specifies that the time at which HSO.0 and HSO.1 get turned off is to be T1 (now) + (5000). Two NOPs provide the 8 state times needed before we can enter the next HSO command into the CAM file. That next command consists of the instruction loading 17 into HSOCOM which specifies that HSO.2 and HSO.3 be turned off together WITH the generation of an HSO interrupt. The turn-off again is to occur (5000) from now in time, as the instruction at 28B4 requests. The interrupt system is re-enabled and we return to "other tasks" at HERE.

Thus, at (5000) from now, HSO.0, HSO.1, HSO.2, and HSO.3 all go off and an interrupt is generated (by the HSO.2, HSO.3 pair going off). We are back in the ISR. Fall-through JBS at 2893 (HSO.3 is low) to 2896 results in REG1 being incremented from 2F to 30. 30 is then loaded into HSOCOM specifying that HSO.0 be turned on (5000) from "now" in time (see ADD at 289B) with the generation of an HSO interrupt. The sequencing pattern starts to repeat.

PROCEDURE

1. Reset the unit and enter BY 09 = 00 to clear the CAM and all pendings. Enter WO 5000 = 0FFFF for 131 msec. time intervals in the sequencing pattern. Execute from 2870 and observe the sequencing pattern at HSO.3, .2, .1, .0 just as depicted in section 1 of the formulation. You should be able to estimate the time intervals to be about 1/8 sec.
2. On-the-fly, enter WO 5000 = 8000 and immediately see the time intervals in the sequencing change to about .066 sec.
3. Etc.

PROBLEMS

1. Modify the program so that you realize an up-down sequencer such that, when the last pin HSO.3 goes on, the pins then go off in reverse order: HSO.3 first, then HSO.2, then HSO.1, then HSO.0, before they start up again.
2. Modify the program so that the sequencer becomes a distributor in which a pin goes on, but then goes off before the next significant bit goes on. When HSO.3 goes on and then off, the situation is to start over from HSO.0. Compare your solution with Expt. 9-8.
3. Modify the program so that an up-down distributor is implemented whereby you change problem 2 above so that when HSO.3 goes on and off, HSO.2 is to go on then off, then HSO.1 is to go on/off, then HSO.0 is to go on/off before the up cycle begins again.

EXPERIMENT 6-18

IMPLEMENTING A PRESCALAR WITH THE HSO UNIT.

FORMULATION

This experiment is based on a modification of the program in Expt. 5-15. In that experiment we had the HSO unit reset Timer 2 when the latter had counted a specified number of events. It is but a short step to the realization of a prescalar, with the specified number of events being the scale factor. (Recall that in Expt. 5-15 the specified number of events was loaded into address 5000 at run-time).

In the program at 2750 in Expt. 5-15 we will enter the following modifications: BY 275C = 0FD, 0FD, 0FD (this cancels out the LDB P1, REG1 instruction at 275C) and BY 276E = 17, 0F. This replaces the NOPs at 276E, 6F in Expt. 5-15 with the instruction INCB P1. In that way we do NOT output every increment of T2 (at 275C) but rather only AFTER the specified number of counts is reached (CMPB instruction at 275F) and T2 has been reset to 0 (LDB HSOCOM and ADD HSOTIME instructions at 2766 and 2769).

PROCEDURE

1. Reset the unit and enter BY 09 = 00.
2. Make the program changes in Expt. 5-15 suggested above.
3. Enter BY 5000 = 06 for a divide by 6 prescalar.
4. Connect a debounced switch to T2CLK at P2.3.
5. Execute Expt. 5-15 from address 2750.
6. Throw the T2CLK switch a number of times. For every 6 transitions at T2CLK the LEDs at P1 go up by 1 in byte value.
7. On-the-fly, enter BY 5000 = 08. Continue throwing the T2CLK switch. This time P1 increments for every 8 transitions at T2CLK.

EXPERIMENT 6-19

WAVEFORM GENERATION USING THE PWM UNIT TOGETHER WITH AN HSO SOFTWARE TIMER.

INTRODUCTION

In Expts. 5-3, 6-2, and 6-3 waveforms (ramps and triangles) and motor speed control profiles (trapezoids) were generated using the PWM register and the analog (integrated) output at pin P2.5 in its PWM function. The profile of the waveform, in particular its slope, depends on several parameters: the number of increments of the PWM register from one time to the next (the larger that number, the larger the slope), and the number of PWM pulses that we allow to be generated of the same width before the next increment(s) of the PWM register is to take place (the larger that number, the smaller the slope, the larger the period). In Expts. 5-3, 6-2, and 6-3 we controlled the number of pulses (64 usec. between pulses) of the same width that were allowed to be generated by simply calling a time delay between successive increment(s) of the PWM register (pulse width). The time delay we employed was based on decrementing registers in sofware loops. On-the-fly we could change the time delay, and hence the number of pulses of identical width that were allowed to be generated, and hence the slope, by simply entering a new word in location 5000 (which was then passed by the program into TREG in Expt. 5-3 and REG2 in Expt. 6-2, 6-3). The delay needed was some multiple of the 64 usec. that transpires between the PWM's output of successive pulses, less the time needed to execute the instructions involved before the next increment(s) of the PWM, including the CALL of the delay routine itself.

Naturally, that approach ties up the processor's time mostly in performing loops over and over again - not a very efficient way to utilize its power, particularly a well endowed microcomputer like the 8096. What we'll do now is have one of the Software Timers associated with the HSO unit take on the job of counting time for us and letting us know when the specified time is over by generating a Software Timer interrupt (vector entry address 200A). The interrupt service routine will then increment the PWM to generate more pulses, but of increased width. In that way we are relieved of the software overhead. The CPU can go on to "other tasks" before being interrupted again by the Software Timer after the desired number of identical pulses of increased width is again generated. Again, we'll have to arrange for the time expiration associated interrupts to be generated at times which are 64 usec. apart, or multiples thereof, so that 1 or 2 or 3 etc. pulses of identical width are produced before the PWM is incremented.

The program at 2900 below solves the problem of sawtooth waveform generation in this manner. Compare it with the program at 2220 in Expt. 5-3 where sawtooth waveforms were generated with the PWM and software time delay loops.

```
        06 00           HSOCOM  EQU     06H
        04 00           HSOTIME EQU     04H
        09 00           PINT    EQU     09H
        08 00           MINT    EQU     08H
        0A 20           INVEC   EQU     200AH
        40 00           REG1    EQU     40H
        17 00           PWM     EQU     17H
        16 00           IOC1    EQU     16H
        0A 00           T1      EQU     0AH
        18 00           SP      EQU     18H
        50 00           TEMP    EQU     50H
                        ;
                        ;
2900                            ORG     2900H
                        ;
2900    A1 C0 00 18             LD      SP,#00C0H         ;Initialize SP to 00C0H.
2904    B1 01 16                LDB     IOC1,#01H         ;Load IOC1 to select PWM function.
2907    FA                      DI                        ;Disable global interrupt bit.
2908    A1 28 29 50             LD      TEMP,#SOFTINT     ;Load address of HSO interrupt
290C    C3 01 0A 20 50          ST      TEMP,INVEC[0]     ;service routine into INT VECT
                                                          ;table.
2911    B1 20 08                LDB     MINT,#20H         ;Enable Software timer intr. source.
2914    B1 00 40                LDB     REG1,#00H         ;Load REG1 with 00.
2917    B0 40 17                LDB     PWM,REG1          ;Initialize PWM reg with REG1.
291A    B1 38 06                LDB     HSOCOM,#38H       ;Enable software timer0 interrupt.
291D    47 01 00 50 0A          ADD     HSOTIME,T1,5000H[0] ;STimer0 is to expire at time in
        04
                                                          ;location 5000H.
2923    11 09                   CLRB    PINT              ;Clear pending interrupts.
2925    FB                      EI                        ;Enable global interrupt bit.
2926    27 FE           HERE:   SJMP    HERE              ;Loop here.
                        ;
                        ;
                        ;       SOFTWARE TIMER INTERRUPT SERVICE ROUTINE
                        ;
                        ;
2928    17 40           SOFTINT:INCB    REG1              ;Increment REG1 for new PWM value.
292A    B0 40 17                LDB     PWM,REG1          ;Load PWM reg with REG1.
292D    B1 38 06                LDB     HSOCOM,#38H       ;Enable software timer0 interrupt.
```

```
2930  47 01 00 50 0A        ADD     HSOTIME,T1,5000H[0] ;STimer0 is to expire at time in
      04
                                                       ;location 5000H.
2936  F0            RETURN: RET                         ;Return to main program.
```

The first 6 lines of code initializes the SP, selects P2.5 in its PWM role, disables the interrupt system, loads #SOFTINT (2928) into the Software Timer vector entry location INVEC (200A), and sets MINT.5 = 1, unmasking the Software Timer interrupt line. The program then loads 00 into REG1 prior to loading it into the PWM (we can not directly increment the latter as it is a write-only SFR, so we'll do that through REG1). 0 "pulse widths" are being specified. Next we load 38 into HSOCOM. This is specifying that Software Timer 0 in the HSO unit count down a certain amount of time and then generate a Software Timer interrupt at its expiration. Timer T1 is to be the reference. The "certain amount of time" is specified in the next instruction, which loads 5000's word contents plus the current value in timer T1 into HSOTIME. That is to say STIMER0 is to count down the amount of time specified in location 5000 and then generate an interrupt, i.e. at (5000) from "now". Pendings, if any, are then cleared, the interrupt system is enabled, and the processor is off to "other tasks" as simulated by the SJMP HERE instruction.

(5000) secs. later an interrupt is generated by STIMER0 and we are vectored to the Software Timer ISR at 2928 (actually it is the HSO unit that generates the STIMER0 interrupt, but to 200A and not to 2006 in this case). In the ISR we increment REG1 and pass that into the PWM to generate an increased pulse width. Since the command written at 291A, 291D in the main program has been executed out of the CAM file, and we need a similar time delay again before the next increment of PWM is to occur, we write the same command for the CAM again at 292D and 2930 in the ISR. This will guarantee that the same number of pulses, but of incremented width, will be generated by the PWM before still another increment is made. The ISR then returns to "other tasks" in the main program at HERE. The PWM keeps generating pulses (of incremented width) while "other tasks" are being executed. (5000) secs. from "now" another Software Timer interrupt to the ISR causes PWM to increment again for a still larger pulse width, and the whole series of events repeats. Eventually REG1 overflows to 00 and another ramp has been done. We start over from baseline 0.

The only question left is: what values are to be placed in location 5000 at run-time or afterwards on-the-fly? To have ONE PWM pulse generated before the PWM is incremented requires 64 usec. less the time needed to execute: a) the interrupt vector call: 24 states - here our stack is in external RAM (see section 2.5.4, p. 2-11 Microcontroller Handbook), b) INCB in the ISR - 4 states, c) two LDB instructions in the ISR - 4 states each, d) the ADD in the ISR - 13 states, and e) the RET in the ISR-16 states. This adds up to a total of 65 states or about 16 usec. Thus we need 64 - 16 = 48 usec. time from STIMER0. This, in turn would require that we load 24 dec. into address 5000 i.e. 24 x 2 usec. per T1 count = 48 usec. Thus 0018H into 5000 is required. This should then produce 256 increments with incremented pulses separated by 64 usec. or a period of 16.38 msec.

Should we desire TWO PWM pulses of identical widths before another PWM increment is made, we'd need 128 - 16 = 112 usec. time, so (5000) = 56 dec. = 0038H would be required. In that case the ramp period would be 128 usec. x 256 increments = 32.8 msec.

For THREE PWM pulses of identical widths to be generated before another PWM increment is made will require 192 - 16 = 176 usec., so (5000) = 88 dec. = 0058H is needed. In this case the ramp period would be 192 usec. x 256 increments or about 49.14 msec.

PROCEDURE

1. Reset the unit and enter BY 09 = 00 to clear out the CAM file and all pendings. Connect filtered output at P2.5 to a scope.
2. Enter WO 5000 = 0018. Execute from 2900 and observe sawtooth waves on the scope. We measured the period to be 16.4 msec. as predicted above.
3. On-the-fly enter WO 5000 = 0038. Observe the ramp slope and period instantly change. The slope is much smaller (about 1/2). We measured a 33 msec. period, again in agreement with the prediction above.
4. Enter WO 5000 = 0058. The slope decreases again. We measured the period to be about 48 msec. in conformity with the previous expectations.

CONCLUSION

This experiment illustrates just some of the large amount of versatility and power that the 8096 is capable of. There is a point to having done waveform generation the classical way in Expts. 5-3, 6-2 and then again here with the HSO unit's software timers. In the former cases the processor was dedicated to waveform generation with almost all its time tied up in software loops. In this experiment we have the 8096 generating waveforms as well as executing "other tasks".

EXPERIMENT 6-20

A SUBHARMONIC GENERATOR IMPLEMENTED WITH THE HSO UNIT [BASED ON EXPT. 5-16 (B)]

FORMULATION

1. In Expt. 5-16(B) we had the HSO unit generate a pulse train at pin HSO.0. The on-time there was determined by the word value loaded into address 5000 at run-time, or changed on-the-fly during execution. We'd now like the same thing to happen at HSO.0 but, in addition, we wish to observe pulses at P1's LEDs whose period is to be an even multiple of the period of the pulses at HSO.0, i.e. one P1 on or off-time is to equal an integral number of HSO.0 periods, thus implementing a subharmonic generator.
2. The program to be executed is the one at 27A0 in Expt. 5-16(B). However, the HSOINT ISR will not be the one at 27D9 in Expt. 5-16(B) but the one presented, and analyzed, below at 27F1. This means we'll have to change the byte D9 at 27A9 in Expt. 5-16(B) to F1. This we'll do by entering BY 27A9 = 0F1. That will establish #HSOINT to be 27F1. The program at 27F1 below should be entered after the last instruction at 27F0 in Expt. 5-17.
3. REG1 (and, initially, REG2) will contain 1/2 the subharmonic period factor, loaded at run-time, or changed on-the-fly thereafter. We'll assign 50 (and 60) as the RAM addresses of REG1 (and REG2). Thus loading 03 into REG1 will give a 6:1 ratio in periods; 07 will give 14:1, 0A will give 20:1, etc.
4. We'll enter WO 5000 = 8000, thereby specifying square waves at HSO.0 of 65 msec. on-time and 131 msec. periods, just as we observed in Expt. 5-16(B) (see (4) in the PROCEDURE section there).
5. We'll display the HSO.0 and P1 pulse trains on a dual channel scope so that we can measure fundamental and subharmonic periods. We'll actually be able to measure P1's periods with a stopwatch in several cases.

The new ISR for Expt. 5-16(B) is shown below at 27F1. It is entered every time ANOTHER HSO.0 pulse is generated [see LOAD CAM routine at 27B9 in Expt. 5-16(B)]. There we decrement the subharmonic factor in REG2 (be it 03 for 6:1 period ratio, or 07 for 14:1 period ratio, etc). If REG2 is not 0, we jump to 27FA (ANOTHER) where a call of LDCAM at 27B9 reloads the CAM in order to produce yet another pulse at HSO.0. The RET returns to the main program [to the HERE loop at 27B7 ("other tasks") in Expt. 5-16(B)]. And indeed another pulse at HSO.0 will be produced with interrupt entry to 27F1 again. In this manner we generate a number of pulses at HSO.0 equal to the initial value in REG2. When REG2 is decremented to 0 we fall-through the DJNZ at 27F1 to the XORB instruction at 27F4. There we complement the state of P1, thus accomplishing 1/2 period at P1 - hence the original value in REG2 is 1/2 the ratio of periods of P1 to HSO.0. The next instruction reloads REG2 with the 1/2 period multiplier (from REG1) so that we're ready for the next 1/2 period when we'll complement P1 again. The next instruction at 27FA calls LDCAM at 27B9 in Expt. 5-16(B)'s program. Thus pulses at HSO.0 will always be generated, as will pulses at P1, with their period ratios an even number.

```
        50 00       REG1     EQU     50H
        60 00       REG2     EQU     60H
        0F 00       P1       EQU     0FH

                    ;
27F1                         ORG     27F1H
                    ;
27F1    E0 60 06             DJNZ    REG2,ANOTHER    ;If REG2 != 0 then do another pulse.
27F4    95 FF 0F             XORB    P1,#0FFH        ;Else complement LEDs to achieve
                                                     ;subharmonic generation.
27F7    B0 50 60             LDB     REG2,REG1       ;Reload REG2.
27FA    EF 03 D8    ANOTHER:CALL     LDCAM           ;Load CAM with new commands.
27FD    F0                   RET                     ;Return to main routine.
```

PROCEDURE

1. Reset the unit and enter BY 09 = 00 to clear the CAM and all pendings. Enter BY 5000 = 8000 for 65 msec. on-time.
2. Enter BY 27A9 = 0F1 at address 27A9 of Expt. 5-16(B). The ISR is now at 27F1. Enter BY 0F = 00 to clear the LEDs at P1. Enter BY 50 = 03 and BY 60 = 03 (REG1 and REG2). Connect HSO.0 and one of the LEDs at P1 to scope inputs.
3. Execute from 27A0 in Expt. 5-16 (B). Observe HSO.0 go on/off with 131 msec. periods as measured on the scope (50% duty cycle). We observed P1's period to be about 6 x HSO.0's i.e. about 3/4 sec.
4. On-the-fly enter BY 50 = 07 and now observe P1 toggle with a period about 14x that of HSO.0. We measured about 1.8 secs. for its period.
5. Enter BY 50 = 0A and observe P1's period increase to about 2.5 sec., or 20x that of HSO.0's which stays constant.
6. Enter BY 50 = 01 and measure P1's period. It is now about 1/4 sec. i.e. 2x that of HSO.0.
7. Change FFFF at 27D2, D3 in Expt. 5-16(B) and HSO.0's on-time (WO 5000). Observe.

EXPERIMENT 6-21

USING THE HIGH SPEED INPUT UNIT TO MEASURE PULSE WIDTHS.

APPROACH

1. A 1 msec. period, 50% duty cycle pulse train (1KHz), TTL level signal will be input to HSI.0.
2. To measure the pulse width, we'll select the HSI MODE such that positive and negative transitions on HSI.0 will be allowed to enter the HSI FIFO. Thus mode 3 for HSI.0 is selected, meaning that 03 is to be loaded into the HSIMODE register.
3. Register "T1HI" (40) will record the time that the first high (leading edge of pulse) entered the FIFO. Register "T1LO" (50) will record the time that the first low (trailing edge of pulse) entered the FIFO right after the first high. These recordings will be achieved by successive readings of HSITIME in our HSI ISR. The HSI ISR will be entered only when the FIFO becomes full i.e. HSI is to generate an interrupt only when its FIFO goes from a non-full to full state. The times of the first two entries in the FIFO will then be read in the ISR. [Possibly three entries will have to be read if the first one was due to a negative transition. In that case the time of the first negative transition will be discarded by reading HSITIME into a dummy register "REG" (70H].
4. Subsequent queries of WO 50 and WO 40 for the T1HI and T1LO time values will allow the pulse width to be calculated from the formula t = (T1LO - T1HI) x 2 usec., where the T1LO and T1HI HEX time values are converted to decimal. 2 usec. is the period of the clock driving T1 (at 12 MHz). We expect the result to be 0.5 msec. for the 1KHz signal.
5. Remember that the time values that enter the HSI FIFO (and ultimately the HSITIME register through the Holding Register) are derived from Timer T1 (see Fig. 2-14 p. 2-12 Microcontroller Handbook or section J chapter 1 this book). Recall also that every time we read HSITIME, we are reading it from the entry in the Holding Register, which got there from the first entry into the FIFO. Reading HSITIME empties the Holding Register and allows the next entry stored in the FIFO (if any) to seep down (8 state times) to the H.R. for subsequent reading, if desired.
6. A "FIFO full" interrupt causes entry to our HSI ISR. The first instruction there is a DI. Thus further "FIFO full" interrupts will not be honored. (The continual stream of

transitions from the input signal into HSI.0 is what fills up the FIFO to cause the "FIFO full" interrupt). Our ISR will examine only the times of the first two, or at most three, FIFO entries. That removes 2 or 3 FIFO entries. The stream of HSI.0 pulses will again fill up the now less than full FIFO but no further interrupts to the ISR will occur.

The program at 2A50 is presented below.

```
        03 00            HSIMODE EQU    03H
        06 00            HSISTAT EQU    06H
        04 00            HSITIME EQU    04H
        09 00            PINT    EQU    09H
        08 00            MINT    EQU    08H
        04 20            INVEC   EQU    2004H
        60 00            TEMP    EQU    60H
        16 00            IOC1    EQU    16H
        18 00            SP      EQU    18H
        15 00            IOC0    EQU    15H
        40 00            T1HI    EQU    40H
        50 00            T1LO    EQU    50H
        70 00            REG     EQU    70H
                         ;
                         ;
2A50                             ORG    2A50H
                         ;
2A50    A1 C0 00 18              LD     SP,#00C0H        ;Initialize SP to 00C0H.
2A54    FA                       DI                      ;Disable global interrupt.
2A55    B1 01 15                 LDB    IOC0,#01H        ;Enable HSI.0 into FIFO.
2A58    B1 80 16                 LDB    IOC1,#80H        ;Enable HSI interrupt when FIFO
                                                         ;becomes Full.
2A5B    B1 03 03                 LDB    HSIMODE,#03H     ;Load FIFO on either transition
                                                         ;of HSI.0.
2A5E    B1 04 08                 LDB    MINT,#04H        ;Enable HSI Data Available
                                                         ;interrupt source.
2A61    A1 6F 2A 60              LD     TEMP,#HSIINT     ;Load address of HSI interrupt
2A65    C3 01 04 20 60           ST     TEMP,INVEC[0]    ;service routine into INT VECT
                                                         ;table.
2A6A    11 09                    CLRB   PINT             ;Clear all pending interrupts.
2A6C    FB                       EI                      ;Enable global interrupt bit.
2A6D    27 FE            HERE:   SJMP   HERE             ;Loop here.
```

```
                    ;       HSI INTERRUPT SERVICE ROUTINE
                    ;
                    ;
2A6F                        ORG     2A6FH
                    ;
2A6F   FA           HSIINT: DI                      ;Disable global interrupt bit.
2A70   39 06 05             JBS     HSISTAT,1,POS   ;If HSI.0 = 1, then goto POS.
2A73   A0 04 70             LD      REG,HSITIME     ;Else pull it out by reading HSITIME.
2A76   FD                   NOP                     ;Delay 4 state times.
2A77   FD                   NOP                     ;Delay 4 state times.
2A78   A0 04 40     POS:    LD      T1HI,HSITIME    ;Read time of positive transition
                                                    ;into T1HI.
2A7B   FD                   NOP                     ;Delay 4 state times.
2A7C   FD                   NOP                     ;Delay 4 state times.
2A7D   A0 04 50             LD      T1LO,HSITIME    ;Read time of negative transition
                                                    ;into T1LO.
2A80   F0           RETURN: RET                     ;Return to main program.
```

The main program accomplishes the following: it initializes SP to 00C0 and disables all interrupts. It then loads IOC0 with 01 to enable HSI.0 transitions to be recorded in the FIFO and loads IOC1 with 80 to allow HSI interrupts to be generated whenever the FIFO in the HSI unit becomes full with recorded events. HSIMODE is then loaded with 03 to ensure that HSI.0 events will enter the FIFO for both positive and negative transitions on HSI.0. MINT.2 is set to 1 to unmask the HSI interrupt mask bit. #HSIINT (2A6F) is loaded into the interrupt vector table at address 2004 (INVEC) appropriate to HSI interrupts - thus establishing our ISR at 2A6F. The program then clears any pendings that may exist and enables the interrupt system. Finally, "busy tasks" at 2A6D, simulated by SJMP HERE, is entered.

The HSI ISR at 2A6F, entered when the FIFO becomes full with positive and negative transitions at the HSI.0 pin, immediately disables the interrupt system. We then poll status bit 1 in the HSISTATUS SFR. This will tell us if HSI.0 was driven high or low BY THE EVENT THAT OCCURRED AT THE RECORDED TIME. If that bit is 1 then a positive transition occurred and the JBS instruction jumps to POS at 2A78 where we read HSITIME into register T1HI. This empties the H.R. and allows the next event entry (a negative transition) to enter the H.R. (it may take up to 8 state times for this to happen, hence the two NOPs, as we don't want the next reading of HSITIME to be invalid). At 2A7D, HSITIME for the negative transition is read into T1LO and a return is made to "busy tasks" in the main program. The FIFO is no longer full, so further positive and negative transitions on HSI.0 will enter the FIFO filling it again but because of the DI, no further interrupts to the ISR will be made. Thus additional events at HSI.0 will not be recorded in the now full

FIFO. We have read all the information we need.

In the event that the JBS at 2A70 indicated that bit 1 in HSI-STATUS was low (a negative transition first entered the FIFO) we do not wish to record its time into T1HI. We fall-through the JBS and read out that time into a dummy register, thereby allowing the next FIFO entry (a positive transition) to seep down into the H.R. The two NOPs at 2A76, 77 allow for the 8 state times that it may take for that next entry to reach the H.R. This is followed by a read of the time of the positive transition into T1HI at POS and the time of the next negative transition into T1LO at 2A7D. We then return to the main program. Examining WO 40 for T1HI's value and WO 50 for T1LO's value will give us the pulse width when those values are subtracted and multiplied by 2 usec.

PROCEDURE

1. Connect a 1KHz TTL level signal to HSI.0 (50% duty cycle).
2. Reset the unit to clean out the FIFO and enter BY 09 = 00 to do away with any pendings.
3. Execute the program. Enter WO 50 and WO 40 to find the values of T1LO and T1HI. We found 8867 and 876C, respectively, on our first run. Subtracting, converting to decimal and multiplying by 2 usec. gives a pulse width of 502 usec. = 0.502 msec.
4. ESC, reset, enter BY 09 = 00 and execute the program again. This time we found 9157 and 905E in 50 and 40, respectively. This works out to 498 usec. = 0.498 msec. for the width.
5. ESC, reset, enter BY 09 = 00 and execute the program again. We found 45F1 and 44F6 in registers 50 and 40. These values lead to a pulse width of 502 usec.
6. ESC, reset, enter BY 09 = 00 and execute the program again. The values in registers 50 and 40 were now found to be 3213 and 3119. These lead to a pulse width of 500 usec.

CONCLUSION

Comparing the above results with the expected 500 usec. width of the 1KHz 50 % duty cycle pulses, we do indeed find perfect agreement TO WITHIN THE 2 USEC. RESOLUTION OF THE HSI UNIT for 12 MHz clock.

EXPERIMENT 6-22

USING THE HIGH SPEED INPUT UNIT TO MEASURE PULSE PERIODS.

This experiment will be realized by a modification of parts of the main program of Expt. 6-21 and the employment of a new HSI ISR (at 2A90 now).

METHOD

1. The HSI ISR address 2A6F, specified at 2A62, 63 in the main part of the program of Expt. 6-21, will now be changed to 2A90 by simply entering BY 2A62 = 90, replacing the previous 6F there.
2. The value 03 loaded into HSIMODE at 2A5C of Expt. 6-21 will now be changed to 01 to specify that HSI.0 event entries into the FIFO are to be made only for positive (leading edge) transitions. This is easily done by entering BY 2A5C = 01, replacing the previous 03 there.
3. The 1 KHz 50% duty cycle TTL signal is again connected to HSI.0's input.
4. The HSI ISR is at 2A90 and is presented below:

```
        03 00       HSIMODE EQU     03H
        06 00       HSISTAT EQU     06H
        04 00       HSITIME EQU     04H
        40 00       T1HI    EQU     40H
        50 00       T1LO    EQU     50H
                    ;
                    ;
                    ;
                    ;       HSI INTERRUPT SERVICE ROUTINE
                    ;
                    ;
2A90                        ORG     2A90H
                    ;
2A90    FA          HSIINT: DI                      ;Disable global interrupt bit.
2A91    A0 04 40            LD      T1HI,HSITIME    ;Read time of positive transition
                                                    ;into T1HI.
2A94    FD                  NOP                     ;Delay 4 state times.
2A95    FD                  NOP                     ;Delay 4 state times.
2A96    A0 04 50            LD      T1LO,HSITIME    ;Read time of next positive
                                                    ;transition into T1LO.
2A99    F0          RETURN: RET                     ;Return to main program.
```

In the new HSI ISR above, we simply disable the interrupt system, read the time of the first positive transition of the pulse train from HSITIME into the T1HI register (40 of Expt. 6-21), and wait 8 state times for the next FIFO entry (the next positive transition of the pulse train) to drop into the H.R. from the full FIFO. We then read the time from HSITIME that that second positive transition occurred into T1LO (register 50 of Expt. 6-21 - we still CALL it T1LO even though we SHOULD have declared the 40 and 50 registers as T1HI1 and T1HI2 for this experiment), and return to "busy tasks" at 2A6D (HERE) of Expt. 6-21. The period will then simply be the value found in WO 50 less the value found in WO 40, with the difference being multiplied by 2 usec.

PROCEDURE

1. After you've made the changes in steps (1) and (2) under METHOD above, reset the unit and enter BY 09 = 00 to clear out the FIFO and eliminate any pendings.
2. Execute the program from 2A50. Enter WO 50 and WO 40 to ascertain the time values in "T1LO" and "T1HI", respectively. We found 978A and 9595. Expressing the difference in decimal and multiplying by 2 usec. gives us a period of 1002 usec. or 1.002 msec. compared with the exact 1 msec. value of the input signal.
3. ESC, reset, enter BY 09 = 00 and again execute from 2A50. This time we found registers 50 and 40 contained the time values B319 and B125, giving a period of 1000 usec. or exactly 1 msec. Again we note the accuracy is to within the 2 usec. HSI unit's time resolution capability.

EXPERIMENT 6-23

(A). USING THE HSI UNIT AND T1OV TO MEASURE THE NUMBER OF SWITCH BOUNCES AND THEIR TIMES OF OCCURRENCE.

(B). CHANGING HSI MODE ON-THE-FLY.

INTRODUCTION

This experiment is divided into two parts. In the first part (A), we use Timer 2 to determine the number of switch bounces (as in Expt. 6-10) and the HSI unit to determine the exact times of their occurrence. The bouncing switch's output is input to HSI.1 which will act both as the source for T2 events and as a source of transitions for the HSI's FIFO. In the second part (B), we demonstrate how the HSI mode can be changed DURING THE PROGRAM so that, for example, after the first positive transition on a 1 KHz pulse signal is recorded in the FIFO, only negative pulse transitions are recorded thereafter. This is a very useful and powerful feature of the HSI unit.

(A). USING THE HSI UNIT AND T1OV TO MEASURE THE NUMBER OF SWITCH BOUNCES AND THEIR TIMES OF OCCURRENCE

Unless you are using a debounce circuit like the one in Fig. 2-2, mechanical switches are naturally bouncing. The number of bounces and the time from first till last bounce naturally depend on the switches' mechanical characteristics and, in our case, on the time we hold the switch down before release. The times between subsequent bounces will turn out to be surprisingly small.

We shall here measure the number of bounces and the exact times at which they occur. Pin HSI.1 and T2 will be used for that purpose, with the switch output connected to HSI1. To realize a bouncing switch from the debounced switch, simply take the output at pin 1 of the 7400 IC in Fig. 2-2 rather than at pin 6. This experiment differs from a similar one performed in Expt. 6-10 in that, there, the times of the FIRST switch contact (high) and the LAST bounce to low were recorded in T1. Total elapsed time could then be calculated. Here, we also record the times of first and last bounce and, IN ADDITION, the times of each bounce. A table of all bounce times, from first to last, is constructed in memory. In that way an extremely accurate history of switch bounce is recorded. In both Expt. 6-10 and 6-23, here, the number of bounces are displayed at P1's LEDs and the number of timer T1 overflows from first switch contact till last bounce is also recorded. (In Expt. 6-10 the number of overflows was necessary to calculate time from first till last bounce. Here that number is not really needed since our table that we construct will reveal the number of T1 overflows, but we nevertheless incorporate the steps in the program to determine it for comparison with what the table reveals.) We'll be connecting the bouncing switch into HSI.1 to record bounce TIMES in the FIFO and ALSO to record NUMBER of bounces in event counter T2 (we'll program HSI.1 to be T2's clock source).

The program at 2AB0 below is analyzed at its conclusion.

```
        03 00        HSIMODE EQU    03H
        06 00        HSISTAT EQU    06H
        04 00        HSITIME EQU    04H
        09 00        PINT    EQU    09H
        08 00        MINT    EQU    08H
        04 20        INVEC   EQU    2004H
        00 20        INVEC1  EQU    2000H
        60 00        TEMP    EQU    60H
        16 00        IOC1    EQU    16H
        18 00        SP      EQU    18H
        15 00        IOCO    EQU    15H
        0C 00        T2      EQU    0CH
        0F 00        P1      EQU    0FH
        70 00        REG     EQU    70H
        80 00        REG1    EQU    80H
        90 00        REG2    EQU    90H
        A0 00        REG3    EQU    0A0H
                     ;
                     ;
2AB0                         ORG    2AB0H
                     ;
2AB0    A1 C0 00 18          LD     SP,#00C0H     ;Initialize SP to 00C0H.
2AB4    FA                   DI                   ;Disable global interrupt.
2AB5    B1 86 15             LDB    IOCO,#86H     ;Enable HSI.1 into FIFO,
                                                  ;and as T2CLK source. Resets T2.
2AB8    B1 00 16             LDB    IOC1,#00H     ;Will generate HSI interrupt
                                                  ;when HOLDING REG becomes full.
                                                  ;Disables T1 and T2 overflow
                                                  ;interrupts.
```

```
2ABB   B1 04 03                     LDB    HSIMODE,#04H      ;Load FIFO on positive transition
                                                             ;of HSI.1.
2ABE   B1 05 08                     LDB    MINT,#05H         ;Unmask HSI interrupt and TOV
                                                             ;interrupt sources.
2AC1   A1 E7 2A 60                  LD     TEMP,#HSIINT      ;Load address of HSI interrupt
2AC5   C3 01 04 20 60               ST     TEMP,INVEC[0]     ;service routine into INT VECT table.
2ACA   A1 F3 2A 60                  LD     TEMP,#T1OVINT     ;Load address of T1OV interrupt
2ACE   C3 01 00 20 60               ST     TEMP,INVEC1[0]    ;service routine into INT VECT table.
2AD3   11 09                        CLRB   PINT              ;Clear all pending interrupts.
2AD5   FB                           EI                       ;Enable global interrupt bit.
2AD6   A1 00 50 80                  LD     REG1,#5000H       ;Initialize REG1 to point to base
                                                             ;address of bounce time table.
2ADA   A0 0C 70           RDCOUNT:LD       REG,T2            ;Read T2 value (COUNT) into REG.
2ADD   07 70                        INC    REG               ;Increment REG.
2ADF   08 01 70                     SHR    REG,#01H          ;Shift count right 1 bit (div. by 2).
2AE2   B0 70 0F                     LDB    P1,REG            ;Output low byte of count to LEDs.
2AE5   27 F3                        SJMP   RDCOUNT           ;Loop back to read and display count.
                          ;
                          ;
                          ;         HSI INTERRUPT SERVICE ROUTINE
                          ;
                          ;
                          ;
2AE7   C2 81 04           HSIINT: ST       HSITIME,[REG1]+   ;Read time of positive transition
                                                             ;and store in time table.
                                                             ;Auto-increment pointer.
2AEA   11 09                        CLRB   PINT              ;Clear pendings, if any.
2AEC   B1 04 16                     LDB    IOC1,#04          ;Enable T1OV interrupt source for
                                                             ;timer overflows.
2AEF   A0 A0 90                     LD     REG2,REG3         ;Read number of T1 overflows from
                                                             ;REG3 into REG2.
2AF2   F0                                  RET               ;Return to main program.

                          ;
                          ;
                          ;         T1OV INTERRUPT SERVICE ROUTINE
                          ;
                          ;
2AF3   07 A0              T1OVINT:INC      REG3              ;Increment REG3. Another T1OV overflow
                                                             ;has occurred.
2AF5   F0                           RET                      ;Return.
```

The main program above sets SP and then loads 86 into IOC0 to: enable HSI.1 transitions into the FIFO; enable it as the source for T2's events; and to reset T2 to 0. 00 is then loaded into IOC1 to request an HSI interrupt whenever the HSI Holding Register becomes full and to disable T1 or T2 overflow interrupts. We next load 04 into HSIMODE to have the FIFO accept only POSITIVE transitions on the HSI.1 line. 05 is loaded into MINT to unmask both the HSI and TOV interrupt sources. The addresses of the HSI ISR (2AE7 = #HSIINT) and the T1OV ISR (2AF3 = #T1OVINT) are then loaded into the vector interrupt location table at, respectively, 2004 (INVEC) and 2000 (INVEC1), appropriate to HSI and TOV interrupts. The program then clears pendings, enables the interrupt system and loads REG1 with 5000 which will be the base address of the table that will record all the times that the switch bounces high (0 to 1 transitions). We next output the number of bounces up to any given time at P1's LEDs (incremented value of T2 is divided by 2, since T2 increments by TWO for each complete bounce hi/lo). The program loops back to RDCOUNT to continue recording numbers of bounces from T2 as they occur.

When the first contact is made, the loop is interrupted because a 0 to 1 transition event enters the FIFO (remember 04 was placed in HSIMODE) and seeps down to the H.R. This causes an HSI interrupt since the H.R. BECAME full. The first HSI ISR instruction, ST, at 2AE7 reads out the time word of this event from HSITIME, stores it into address 5000, 5001, and auto-increments REG1, the pointer, to prepare it for the next word address in the table that will soon be needed. The reading of HSITIME by ST empties the H.R. The next two instructions remove any previous T1 overflow interrupts that may be pending and THEN enables the T1OV interrupt source for timer overflows (TOV interrupts). Thus T1 overflows will be counted FROM THE TIME THAT SWITCH CONTACT WAS FIRST MADE. Free-running T1 would certainly have a pending that would have been serviced had we not done this, and this would lead to an error in a reading of the true number of overflows that might occur AFTER the switch went high. The number of T1 overflows, counted up in REG3 (see T1OV's ISR), is next passed to REG2, for reasons we'll soon see. A return is then made to RDCOUNT loop in the main program.

The next time a 0 to 1 bounce is made at the switch, the event is again recorded in the FIFO and moves down to the NOW EMPTY H.R., FILLING IT and thereby causing ANOTHER HSI interrupt. Everything repeats, except that the time of this occurrence is stored at the next word address in the table since REG1, the pointer, was previously doubly incremented. The latest count of overflows (in REG3) is updated in REG2. Thus an expanding table of leading edge bounce times is unfolding. Meanwhile, the background RDCOUNT loop in the main program is recording the number of bounces of the switch and displaying same at P1's LEDs.

All the while the above is happening, T1 creates overflow interrupts every 131 msec. (after the first overflow occurred). This causes successive entries into T1OV's ISR at 2AF3 where REG3 is incremented each time, to keep a record of the number of overflows. When the switch stops bouncing we remain in the RDCOUNT loop with the table of bounce times established and P1 displaying the total number of bounces. Every 131 msec. thereafter a brief excursion to the T1OV ISR occurs where REG3 CONTINUES to increment. But that doesn't bother us. We nailed down the value of REG3 at the time of the LAST 0 to 1 bounce in the HSI ISR at 2AEF and passed it to REG2. Thus REG2 has the number of T1 overflows that occurred from the time of the first high on the switch to the time of its last bounce. One cannot simply subtract two values recorded by HSITIME and say that represents the correct time interval. Overflows of T1 may have occurred and multiples of 0.131 sec. may have to be added to that interval. Hence the need for a T1OV ISR.

PROCEDURE

1. Connect the bouncing switch (output from pin 1 of IC 7400 in Fig. 2-2) to HSI.1. HSI.1 will trigger the recording of events into the HSI FIFO AND into T2.
2. Reset the unit to clear out the FIFO. Enter BY 09 = 00 to clear pendings. Enter WO 0A0 = 0000 to clear REG3 (counter for number of T1 overflows).
3. Enter WO 5000 TO 5100 = 0000, initializing our table. This will allow us to see shere the time entries for the bounces end i.e. the table's end will be clearly delineated in that way.
4. Execute from 2AB0 and throw the switch, quickly releasing it.
5. Record the number of bounces displayed at P1. We found P1 = 13 dec.
6. Enter WO 5000 TO 5100 and examine the table. Here were our results (bounce times): 9038, 4F9D, 4FAA, 4FAC, 4FDB, 5095, 50A3, 50D2, 50F3, 510D, 51A5, 5215, 5236 (at 5018) (13 entries, equal to the number of bounces, as expected). The table indicates one overflow. When we queried REG2 for the number of overflows (WO 90), we found 0001 there, in agreement with what the table indicates. Note that the longest time is from first contact high to next contact high, as expected, since that is determined by how long we kept the switch depressed before release. The subsequent time intervals are VERY short. Thus, the time from 9038 to 4F9D (taking account of the T1 overflow) is about 98 msec., while times between later bounces vary from .025 msec. to about .065 msec., indeed short compared to the initial depress to release time. The total time from first high to last high is 99.32 msec. i.e. (FFFF - 9038) + 5236 converted to decimal and then multiplied by 2 usec. (see (9) below for formula).

7. Examine REG1 i.e. WO 80. REG1 is the pointer. It should be pointing to the address just after the address of the last entry in the table since it is always auto-incremented. We found WO 80 read 501A, as expected. Note the listing of the table entries in step (6) above starts at 5000 and ends at 5018.
8. ESC and repeat steps (2)-(7) several times for different throws of the switch. Try to release the switch extremely quickly in one case and then keep the switch depressed for a relatively long time before release in another case. Our result of about 99 msec. indicates a relatively long time of first contact before our release. We were getting a range of about 40-60 msec. for bounce time in Expt. 6-10. There we specifically had in mind to release the switch quickly. Here we were more natural about the release time (see (10) below).
9. Don't forget to use the correct formula for total bounce time i.e. T = (LAST - FIRST) x 2 usec. if REG2 = 0 (no overflows) or T = [(65,536 - FIRST) + LAST + (REG2 - 1) x 65,536] x 2 usec. if REG2 is greater than 0. FIRST and LAST are the first and last table entries made by the bouncing switch on 0 to 1 transitions.
10. We repeated the experiment (steps 2-7), this time releasing the lever switch very quickly. We found the following results: P1 = 17 bounces, WO 90 = 0000 (no overflows), and the table entries starting at 5000 were: 687F, E527, E53A, E54A, E55E, E565, E615, E61B, E635, E6A2, E6EE, E6F4, E6FB, E71C, E735, E73A, E764 (at 5020). WO 80 gave 5022 (pointing to the next address after the last entry). The table confirms no overflows. Typical times between bounces after release are e.g. (E565 - E55E) x 2 usec. = 14 usec.!, (E635 - E61B) x 2 usec. = 52 usec., etc. The time from first contact to release was, in this case, (E527 - 687F) x 2 usec. = 63.82 msec., while the time from first contact to last bounce was (E764 - 687F) x 2 usec. = 64.97 msec.
11. We then repeated the experiment on the DEBOUNCED SWITCH (output taken from pin 6 of IC 7400 in Fig. 2-2), in which we threw the switch 4 times at estimated 1 sec. intervals between throws. Here were our results: P1 = 4, WO 90 = 19H (overflows), table starting at 5000 = 4BB1, 6A44, 9532, 2857, WO 80 = 5008 (address after last table entry). Using the second of the two formulas in (9) above on this data gave 3.26 sec. from first contact till last contact (3 intervals of estimated 1 sec. durations). This is excellent agreement considering our 1 sec. estimates between throws.

(B). CHANGING HSI MODE ON-THE-FLY

To demonstrate the HSI's ability to change mode during the program, we connected a 1KHz, 50% duty cycle, TTL source to HSI.1 and ran the program of part (A) as is. VERY QUICKLY after entering G FR 2AB0, carriage return, (less than 1/4 sec.), we pressed the ESC key, effectively cutting off any further entries into the FIFO and guaranteeing a read-out of "bounces" at P1 of less than FF (255) (and a table of no more than 255 entries). Remember, the program as it stands in part (A) works with the mode that allows only positive transitions to enter the FIFO. Hence our table should show 1 msec. spacings between ALL entries. Before running we reset, entered BY 09 = 00, WO 0A0 = 0000, and WO 5000 TO 5200 = 0000 (just as we did in the procedure section of part (A), only a 5000 to 5200 table span was now provided). Then executing, with a quick ensuing ESC, and inspecting WO 5000 TO 5200, revealed a table of 253 words, matching EXACTLY the value FD that we observed at P1's LEDs. The last entry address was 51F8 and WO 80 revealed 51FA, as it should. Importantly, the difference in times between the FIRST two entries, and between ALL successive entries, was observed to be either 998 usec., 1000 usec., or 1002 usec. -- just as we'd expect for a mode that allows only positive transitions of the 1KHz input to be recorded in the FIFO.

What we did next was to enter the instruction LDB HSIMODE, #08H at 2AEF in the HSI ISR and push down all the rest by 3 addresses (LD REG2, REG3; RET; ING REG3; and RET). What this does is ensure that the first positive transition from the 1KHz pulse train gets into the FIFO (with an interrupt generated). The ISR then reads the time of that first positive transition into the base address, 5000, of the table and then changes the mode from 04 to 08. This stipulates that, HENCEFORTH, only negative going pulse edges will enter the FIFO (with interrupt). The ISR then stores the times of those entries into the table. An examination of the table should then reveal 1/2 msec. between first (high) and second (low) entries in the table, and then 1 msec. between all consecutive (low) entries.

To see if the above is so, we modified the program by entering BY 2AEF = 0B1, 08, 03, 0A0, 0A0, 90, 0F0, 07, 0A0, 0F0. The first three bytes are code for LDB HSIMODE, #08H. The others are the former instructions displaced 3 addresses. Since T1OVINT will now appear at 2AF6, we need to change F3 at 2ACB in the program to F6, which we do by entering BY 2ACB = 0F6. Reset and enter BY 09 = 00, WO 0A0 = 0000, WO 5000 TO 5200 = 0000, as before. Execute from 2AB0 and quickly depress the ESC key (in less than about 1/4 sec.). Inspect WO 5000 TO 5200. We found a table of 211 entries matching the value of counts displayed at port 1's LEDs, namely D3. The last entry address was 51A4 and WO 80 revealed 51A6, as it should. This time the difference in times between the first two entries was observed to be 502 usec. while the difference in times between all successive consecutive entries was observed tos be either 998 or 1000 or 1002 usec., just as we'd expect for this changing mode example.

We have demonstrated in part (B) the HSI Unit's ability to change mode programmably and record transitions accordingly. A very useful feature.

EXPERIMENT 6-24

USING THE HSI UNIT IN A "ROTATING MACHINERY" SIMULATION APPLICATION.

This experiment would have importance in many areas of science and technology. In the area of rotating machinery or precision cutting and tooling we might, for example, need to monitor RPM at "instantaneous" times to ensure that variations in RPM do not occur beyond tolerable limits. In that way precision quality control, for example, can be assured on parts being produced. The formulation below describes the problem in detail and how we propose to simulate it and solve it with the HSI unit.

FORMULATION

1. Imagine a rotating part with a large number of teeth or cogs provided, so that a source of light is blocked as each cog passes the source. A photodiode circuit on the other side could then provide 0 to 1 transitions due to each non-transmit/transmit event as cogs pass by. The transitions could be input to HSI.1, say, for event/time entries into the HSI FIFO. Those times could then be read from the FIFO to create a table of the times as to when successive cogs passed by. Examining or reading out successive entries in the table would then give us a very fine, instantaneous, and continuous monitoring of rotational speed -- not merely an average RPM. In other words, a tachometer.
2. In addition to using HSI.1 to input event/times of the 0 to 1 transitions to the FIFO, we'll have it used also as the source for events in timer T2 and read out the number of those events at port P1's LEDs. This will tell us how many cogs have passed by up to any given moment.
3. Imagine, also, an opening on the body of the rotating part where another source of light can pass through once every revolution, creating a 0 to 1 transition at another photodiode crcuit on the other side of the rotating part. The latter output could then be input to HSI.0 which might be used BOTH as the source for resetting T2 (when the opening passes the light source after one revolution) AND as the source of an external interrupt. The HSI.0 ISR will simply read out the time of the last event in the table (last cog that passed the other light source described in (1) above), disable HSI.1 as the source to T2 so that no more cog events will enter T2, and disable the interrupt system so that no further HSI.0 or HSI "Holding Register Loaded" interrupts will be honored. The time read out for the

last event minus the time of the first event in the table will thus give us the time for one rotation of the part.

4. We'll specify that an "HSI Data Available" interrupt be generated EACH time a cog-created event at HSI.1 occurs and enters the Holding Register through the FIFO i.e. "HSI INTERRUPT, HOLDING REGISTER LOADED". The HSI Data Available ISR will display the total number of cog events to now at HSI.1 (recorded in T2) at port 1's LEDs. It will also read the time of the cog event that took us into the ISR and store it as another entry in the table of event times we'll be creating. Times between successive entries in the table give the times between successive cog events. When we said in (3) above that the HSI.0 ISR disables the interrupt system, among other things, it means that further HSI.1 events created by the still rotating cogs will enter and fill up the FIFO (not T2), but that we'll not be going back to the HSI ISR to read the times of those further events. One revolution has been made and we have sufficient data for the pruposes of this experiment. This restriction can be easily removed and continuing events can be monitored and recorded if desired.
5. The simulation will consist in using a 1KHz, 50% duty cycle, TTL output as the transition source for HSI.1. This would be equivalent to 1 msec. separation in time between an event into HSI.1 from one cog and an event into HSI.1 from the previous cog. Thus if we had 10 or 20 teeth on the rotating part, one revolution would have to be accomplished in 10 or 20 msec. to be equivalent to our simulation. That would correspond to 100 or 50 RPS and hence 6000 or 3000 RPM, just to give an idea of the reality of our approach. The simulation will also consist in using a debounced switch as input to HSO.0. Throwing it low to high will cause a reset of the count in T2 to 0 and an HSI.0 interrupt to the HSI.0 ISR where the time of the last event is recorded and HSI.1 is disabled from T2. That time minus the time of the first event in the table gives the time for one rotation of the part, as already mentioned. Thus our debounced switch at HSI.0 will, when thrown low to high, simulate the sudden passage of the light source through the opening in the part after another revolution of the part has been made (see (3) above).
6. From a programming stand-point, the essentials to keep in mind are the following: a) IOC0.2 will be set to 1 to enable events at HSI.1 to enter the FIFO; b) IOC0.7 will be set to 1 (0) to enable (disable) HSI.1 as the source for T2 clock events; c) IOC1.7 will be set to 0 to allow HSI Data Available interrupts to be generated each time the Holding Register gets loaded with an event/time; d) IOC0.3 will be set to 1 to enable the T2 external reset facility; e)

IOC0.5 will be set to 1 to enable HSI.0 as the source for an external T2 reset; f) MINT.4 and MINT.2 will be set to 1 to unmask the HSI.0 external interrupt source and the HSI interrupt source; g) IOC0.0 will be set to 0 to disable HSI.0 as an input to the FIFO; h) HSIMODE will be loaded with 04 so that only positive transitions at HSI.1 will enter the FIFO.

7. This experiment should illustrate clearly not only how powerful the HSI unit is, but the additional power and versatility available as a result of the multi-function nature of the HSI.0 and HSI.1 pins: HSI.0 can be used as a source for T2's reset, and as a source of external interrupt, as well as a source of events for the FIFO (we're not using the latter here). HSI.1 can be used as a source of events for the FIFO AND as a source of events for counter T2.

The program at 2B00 is presented below.

```
        03 00           HSIMODE EQU     03H
        04 00           HSITIME EQU     04H
        09 00           PINT    EQU     09H
        08 00           MINT    EQU     08H
        04 20           INVEC1  EQU     2004H
        08 20           INVEC2  EQU     2008H
        40 00           TEMP    EQU     40H
        50 00           REG1    EQU     50H
        60 00           REG2    EQU     60H
        70 00           REG3    EQU     70H
        16 00           IOC1    EQU     16H
        18 00           SP      EQU     18H
        15 00           IOCO    EQU     15H
        0C 00           T2      EQU     0CH
        0F 00           P1      EQU     0FH
                        ;
                        ;
2B00                            ORG     2B00H
                        ;
2B00    A1 C0 00 18             LD      SP,#00C0H       ;Initialize SP to 00C0H.
2B04    FA                      DI                      ;Disable global interrupt.
2B05    11 0F                   CLRB    P1              ;Clear LEDs.
2B07    A1 2E 2B 40             LD      TEMP,#HSIINT    ;Load address of HSI interrupt
2B0B    C3 01 04 20 40          ST      TEMP,INVEC1[0]  ;service routine into INT VECT
                                                        ;table.
2B10    A1 3D 2B 40             LD      TEMP,#HSI0INT   ;Load address of HSI.0 interrupt
2B14    C3 01 08 20 40          ST      TEMP,INVEC2[0]  ;service routine into INT VECT
                                                        ;table.
```

```
2B19   B1 AE 15                 LDB    IOC0,#0AEH        ;Selects HSI.1 as source
                                                         ;for T2CLK, HSI.0 as T2RST,
                                                         ;enables Ext. reset, and  HSI.1
                                                         ;input to FIFO and resets T2 to 0.
2B1C   B1 00 16                 LDB    IOC1,#00H         ;Enable HSI interrupt when HLDG. REG.
                                                         ;is loaded.
2B1F   B1 14 08                 LDB    MINT,#14H         ;Enable HSI.0 and HSI interrupt
                                                         ;sources.
2B22   B1 04 03                 LDB    HSIMODE,#04H      ;Load FIFO on positive transitions
                                                         ;of HSI.1.
2B25   A1 00 50 50              LD     REG1,#5000H       ;Load address of event table into
                                                         ;REG1.
2B29   11 09                    CLRB   PINT              ;Clear all pending interrupts.
2B2B   FB                       EI                       ;Enable global interrupt bit.
2B2C   27 FE           HERE:    SJMP   HERE              ;Loop here.

                       ;        HSI INTERRUPT SERVICE ROUTINE
                       ;
                       ;
                       ;
2B2E   A0 0C 60        HSIINT:  LD     REG2,T2           ;Load #EVENTS into REG2.
2B31   07 60                    INC    REG2              ;Increment it.
2B33   08 01 60                 SHR    REG2,#01          ;'Divide' REG2 by 2 to define an
                                                         ;event.
2B36   B0 60 0F                 LDB    P1,REG2           ;Output #EVENTS to LEDs.
2B39   C2 51 04                 ST     HSITIME,[REG1]+   ;Store the time of this event into
                                                         ;table pointed to by REG1. Increment
                                                         ;REG1 by 2.
2B3C   F0                       RET                      ;return to main.

                       ;
                       ;        HSI.0 INTERRUPT SERVICE ROUTINE
                       ;
                       ;
2B3D   FA              HSI0INT:DI                        ;Disable global interrupt bit.
2B3E   05 50                    DEC    REG1              ;Decrement REG1 twice to adjust table
2B40   05 50                    DEC    REG1              ;pointer to last event.
2B42   A2 50 70                 LD     REG3,[REG1]       ;Retrieve time of last entry.
2B45   B1 2C 15                 LDB    IOC0,#2CH         ;Disables HSI.1 as T2 source.
2B48   F0                       RET                      ;return to main routine.
```

The main program accomplishes the necessary initializations as follows: after setting the SP and disabling the interrupt system, the LEDs, where number of events will be displayed, are cleared at P1. The address of the HSIINT routine (2B2E) is loaded into 2004 (INVEC1), the location in the interrupt vector table appropriate to an HSI interrupt. The address of the

HSI0INT routine (2B3D) is then loaded into 2008 (INVEC2), the location in the interrupt vector table appropriate to an HSI.0 external interrupt. 0AE is then loaded into control register IOC0. This accomplishes the following: selects HSI.1 as source of events for T2, selects HSI.0 as source for a T2 reset, enables the external reset facility, enables HSI.1's input to the FIFO, resets (by software) T2 to 0, and disables HSI.0's input to the FIFO. Next 00 is loaded into IOC1 to allow for HSI interrupts each time the Holding Register is loaded with another event. 14 into MINT will unmask the HSI.0 and HSI interrupt sources (the former external, the latter internal). 04 into HSIMODE ensures that only + transitions on HSI.1 will enter the FIFO. 5000 is loaded into REG1 to establish the base address of the table of event times to be created. Any existing pendings are then cleared before the global interrupt bit is enabled. Finally the CPU enters "other tasks" simulated by SJMP HERE.

As HSI interrupts are created by the rotating cogs (i.e. positive transitions into HSI.1 from the 1KHz input signal every 1 msec. enter the FIFO and then the H.R. to create the interrupts), we are vectored to the HSIINT ISR at 2B2E. There we read the number of events from T2 (fed by HSI.1) into REG2 and then normalize it (INC and SHR), so that each positive transition will correspond to one event (remember T2 increments on both positive and negative transitions). The number of events is then displayed at port 1's LEDs. The value of T1 in HSITIME for that event (cog interrupt) is then stored in the location pointed to by REG1 (5000 for the first event). REG1 is auto-incremented (by two) to get ready to store the time (word) value of the next event when we again enter the HSI ISR. The RET returns us to "other tasks" at HERE in the main program. When the next cog passes (1 msec. later in our simulation) another event enters the FIFO from HSI.1 and finds its way down to the H.R. (remember the previous read of HSITIME by the ST instruction at 2B39 emptied the H.R.). That creates another HSI interrupt and we're back into the HSI ISR where P1's display is incremented by 1 to indicate another cog has passed by. ST stores the time of this latest event into the next word address in the table (pointed to by the doubly incremented REG1), auto-increments REG1 again, and empties the H.R. Thus you can see how a table of all cog events is being formed and how P1 will display the number of such events as they occur.

When the rotating part has made one revolution the second light source "gets through the opening in the part" and creates an HSI.0 interrupt (simulated by our throwing the debounced switch at HSI.0 low to high). We are vectored to the HSI.0 ISR at 283D. Since HSI.0 is also the source of a T2 reset, we enter the HSI.0 ISR with T2 cleared. There, we disable the system (we have our data -- no more interrupts needed or wanted). We then decrement REG1 twice to bring the pointer back to the last entry in the table. We fetch that last entry's time value from the table and store it in REG3 so that (REG3) minus the first entry in the table at 5000, 5001 (plus any T1 overflows) will tell us the time for one rotation. Next 2C is loaded into IOC0 to disable HSI.1 as the source of T2 events, so that T2 will remain cleared (although P1 will continue to display the final total number of events at HSI.1). The RET takes us back to "other tasks" at HERE and no further interrupts are accepted.

PROCEDURE

1. Connect the 1KHz input signal to HSI.1 and a debounced switch to HSI.0. Reset the unit to clear out the FIFO and enter BY 09 = 00 to clear pendings.
2. Enter WO 5000 TO 5200 = 0000. This will allow our table to indicate where the last event entry was made when we later examine it i.e. where does the table end?
3. Execute from 2B00 and very quickly (in less than 1/4 sec.) throw HSI.0 high (so that less than 256 positive transitions at 1 msec. intervals in HSI.1 will be made from the input signal, allowing us to see the count at P1's 8 LEDs WITHOUT OVERFLOW).
4. Read the number of events at P1's LEDs (the last value in T2 before it was cleared by the throw of HSI.0). We found P1 = 46H = 70 dec.
5. Now examine the table of event times by entering WO 5000 TO 5200. Calculate the differences of several pairs of contiguous events i.e. WO 5002 - WO 5000; WO 5004 - WO 5002; WO 5006 - WO 5004, etc. We found, respectively, the following results: first pair gave a difference ED1F - EB2A = 1F5 = 501 = 1.002 msec.; second pair gave EF13 - ED1F = 1F4 = 500 = 1.000 msec., third pair gave F107 - EF13 = 1F4 = 500 = 1.000 msec., etc. The last pair in the table gave 7204 - 7010 = 1F4 = 500 = 1.000 msec. All as expected.
6. At what address in the table was the last event recorded? We found it to be at 508A corresponding to 1 + (138/2) = 70 events (words) recorded. This is in perfect keeping with the number of events observed at P1 in (4) above. What is the time value at that last address? In our case it was 7204H. Calculate the difference between T1 at 5000 (first event: EB2A) and T1 at that last address. In our case it was 7204H - EB2AH (time for "one rotation"). Careful! Watch out for overflows of T1 in the table and take them into account. Thus, in our case, we observed 1 T1 overflow from the table. Hence time for 1 rotation = (FFFF - EB2A + 7204) x 2 usec. = 34,521 x 2 usec. = 69.04 msec. This agrees with the result in (4) above i.e. 70 events implies

69 INTERVALS at 1 msec. each, or 69 msec. total.

7. Now examine WO 70 (REG3) and verify that it is the time value of the last event in that it equals the value of T1 in the last entry in the table. We found 7204 in agreement with the last value in the table (see HSI.0 ISR).
8. The final value of the pointer, REG1, should be the address of the last entry in the table (see HSI.0 ISR). Query WO 50. We found 508A, as expected.
9. Read the present value in T2 by entering WO 000C. It should be 0 because of the reset of T2 that occurred when HSI.0 was thrown high. We found it to be 0000. Remember, the loading of 2C into IOC0 in the HSI.0 ISR inhibits HSI.1 events from being input to T2, so T2 stays at its last value, the reset value that throwing HSI.0 high produced.

EXPERIMENT 6-25

D TO A CONVERSION USING THE HSO UNIT AS AN ALTERNATIVE TO PWM.

We have implemented D to A conversion in a number of experiments in which the PWM SFR was used to drive output pin P2.5 with PWM pulses. We had an RC filter circuit integrate that output to a smooth analog voltage (see Expts. 5-2, 5-3, 6-1, 6-2, 6-3, 6-19). We can also accomplish D to A conversion by having the HSO unit create pulses of constant or varying widths. The former will be called the "static case". It will generate fixed d.c. filtered voltages at an HSO pin. Their magnitude will be controlled as different bytes are entered from the keyboard on-the-fly. The constantly varying width case leads to waveform generation at the HSO pin, e.g. ramps, and will be denoted as the "dynamic case". Whereas the period of the PWM-generated pulses is a fixed 64 usec., the periods of the HSO-produced pulses can be anything from 0 to 131 msec. as we've seen in all the previous work with the HSO unit.

FORMULATION

1. The program that is given later will contain within it two cases (depending on whether we put NOPs in place of certain instructions or not):
2. The first case is the "static case", in which the time between HSO pulses generated at pin HSO.0 will be a fixed 510 usec. = 0.510 msec. Their pulse widths can be anything between 0 and 498 usec. = 0.498 msec., depending on the size of the word entered into REG1 (address 50H) at run-time (which can be changed on-the-fly thereafter). This case will, therefore, produce static d.c. voltages at HSO.0 ranging from 0 to about 5 volts, depending on the instantaneous word entered into REG1. Thus the low byte of the digital word entered into REG1 from the keyboard will be converted to an analog output at HSO.0.
3. The second case is the "dynamic case", in which the time between pulses will again be a fixed 510 usec. (by choice. We're not restricted to that value in either case 2 above or here.). This time the width of each successive pulse at HSO.0 is incremented by 1 (on a scale of 0 to 255) relative to the pulse just preceding it. In that way we'll generate a ramp output at HSO.0 whose period will clearly be 0.51 msec. x 256 = about 131msec. The ramp then repeats.
4. The HSO.0 outputs in cases (2) and (3) above will be integrated by the same filter circuit we've been employing at

the output to P2.5 in its PWM mode. We'll then measure the smooth analog voltage at the output of that filter with a VTVM in case (2) above, or we'll observe the output on a scope in case (3) above.

Let us proceed directly to the program and then analyze it. It is presented below at 2D00.

```
        06 00             HSOCOM  EQU     06H
        04 00             HSOTIME EQU     04H
        09 00             PINT    EQU     09H
        08 00             MINT    EQU     08H
        06 20             INVEC   EQU     2006H
        40 00             TEMP    EQU     40H
        0A 00             T1      EQU     0AH
        18 00             SP      EQU     18H
        50 00             REG1    EQU     50H
                          ;
                          ;
2D00                              ORG     2D00H
                          ;
2D00    A1 C0 00 18               LD      SP,#00C0H         ;Initialize SP to 00C0H.
2D04    FA                        DI                        ;Disable global interrupt.
2D05    B1 08 08                  LDB     MINT,#08H         ;Enable HSO interrupt source.
2D08    A1 1D 2D 40               LD      TEMP,#HSOINT      ;Load address of HSO interrupt
2D0C    C3 01 06 20 40            ST      TEMP,INVEC[0]     ;service routine into INT VECT
                                                            ;table.
2D11    A1 06 00 50               LD      REG1,#0006H       ;Load REG1 with 0006.
2D15    11 09                     CLRB    PINT              ;Clear ALL pending interrupts.
2D17    EF 13 00                  CALL    LDCAM             ;Call load CAM routine.
2D1A    FB                        EI                        ;Enable global interrupt bit.
2D1B    27 FE             HERE:   SJMP    HERE              ;loop here.

                          ;
                          ;
                          ;
                          ;       HSO INTERRUPT SERVICE ROUTINE
                          ;
2D1D    07 50             HSOINT: INC     REG1              ;Incr. REG1.
2D1F    89 F9 00 50               CMP     REG1,#00F9H       ;Compare with 00F9H
2D23    D7 04                     JNE     LDRET             ;If not equal jump to load cam
                                                            ;routine then return.
2D25    A1 06 00 50               LD      REG1,#0006H       ;Else reload REG1.
2D29    EF 01 00          LDRET:  CALL    LDCAM             ;Load CAM to repeat pulses.
2D2C    F0                        RET                       ;Return to main routine.

                          ;       LOAD CAM ROUTINE
```

```
2D2D   B1 20 06        LDCAM:  LDB   HSOCOM,#20H      ;Load HSO command with 20H for HSO.0
                                                      ;to go on. (no interrupt)
2D30   45 03 00 0A 04          ADD   HSOTIME,T1,#0003H;Execute approx. NOW.
2D35   FD                      NOP                    ;Delay 4 state times
2D36   FD                      NOP                    ;Delay 4 state times.
2D37   B1 00 06                LDB   HSOCOM,#00H      ;Load HSO command with 00H for HSO.0
                                                      ;to go off. (no interrupt)
2D3A   44 50 0A 04             ADD   HSOTIME,T1,REG1  ;Execute at time in REG1 + T1.
2D3E   FD                      NOP                    ;Delay 4 state times
2D3F   FD                      NOP                    ;Delay 4 state times.
2D40   B1 30 06                LDB   HSOCOM,#30H      ;Load HSO command with 30H for HSO.0
                                                      ;to go on.
2D43   45 FF 00 0A 04          ADD   HSOTIME,T1,#00FFH;Execute at time = T1 + 00FF, with
                                                      ;interrupt.
?D48   F0                      RET                    ;Return to main routine.
```

The main part of the program is concerned mostly with initializations, as usual. Thus the SP is initialized; the interrupt system is disabled,; the HSO interrupt source is unmasked in preparation for generating HSO pulses at HSO.0 with interrupts; the address of our HSO ISR (2DID) is entered into the vector interrupt table location (2006) appropriate to an HSO interrupt; REG1 is initially loaded with 0006 to specify the INITIAL pulse width BEFORE any changes in pulse widths are made EITHER by program incrementations of REG1 OR through keyboard entries to REG1 on-the-fly; pendings (if any) are cleared; the LOAD CAM routine at 2D2D is called in order to generate the FIRST pulse of PERIOD 512 usec. and WIDTH 12 usec. (0006 x 2 usec.); the interrupt system is enabled to receive HSO interrupts (which will be generated every time ANOTHER pulse at HSO.0 is generated); and finally the processor goes on to "other tasks" at 2D1B (simulated by SJMP HERE).

Let us now look at the LDCAM routine, located at 2D2D, which was first called at 2D17 in the main program above. 20 into HSOCOM asks that HSO.0 be turned on without HSO interrupt generation. Then 0003 + T1 is loaded into HSOTIME specifying that it be turned on essentially "now". NOPs are required for 8 state times before another entry can be made into the H.R. while the previous entry to H.R. is getting into the CAM. 00 loaded into HSOCOM then specifies that HSO.0 be turned off without HSO interrupt generation. (REG1) + T1 loaded into HSOTIME then specifies that HSO.0 is to be turned off at a time (REG1) from "now". Hence (REG1) will determine the pulse width. Right now (REG1) is 0006 (for 12 usec. width), but in the HSO ISR, REG1 will be incremented to produce ramp waveforms, OR (with NOPs there) REG1 will be determined by word values entered into REG1 (50) from the keyboard at run-time (or on-the-fly as the program is executing). After 8 more state times, 30 is loaded into HSOCOM specifying that HSO.0 be turned on again (completion of one pulse) WITH generation of an HSO interrupt. T1 + 00FF loaded into HSOTIME specifies that HSO.0 is to be turned on again 510 usec. from "now", i.e. the periods of the generated pulses will be the fixed value 510 usec. Clearly, we can make that period anything we wish from 2 usec. to 131 msec. by simply changing the word 00FF at address 2D44,45 in LDCAM to any value between 0001 and FFFF, as long as (REG1) (pulse width) is less than that period value.

It should now be clear that the HSO ISR is entered every time another complete pulse is generated because we've arranged that LDCAM put out an HSO interrupt only AFTER one ADDITIONAL pulse has been generated. Let's analyze the HSO ISR at 2D1D. There we increment REG1 (pulse width) for the "dynamic case" of ramp waveform generation (that, and certain ensuing instructions, will be replaced with NOPs at run-time for the "static case" to be discussed). CMP then asks whether REG1 has reached 00F9 i.e. a pulse width JUST BELOW the period 00FF that LDCAM specified. (This will correspond to a voltage peak of close to 5 volts.) If not, JNE causes a jump to LDRET where we call LDCAM to produce another pulse of INCREMENTED width (REG1 has just been incremented) with subsequent return to "other tasks" at HERE in the main program. When further entries into HSO ISR increment REG1 to 00F9, we fall through the JNE at 2D23. Approximately 5 volts peak has been reached and the fall-through reloads REG1 to its initial width of 0006. The ramp will start all over. LDCAM is then called to generate a pulse of this new (minimal) width, again followed by a return to "other tasks" in the main program. All repeats -- new ramps will be generated. We again bring to your attention that with certain NOPs in the HSO ISR routine (to be described in the PROCEDURE section below), the ramp waveforms at HSO.0 will change to d.c. static levels at the filtered HSO.0 output, of magnitude dependent on REG1 values entered from the keyboard at run-time, or after execution.

PROCEDURE

1. We treat the "dynamic case" first in which the program remains just as is. Connect the output at HSO.0 to the RC filter used previously at P2.5's PWM output. Connect the filter output to a scope. Reset the unit to clear the CAM and H.R. Enter BY 09 = 00 to clear any pendings. Execute the program from 2D00. We observed ramps on the scope. We measured a period of about 120 msec. There was considerable rounding at the troughs of successive ramps due, no doubt, to the fixed RC value of the filter used, hence the disagreement with the expected 131 msec. See section (3) FORMULATION. The peak voltage of the ramps was measured to be about 4.65 volts, again probably the result of the fixed RC value.

2. ESC. We now treat the "static case". If we enter NOPs at addresses 2D1D through 2D28 in the HSO ISR, we'll be eliminating the increments of REG1 (and hence also of the pulse widths). Ramps at HSO.0 will no longer occur. Instead the pulse width of all the pulses will be determined by whatever is in REG1 (see instruction at address 2D3A). The latter can be simply set to any value by entering a word into it (address 50) from the keyboard at run-time and, subsequently, on-the-fly. Of course, the size of the word should be less than 00FF which is our period (see instruction at address 2D43 in LDCAM). Hence, the filtered output voltage at HSO.0 will have a magnitude proportional to the size of the word (actually to the low byte of the word). D to A conversion results.
3. Reset the unit and enter BY 09 = 00. Connect the filtered voltage output at HSO.0 to a VTVM. Place NOPs at 2D1D through 2D28 by entering BY 2D1D TO 2D28 = 0FD. Execute from 2D00. Enter, in turn, the following word values at 50 (REG1): WO 50 = 0011, then 0022, 0033, 0044, 0055, 0066, 0077, 0088, 0099, 00AA, 00BB, 00CC, 00DD, 00EE, 00FF. For each entry measure the corresponding voltage at HSO.0 with the VTVM. We found, respectively, 0.52 volts, 0.81V, 1.10V, 1.38V, 1.68V, 1.97V, 2.26V, 2.57V, 2.86V, 3.17V, 3.48V, 3.79V, 4.11V, 4.42V, and 4.74V.

PROBLEM

Modify the program so that the time between pulses is not fixed at 510 usec. but can be anything entered from the keyboard into REG2 (address 60H).

EXPERIMENT 6-26

MEASURING THE TIME INTERVAL BETWEEN INCOMING EVENTS ON TWO DIFFERENT HSI PINS. CALIBRATING THE HSI UNIT.

INTRODUCTION

The HSI Unit, through its HSI STATUS and TIME Registers, can tell: 1. WHEN an incoming EVENT (transition) on an HSI pin occurred as recorded in HSITIME by timer T1 (taking account of T1 overflows, if necessary, to establish time intervals), 2. at WHICH of the four HSI pins the EVENT occurred, 3. what the CURRENT STATUS at that (or any other) pin is. Remember, the HSI STATUS Register's four 2-bit pairs associated with each HSI pin tell us the CURRENT STATUS of that pin (upper bit), and whether a TRANSITION (EVENT) occurred at that pin (lower bit) AT THE TIME RECORDED IN THE FIFO (the 20-bit FIFO registers hold the 16-bit times and the four pin TRANSITION bits). In the experiments with the HSI Unit in Chapters 5 and 6 we have concerned ourselves with incoming events at only one pin in any given experiment. Hence, at most, we were concerned with the upper of the 2-bit pairs in the HSI STATUS Register associated with any given pin, namely the CURRENT STATUS of the pin, knowing ahead of time that an event would sooner or later occur at THAT pin. Thus if the HSI MODE Register was set to have the FIFO accept positive AND negative transitions on one pin, it was necessary and sufficient in the HSI ISR routine to poll only the CURRENT STATUS bit of that pin -- if it was high a positive transition occurred, if low a negative transition occurred. Polling in the ISR to ascertain if an EVENT occurred on that pin would be redundant - it did! Or, in a number of cases, no polling of HSI STATUS was at all necessary where the mode was set for the FIFO to accept ONLY positive or ONLY negative transitions on ONE pin. In that case, entering the HSI ISR made it a foregone conclusion that a positive or negative transition occurred on that pin, so why poll the CURRENT status bit or EVENT bit for that pin?

Now, however, we are going to have two HSI pins carry incoming events and we wish to measure the time between the arrival of the two events on the DIFFERENT pins. In that case it is essential that we poll the LOWER bit of the current status/event bit-pairs to determine at which pin the EVENT arrived, at the recorded time. And we'll have to poll that bit for each of the pins in contention. In our case, we are allowing events to occur at HSI.0 and HSI.1, to illustrate the method. Thus we'll poll HSI STATUS bits 0 and 2 in the HSI ISR routine to determine

WHERE the EVENT occurred AT THE RECORDED TIME. A 1 found at HSI STATUS.0 would indicate the event occurred at HSI.0, while a 1 found at HSI STATUS.2 would indicate the event occurred at HSI.1, AT THE RECORDED TIME.

FORMULATION

1. The two events (positive transitions) will be generated by our program at precise times. Thus we'll have the program create a 0 to 1 transition at P1.0 at a GIVEN time and THEN a 0 to 1 transition at P1.1 at a PRECISE TIME LATER (a simple 576 usec. delay loop is entered in the program between events for this purpose. Any other delay time is easily selected. We do that too: see PROCEDURE).
2. P1.0 and P1.1 are connected first to HSI.0 and HSI.1, respectively, and then, in another run of the program, the connections are reversed with P1.0 driving HSI.1 and P1.1 driving HSI.0.
3. REG0 (WO 50) and REG1 (WO 60) will store the times of the events recorded in the FIFO for HSI.0 and HSI.1, respectively.
4. The time interval between events will be t = (REG1 - REG0) x 2 usec. when P1.0 is connected to HSI.0 and P1.1 to HSI.1.
5. When the connections from P1 to HSI are reversed, the time will be found from t = (REG0 - REG1) x 2 usec.
6. In either case, (4 or 5), the results should agree with the expected 576 usec. time interval generated by our loop, or with whatever other delay time is programmed.

The program at 2E00 is presented below.

```
18 00        SP       EQU    18H
08 00        MINT     EQU    08H
09 00        PINT     EQU    09H
03 00        HSIMODE  EQU    03H
04 00        HSITIME  EQU    04H
06 00        HSISTAT  EQU    06H
04 20        INVEC    EQU    2004H
90 00        TEMP     EQU    90H
0F 00        P1       EQU    0FH
15 00        IOC0     EQU    15H
16 00        IOC1     EQU    16H
40 00        REG      EQU    40H
50 00        REG0     EQU    50H
60 00        REG1     EQU    60H
```

```
2E00                              ORG     2E00H
                        ;
2E00   A1 C0 00 18                LD      SP,#00C0H          ;Initialize SP.
2E04   FA                         DI                         ;Disable global interrupt.
2E05   A1 00 10 90                LD      TEMP,#1000H        ;Delay allows for iSBE-96 overhead
2E09   05 90            LOOP:     DEC     TEMP               ;when using the GO command.
2E0B   D7 FC                      JNE     LOOP               ;
2E0D   11 0F                      CLRB    P1                 ;Clear LEDs at P1.
2E0F   B1 04 08                   LDB     MINT,#04H          ;Unmask HSI interrupt.
2E12   B1 05 03                   LDB     HSIMODE,#05H       ;Only positive transitions on
                                                             ;HSI.0 AND HSI.1 lines will enter
                                                             ;FIFO.
2E15   B1 05 15                   LDB     IOC0,#05H          ;Enable HSI.0,HSI.1 lines into FIFO.
2E18   B1 00 16                   LDB     IOC1,#00H          ;Program HSI interrupt to occur when
                                                             ;Holding Register becomes loaded.
2E1B   A1 35 2E 90                LD      TEMP,#HSIINT       ;Load address of HSI interrupt service
2E1F   C3 01 04 20 90             ST      TEMP,INVEC[0]      ;routine into INT.VECT table.
2E24   11 09                      CLRB    PINT               ;Clear ant pending interrupts.
2E26   B1 01 0F                   LDB     P1,#01H            ;Initiate positive transition at
                                                             ;HSI.0 (via P1.0).
2E29   B1 FF 40                   LDB     REG,#0FFH          ;Load REG with FFH for 576 usec. delay.
2E2C   E0 40 FD         MORE:     DJNZ    REG,MORE           ;Decrement REG and jump if != 0 to
                                                             ;MORE.
2E2F   B1 03 0F                   LDB     P1,#03H            ;Else initiate positive transition
                                                             ;at HSI.1 (via P1.1).  Maintains HSI.0
                                                             ;high.
2E32   FB                         EI                         ;Enable global interrupt.
2E33   27 FE            HERE:     SJMP    HERE               ;Loop here.
                        ;         HSI INTERRUPT SERVICE ROUTINE
                        ;
2E35   38 06 05         HSIINT:   JBS     HSISTAT,0,HSI0     ;If event occurred on HSI.0,jump to
                                                             ;HSI0.
2E38   3A 06 07                   JBS     HSISTAT,2,HSI1     ;Else, if event occurred on HSI.1,
                                                             ;jump to HSI1.
2E3B   20 08                      SJMP    RETURN             ;Jump to RETURN to main program.
2E3D   A0 04 50         HSI0:     LD      REG0,HSITIME       ;Read time of HSI.0 transition into
                                                             ;REG0.
2E40   20 03                      SJMP    RETURN             ;Jump to RETURN to main program.
2E42   A0 04 60         HSI1:     LD      REG1,HSITIME       ;Read time of HSI.1 transition into
                                                             ;REG1.
2E45   F0               RETURN:   RET                        ;Return to main program.
```

The main part of the program initializes the stack pointer and disables the interrupt system. Now something "new" has been added. A (roughly) 12 msec. time delay loop is included with the LD TEMP, DEC TEMP, JNE LOOP instructions. We shall be introducng a 576 usec. delay loop at 2E29 for the purpose of precisely separating our HSI.0, HSI.1 events. After user enters G FR UVWX, carriage return (to execute a program from UVWX), the

SBE echoes the Return, sends out a Line Feed, then four NULLs, and then the carrot prompt. This SBE overhead will steal time from your program (not much), by means of its monitor's NMI interrupts, to accomplish those final tasks before allowing your program to execute. In our case, that would be bad news: our 576 usec. delay loop (used to separate HSI.0, HSI.1 events later) would be LENGTHENED CONSIDERABLY, at our program's expense, by the iSBE's required overhead, as its NMI jabs in and out of our delay loop to steal time for its overhead. Since we are trying for a precise 576 usec. loop to "calibrate" the HSI Unit, we give the SBE more than its required time for executing its up-front overhead with our own up-front 12 msec. delay loop. After that, iSBE won't bother us or corrupt our 576 usec. delay. (Without it, we found the 576 usec. delay between HSI.0.1 events became a 732 usec. "delay" -- to give you an idea of what the iSBE steals from you immediately after you execute your program. This has never been critical in any of the experiments done heretofore, but it will be here if we don't include the up-front delay loop at 2E05.)

The program then continues by clearing the LEDs at P1, unmasking the HSI interrupt source and setting the HSIMODE for only positive transitions on HSI.0 and HSI.1 to be accepted into the FIFO. Loading 05 into HSIMODE accomplishes the latter. Similarly, loading 05 into IOC0 enables the HSI.0 and HSI.1 lines into the FIFO. The program then clears IOC1.7 to allow for HSI interrupts whenever the HSI Holding Register BECOMES loaded. The address HSIINT (2E35) of the HSI ISR is next entered into INVEC (2004 for HSI interrupts) and any pendings are cleared. At this point we raise P1.0 high so that HSI.0 goes high (assuming P1.0 is connected to HSI.0). This creates an event/time transition into the FIFO, which seeps down into the H.R. thereby creating an HSI interrupt. This interrupt becomes pending since EI has not yet been programmed. The two lines at 2E29, 2E2C provide the 576 usec. delay loop (FF at 2E2A can be changed to arrive at smaller delays) before 03 is output to P1, raising P1.1 high and maintaining P1.0 high. 9 state times for DJNZ times 256 times 1/4 usec. = 576 usec. This causes a positive transition on HSI.1 (assuming P1.1 is connected to HSI.1) and another event/time enters the FIFO. So far there are two entries in the FIFO (one in H.R.) and one outstanding pending interrupt (due to the first transition on HSI.0).

At this point we enable the global bit and then enter "other tasks" at SJMP HERE. It is at this point that the HSI pending interrupt is serviced. We are vectored to the HSI ISR at 2E35. There we poll bit 0 of HSISTATUS register. This bit, if 1, would indicate that an event occurred on the HSI.0 line AT THE TIME RECORDED IN THE FIFO (in this case "event" was a positive transition on HSI.0). In that case JBS would cause a jump to HSI0 at 2E3D where the time of that event is read out from HSITIME and stored in REG0. This is followed by SJMP RETURN which gets us back to SJMP HERE via RET at 2E45. The reading of HSITIME empties the H.R. and allows the second entry in the FIFO (from the transition on HSI.1) to enter H.R. This creates another HSI interrupt. This time JBS at 2E35 finds NO EVENT AT BIT 0 OF HSISTAT AT THE RECORDED TIME i.e. at the time HSI.1 went high. So we fall through to the second JBS at 2E38 where we test for an event on HSI.1 i.e. we test bit 2 of HSISTATUS. Finding a 1 there (event at HSI.1 occurred at the recorded time), the jump to HSI1 is taken where the time of the HSI.1 event is read into REG1, emptying H.R. Return to the main program loop then occurs.

The difference REG1 - REG0 should give the separation in time of the events at HSI.0 and HSI.1, namely 576 usec. in this case. If the P1.1 and P1.0 connections to HSI.1 and HSI.0, respectively, were reversed, then the first entry into the ISR would find HSISTAT.0 to be 0 (no event transpired on HSI.0 as yet, only at HSI.1). Fall-through the JBS at 2E35 to JBS at 2E38 would take place. There we'd find HSISTAT.2 to be 1, as an event occurred at HSI.1. In that case the jump to HSI1 is taken where the time that HSI.1 went high is recorded into REG1. H.R. empties. Return to HERE then transpires. The next HSI interrupt (when the HSI.0 event entry in the FIFO enters the H.R.) enters 2E35 where HSISTAT.0=1 is this time found since the second entry corresponds now to an event that happened on HSI.0, not HSI.1. The jump to HSI0 is taken where the time that HSI.0 went high is recorded into REG0 and SJMP to RETURN then takes place. Clearly, in this case, the time separation between events is now given by REG0 - REG1 and should be 576 usec. again (see PROBLEM below).

Finally, note that we may change FF at 2E2A to eg. 80H. This should give time separation equal to 288 usec. 40 should give 144 usec., etc. Thus we have a handy, precise way of calibrating, if you like, the HSI unit.

PROCEDURE

1. Reset the unit and enter BY 09 = 00. Connect P1.0 to HSI.0 and P1.1 to HSI.1. Execute the program from 2E00. Examine WO 60 and WO 50 i.e. REG1 and REG0, respectively. We found 399D and 387D leading to a difference of 120H = 288 dec. Multiplying by 2 usec. gives 576 usec., exact agreement.
2. Reset and enter BY 09 = 00, BY 2E2A = 80. Execute again. This time we found WO 60 = 7AA6 and WO 50 = 7A15 giving a difference of 91H = 145 dec., or 290 usec. The delay loop

at 2E2C was reduced to 288 usec. with 80 at 2E2A.

3. Reset and enter BY 09 = 00, BY 2E2A = 40. Execute. We read WO 60 and WO 50 to be 0A29 and 09E1 giving a difference of 48H 72 dec., or 144 usec. 40 at 2E2A corresponds to a delay of 144 usec.
4. In the same way we found REG1 - REG0 = 72 usec. and 36 usec. when (2E2A) was changed to 20H and 10H, respectively. Excellent agreement.
5. Reset and enter BY 09 = 00. Reverse connections so that P1.0 feeds HSI.1 and P1.1 feeds HSI.0. Repeat steps 1, 2, and 3 above with FF, 80, and 40, respectively, at 2E2A. We found, in each case, the following: With FF, WO 50 = 9D63, WO 60 = 9C44 leading to a difference of 11FH or 287 dec. or 574 usec. With 80, we found WO 50 = 3207 and WO 60 = 3177 leadng to 90H = 144 dec. = 288 usec. 40 gave 0468 - 0420 = 48H = 72 dec. = 144 usec. Perfect agreement.

PROBLEM

Modify the program so that a register will read out the absolute difference of the HSI.1, HSI.0 times regardless of which occurred first. Employ another register as a semaphor to indicate which event occurred first and develop the algorithm accordingly.

CHAPTER 7

ARITHMETIC FEATURES OF THE 8096.

INTRODUCTION

Some of the unique arithmetic features of the 8096 make it formidable in the area where arithmetic versatility, speed, accuracy, and reductions in software overhead are essential. For a microcontroller, it is quite surprising to see an arithmetic capability that rivals some of the big-name 16-bit microprocessors (e.g. the 80186 -- without the 8087 numerical processor, that is).

The purpose of this chapter is to bring to your attention the powerful arithmetic features of the 8096. It is not our intention here to develop applications using those arithmetic features, nor to develop "math packages". Some of the applications experiments in chapter 9 and 10 will be using these arithmetic features. Rather we are here interested in pointing out the use and advantages of the normalization, sign extend, and multiply and divide instructions, in particular, and how the availability of the "sticky bit", ST, and "overflow trap", VT, flags facilitates arithmetic procedures. The discussions will point out how substantial software overhead would have to be incurred by the programmer if these instructions or flags did not exist in hardware. The N (negative) flag is also discussed.

As far as math packages and applications involving the 8096's arithmetic facilities, we refer you to 1) PL/M-96 User's Guide, Intel, 1983; 2) The Intel FPAL96 library (Floating Point Arithmetic Library); 3) 8096 Floating Point Arithmetic Library

User's Guide (order number 122133) for a detailed explanation of the FPAL96 library; 4) Intel's REAL MATH standard as applied to PL/M-96.

The approach we've taken in THIS chapter is one more of discussion of the arithmetic facilities available with the 8096 than of developing applications experiments using those facilities. That could be a book unto itself (see references mentioned above). WE DO INCORPORATE A NUMBER OF THOSE ARITHMETIC FACILITIES, HOWEVER, IN VARIOUS APPLICATIONS EXPERIMENTS IN CHAPTER 9 AND AGAIN IN CHAPTER 10 (USING PL/M-96), WHERE FRACTIONAL MULTIPLY, MULTIPLY AND DIVIDE, ADD, AND SQUARE ROOTS ARE INVOLVED. The experiments in this chapter are short ones illustrating the sign extend instruction and the sticky bit and N flag. While we discuss normalization and its relationship to floating point arithmetic, we do not here develop programs or applications involving them. That is best left to the four references cited above to which the reader is referred.

A. THE 8096 AND MATHEMATICAL OPERATIONS.

In the area of mathematical operations with microprocessors or microcomputers, there are two major capabilities that play an important role. These are speed of instruction execution and the number of bits available to hold operands and results. "Number Crunching" ability is in direct proportion to these two capabilities. In looking at the 8096 arithmetical capabilities, one immediately notes the support of 16-bit operands and 32-bit results (in the case of two divide instructions, a 32-bit operand is involved). Along with this large bit length, the 8096's arithmetical operations execute remarkably fast for this low cost, highly integrated device.

One of the major errors in numerical calculations using fixed length binary integers is truncation. While it is impossible to totally eliminate truncation, the effect of round-off can be minimized by increasing the bit length of the numbers representation. The 8096 provides for 32-bit results in its 16 x 16 bit multiply instructions and in its 32/16 bit divide instructions. It also provides for the shifting of 32-bit quantities directly. This represents a significant enhancement over other microcontrollers and even over the 16-bit 8086 family of microprocessors (not counting that family's numeric co-processor 8087). Besides increased bit length capability, the 8096 provides for fast execution when using its multiply and divide operations, requiring, on average, only 6.5 usec. Additionally, while providing support for 32-bit operands, the 8096 has not sacrificed the ability to manipulate bits (see bit manipulation instructions in chapter 3's experiments).

The 8096 goes further in support of mathematical operations by providing a number of single instructions that adjust and prepare operands before and after calculations.

B. THE EXTB INSTRUCTION.

The first of these instructions is the EXTB instruction ("Sign Extend Short Integer Into Integer"). This performs a sign extension of a byte operand into an integer (word) operand. This is required when attempting to add or subtract a short integer and an integer, to put them on the same bit length basis. The experiment below (at 4000) demonstrates the use of the EXTB instruction.

EXPERIMENT 7-1

THE EXTB (SIGN EXTEND) INSTRUCTION. ADVANTAGES.

```
        40 00          REG1    EQU     40H
        50 00          REG2    EQU     50H
        60 00          REG3    EQU     60H

4000                           ORG     4000H

                       ;
4000    16 40                  EXTB    REG1             ;Sign-extend REG1 to 16 bits.
4002    44 50 40 60            ADD     REG3,REG1,REG2   ;Add REG1 and REG2 put result in
                                                        ;REG3.
4006    27 FE          HALT:   SJMP    HALT             ;Loop here.

4008                           END
```

Here the original byte (short integer) is in byte address 40 and its sign extension will be INTO byte address 41. The resultant 16-bit (sign extended) integer is at word address 40. It is then added to the word in REG2 with the result placed in word register REG3.

CASE 1: Take REG1 = 08H and REG2 = 3000H at run-time i.e. BY 40 = 08, WO 50 = 3000. Execute from 4000. Examine REG3 i.e. WO 60. Find 3008 as the result. Examine WO 40. Find 0008, as expected.

CASE 2: ESC. Enter BY 40 = F8 (for REG1) and WO 50 = 3008 (for REG2). Execute from 4000. Examine WO 40. Find FFF8, as expected. Examine WO 60 and find 3000. Note that REG1 + REG2 = FFF8 + 3008 = 3000. Note, also, that PRIOR to the extension, you would have found 00F8 at WO 40. Why? (See CASE 1).

By having the single instruction, Sign Extend, the 8096 eliminates the following MULTI-INSTRUCTION sign extension:

```
        LDB REG - HI, #00H
        JBC REG, 7, NO EXT
        LDB REG - HI, #0FFH
NOEXT:
```

The EXTB instruction requires 4 state times for execution. The above instructions require a total of either 13 state times (JBC not taken) or 17 state times (JBC taken). The savings is, therefore, as much as 13 state times.

There is also the EXT instruction for sign extending an integer into a double integer. The 8096 also provides greater execution time savings by combining the load operation and the EXTB operation into a single instruction: LDBSE (Load Integer With Short Integer), which sign extends a short-integer operand and then loads it into a destination word location (see Expt. 3-12 on the LDBSE and LDBZE instructions in chatper 3). This is extremely useful as it allows the employment of the variety of 8096's addressing modes to obtain the operand i.e. LDBSE wreg, baop vs. EXTB wreg.

C. THE NORML INSTRUCTION AND FLOATING POINT ARITHMETIC.

The next single instruction operation that is extremely useful is the NORML (Normalize Long-Integer) instruction. We refer to it as the Normalization instruction for short. This instruction allows the 8096 to support a library of floating point routines (FPAL 96) that have been coded very efficiently using NORML. (See Expt. 3-15 in chapter 3 using the NORML instruction).

The use of floating point format in microprocessor mathematical operations is made simpler if the normalization operation is done efficiently. This traces to the fact that prior to, or following, a floating point arithmetical operation, the operands/result must be normalized. This means the mantissa field of the FP-represented number must have a 1 in its high order bit (with the exception of the number 0). However, to provide this format, the shift operation used must allow the program to adjust the exponent field by the number of shifts of the mantissa.

Therefore, normalization requires shifting the mantissa LEFT until a one is shifted into the high order bit. This must then be followed by the exponent being decremented for EACH shift required. Equivalently, the number of shifts can be SUBTRACTED from the exponent field.

For certain floating point operations, such as addition and subtraction, the de-normalization operation is also necessary. De-normalization involves adjusting the mantissa of one or both of the floating point operands to make the exponents equal. The addition and subtraction operation then reduces to a simple add or subtract of the mantissa and assignment of the common exponent to the result. This would then be followed by normalization of the result. Floating point multiplication and division do not require de-normalization and are performed by multiplying or dividing the mantissas of the two operands. The exponents of the multiplied or divided operands are added or subtracted, respectively.

The concept of REAL number representation is another way of referring to the use of floating point representation of a number. The use of floating point allows the programmer to implement an arithmetic operation with greater accuracy. Otherwise, the programmer is left to use integer arithmetic and suffer its inaccuracies as in, for example, 7 divided by 2 yielding 3. Floating point representation allows one to represent a number as an integer portion AND FRACTIONAL PORTION. Thus REAL would yield the real answer 3.5, which can be properly represented in floating point.

The FPAL96 library for 8096 uses the form which contains a fraction and an exponent. This representation is shown below (see p. 13-1 of PL/M-96 User's Guide, 1983, Intel Corp). The number occupies 4 consecutive bytes. There are several rules regarding how these 4 bytes represent a number. They are given below.

A REAL value occupies four contiguous memory bytes, starting on a word boundary. The four bytes may be viewed as 32 contiguous bits. The bits are divided into fields, as follows:

sign (1 bit)	exponent (8 bits)	fraction (23 bits)

where

- the byte with the lowest address contains the least significant eight bits of the fraction field, and the byte with the highest address contains the sign bit and the most significant seven bits of the exponent field.
- the sign bit is zero if the REAL value is positive, and one if the REAL value is negative. The value of zero can be either positive or negative.
- the exponent field contains a value offset by 127—in other words, the actual exponent can be obtained from the exponent field value by subtracting 127. An exponent field of all zeroes or all ones represents special cases. See the Denormal Operand Exception in section 13.3.
- the fraction field contains the binary digits of the fractional part of the REAL value when it is represented in binary scientific notation (see below). A zero is represented by a value that has all zeroes in both the exponent and fraction fields.

It is important to point out that the format described above is used for STORAGE of floating point (REAL) numbers prior to, and after, a mathematical operation. When actually performing the operation, the operands are expanded to a 6-BYTE representation consisting of a byte for the sign, a byte for the exponent, and 4 bytes for the mantissa. Thus

SIGN	EXPONENT	MANTISSA
(8 bits)	(8 bits)	(32 bits)

The exponent is represented as a value offset by 127, or what is referred to as "excess - 128 notation". This simply means that a NEGATIVE exponent is subtracted from 127 to obtain the exponent field of the floating point number, and a POSITIVE exponent is added to 127 to obtain its value. An example of floating point number representation is as follows:

3.1875 (dec) is represented as 11.0011(B) in fixed point binary representation. To obtain the floating point representation, the following operations are performed (for clarity the number will be represented using binary scientific notation e.g. 1.10011 x 2'):

1. The sign bit is 0 since the number is positive.
2. The exponent becomes 128 since it represents a +1 (127 + 1).
3. The mantissa is 100110.....0.

This would be STORED in the following way

01000000	highest location in memory.
01001100	
00000000	
00000000	lowest location in memory.

The operation of adjusting the number so that it has a 1 in the MSB of the mantissa is the job of NORML. This 1 is actually not STORED with the number. It is ASSUMED to alway be there since the number has been assumed to be normalized. However, as noted before, during the actual calculations using floating point numbers, the "hidden bit", as it is referred to, is brought back into play in the 6 BYTE format. In this operating format we can see why the 8096 is efficient in handling floating point numbers. The mantissa is now represented by 4 BYTES (a long integer). Thus the NORML instruction can operate directly on THAT portion of the number. This would not be the case if we used the 4 BYTE STORAGE representation of the number. After an operation, the number's mantissa would be normalized and the storage format constructed using the shifted mantissa and the count (number of shifts performed). The latter is then subtracted from the exponent.

A detailed description of these FP calculations is beyond the scope of this chapter. The reader is referred again to the FPAL96 REAL MATH library routines for detailed descriptions. Our intention here was to point out the role of the NORML instruction in floating point arithmetic and the advantages that accrue to the programmer when working with the powerful 8096 instruction set in floating point applications because of the existence of that instruction.

D. THE STICKY BIT, ST, AND ROUNDING.

The next area we'll examine is the use of the "STICKY BIT" (the ST flag). (Consult your Microcontroller Handbook and Expt. 3-9 as to how the SHIFT instructions affect C and ST). It greatly helps facilitate reducing round-off error in arithmetical operations. Very often a number is shifted to allow its representation by a smaller number of bits. An exmple would be storing the 10-bit result of an 8096 A/D conversion as an 8-bit quantity. Another common operation is arithmetic shifting right to perform division by powers of 2. If these operations are done using a single instruction that performs multiple shifts, a problem of round-off arises.

Round-off occurs from the use of a finite set of binary bits to represent infinite granularity. Typically, the C (Carry) flag is used to determine the rounding off of a quantity during the shifting operation. However, to insure that there is no loss of knowledge when a 1 bit is shifted OUT (lost), a test must be made after EACH shift operation to see if that occurred. This does not allow using SINGLE instructions that perform multiple shifts. This would reduce the speed of execution considerably.

In using the sticky bit available with the 8096, one can make use of its multiple shift instructions and yet test the state of BOTH the C bit AND the ST bit directly AFTER ALL the shifts are complete. An example of the greater accuracy obtained through the use of the sticky bit flag (ST) is demonstrated in the experiment below at 4100.

EXPERIMENT 7-2

THE STICKY BIT AND ROUNDING.

```
        40 00      REG1    EQU    40H
        50 00      REG2    EQU    50H

4100                       ORG    4100H
                   ;
4100    A0 40 50           LD     REG2,REG1     ;Copy original number into REG2.
4103    0A 04 50           SHRA   REG2,#4       ;Shift REG2 right 4 times divide
                                                ;by 16.
4106    27 FE      HALT:   SJMP   HALT          ;Loop here.

4108                       END
```

Review the EXACT definition of the SHRA instruction in your Microcontroller Handbook with its consequences on the C and ST flags. Also see our Expt. 3-9.

PROCEDURE

1. Enter WO 40 = 0050 (= 80 dec).
2. Execute from 4100.
3. Examine WO 50 and find 0005, as expected.
4. Examine PSW and find C = 0, ST = 0, as expected.
5. ESC. Enter WO 40 = 0047.
6. Execute from 4100.
7. Examine WO 50 and find 0004, as expected.
8. Examine the PSW and find C = 0, ST = 1. The actual value after the shifts would have been 4.4375 had three 1s NOT been lost. Instead we find 0004 = 4.0000. The error incurred is 0.4375 (LESS than 1/2 the value of the original LSB). Remember 0047 = 0100.0111 = 4.4375. Without the availability of the ST flag, the knowledge of this error would have been lost. C = 0 and ST = 1 reminds us of the size of the error. The programmer would be left to consider whether to round up or down without having the proper information.

9. ESC. Enter WO 40 = 0068.
10. Execute from 4100.
11. Examine WO 50 and find 0006, as expected.
12. Examine PSW and find C = 1, ST = 0. In this case the actual value after the shifts would have been 6.5 had bit 3's 1 not been lost i.e. 0110.1000 = 6.5. Actually, we have 6 so the error is 0.5 which is EQUAL to 1/2 the LSB. This case and size of error was foretold and handled by the C flag alone (C = 1).
13. ESC. Enter WO 40 = 006C.
14. Execute from 4100.
15. Examine WO 50 and find 0006 as expected.
16. Examine PSW and find C = 1, ST = 1. In this case the actual value after the shifts would have been 6.75 (i.e. 0110.1100) had two 1s not been lost from bits 2 and 3. Actually, we have 6, so the error is 0.75 which is GREATER than 1/2 LSB. This time both C = 1 and ST = 1 alert us to the size of the error (GREATER than 1/2 LSB). Again, the presence of the ST flag provides important information to the program which then has to use the resulting numerical data.

This insight provided by C and ST is extremely important when operating on floating point numbers, since the fractional information that would be lost in the absence of the ST bit can now be properly used to enhance the accuracy of the calculation.

Another example of the power of the sticky bit would be in adjusting the result of a 10-bit A/D conversion to be held in byte format. A shift right by 2 would be a divide by 4 of the 10-bit quantity. However, that information plus the state of the carry bit would still give only PART of the real story. For example: take 10-bit A/D result = 10110111 = 2DFH. This equals 735 x 5V/1024 or 3.587 volts. If we now shift the result right by 2 positions, the byte would be 10110111 = 0B7H = 183 x 5/1024 = 0.893 volts. The actual result should have been 0.897 volts, an error of 4 millivolts (i.e. 183.75 x 5/1024 = 0.897V, taking account of the 2 lost bits). The C flag would alert the programmer of a loss of 1/2 LSB (or 2.44 millivolts) but the shifting ACTUALLY lost 4.0 millivolts as would be shown by the setting of the ST flag. In certain applications the loss of the 1.6 millivolts could have a significant effect. This is especially true if this result is further processed where other errors might be introduced to compound the inaccuracies. This error could be detected without the sticky bit by testing the C flag after EACH shift operation (remember the LSB after each shift goes to the Carry). But, as mentioned earlier, this leads to a significant reduction in the speed of the operation. As part of a STRING of mathematical operations, this inefficiency could prove to be costly. Hence the great advantage and usefulness of the sticky bit.

E. THE OVERFLOW TRAP FLAG, VT, AND ITS ADVANTAGES.

Analogous to the support provided by the ST flag, the VT (oVerflow Trap) flag provides information that is often lost in multiple operations. The VT flag is set whenever there is an overflow out of the MSB of the result operand. This is identical to the operation of the V (oVerflow) flag, except that the VT flag, once set, will not reset except if cleared by a CLRVT, JVT, JNVT, RST or PUSHF instruction. Therefore, if an arithmetic operation caused an overflow, both V and VT would be set. If the following operation does NOT cause an overflow, V is cleared but VT remains set until specifically cleared. This allows the program to be written more efficiently since there is only ONE test of the VT flag that need be made (at the end of a multiple string of arithmetic operations) as opposed to a test of the V flag after EACH operation in the string.

While these efficiencies may not appear to be massive, when considered individually, they have profound impact when used in concert with the other efficient operations of the 8096. (See also Expt. 3-7 on the V, VT flags).

F. THE USE AND ADVANTAGES OF THE N (NEGATIVE) FLAG IN ARITHMETIC.

The N flag is also a powerful addition to the arithmetic processing of numbers using the 8096. This flag is used to declare if the result of the last arithmetic or logical operation is negative. The important feature of the N flag is its ability to reflect a negative value EVEN IF THERE WAS AN OVERFLOW OUT OF THE MSB OF THE RESULT. This is important since the MSB is typically used to define whether the operand is a negative (MSB = 1) or positive (MSB = 0) number. WITHOUT the N flag, a result that had its MSB OVERFLOW would have indicated a 0 for the MSB (positive result). We would thus interpret the result as a positive number, when in reality it was negative.

EXPERIMENT 7-3

USING THE 8096's N FLAG.

```
        40 00          REG1    EQU     40H
        50 00          REG2    EQU     50H

4200                           ORG     4200H
                       ;
4200    74 50 40               ADDB    REG1,REG2       ;Add REG2 to REG1.
4203    27 FE          HALT:   SJMP    HALT            ;Loop here.

4205                           END
```

PROCEDURE

1. Enter BY 40 = 9CH = -28 (dec) (signed magnitude).
2. Enter BY 50 = 9CH = -28 (dec) (signed magnitude).
3. Execute from 4200.
4. Examine the result in REG1 and find BY 40 = 38H = +56 (dec). Bit 7 = 0 but N flag = 1 i.e. ....
5. Examine the PSW and find bit 14 = N = 1.

As can be seen the result is incorrectly represented as a positive number (bit 7 in 38H is 0), but the N flag tells us otherwise. It says the result is not +56 (dec) but -56 (dec) as it clearly should be: (-28) + (-28) = -56 dec.

CONCLUSION

The intent of this chapter was to present the aspects of the 8096 that enhance its ability to perform mathematical operations. As pointed out, the 8096's speed and ability to manipulate 32-bit quantities (including multiply and divide) set it apart from other microcontrollers. But it's the addition of the Sticky Bit facility, and the EXT, EXTB, LDBSE, and NORML instructions that make the 8096 an efficient engine for floating point operations. We come back to applications with arithmetic in some of the experiments in chapters 9 and 10.

CHAPTER 8

SERIAL I/O WITH THE 8096. APPLICATIONS.

INTRODUCTION

We now turn our attention to Serial Communications with the 8096. This will bring us into direct involvement with the 8096's Serial I/O SFRs which, so far, we have not studied or been involved with. As we indicated in Chapters 5 and 6, where the study of the 8096's SFRs and applications with them were made, we were going to defer the study of, and applications with, the Serial I/O SFRs to this chapter. These are the byte SFRs:

SBUF(TX), with SFR address 07H (write only);
SBUF(RX), with SFR address 07H (read only);
BAUD-RATE, with SFR address 0EH (write only);
SP-CON, with SFR address 11H (write only);
SP-STAT, with SFR address 11H (read only).

SBUF(TX) is the transmit buffer for the serial port. The contents of the byte to be outputted serailly at TXD must be written into SBUF(TX) at 07. SBUF(RX) is the receive buffer for the serial port. It will hold the byte serially received at RXD, if any, and must eventually be read from 07. BAUD-RATE is the SFR which determines the baud rate based on the two bytes written to it sequentially at 0EH. SP-CON is the SFR that CONTROLS the type of action desired at the serial port. It is written to at 11H. SP-STAT, when read at 11H, reveals certain aspects of the serial port's STATUS. We'll go into more details as we meet them later.

Our approach will be to study, carefully explain, and use all of these SFRs in the context of each of the six applications experiments involving Serial I/O in this chapter.

The serial port on the 8096 consists of the output TXD (serial port transmit) and input RXD (serial port receive) pins. They are pins 60 and 61, respectively, on the 68-pin version. Please note that TXD is the ALTERNATE FUNCTION for P2.0 (bit 0 of port 2) and RXD is the ALTERNATE FUNCTION for P2.1 (bit 1 of port 2). IOC1.5 is the bit in control register IOC1 that must be set to 1 to select the TXD alternate roll for P2.0 (0 would select P2.0 in its straight digital output function). On the other hand P2.1 serves as an input line (always) and, therefore, it serves equally as RXD WITHOUT the need to set or reset any bit in any of the control registers, although REN (bit 3 in SPCON) must be set to 1 to enable the receive FUNCTION. (Note that port P2 in its regular, non-alternate mode was studied in Expt. 5-6). Setting REN to 1 in SP-CON does NOT disable the transmit function, except in MODE 0.

For those familiar with the 8051 single-chip microcontroller, be it noted that the 8096's serial port has many similarities with its 8051 counter-part. There are also some differences. However, we are not assuming any prior knowledge with the 8051's serial port in what follows in this chapter.

IMPORTANT NOTE

As you go through this chapter, you are referred to pp. 2-17, 2-18, 2-19, 3-16, 4-9, 4-10, 4-11, and 4-12 of the Microcontroller Handbook (1985). Except for pp. 4-9, 4-11, 4-12, and 3-16, all of this material is reproduced in section H (pp. 24, 25, 26) of chapter 1 of this book. Very good coverage can also be found on pp. 13-16 of Intel's AP Note 248 by Ira Horden, 1985 ("Using the 8096"). We will be covering and explaining all of this material quite carefully as we proceed through chapter 8, but it might be a good idea to read the above material first before going on, especially pp. 2-17, 2-18, 2-19, and 4-10 of the handbook (see section H chapter 1). After finishing this chapter you may want to refer to p. 3-16 of the Handbook for another example "Programming the Serial I/O Channel".

A. CRUCIAL POINTS TO REMEMBER IN WORKING WITH AND PROGRAMMING THE 8096'S SERIAL PORT AND ITS SFRs (CAUSE AND EFFECT). HOW TO AND WHY.

1. The baud rate selected for the communication is achieved by writing two bytes sequentially into the BAUD-RATE SFR at 0EH. The word is then automatically stored in an internal 16-bit baud rate register. The first byte entered becomes the low byte in the 16-bit baud register and the second becomes the high byte. MSB of the high byte determines which of two sources will supply the input frequency to the baud rate generator on chip. If it is 1, the frequency on the XTAL1 pin is chosen. If it is 0, the external frequency from the T2CLK pin is selected. The remaining (lower) 15 bits written into the baud rate register define an unsigned number B (max. value 32,767 = 7FFFH) which, when used in certain equations, will yield the operative baud rate. Those equations are given on p. 2-19 of the Microcontroller Handbook (1985) or on p. 26 in chapter 1 of this book. From those equations, the following results are inferred, relevant for a 12MHz clock at XTAL1 (see p. 2-19 Microcontroller Handbook):

BAUD RATE (BAUD)	B VALUE (MODE 0)	B VALUE (MODES 1, 2, or 3)
9600	8137H	8013H
4800	8270H	8026H
2400	84E1H	804DH
1200	89C3H	809BH
300	A70FH	8270H

It should be noted that the B value of 8013H above really works out to a baud rate of about 9400 rather then 9600. However, Intel's AP Note 248 (pp. 14, 15) states: "in most cases a serial link will work if there is less than a 2.5% difference between the baud rates of the two systems".

The equations that pertain when T2CLK is the frequency source for the baud rate generator (see p. 26) will give a different BAUD RATE vs. B value table. We do not list it here. The equations pertinent to T2CLK and to XTAL1 on p. 26 are presented in the form which gives baud rate as a function of the 15-bit number B for the various modes. They can easily be inverted to give the necessary value of B (to be loaded into BAUD-RATE SFR 0EH as two sequential bytes) as a function of the desired baud rate (for any input frequency to the baud rate generator). Thus we find:

Modes 1,2,3: B = [XTAL1 frequency/64 x Baud Rate] -1.

Mode 0: B = [XTAL1 frequency/4 x Baud Rate] -1, B $\neq$ 0.

Modes 1,2,3: B = T2CLK frequency/16 x Baud Rate, B $\neq$ 0.

Mode 0: B = T2CLK frequency/Baud Rate, B $\neq$ 0.

Remember, these equations are useful in determining the necessary value of B to be written into SFR 0EH [low byte of B first, high byte of B next (with MSB of high byte = 1 for XTAL1 as the source, or = 0 for T2CLK as the source)]. That B value will produce the desired baud rate. Note that the baud rate generator on chip is independent of Timers 1 and 2 so that the HSI/O units are not interfered with in Serial I/O operation.

2. When a byte is loaded into SBUF(TX) for transmission, a Serial I/O interrupt will be generated (vectoring to 200CH in the VECT. INT. location table) ONLY after the byte has been COMPLETELY shifted out of SBUF(TX) via the TXD pin. That interrupt may be honored immediately [if interrupt mask bit .6 was set to 1 and PSW.9 was set to 1 (EI)] or it will become pending (if either mask bit .6 or PSW.9 or both were not set to 1). In EITHER case the TI bit (5) in SP-STAT (see p. 24, chapter 1) is set to 1 as a flag indicating that transmission out of SBUF(TX) was completed (TI stands for "transmit interrupt") and was accompanied by a Serial I/O interrupt (serviced or pending).

3. When a complete byte has entered SBUF(RX) via the RXD pin (reception), a Serial I/O interrupt is generated (to SAME vector location 200CH). Whether honored or pending, the RI bit (6) in SP-STAT is set to 1 as a flag indicating that reception of a complete byte into SBUF(RX) was made (RI stands for "receive interrupt") and that it was accompanied by a Serial I/O interrupt (serviced or pending).

4. Since "transmission out through TXD complete" and "reception in through RXD complete" both cause interrupts with the SAME vector entry location 200CH, it becomes necessary to ascertain whether it was reception of a byte or transmission of a byte (or both in full duplex) that was responsible. So now you see why the RI and TI bits in SP-STAT are valuable as flags. You will have to poll SP-STAT (SFR 11H) to determine which of the two bits is high to be able to infer if it was a completed transmission or a completed reception (or both in full duplex) that occurred. Since a reading of SP-STAT CLEARS the TI and RI flags (very im-

portant and useful in itself in ANOTHER context to be discussed shortly - see 7c below), it becomes incumbent on the user to read SP-STAT into a register in the RAM file where those bits can be tested without their being automatically cleared by the reading, SHOULD THEY NEED TO BE READ AGAIN.

5. Note that if reading SP-STAT did NOT clear the RI and TI flags, then the next time you read SP-STAT to see if a new transmission or reception was completed, you'd find RI or TI still 1, even if no new transmission or reception was completed, and this would falsely tell us that another transmission or reception did occur, when it didn't. This latter statement applies if you're using the POLLING mode in the main program re: SP-STAT i.e. WAITING till RI or TI goes hi to indicate a completed reception or transmission. But even if you're using the INTERRUPT mode and are testing SP-STAT in the ISR for the state of RI and TI, a completed RECEPTION would have vectored us to the ISR where a test of SP-STAT would find RI = 1. If reading SP-STAT did not clear RI, then a SUBSEQUENT COMPLETED TRANSMISSION would again vector us to the ISR where we'd now find BOTH RI and TI set upon reading SP-STAT. That would infer that a new reception AS WELL AS transmission occurred, when in reality only a transmission occurred this time. HENCE THE NEED FOR THE CPU TO CLEAR SP-STAT ANY TIME IT IS READ AND FOR US TO READ IT INTO A TEMP TO KEEP A COPY OF THE RI, TI STATUS SHOULD WE NEED TO TEST THE PREVIOUS SP-STAT STATUS AGAIN.

6. The USER must ALSO clear the flag bit(s) in TEMP. This needs some amplification. After testing TEMP for the status of RI or TI to ascertain whether a completed reception or completed transmission occured, WE should clear THAT bit in TEMP, otherwise the NEXT time we read TEMP it will indicate that a NEW reception or transmission occurred (RI or TI still high) when in fact none may have occurred. Thus, if we are testing for, say, reception in a polling mode and reception is finally indicated by RI going high, we'll fall through to read the received byte out of SBUF(RX). We should then immediately clear bit 6 of TEMP (the RI flag indicator) so that NEXT time around, a poll of bit 6 will NOT reveal a NEW reception when in fact none may have yet occurred. All during this time a transmission may have occurred, setting bit 5 of TEMP high (the TI flag indicator), so we DON'T yet clear bit 5 of TEMP UNTIL AFTER we poll it. If bit 5 is high, transmission of the old byte out of SBUF(TX) must have occurred and we fall through to load SBUF(TX) with the NEXT charac-

ter to be transmitted. We then immediately clear bit 5 of TEMP, so that NEXT time around we don't get a false indication that the NEW byte in SBUF(TX) has been completely transmitted, when in fact it may not have been yet. We WAIT till TI (bit 5 in TEMP) again goes high to let us know that, indeed, a NEW transmission has occurred and THEN clear that bit. The best way to clear the RI or TI bits in TEMP is simply to use ANDB TEMP, #0BFH or ANDB TEMP, #0DFH, instructions, respectively.

7. NOW COMES THE HEART OF THE MATTER: WHAT ARE THE CONDITIONS THAT THE USER MUST SET UP, PROGRAMMABLY, TO START RECEPTION FROM RXD AND/OR TO START TRANSMISSION OUT OF TXD? Let us first present them as they pertain to modes 1, 2, 3 and then, SEPARATELY, as they apply to mode 0. [We discuss the subject of MODES in part (B) of the INTRODUCTION which follows the conclusion of this section (A)]. IN ALL CASES BELOW INITIALIZE BAUD RATES.

7a. TO START RECEPTION IN MODES 1, 2, OR 3: 1) Set REN (bit 3 in SP-CON at 11H) to 1 to enable the receive function. 2) Write the correct mode bits 0,1 or 1,0 or 1,1 at the M2,M1 bits in SP-CON to specify mode 1, or mode 2, or mode 3. 3) The first trailing edge (1 to 0 transition i.e stop to start bit) arriving at the RXD pin initiates reception from RXD into SBUF(RX), WHOSE COMPLETELY RECEIVED BYTE CAN LATER BE READ FROM 07H. When reception of the byte is complete a Serial I/O interrupt is generated (vector entry at 200CH, if serviced). The RI flag in SP-STAT then goes high.

7b. TO START TRANSMISSION IN MODES 1, 2, OR 3: 1) Set IOC1.5 = 1 to enable TXD at P2.0. 2) Set REN (bit 3 in SP-CON at 11H) to either 1 or 0, (FOR FULL DUPLEX REN MUST BE SET TO 1). 3) Write the correct mode bits M2,M1 into SP-CON to select either mode 1, 2, or 3. 4) Write the byte to be transmitted into SBUF(TX) (07H). Transmission then starts at TXD. A Serial I/O interrupt is generated when transmission is complete (vector entry at 200CH, if serviced). The TI flag in SP-STAT then goes high.

7c. TO START RECEPTION IN MODE 0: 1) Set IOC1.5 to 1 to enable TXD at P2.0. 2) Cause a rising edge on REN (write a 1 to bit 3, Receiver Enable, in SP-CON), OR 3) Clear the RI flag (bit 6 in SP-STAT) with REN = 1. In the latter case a simple read of SP-STAT will clear RI. When reception on RXD into SBUF(RX) is complete, a Serial I/O interrupt is generated (to 200CH, if serviced) and the RI bit in SP-STAT is set to 1. The above conditions, when met, automatically start the output of 8 shift clocks from TXD to CLOCK of an external shift register to clock 8 bits of data FROM it INTO SBUF(RX) through RXD.

7d. TO START TRANSMISSION IN MODE 0: 1) Set IOC1.5 to 1 to select the TXD function for P2.0. 2) Set REN to 0 (write a 0 to bit 3 in SP-CON). 3) Write the byte to be transmitted into SBUF(TX). These conditions will cause 8 shift clocks to be generated at TXD which can then be connected to CLOCK of an external shift register to clock 8 bits of data FROM SBUF(TX) into the external shift register VIA THE RXD PIN. PLEASE NOTE THAT IN MODE 0, OUTPUTTING OR INPUTTING OF THE DATA OCCURS ON THE RXD PIN WHILE THE TXD PIN SERVES TO OUTPUT THE SHIFT CLOCKS TO THE EXTERNAL SHIFT REGISTER IN BOTH CASES. Again, when transmission out of SBUF(TX) is complete, a Serial I/O interrupt is generated (to 200CH, if serviced) and the TI bit in SP-STAT is set to 1. In both 7c and 7d we must, of course, make sure that we've written M2 = M1 = 0 into SP-CON to select MODE 0. Mode 0 serves for I/O port expansion (7c IN, 7d OUT).

8. Further remarks about SP-STAT and SP-CON that should be made here are the following (they'll be expanded upon when we discuss the MODES in more detail in section (B) below): 1) Writing the proper M2,M1 control bit combinations into bits 1,0 of SP-CON will specify the MODE for the serial communcation. 2) The PEN control bit (Parity Enable, bit 2 in SP-CON) enables the parity function in MODES 1 and 3 (even parity only) if it's 1, otherwise the parity function is not operative. 3) TB8 (control bit 4 in SP-CON) programs the 9th data bit to 1 or 0 (in MODES 2 or 3) on transmit (if parity has not been chosen for the 9th bit in mode 3). TB8 clears after transmission in MODES 2 and 3. As with REN and the M2,M1 mode bits, the PEN and TB8 bits are controlled by simply writing the desired byte into SP-CON. 4) Finally, status bit 7 in SP-STAT serves two functions. As RB8, it reveals the status of the 9th bit RECEIVED (if PEN = 0 i.e. parity disabled). As RPE, it is the parity error indicator (if parity is operative i.e. PEN = 1). RPE stands for Receive Parity Error.

B. THE FOUR SERIAL I/O MODES AND THEIR COMMUNICATIONS FEATURES.

1. MODE 0: This synchronous mode is selected when bits M2,M1 (1,0 bits) in SP-CON are both set to 0. In this mode, RXD and TXD are used to implement I/O expansion whereby exter-

nal shift registers are used as additional parallel output or input ports. Refer to Fig. 4-13 p. 4-10 of the 1985 Microcontroller Handbook (also p. 26, chapter 1 in this book) where a typical serial port interface to implement I/O expansion is given. Inputting from an external parallel port to the serial port is accomplished when the 8 shift clocks emanating from TXD are used to serially clock the 8 bit parallel input data stored in the external shift register (e.g. the 74165) via RXD into SBUF(RX). There it can be read as a parallel byte. The program conditions for this to occur were given in section 7c of the previous part (A), where starting reception (inputting) in MODE 0 was discussed. We cover the case of I/O expansion for inputting in Expt. 8-2 and also present a figure there showing the serial port connections to the external shift register which we used in that experiment. Outputting to a parallel port from the serial port is accomplished when 8 shift clocks from TXD are used to clock the serial bits output at RXD [from SBUF(TX)] into the external shift register (e.g. 74164 or CD4094) where they will then reside as a parallel output byte. The program conditions for this to occur were given in section 7d of part (A), where starting transmission (outputting) in MODE 0 was discussed. We cover the case of I/O expansion for outputting in Expt. 8-1 and give a diagram there showing the serial port connections to the external shift register (CD4094) which we used in that experiment. Note that in MODE 0 TXD is used exclusively for outputting the 8 shift pulses to the external shift register while RXD is used to serially OUTPUT from SBUF(TX) OR to serially INPUT into SBUF(RX). See p. 25, chapter 1 for MODE 0 timings or p. 4-10 Fig. 4-12 of the Microcontroller Handbook (1985).

2. MODE 1: This asynchronous mode is selected when M2 = 0 and M1 = 1 are written into SP-CON. The frames are 10 bits for both transmit and receive consisting of a start bit (0), 8 data bits (LSB first), and a stop bit (1). These frames are transmitted through TXD and received via RXD. The 8th data bit becomes an even parity bit, which is transmitted, if PEN = 1 is written into SP-CON. The parity calculation is done in hardware for even parity. MODE 1 is often used when linking the serial port to a CRT terminal. The software steps required to start transmission or reception in MODE 1 were covered in sections 7a and 7b of part (A). See p. 25, chapter 1 for the data frame in MODE 1. MODE 1 is covered in Expts. 8-3, 4, and 5.

3. MODE 2: This asynchronous mode is selected when M2 = 1 and M1 = 0 are written into SP-CON. It supports 11 bit frames that can be transmitted through TXD and received through RXD: start bit (0), 8 data bits (LSB first), a programmable 9th data bit, and a stop bit (1). The value written into TB8 of SP-CON is the value assigned to the 9th data bit on transmission. It is cleared after transmission. When receiving, the 9th data bit controls whether a serial I/O interrupt will be generated or not on complete reception into SBUF(RX). If that received 9th bit is 1 a serial I/O interrupt will be generated, if 0 there will be no such interrupt. This is very useful in master - slave applications. The data frame for this mode is shown on p. 25 of chapter 1. The software steps required to start transmission or reception in MODE 2 were covered in sections 7a and 7b of part (A). MODE 2 is very important when used with MODE 3 (discussed below) in Multiprocessor (Interprocessor/master-slave) Communications. See Expt. 8-6.

4. MODE 3: This asynchronous mode is selected when M2 = 1 and M1 = 1 are written into SP-CON. It supports 11 bit frames that can be transmitted over TXD and received via RXD. Again the start bit is 0, then follow 8 data bits (LSB first), then a programmable 9th bit which equals the value written to TB8 in SP-CON (if PEN = 0), and then the stop bit (1). (If PEN = 1 in SP-CON, the 9th bit will be a parity check bit). But now note that, on complete reception, the received 9th data bit is stored and the serial port interrupt is generated REGARDLESS of its value. This has importance when we describe Multiprocessor Communications in 5 below. The data frame for MODE 3 is shown on p. 25, chapter 1. The software steps required to start transmission or reception were covered in sections 7a and 7b of part (A). See Expt. 8-6.

5. USING MODES 2 AND 3 IN MULTIPROCESSOR COMMUNICATIONS: We are quoting here from section 2.11.2 on p. 2-18 of the Microcontroller Handbook (1985), also found on p. 25 of our chapter 1: "When the master processor wants to transmit a block of data to one of several slaves, it first sends out an ADDRESS frame which identifies the target slave. An address frame will differ from a data frame in that the 9th bit is 1 in an address frame and 0 in a data frame. No slave in Mode 2 will be interrupted by a data frame. An address frame, however, will interrupt all slaves (in mode 2) so that each slave can examine the received byte to see if it is being addressed. The addressed slave then switches to mode 3 to receive the coming

DATA FRAMES, while the slaves that were not addressed stay in mode 2 and go on about their business". Note added by authors in parenthesis.

Or to quote p. 15 of Intel's AP Note 248 (1985): "The software used to communicate between processors is simplified by making use of Modes 2 and 3. In a basic protocol the 9th bit is called the address bit. If it is set high then the information in that byte is either the address of one of the processors on the link, or a command for all the processors. If the bit is 0, the byte contains (data) information for the processor or processors previously addressed. In standby mode all processors wait in Mode 2 for a byte with the address bit set. When they receive that byte the software determines if the next (data) message is for them. The processor that is to receive the message switches to Mode 3 and receives the information. Since this information is sent with the 9th bit set to 0 none of the processors set to Mode 2 will be interrupted. By using this scheme, the overall CPU time required for the serial port is minimized". Note added by authors in parenthesis.

Fig. 2-18, p. 16 of AP Note 248 gives a typical connection diagram for the multiprocessor communication mode showing an optional 80186/80286 main system interacting with a master 8096 which then communicates with 8096 and 8051 slaves assigned to various tasks. The master 8096 converts vectors to individual axis commands, controls the serial link, and monitors the entire system for faults. The slaves are assigned tasks such as axis control, process control, limit checking, and printer interface. The optional 80186/286 main system would e.g. calculate coordinate transforms, determine vector exponents and travel times, and provide user interface. See also our Expt. 8-6 for the program and interface for an 8096/8096 master - slave application we implement.

This concludes our introduction to, and discussion of, the important foundations of 8096 Serial I/O and its associated SFRs. The experiments that we now undertake in this chapter will illustrate most of the points we've covered so far with real applications.

EXPERIMENT 8-1

OUTPUT PORT EXPANSION USING THE 8096 SERIAL PORT IN MODE 0: TRANSMISSION

INTRODUCTION

We refer you to sections 7c and 7d of part (A) and to section 1 of part (B) which pertain specifically to MODE 0. A re-reading of sections 1 through 6 in part (A) will also prove useful.

In this experiment we shall be POLLING the TI flag in SP-STAT to indicate when transmission out of the 8096 serial port to the output port is complete.

Figure 8-1 on the next page shows our serial port interface to the serial-in to parallel-out shift register (CMOS CD4094). There the serial bits sent out from SBUF(TX) through RXD are shifted and collected as a parallel byte at the output port Q8, Q7 ... Q1 of the CD4094. The 74LS244 is used as a buffer (octal, non-inverting) to have Q8 ... Q1 at CD4094 drive LEDs which we have available at port 1 of the 8096.

It is very important to note that in order for the CD4094 to shift the transmitted bits received at SERIAL DATA IN via RXD into a parallel byte at Q8 ... Q1, several conditions are necessary: 1) the CD4094 must be in the "shift mode"; 2) SBUF (TX) must be loaded with the data to be transmitted in order to generate the shift clocks at TXD; 3) the latter must be connected to CLOCK of the CD4094 in order to shift in the data; 4) the data must be output (transmitted) at RXD (with REN = 0) with RXD connected to SERIAL DATA IN of the CD4094; 5) and finally, when transmission is complete, as indicated by TI in TEMP going high, we must latch the 4094's received parallel data into its output register to make it available at Q8 .... Q1 (see Fig. 8-1). Point (1) above is accomplished by connecting P2.7's output to STROBE on the CD4094 and DRIVING IT LOW JUST BEFORE LOADING SBUF(TX) WITH THE DATA TO BE TRANSMITTED. Point (5) above (latching) is accomplished by simply raising P2.7 high i.e. for the 4094 a leading edge transition at STROBE does the latching in. In other words, STROBE at a LOW LEVEL sets the SHIFT MODE for the 4094, while a subsequent POSITIVE LEADING EDGE on STROBE does the LATCHING. The shift mode condition will be achieved by a simple ANDB P2, #7FH instruction in our program, and the latching will occur after an ORB P2, #80H instruction is executed. The latter will occur only AFTER: a) a polling of SP-STAT reveals that trans-

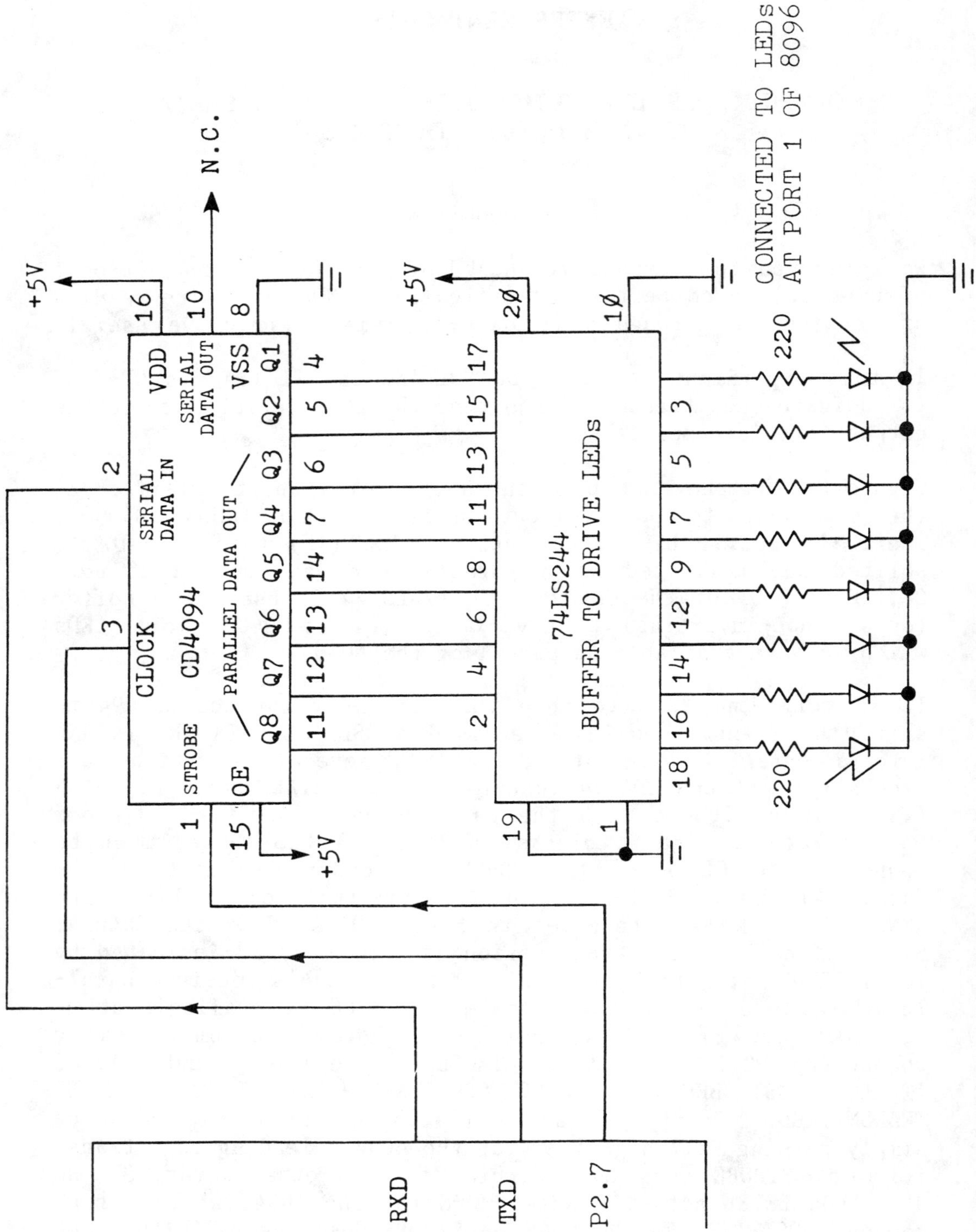

FIGURE 8-1: Output expansion port interface to the 8096's serial port used in Expt. 8-1. CD4094 is a serial-in to parallel-out shift register. The 74244 is an octal buffer (non-inverted).

mission out of SBUF(TX) via RXD is COMPLETE, as evidenced by the TI flag in SP-STAT going high, and b) we clear that flag in TEMP. The serially transmitted data is now available at the CD4094's parallel output register.

In the experiment, we'll set the switches at the 8096's port 0 for the byte to be transmitted to the output expansion port at the CD4094 shift register. As their bits are varied we should see their corresponding byte value reflected at the LEDs being driven by the 74LS244's output, the latter buffer being driven by the CD4094's output. LEDs at the 8096's port 1 are used.

The program at 4100 is shown below. It is then analyzed. Review part (A) of the introduction and also "MODE 0" in part (B).

```
        18 00        SP       EQU    18H
        11 00        SP_CON   EQU    11H
        11 00        SP_STAT  EQU    11H
        07 00        SBUF     EQU    07H
        0E 00        BAUD     EQU    0EH
        01 00        BAUD_LO  EQU    01H
        80 00        BAUD_HI  EQU    80H          ;Baud value of 8001H = 1.5Mbits.
        60 00        TEMP     EQU    60H
        80 00        XDATA_0  EQU    80H
        16 00        IOC1     EQU    16H
        0E 00        P0       EQU    0EH          ;Switches
        0F 00        P1       EQU    0FH
        10 00        P2       EQU    10H
                     :
                     ;
4100                          ORG    4100H
                     ;
4100    A1 C0 00 18           LD     SP,#0C0H     ;Initialize SP.
4104    FA                    DI                  ;Disable interrupts.
4105    91 20 16              ORB    IOC1,#20H    ;Select TxD output for P2.0.
4108    B1 00 60              LDB    TEMP,#00H    ;Initialize TEMP.
410B    B1 FF 0F              LDB    P1,#0FFH     ;Load 0FFH to force P1 to no drive
                                                  ;condition.
410F    B1 01 0E              LDB    BAUD,#BAUD_LO ;Load low byte of baud value.
4111    B1 80 0E              LDB    BAUD,#BAUD_HI ;Load high byte of buad value.
4114    B1 00 11              LDB    SP_CON,#00H  ;Initialize serial port; mode 0,
                                                  ;REN = 0, PEN = 0.
4117    B0 0E 80     LOOP1:   LDB    XDATA_0,P0   ;Load data to be output into XDATA_0
                                                  ;from switches at P0.
411A    EF 02 00              CALL   OXPORT       ;Call output expansion port routine.
411D    27 F8                 SJMP   LOOP1        ;Jump to LOOP1.
```

```
                        ;       OXPORT ROUTINE

411F   F2               OXPORT: PUSHF                       ;Save flags.
4120   71 7F 10                 ANDB    P2,#7FH             ;Clear port load signal for shifting.
4123   B0 80 07                 LDB     SBUF,XDATA_0        ;Load byte into SBUF to transmit.
4126   90 11 60         LOOP2:  ORB     TEMP,SP_STAT        ;Copy serial port status into TEMP.
4129   35 60 FA                 JBC     TEMP,5,LOOP2        ;If TI = 0, goto LOOP2
412C   71 DF 60                 ANDB    TEMP,#0DFH          ;Clear TI flag in TEMP.
412F   91 80 10                 ORB     P2,#80H             ;Raise port load signal to latch data
                                                            ;into external shift reaister.

4132   F3                       POPF                        ;Restore flags.
4133   F0                       RET                         ;Return to main program.
```

In the above program we first initialize the stack pointer to our usual location 00C0 and then disable the interrupt system to stress that we'll use a polling mode to determine when transmission out is complete i.e. when TI goes high. We then select the TXD function for P2.0 by setting bit 5 in IOC1 to 1. TEMP is then initialized to 0. It will later hold a copy of the flags from SP-STAT for testing. Port P1 is then loaded with FF. Writing all 1s out to P1 will cause the internal drives of this quasi-bidirectional port to be left off rather than turned on. Remember our LEDs are also connected to P1 of the 8096. This will allow the LEDs to be driven by the CD4094/74LS244 combination (the output port) without interference from P1. Next, we load the BAUD SFR at 0EH with two sequential bytes: #BAUD-LO = 01H and #BAUD-HI = 80H. This selects the XTAL1 pin (12MHz) and sets the baud rate to its maximum in MODE 0 : 1.5 Mbits (see the equation for MODE 0 giving baud rate vs. the lower 15 bit quantity (B) loaded into SFR 0E, on p. 2-19 Microcontroller Handbook (1985) or on p. 26 of chapter 1 in this book). We then initialize SP-CON to 00. This selects MODE 0 and sets REN to 0. Setting REN to 0 is necessary for TRANSMISSION (OUTPUT) in MODE 0 (REN = 1 enables reception (input) and that would conflict with transmission on the RXD line which serves in both capacities in MODE 0). Remember, the condition for transmission in MODE 0 is REN = 0 and a loading of SBUF(TX) with the byte to be transmitted (see section 7d in part (A) of the introduction).

At this point, we load the data to be output into XDATA-0 (register 80H in RAM file) from the switch values input to port P0. We then call the OXPORT routine at 411FH (Output to eXpansion PORT). The latter routine is the heart of the matter.

The first instruction in the OXPORT routine is PUSHF which saves the PSW on the stack and then sets the PSW to 0 (not necessary here, but recommended good practice). The next instruction, ANDB, lowers P2.7 to 0 to enable the "shift mode" at the CD4094. Next, we load SBUF(TX) with the switch byte now residing in XDATA-0. This is the byte to be transmitted to the output port at CD4094. The crucial steps are now at LOOP2. The first instruction in that loop copies the status bits RBE/RPE, RI, and TI into register TEMP's most significant three bits using the ORB instruction. (Remember, reading SP-STAT clears its RI and TI bits but TEMP now has a permanent copy of those bits). The JBC TEMP, 5, LOOP2 instruction keeps polling SP-STAT.5 (TI) until the TI bit read from SP-STAT goes high. If it's not high, transmission out of SBUF(TX) is not over and we are tied up in the JBC loop. When all 8 bits have been transmitted out of SBUF(TX), TI will go high and we fall through JBC to the instruction that clears bit 5 (TI) in TEMP so that we can make a fair test next time we enter OXPORT as to whether a NEW byte has been transmitted out of SBUF(TX). ANDB TEMP, #0DFH clears the TEMP TI flag (bit 5 in TEMP) for that purpose. We now create the low to high transition at P2.7 which will latch the data (parallel byte at the external CD4094 shift register) into its output register. Remember, P2.7 is connected to STROBE (pin 1) of CD4094. This is accomplished with the instruction ORB P2, #80H. The PSW is then popped back from the stack and a return is made to the main program at SJMP. From there we are taken back to LOOP1 where new (or the same) switch data is read and loaded into XDATA-0 for subsequent loading into SBUF(TX) the NEXT time OXPORT is called. This new (or old) byte will be output to the external shift register in the same ways as just explained. Thus the LEDs at the new I/O output expansion port (CD4094) will reflect whatever bytes the 8096 outputs to it, in this case from the input switches at its port P0.

PROCEDURE

1. Reset and enter BY 09 = 00.
2. Set the switches at P0 to XX.
3. Execute from 4100.
4. Observe the LEDs at OXPORT(shared with port 1) display XX.
5. On-the-fly change the switch data at P0 and observe the LEDs at OXPORT reflect the change.

FURTHER DISCUSSION

To expand MODE 0's I/O expansion facility to more than one output port, the following should be implemented: for outputting, additional serial-to-parallel shift registers are included by connecting the serial OUTPUT of the shift register (pin 10 of CD4094) to the serial INPUT (pin 2) of the NEXT shift register, etc. The external control lead P2.7 can then be connected to pin 1 of EACH additional external shift register. Additionally, the TXD pin, with its shift clock output, can be connected to pin 3 of EACH additional output device. The software must be modified to access these additional devices. This can be accomplished in a number of ways. One method is now described. We start by mapping each expansion port to a register in the 8096's RAM register file. This provides a convenient means for any routine to write to the out-port, as well as providing a copy (read) of the data written. If there are N ports, then N associated bytes must be mapped on the RAM table. In that case, the OXPORT routine must now be modified to take each byte from the RAM register array and output it to the appropriate output expansion port. Since the external shift registers are connected in series and we simply write out each byte one after the other, the correct data will be shifted through EACH cascaded stage. AFTER all the bytes are shifted out, the common load control line (here P2.7) is raised to load the newly shifted data into the parallel outputs of all the external shift registers.

The additions to the present OXPORT routine needed to implement the above expansion of output ports would consist of: a) initialization of a register NPORT with the number N (number of output ports desired) early in the main program, and b) after the ANDB TEMP, #0DFH in the present OXPORT routine the addition of the instructions DEC NPORT and JNE THERE, where THERE would be the label to be associated with a LDB SBUF, [BUF]+ instruction that now replaces the LDB SBUF, XDATA-0 instruction (so as to read the next entry from the RAM table). BUF would be the base address of the table.

EXPERIMENT 8-2

INPUT PORT EXPANSION USING THE 8096 SERIAL PORT IN MODE 0: RECEPTION.

INTRODUCTION

We again refer you to sections 7c and 7d of part (A) and to section 1 of part (B) which pertain to MODE 0. Also refer back to sections 1 through 6 in part (A) if you need clarification on related points in serial I/O.

In this experiment we shall be POLLING the RI flag in SP-STAT to indicate when reception from the input port into the 8096 serial port is complete.

Figure 8-2 on the next page shows the serial port interface to the parallel-in to serial-out shift register (74LS165) which we used for this experiment. The parallel bits input by the switches at I8 .... I1 of the 74165 are shifted out from pin 9 "SERIAL DATA OUT" on to the RXD line for inputting into SBUF (RX) of the 8096. The shifting is done by the 8 shift pulses from TXD that is connected to CLOCK (pin 2) of the 74165.

Before this can be done, however, the control lead at "SHIFT/ LOAD" of the 74165 (pin 1) must be brought HIGH/LOW to first LOAD the parallel input data at I8 .... I1 into the INTERNAL SHIFT REGISTER of the 74165. Then RAISING that lead high sets the 74165 in the "shift mode". This high/low/high signal to the "shift/load" control lead of the 74165 will be furnished programmably by having pin P2.7 of the 8096 raised high, then set low, and then raised high again. We have connected P2.7 to "SHIFT/LOAD". However, note that this time, unlike the outputting situation in Expt. 8-1, this control lead pulse must occur BEFORE shifting out to RXD starts and BEFORE we start testing SP-STAT's RI flag for completed reception in SBUF(RX), otherwise there'd be INVALID data in the 74165's internal shift register that would be shifted out to RXD for reception. This negative pulse on the control lead assures that valid data from the switches gets loaded into the 74165 for serial shifting into the 8096. In the outputting case of Expt. 8-1, only AFTER TI = 1 confirmed that the byte in SBUF(TX) was completely transmitted to the serial-in, parallel-out shift register (CD4094), did we provide a control lead low to high signal to allow the 8 parallel bits collected at the external shift register's buffer to be LATCHED into its parallel output port register. You will note that difference in the IXPORT subroutine in the

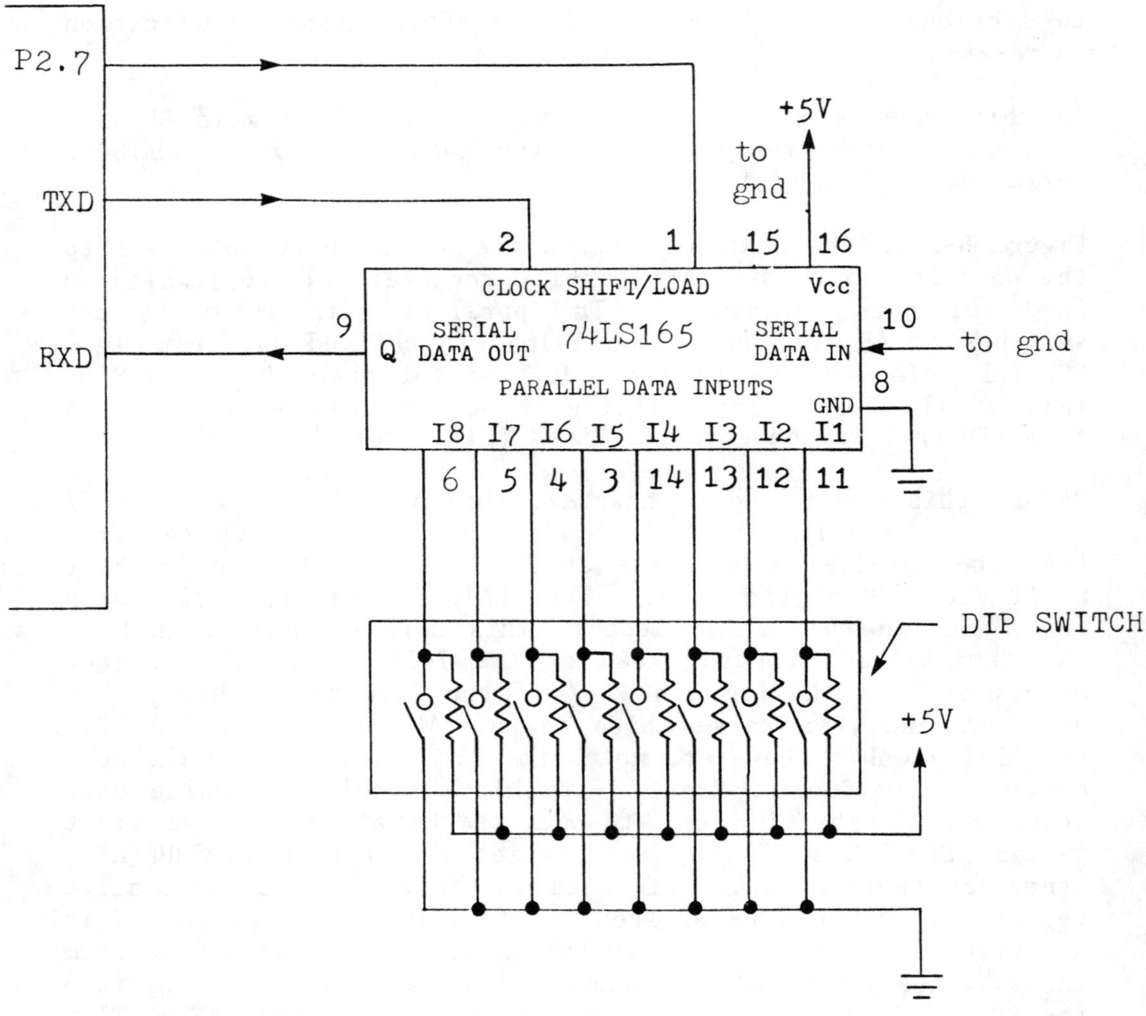

FIGURE 8-2: Input expansion port to the 8096's serial port used in Expt. 8-2. Pin 15 (Clock Inhibit) is grounded, together with pin 10 (Serial Data In). The 74165 is a parallel-in to serial-out shift register.

program that follows vs. the OXPORT subroutine in the program of Expt. 8-1. ORB P2, #80H followed by ANDB P2, #7FH and ORB P2, #80H instructions will provide the required pulse.

In this experiment we'll employ the switches that we've connected to the 74165 input port for the byte to be transmitted into the 8096 via RXD. We'll then output that input switch data for display at our LEDs at the 8096's port P1. As the program runs we'll vary the switch byte at the 74165 and see its new values mirrored at P1's LEDs.

The program at 4000 is presented below and then analyzed. Again, the analysis rests on the discussions in parts (A) and (B) (MODE 0) presented in the introduction.

```
        18 00           SP       EQU    18H
        11 00           SP_CON   EQU    11H
        11 00           SP_STAT  EQU    11H
        07 00           SBUF     EQU    07H
        0E 00           BAUD     EQU    0EH
        01 00           BAUD_LO  EQU    01H                 ;Baud rate value 8001H = 1.5Mbits
        80 00           BAUD_HI  EQU    80H
        60 00           TEMP     EQU    60H
        80 00           XDATA_I  EQU    80H
        16 00           IOC1     EQU    16H
        0F 00           P1       EQU    0FH                 ;LEDs
        10 00           P2       EQU    10H
                        :
                        ;
4000                             ORG    4000H
                        ;
4000    A1 C0 00 18              LD     SP,#0C0H            ;Initialize SP.
4004    FA                       DI                         ;Disable interrupts.
4005    B1 00 60                 LDB    TEMP,#00H           ;Initialize TEMP.
4008    91 20 16                 ORB    IOC1,#20H           ;Select TxD output for P2.0.
400B    B1 01 0E                 LDB    BAUD,#BAUD_LO       ;Load low byte into BAUD rate register.
400E    B1 80 0E                 LDB    BAUD,#BAUD_HI       ;Load high byte into BAUD register.
4011    B1 08 11                 LDB    SP_CON,#08H         ;Initialize serial port; mode 0,
                                                            ;REN = 1, PEN = 0.
4014    B1 00 0F                 LDB    P1,#00H             ;init LEDs.
4017    EF 05 00        LOOP1:   CALL   IXPORT              ;Call input expansion port routine.
401A    B0 80 0F                 LDB    P1,XDATA_I          ;Output input data from xport to
                                                            ;LEDs.
401D    27 F8                    SJMP   LOOP1               ;Loop back to repeat read of XPORT.
```

```
                        ;       IXPORT ROUTINE

401F   F2               IXPORT: PUSHF                       ;Save flags.
4020   B1 00 60                 LDB     TEMP,#00H           ;Initialize temporary serial
4023   91 80 10                 ORB     P2,#80H             ;Initialize load/shift control lead.
4026   71 7F 10                 ANDB    P2,#07FH            ;Clear port load signal to latch data.
4029   91 80 10                 ORB     P2,#80H             ;Bring control lead high for shift
                                                            ;mode of 74LS165.
402C   90 11 60         LOOP2:  ORB     TEMP,SP_STAT        ;Copy serial port status into TEMP.
                                                            ;This will start shifting data in.
402F   36 60 FA                 JBC     TEMP,6,LOOP2        ;If RI = 0, then goto LOOP2,
4032   B0 07 80                 LDB     XDATA_I,SBUF        ;Else read input byte into XDATA_I.
4035   71 BF 60                 ANDB    TEMP,#0BFH          ;Clear RI flag in TEMP.
4038   F3                       POPF                        ;Restore flags.
4039   F0                       RET                         ;Return to main program.
```

The program starts with initialization of the stack pointer and disabling of the interrupt system. We disable interrupts to stress we'll be using the polling mode to ascertain when reception of the input data into SBUF(RX) is complete i.e. a polling of the RI bit in SP-STAT will indicate reception into SBUF(RX) is complete when it goes high. IOC1.5 is then set to 1 to enable the TXD function at P2.0. TEMP is initialized to 0. It will later hold a copy of the flags from SP-STAT for testing. A 1.5 Mbit baud rate is selected by loading BAUD SFR at 0EH with, FIRST, 01 and THEN with 80. The latter's MSB selects XTAL1 pin for its 12MHz clock input to the 8096's baud rate generator. The former sets the Baud Rate in the MODE 0, XTAL1 equation on p. 26 (or p. 2-19 Microcontroller Handbook, 1985). Verify that 8001 does indeed yield 1.5 M bits/sec. SP-CON is next loaded with 08 to select MODE 0 and to enable reception (REN = 1). Section 7c of part (A) indicated that a rising edge on REN in MODE 0 will generate TXD shift clocks and start reception (in our case of the initial random values in the external shift register). After reception is complete RI in SP-STAT goes high. We then initialize the LEDs at P1 to 0 (they will reflect the inputted byte from the switches at the 74165 input port).

The crucial part of the program starts with the next instruction at LOOP1, the call to the IXPORT routine (Input from eXpansion PORT) at 401F. That routine starts with a push of the flags (PSW) (good subroutine practice.) We then immediately latch the switch data at the 74165 into the latter's internal shift register prior to transmitting it out to the RXD line for reception at the 8096. This is accomplished by raising P2.7 high (ORB instruction), then sending it low (ANDB), then raising it back high (ORB). The first two of these instructions latch the input data at the switches into the 74165 and the third puts the 74165 into the "shift mode". Shifting will start when the TXD clocks AGAIN arrive at the CLOCK pin of 74165 (see below). Remember, P2.7 is the drive for the control lead on the 74165 ("SHIFT/LOAD"). We are now ready to test whether reception of the data into SBUF(RX) is complete. We ORB SP-STAT into TEMP. Remember, TEMP was initialized to 0. That reads in bits 7, 6, 5 of SP-STAT into TEMP (6 being RI, 5 TI) and also CLEARS the RI and TI flags in SP-STAT. Now section 7c of part (A) in the introduction indicated that one method of STARTING reception in MODE 0 on the RXD line was to clear the RI flag with REN high. Clearly, that's accomplished with the ORB TEMP, SP-STAT read instruction, since RI in SP-STAT went high from the reception in SBUF(RX) of the PREVIOUS RANDOM DATA. The reading of SP-STAT makes RI go low and, with REN high, this starts 8 NEW TXD clocks to shift in the (by now) valid byte at the external shift register. Those 8 shift clocks connected to the CLOCK pin (2) of the 74165 start the serial outputting of the valid input data through the "SERIAL DATA OUT (Q)" pin on to the RXD line into SBUF(RX). (NOTE: LDB TEMP at 4020 not needed. See 4005).

Now that valid serial reception has started, the LOOP2 polling of bit 6 in TEMP (RI flag) will continue so long as RI is low. It will go high when reception of the full byte in SBUF (RX) is indicated. When it does, fall-through JBC to LDB XDATA-I, SBUF occurs. There, we load the received byte in SBUF (RX) into our "XDATA-I" register (80H) for subsequent outputting to the LEDs at P1. We then clear the RI flag in TEMP with the ANDB TEMP, #0BFH instruction, so that we don't get a false indication of reception of a new byte next time we enter IXPORT, when in fact one may not have occurred. The PSW is then restored. A return to the LDB P1, XDATA - I instruction in the main program outputs the inputted data to P1's LEDs. The last instruction in the main program jumps back to LOOP1 where IXPORT is again called. Any change in data at the switches will then be displayed at P1's LEDs. The cycle of events repeats.

PROCEDURE

1. Reset and enter BY 09 = 00.
2. Set the switches at IXPORT (74165) to XX.
3. Execute from 4000.
4. The LEDs at port 1 should display the value XX.
5. While the program is running change the input switches and observe the LEDs always reflect the change.

NOTE

This experiment could not be verified in hardware because of a bug in our 8096 (one of the earlier production units). [As this book goes to print a new version of the 8096 is being sampled which does not have the bug]. We are confident our interfacing and software are correct, as a similar experiment with the same interface and essentially the same software was performed successfully and presented in the 8051 book by the authors. Intel has also verified the logical flow of the experiment.

LATE NOTES AT PRESS TIME

1. In Mode 0 you can not set the mode and START RECEPTION with one instruction i.e. LDB SPCON, #08. You must set the mode first (LDB SPCON, #00), THEN set REN to 1 (LDB SPCON, #08). Expt. 8-2 should work on your 8096 part with this two-stage loading.

2. An alternative, and possibly clearer, way of stating the last paragraph on p. 416 and the material on p. 417 up to the PROCEDURE, would go as follows: The first time that the ORB TEMP, SPSTAT instruction is executed, RI is a 1 from the initial reception of random data. Reading RI clears RI but TEMP bit 6 will be a 1. Therefore, the JBC command will not cause a jump, and the random data that was received will be loaded into XDATA-I. The second time through the subroutine occurs when the first VALID data byte gets loaded into XDATA-I. Basically, calling IXPORT results in SBUF(RX) being put into XDATA-I and a new reception being started, which results in a new data byte being put into SBUF(RX) for a subsequent IXPORT call.

3. The 10th line down after the program on p. 416 should read: "The latter's MSB selects the XTAL1 pin as the clock source for the 8096's baud rate generator. The former, along with bits 0 to 6 of the latter, make up a 15-bit number that selects the baud rate in Mode 0."

EXPERIMENT 8-3

ASYNCHRONOUS MODE 1 COMMUNICATION WITH A CRT TERMINAL: RECEPTION AND TRANSMISSION INVOLVING SIMPLE ECHO.

INTRODUCTION AND FORMULATION

In this experiment we shall have a CRT terminal interfaced to the serial port of the 8096. Characters entered from the keyboard at the terminal will be input to SBUF(RX) of the 8096 via the RXD serial receive pin and then sent back from SBUF(TX) of the 8096 to the CRT terminal via the TXD serial transmit pin. Thus, characters entered at the terminal will be echoed back by the 8096 for display on the terminal.

In this experiment we POLL the RI and TI flags to determine when reception or re-transmission of a character are complete.

The experiment demonstrates the use of the 8096's serial port operating in MODE 1. This is also referred to as UART mode of operation i.e. asynchronous receive/transmit. The 10-bit frame provided by MODE 1 is a common format used for communicating with ASCII CRT terminals. In this mode full duplex operation is supported, meaning that transmitter (TXD) and receiver (RXD) can operate simultaneously.

In this application we require the connection of a standard ASCII CRT terminal with an RS232 interface. The physical connection is made using connector J6 of the SBE-96. Since the signal levels of the 8096 RXD and TXD pins are TTL, RS232 to TTL and TTL to RS232 level connectors are required. These connections and level conversions can be achieved by lifting two pins of the converters used to drive the SBE-96's J6 connector. The procedure is to lift pin 2 of IC U46 and connect a jumper from this pin to pin 20 of J3 (TXD). Then pin 8 of IC U47 should be lifted and a jumper connected from this pin to pin 19 of J3 (RXD). A standard RS232 cable is then connected between J6 and the CRT terminal.

The program at 4300 for this experiment is presented below. It is analyzed and discussed afterward.

```
                18 00         SP      EQU     18H
                11 00         SP_CON  EQU     11H
                11 00         SP_STAT EQU     11H
                07 00         SBUF    EQU     07H
                0E 00         BAUD    EQU     0EH
                80 00         BAUD_HI EQU     80H
                9B 00         BAUD_LO EQU     9BH                ;1200 BAUD
                60 00         TEMP    EQU     60H
                16 00         IOC1    EQU     16H
                70 00         CHAR_I  EQU     70H
                90 00         CHAR_O  EQU     90H
4300                                  ORG     4300H
                          ;
4300  A1 C0 00 18                     LD      SP,#0C0H           ;Initialize SP.
4304  FA                              DI                         ;Disable interrutps.
4305  91 20 16                        ORB     IOC1,#20H          ;Select TxD output for P2.0.
4308  B1 20 60                        LDB     TEMP,#20H          ;Initialize TEMP, set TI = 1.
430B  B1 9B 0E                        LDB     BAUD,#BAUD_LO      ;Load low byte of baud rate into BAUD.
430E  B1 80 0E                        LDB     BAUD,#BAUD_HI      ;Load high byte of baud into BAUD reg.
4311  B1 09 11                        LDB     SP_CON,#09H        ;Initialize serial port; mode 1,
                                                                 ;REN = 1, PEN = 0.
4314  EF 0B 00            LOOP:       CALL    GET_CHR            ;Call routine to read character from
                                                                 ;serial port. (character is returned
                                                                 ;in CHAR_I register).
4317  FD                              NOP                        ;NOPs will be modified at runtime.
4318  FD                              NOP                        ;
4319  FD                              NOP                        ;
431A  B0 70 90                        LDB     CHAR_O,CHAR_I      ;Copy character from input register
                                                                 ;(CHAR_I) to output register (CHAR_O).
431D  EF 0F 00                        CALL    PUT_CHR            ;Call routine to output character to
                                                                 ;serial port (character in CHAR_O reg).
4320  27 F2                           SJMP    LOOP               ;Go back to LOOP.
                          ;
                          ;
                          ;           INPUT CHARACTER ROUTINE: GET_CHR
                          ;
4322  90 11 60            GET_CHR:ORB         TEMP,SP_STAT       ;Copy serial port status into TEMP.
4325  36 60 FA                        JBC     TEMP,6,GET_CHR     ;If RI = 0, goto GET_CHR.
4328  71 BF 60                        ANDB    TEMP,#0BFH         ;ELse clear RI flag in TEMP.
432B  B0 07 70                        LDB     CHAR_I,SBUF        ;Read character from SBUF into CHAR_I.
432E  F0                              RET                        ;Return to main program.
                          ;           OUTPUT CHARACTER ROUTINE: PUT_CHR
                          ;
432F  90 11 60            PUT_CHR:ORB         TEMP,SP_STAT       ;Copy serial port status into TEMP.
4332  35 60 FA                        JBC     TEMP,5,PUT_CHR     ;If TI = 0, goto PUT_CHR.
4335  B0 90 07                        LDB     SBUF,CHAR_O        ;Else load character from CHAR_O
                                                                 ;into SBUF for transmission.
4338  71 DF 60                        ANDB    TEMP,#0DFH         ;Clear temp TI flag.
433B  F0                              RET                        ;Return to main program.
```

The main part of the program initializes the stack pointer, disables all interrupts and selects the TXD function for P2.0 by loading 20H into IOC1. Interrupts are disabled to stress that we'll use a POLLING mode re: SP-STAT's RI and TI flags to determine when reception or transmission is complete. TEMP is then initialized to 20H for reasons we'll see when we analyze the PUT-CHR routine later. TEMP will hold a copy of SP-STAT. The baud rate is then set to 1200 baud (our terminal) by loading 9BH and then 80 into the BAUD SFR at 0EH. (See table on p. 2-19 of Microcontroller Handbook (1985) or p. 26, chapter 1 of this book). The 80 sets MSB to 1 thereby selecting the 12MHz clock at XTAL1 to drive the 8096's baud rate generator. 09 is then loaded into SP-CON. This selects MODE 1 operation without the parity function and with the receiver enabled (REN = 1) (the transmitter is automatically enabled when a byte is written to SBUF(TX) for transmission, provided IOC1.5 = 1). It also sets TB8 to 0 (not applicable to MODE 1 anyway). Please note that, unlike SYNCHRONOUS MODE 0 where a rising edge on REN automatically starts reception with 8 shift clocks going out of TXD, REN = 1 in the ASYNCHRONOUS MODES 1, 2, 3 enables the receiver but does NOT start reception till the first high to low transition appears on the RXD line.

The next part of the main program, starting at LOOP is crucial. A call is made to the routine GET-CHR (Get Character) at 4322. That routine is the Input Character Routine. Let's analyze it. SP-STAT is copied into TEMP (remember, a reading of SP-STAT clears the RI and TI flags, hence the need for a copy in TEMP). The RI bit (6) in the copy is then tested with the JBC instruction. If RI is low (no character yet received from the terminal) the JBC keeps looping on GET-CHR. However, when RI goes high in SP-STAT it is an indication that a complete character has been received from the terminal via RXD and stored in SBUF (RX). In that case we fall through JBC and immediately clear bit 6 (the RI indicator) in TEMP with the ANDB TEMP, #0BFH. This is necessary so that next time around, when we look for another character transmitted from the terminal, we don't find RI = 1 in TEMP. That would falsely indicate that another character has been received when in fact it may not have been. We have to start afresh as far as the RI bit in TEMP is concerned. RI was reset AUTOMATICALLY in SP-STAT after being copied into TEMP, but the ORB TEMP, SP-STAT will not clear bit 6 in TEMP, as long as the latter is high. Bit 6 of TEMP is our indicator as far as the JBC test is concerned. Having cleared RI in TEMP, we now gather in the byte received from the terminal by reading SBUF(RX) into a register CHAR-I (70H) (Input Character). The GET-CHR routine then returns to the main program where it executes three NOPs (placed there for Expt. 8-4 where they'll be modified). The main routine then loads the character received in CHAR-I into a register CHAR-O (90H) (Output Character). It is from CHAR-O that we'll load SBUF(TX) with the received character for transmission back to the terminal via TXD. That will be done in the PUT-CHR routine.

After the LDB CHAR-O, CHAR-I instruction just discussed, a call to the routine PUT-CHR (Put Character) at 432F is made. That routine is the Output Character Routine. The first instruction in that routine reads SP-STAT into TEMP for a test, this time, of its bit 5 - a copy of the TI flag from SP-STAT. Now bit 5 in TEMP was set to 1 in the initialization of TEMP in the main program (LDB TEMP, #20H). Hence the FIRST test of TEMP.5 by the JBC instruction finds TI high and fall-through to LDB SBUF, CHAR-O occurs. That succeeds in taking the FIRST received character from CHAR-O and loading into SBUF(TX) for transmission. Had we not set TEMP.5 initially high we'd NEVER get out of the JBC loop to transmit that first character. ANDB TEMP, #0DFH then resets TEMP.5 to 0 so that the next time we enter PUT-CHR we indeed WAIT in the JBC loop till the PREVIOUS character that was just loaded into SBUF(TX) has been transmitted out. When that happens TEMP.5 will go high because TI in SP-STAT went high. We fall through JBC to load the NEXT received character into SBUF(TX) for transmission back to the terminal. We again clear TEMP.5 for the next time around. The cycle of events in the PUT-CHR routine keeps repeating after each received character is placed in CHAR-O for transmission. In each case the RET from PUT-CHR is to SJMP LOOP which again calls GET-CHR to poll for the arrival of another character from the terminal before transmitting same back to the terminal in the PUT-CHR routine. Note how PUT-CHR never loads SBUF(TX) with the NEXT received character till the PREVIOUS one has been transmitted as signaled by TI going high. Otherwise we'd corrupt the previous received character that was placed in SBUF(TX). You now see how important the initialization of TEMP to 20H was to allow transmission of the FIRST received byte. As you can see, the GET-CHR and PUT-CHR routines provide a simple software interface to the serial port's input and output operation in MODE 1.

PROCEDURE

1. Re-read the last part of the introduction on the necessary modifications and connections so that a link between the iSBE-96 and the CRT terminal is created.
2. Reset. Enter BY 09 = 0.
3. Execute from 4300. Enter lower case characters at the terminal and immediately see the characters displayed (echoed back) at the terminal's CRT. The key code of the character entered at the terminal was received in SBUF (RX) of the 8096 via RXD and transmitted back to the terminal from SBUF(TX) via TXD for display there. (The displayed characters are lower case).

EXPERIMENT 8-4

ASYNCHRONOUS MODE 1 COMMUNICATION WITH A CRT TERMINAL: RECEPTION AND TRANSMISSION INVOLVING CHARACTER PROCESSING.

This experiment is based on a modification of the program in Expt. 8-3. To allow for such modification we entered three NOPs at addresses 4317, 18, and 19 in that program. If we were to replace the NOPs by the three-byte instruction ANDB CHAR-I, #0DF (71, DF, 70) we'd be changing the ASCII code of the character entered at the terminal's keyboard and subsequently loaded into the CHAR-I register from SBUF(RX) when received by the latter. Bit 5 of the ASCII code stored in CHAR-I would be changed to 0 by that instruction. That would transform a lower case character to upper case e.g. ASCII code 61H for "a" would become 41H for "A". We have PROCESSED the received character by operating on CHAR-I. The LDB instruction at 431A in Expt. 8-3 loads the processed character into CHAR-O so that when the CALL PUT-CHR instruction is next executed, SBUF(TX) will be loaded with this processed character for transmission back to the terminal's CRT. Thus when lower case characters are entered at the terminal's keyboard we should immediately see the processed (upper case) characters echoed on the CRT.

PROCEDURE

1. Reset. Enter BY 09 = 0.
2. Enter BY 4317 = 71, 0DF, 70 carriage return. This inserts the instruction ANDB CHAR-I, #0DF in place of the three NOPs.
3. Execute from 4300. Enter lower case characters at the terminal's keyboard. Immediately see the echoed character in upper case on the CRT. Character processing has been demonstrated with the serial link of the 8096.

PROBLEM

In either Expt. 8-3 or Expt. 8-4, what happens if you: a) place NOPs at 4328, 29, 2A i.e. no clearing of the RI flag, or b) place NOPs at 4338, 39, 3A i.e. no clearing of TI flag, or c) place NOPs at both these locations i.e. no clearing of either flag? Run the experiment under each of these three modified conditions and see what happens (follow the Procedure section in the pertinent experiment). How do you explain the results you see on the CRT? This problem is crucial to gaining insight into the importance of the RI and TI flags and the need to clear them.

EXPERIMENT 8-5

ASYNCHRONOUS COMMUNCATION IN MODE 1. RECEPTION AND TRANSMISSION BASED ON SERIAL I/O INTERRUPTS.

INTRODUCTION

The last two experiments demonstrated the use of the 8096's serial port in MODE 1 operation. The implementation of those experiments were based on a continuous polling of the serial port for a completely received character before re-transmission of the character in processed or un-processed form was undertaken. More specifically, the polling of the port for reception of a character involved a continuous reading of bit 6 (RI flag) in SP-STAT till it indicated RI went high. At that point the flag (bit 6) in TEMP was cleared for next time around and the received byte in SBUF(RX) was read into a register (CHAR-I) for loading (processed or un-processed) into SBUF(TX) to start transmission of same. Polling of SPSTAT.5 was then undertaken to see when TRANSMISSION of the PREVIOUS data was complete before loading SBUF(TX) with NEXT received byte for transmission.

Very often this is not a desirable or realistic situation, either because there needs to be other processing while awaiting serial input, or the speed at which the data is arriving is extremely fast. Waiting around (polling) for the arrival of a character or data is extremely inefficient when there is no prior way of knowing when such information will arrive via the RXD line.

In that case we can use the 8096's ability to generate an interrupt upon receipt of a complete character in the SBUF(RX) receiver register. This has been covered in part (A) of the introduction to this chapter. The interrupt would cause flow from the main program (dedicated to "other tasks") to vector to the serial port's interrupt service routine (ISR) where the character can be read from SBUF(RX). There it can be processed immediately or it can be placed in a buffer or table for later processing by a different routine which might be called. The efficiency of such an approach is clear. We will not, however, in this experiment invoke the interrupt system during the re-transmission of the processed received information, although we certainly could. The reason we won't is simply that the transmission of data will occur at a time SPECIFIED BY THE USER and it will occur in RAPID ORDER as one character after the other is let out from the buffer or table where the received information was stored in processed or un-processed form. Hence the time devoted to that transmission is nowhere near the time we'd spend polling for received characters if we did not use the interrupt approach in the case of reception. In other words, polling TI as to when a character has been completely transmitted out of SBUF(TX) after we placed it there at a DEFINITE time is much, much faster than sitting around polling RI for the arrival of characters at unknown times.

Recall that as soon as the receiver register SBUF(RX) is filled with a received character, a serial I/O interrupt will be generated. The vector is to location 200CH in the interrupt vector table. The actual loading operation involves moving the complete 8-bit entity from the receiver buffer into the receiver register. Once this byte has been transferred, a new character can be shifted into the receiver buffer. This is known as DOUBLE BUFFERING since the CPU need not remove the previously received character from the receiver register before a new character can be shifted in. However, the program (CPU) is required to remove the character from the receiver register BEFORE the last bit has been shifted into the receiver buffer. If this is not done the receipt of the last bit will AUTOMATICALLY cause the 8 bits in the receiver buffer to be loaded into the receiver register. Hence, if the previous character has not been read from the receiver register, SBUF(RX), it will be over-written and its information lost. And this we always do as soon as SP-STAT indicates RI went high.

Remember, also, that the serial port interrupt is shared between the receiver and transmitter, so that either complete transmission out of SBUF(TX) or complete reception into SBUF(RX) will cause the same interrupt vector to 200C. Hence, the first operation in the serial port's ISR is to test the cause of the interrupt by copying SP-STAT into a register TEMP. There we can test the RI and/or the TI bits (6 and 5 in SP-STAT). The transmitter causes an interrupt (and sets the TI bit) as soon as the last bit of the character loaded into SBUF(TX) is shifted out of the TXD lead. If the program were to write to SBUF(TX) before all the bits of the previous character were shifted out, the transmission would be corrupted. And, of course, that's just the purpose of the serial I/O interrupt - to let us know when the previous character has been shifted out so that we can load SBUF(TX) with a new one for transmission.

One application that would require the use of the transmit interrupt is the case where a buffer (a number of characters stored in memory) is to be transmitted and the "other tasks" that the CPU must be concerned with IS VERY TIME CRITICAL

IN NATURE. In that case we would not want the CPU to hang around polling TI as to when another character has been transmitted. Better that it go on to "other tasks" and have the interrupt system let it know when the previous character has been totally transmitted. Thus, the ISR would take a character from the transmit buffer (table) in memory and load it into SBUF(TX) for transmission. The ISR would then decrement a count length register (holding the number of characters left in the buffer) and simply return to "other tasks" in the main program at the point where interrupted. "Other tasks" proceeds while the character is being transmitted. The next interrupt, caused by the complete transmission of the character PREVIOUSLY loaded into SBUF(TX) in the ISR, would cause the cycle to repeat i.e. another entry into the ISR would be made and this would continue until the count length register indicated that the last character from the table was transmitted. We repeat that IN GENERAL it is the reception problem that can waste most of the time if we were polling RI for "received byte complete" and that the transmission problem is not, generally, that wasteful of time if we were to poll TI. That's because there's no way of knowing when to expect the arrival of a receive character.

In this experiment we'll not use the transmit interrupt but instead POLL TI for knowledge as to when transmission of a character is complete. We will, however, use the receiver interrupt so that "other tasks" can be processed while awaiting the arrival of each new character. Of course, the ISR will have to TEST SP-STAT as to whether the interrupt was caused by reception or transmission of a character and take action accordingly. In the latter case, we'll ignore it and simply return out of the ISR to the main program. A SEPARATE routine (PUT-CHR), based on polling TI, will be dedicated to the transmission of characters. On the other hand, the ISR will NOT ignore the RECEPTION of characters. As soon as one is received the ensuing interrupt will vector to the ISR where the character is read and stored in a table in memory for later processing prior to transmission. Return to main program is then made.

As an aside we note a most useful facility with the 8096 that could be used in the application discussed above: its ability to generate an interrupt by simply having the program set a bit in the interrupt pending register (SFR 09). We explored this facility in Expts. 4-3 and 4-8 in chapter 4. In the above application, when ANOTHER buffer of characters became available in the table for transmission, the PROGRAM could invoke its transmission by SETTING the TI flag in TEMP (bit 6) (copy of SP-STAT) and then setting bit 6 in the interrupt pending register at 09. Bit 6 in both the pending and mask (08) registers is associated with serial port interrupts. This software artifice will cause a vectoring to the ISR where the moving of the new characters from the buffer into the transmit register could be initiated. The above setting of TI high in TEMP will allow us to fall through our polling instructions so that the FIRST character from the new table can be loaded into SBUF(TX) for transmission. We would then clear TI in TEMP and our subsequent pollings would then take care of the transmission of all the table's data. We do not do this in this experiment, but it is important to bring this concept and possibility to your attention.

FORMULATION

1. When the program is executed (from 4400), we'll enter 5 numbers from the CRT terminal's keyboard.
2. Nothing will be seen on the terminal's CRT till the 5th number is entered.
3. When the 5th number is entered, the CRT will display 5 numbers, each being one higher in value than the corresponding one entered.
4. A reading of the buffer table starting at 5000, where we store the received, processed data, should reveal the ASCII codes for the INCREMENTED numbers e.g. 31 for 1, 32 for 2, etc., (1, 2 being the incremented numbers).
5. Entering 5 letters from the alphabet should show 5 letters on the display, each one place higher in the alphabet than the letter keyed in. Again, their incremented ASCII codes would be revealed on examination of memory starting from 5000.
6. Thus we are simulating an application where a 5-character buffer is received from some external device (here a CRT terminal). The initial buffer will thus contain the ASCII representation of the numbers 0 to 9 i.e. 30 to 39. Once a complete buffer is received a subroutine INC-BUF is called which processes the data (in our case a simple increment of each ASCII code in the buffer). Our goal is to simulate character processing and not to suggest that our simple incrementation represents, in itself, a real application. Once the codes in the buffer have been incremented by the INC-BUF routine, the new buffer table is transmitted by the calling of the PUT-BUF subroutine. This will result in the incremented characters being seen on the CRT display. The setting up of the table, the processing of it, and the transmission of the processed data is done in the ISR by means of calls from the ISR to the GET-CHR, INC-BUF, and PUT-BUF routines, as we'll see. The ISR is entered every time a newly received character arrives in SBUF(RX) and ALSO upon transmission of another character

out of SBUF(TX). In the latter case we'll race around the ISR to its last instruction, RET. In either case the last RET instruction in the ISR takes us back to LOOP in the main program where "other tasks" can continue to be performed while waiting for the receipt of a new 5-character buffer. In our case, we process the data only AFTER all 5 characters are received.

The program for this experiment starts at 4400 and is given below. We analyze it after it is presented.

```
        18 00          SP       EQU     18H
        11 00          SP_CON   EQU     11H
        11 00          SP_STAT  EQU     11H
        07 00          SBUF     EQU     07H
        08 00          INT_MSK  EQU     08H
        0C 20          INVEC    EQU     200CH
        0E 00          BAUD     EQU     0EH
        80 00          BAUD_HI  EQU     80H
        9B 00          BAUD_LO  EQU     9BH               ;1200 BAUD
        50 00          REG      EQU     50H
        00 50          BUF      EQU     5000H
        60 00          TEMP     EQU     60H
        A0 00          TEMP1    EQU     0A0H
        16 00          IOC1     EQU     16H
        40 00          TCHAR    EQU     40H
        70 00          CHAR_I   EQU     70H
        90 00          CHAR_O   EQU     90H
                       ;
                       ;
4400                            ORG     4400H
                       ;
4400    A1 C0 00 18             LD      SP,#0C0H          ;Initialize SP.
4404    FA                      DI                        ;Disable interrupts.
4405    91 20 16                ORB     IOC1,#20H         ;Select TxD output for P2.0.
4408    B1 20 60                LDB     TEMP,#20H         ;Initialize TEMP, set TI = 1.
440B    B1 9B 0E                LDB     BAUD,#BAUD_LO     ;Load low byte of baud rate into BAUD.
440E    B1 80 0E                LDB     BAUD,#BAUD_HI     ;Load high byte of baud into BAUD reg.
4411    B1 09 11                LDB     SP_CON,#09H       ;Initialize serial port; mode 1,
                                                          ;REN = 1, PEN = 0.
4414    A1 00 00 50             LD      REG,#00H          ;Set character pointer to zero.


4418    A1 76 44 A0             LD      TEMP1,#SERINT     ;Load the address of the serial port
441C    C3 01 0C 20 A0          ST      TEMP1,INVEC[0]    ;interrupt service routine into INT
                                                          ;VECT table.
4421    91 40 08                ORB     INT_MSK,#40H      ;Set serial port interrupt mask bit
                                                          :to enable its interrupt.
```

```
4424  FB                          EI                          ;Enable interrupts.
4425  27 FE             LOOP:     SJMP    LOOP                ;Loop here ("other tasks").

                        ;
                        :
                        ;         INC_BUF - Processes buffer.
4427  A1 00 00 50       INC_BUF:LD        REG,#00H            ;Load character pointer with 0 to point
                                                              ;to first character.
442B  B3 51 00 50 40 LOOP2:  LDB          TCHAR,BUF[REG]      ;Get character from the buffer.
4430  17 40                     INCB      TCHAR               ;Increment character.
4432  C7 51 00 50 40            STB       TCHAR,BUF[REG]      ;Reload processed char. into buffer.
4437  07 50                     INC       REG                 ;Increment character pointer.
4439  89 05 00 50               CMP       REG,#5H             ;Compare REG TO 5.
443D  D7 EC                     JNE       LOOP2               ;If REG != 5, goto LOOP2.
443F  F0                        RET                           ;Else return.
                        :
                        :         PUT_BUF - Outputs buffer to serial port.
                        ;
4440  A1 00 00 50       PUT_BUF:LD        REG,#00H            ;Load character pointer with 0 to
                                                              ;point to first character in buffer.
4444  A1 0D 00 90               LD        CHAR_O,#0DH         ;Load carriage return for output.
4448  EF 1E 00                  CALL      PUT_CHR             ;Output carriage return.
444B  B3 51 00 50 90 LOOP3:  LDB          CHAR_O,BUF[REG]     ;Get character from the buffer.
4450  EF 16 00                  CALL      PUT_CHR             ;Output character to serial port.
4453  07 50                     INC       REG                 ;Increment character pointer.
4455  89 05 00 50               CMP       REG,#5H             ;Compare REG TO 5.
4459  D7 F0                     JNE       LOOP3               ;If REG != 5, goto LOOP3.
445B  F0                        RET                           ;Else return.
                        ;
                        ;
                        ;         INPUT CHARACTER ROUTINE: GET_CHR
                        ;
445C  90 11 60          GET_CHR:ORB       TEMP,SP_STAT        ;Copy serial port status into TEMP.
445F  36 60 FA                  JBC       TEMP,6,GET_CHR      ;If RI = 0, goto GET_CHR.
4462  71 BF 60                  ANDB      TEMP,#0BFH          ;ELse clear RI flag in TEMP.
4465  B0 07 70                  LDB       CHAR_I,SBUF         ;Read character from SBUF into CHAR_I.
4468  F0                        RET                           ;Return to main program.

                        ;
                        ;
                        ;         OUTPUT CHARACTER ROUTINE: PUT_CHR
                        ;
4469  90 11 60          PUT_CHR:ORB       TEMP,SP_STAT        ;Copy serial port status into TEMP.
446C  35 60 FA                  JBC       TEMP,5,PUT_CHR      ;If TI = 0, goto PUT_CHR.
446F  B0 90 07                  LDB       SBUF,CHAR_O         ;Else load character from CHAR_O
                                                              ;into SBUF for transmission.
4472  71 DF 60                  ANDB      TEMP,#0DFH          ;Clear TI flag in TEMP.
4475  F0                        RET                           ;Return to main program.
```

```
                        ;          SERIAL PORT INTERRUPT SERVICE ROUTINE
                        ;
4476   F2               SERINT: PUSHF                          ;Save flags.
4477   90 11 60                 ORB    TEMP,SP_STAT            ;Copy serial port status into TEMP.
447A   36 60 17                 JBC    TEMP,6,NO_CHAR          ;If RI = 0, goto NO_CHAR.
447D   2F DD                    CALL   GET_CHR                 ;Else call GET_CHAR to read character.
447F   C7 51 00 50 70           STB    CHAR_I,BUF[REG]         ;Store character in table and
4484   07 50                    INC    REG                     ;increment character pointer.
4486   89 05 00 50              CMP    REG,#5H                 ;Test if 5 characters received.
448A   D7 08                    JNE    NO_CHAR                 ;If REG != 5, goto NO_CHAR.
448C   2F 99                    CALL   INC_BUF                 ;Else call INC_BUF to process buffer.
448E   2F B0                    CALL   PUT_BUF                 ;Call PUT_BUF to output buffer.

4490   A1 00 00 50              LD     REG,#00H                ;Re-initialize character counter (REG
4494   F3               NO_CHAR:POPF                           ;Restore flags.
4495   F0                       RET                            ;Return to main program.
                        ;
4496                            END
```

The main program initializes SP and temporarily disables the global interrupt bit. IOC1.5 is then set to 1 to select the TXD function for P2.0. 20H is next loaded into TEMP for the following reasons: TEMP will hold a copy of SP-STAT and we want to start with the RI flag in TEMP set to 0 and the TI flag in TEMP set to 1 so that our GET-CHR routine, which polls TEMP.6 for reception, will wait till RI goes high before falling through to reset TEMP.6 to 0 and to read the newly received character. BY THE SAME TOKEN we want to start with TI = 1 so that when we call our PUT-CHR routine to START transmission of the FIRST character out of the buffer table, we'll IMMEDIATELY fall through the JBC test of TEMP.5 to load SBUF(TX) with the FIRST character to be transmitted before resetting TI in TEMP to 0. Otherwise we'd FOREVER be in the JBC loop and could never transmit characters. The NEXT time PUT-CHR is called we WILL be held up in the JBC loop till the PREVIOUS character has been transmitted out of SBUF(TX). Then TI will go high and fall through JBC. At that point we load SBUF(TX) with the NEXT character to be transmitted.

Next we set the baud rate to 1200 by loading SFR 0EH first with 9BH, then with 80H (see p. 26 chapter 1). 09 is then loaded into SP-CON to enable the receiver (REN = 1) and select MODE 1 (transmission will automatically occur when SBUF(TX) is loaded with data, provided IOC1.5 = 1). PEN = 0 disables the parity function for the 8th bit on transmission. We then set our offset (REG) to 0. It will be the pointer into the character table (buffer) we'll be constructing for the received characters. Since we'll be working in the serial I/O interrupt mode we specify the ISR address at # SERINT (in our case at 4476) by loading # SERINT into TEMP1 and then storing TEMP1 at INVEC (200C for serial I/O interrupts). Bit 6 in the interrupt mask register is then set to 1 to unmask the serial I/O interrupt source. EI then anables the global bit and the loop SJMP LOOP simulates "other processor tasks". Only after EI will a serial port interrupt be serviced.

Once a character is received into SBUF(RX), the Serial Port Interrupt Service Routine (SERINT) at 4476 is entered. There we save 8096 status flags with the PUSHF instruction. This not only saves flags but also the interrupt mask register (08). It also resets PSW to 0 so the interrupt mask and flags are both 0. No further interrupts will be honored during the ISR (if they occur they'll become pending) till after the next to last instruction in the ISR, POPF, is executed, restoring flags and the interrupt mask. We then copy SP-STAT into TEMP by means of the ORB instruction. The RI flag at TEMP.6 is then tested to determine if the interrupt is due to the receipt of a character or the transmission of a character. If the latter is the case, RI would be 0 and JBC TEMP.6, NO-CHAR short circuits the ISR by jumping to NO-CHAR where POPF and RET are executed. We're back at LOOP in the main program. If, however, the interrupt was caused by the reception of a character, then RI is high and the test of RI in TEMP.6 would show a 1, so fall-through the JBC test would occur where a call to GET-CHR at 445C is made. There we want to read the received character from SBUF (RX) into a register CHAR-I for storage in the buffer table. The first two instructions in the GET-CHR routine may seem superfluous since TEMP.6 is by now 1 and so we'll immediately fall through JBC TEMP.6, GET-CHR to clear TEMP.6 (ANDB) and read SBUF(RX)'s received character into CHAR-I. The reason we write the GET-CHR routine that way is to make it as general as possible should another application of this program REALLY require a polling of TEMP.6 in the GET-CHR routine to ascertain when a character was received. (Here we KNOW it was received by the test of TEMP.6 in the ISR). This is an example of the portability of the GET-CHR routine used through-out the experiments in this chapter.

A return from GET-CHR takes us back to the STB CHAR-I, BUF [REG] instruction in the ISR. BUF has been defined as 5000H and REG, previously initialized to 00, will be the offset into the table. Thus the first CHAR-I is stored at 5000 in the table. The offset, (REG), is then incremented and its value compared to 5 to see whether 5 characters have been received and stored in the table (CMP REG, #5H followed by JNE NO-CHAR). The latter test dictates that, if less than 5 characters have been received, we jump to NO-CHAR where flags and interrupt mask are restored and a return to "other tasks" at LOOP in the main program is executed. We are not yet ready to process the table because it is as yet incomplete. Eventually the reception of 5 characters (5 interrupts into the ISR) will force a fall through the JNE NO-CHAR instruction where a call to the INC-BUF routine at 4427 is made.

The INC-BUF routine starts with a re-initialization of the offset for the table pointer to 0. The first character, or number, in the table is fetched into the TCHAR register (40H) with the LDB TCHAR, BUF [REG] instruction. Its code value is then incremented. This incremented code value is then stored back into the table by means of the STB TCHAR, BUF [REG] instruction (we could have created two tables had we wished - an original reception table and a processed table). After the offset, (REG), is incremented to point to the next location in the table where the next processed character will be stored, a test is made as to whether 5 characters in the original buffer have been processed (incremented). If not, a jump back to LOOP2 retrieves the NEXT original character code, processes it, and stores it into the next location in the table. If, however, the test shows that 5 characters have been processed from the original table (REG = 5) we fall through JNE LOOP2 to a return to the CALL PUT-BUF instruction back in the ISR.

The first instruction in the PUT-BUF routine at 4440 sets the offset, (REG), back to 0 to point to the first processed character in the PROCESSED table. The code for the carriage return, ODH, is next loaded into CHAR-O and the PUT-CHR routine at 4469 is then called to output the carriage return to the CRT terminal. This will move the cursor of the CRT terminal to the beginning of the line position on the terminal's display. PLEASE NOTE THAT THE ORIGINAL INITIALIZATION OF TEMP TO 20H NOW SERVES US WELL, for when we enter PUT-CHR with ODH in CHAR-O, the FIRST test on TEMP.5 (the TI flag was copied from SP-STAT with the ORB instruction) will show TI high. This results in a fall-through the JBC TEMP, 5, PUT-CHAR instruction to the LDB SBUF, CHAR-O instruction which loads ODH into SBUF (TX) for transmission. Were TI not 1, we'd be locked in the JBC loop forever and could never get OD out for transmission. The ANDB TEMP, ODFH instruction then clears the TI flag at TEMP.5 so that the next time we enter PUT-CHR we DO wait in the JBC loop till the previous character, OD, is completely transmitted out of SBUF(TX). At that point TI goes high and we fall through JBC to load SBUF(TX) with the NEXT character to be transmitted. The return, after OD was loaded into SBUF (TX) and TEMP.5 was cleared, is back to the LDB CHAR-O, BUF

[REG] instruction in the PUT-BUF routine. This fetches the first character from the processed table into CHAR-0. Another call of PUT-CHR results in a wait at PUT-CHR's JBC till the PREVIOUS character was transmitted out to the CRT. At that point TI goes high again and the fall-through to LDB SBUF, CHAR-0 in PUT-CHR loads that next character into SBUF(TX) for transmission. TEMP.5 is again cleared and the return to the PUT-BUF routine results in an incrementation of the offset pointer REG. The CMP and JNE instructions then test as to whether 5 characters have been transmitted from the table. If not, JNE causes a jump back to LOOP3 where the next processed character in the table is fetched for transmission in the PUT-CHR routine. Finally, 5 processed characters will have been transmitted in the PUT-CHR routine and the return to the CMP, JNE instructions in the PUT-BUF routine falls through to a RET to the ISR at the LD REG, #00H instruction which re-initializes the table pointer offset to 0 (pointer to 5000). Processing and transmission of the table buffer to the CRT display are complete. POPF in the ISR restores flags and interrupt mask. Serial I/O interrupts can now again be serviced after the RET instruction at the end of the ISR takes us back to LOOP in the main program ("other tasks"). Entry of 5 new characters can now take place at any time. Interrupts to the ISR will result in the same cycle of events repeating as has just been described.

This program demonstrates the key elements, framework, (subroutines), and methods needed to implement interrupt-driven Serial I/O operation. The reader should be able to modify parts of the program to make it applicable to any situation pertinent to his/her needs.

PROCEDURE

1. Reset and enter BY 09 = 0.
2. Execute from 4400.
3. Enter 5 numbers.
4. After the 5th number is entered the display should show 5 numbers that are each 1 higher than the corresponding numbers entered.
5. Enter BY 5000 TO 5004 to examine the table buffer created in memory. You should see the ASCII codes of the processed (incremented) numbers.
6. Enter 5 new alphanumerics - this time e.g. the letters a, b, c, d, e. The display should show b, c, d, e, f. Examine locations 5000 to 5004 for the processed ASCII results.

PROBLEM

In this experiment we used serial I/O interrupts to vector us to the ISR to RECEIVE and process the data. TRANSMISSION of the data relied on a polling of TI - its interrupts ALSO took us to the ISR but we "short-circuited" them by a quick return to LOOP in the main program. Modify the ISR and any other parts of the program to demonstrate how TRANSMISSION can ALSO be accomplished based on the vectoring of "transmission out of SBUF(TX) complete" INTERRUPTS to the ISR. This adds even more to the efficiency of CPU processing, as NO POLLING of TI would be required. A quick TEST of SP-STAT in the ISR will indicate if the interrupt was due to reception complete or transmission complete.

EXPERIMENT 8-6

INTERPROCESSOR COMMUNICATIONS BETWEEN AN 8096 MASTER AND AN 8096 SLAVE. EMPLOYMENT OF MODES 2 AND 3.

INTRODUCTION

In this experiment two iSBE-96s are employed in a master-slave communications application. We have kept the application simple for purposes of bringing out the important features associated with 8096 to 8096 multiprocessor communications. However, the formulation and the master/slave programs are general enough to easily allow for simple modifications so as to incorporate more complexity into the application. In this regard, several problems are suggested at the end of the experiment. While we are illustrating the method with one 8096 slave, the method can easily be extended to more than one slave. Again, see suggested problems at the end of the experiment.

The experiment is based on serial port interrupts on both master and slave sides. On the slave side the serial receive interrupt's primary purpose is to "wake up" all slaves to check the forthcoming address to see if it's theirs.

A time delay routine based on T1OV interrupts is employed on both the master and slave sides. That routine is just about identical with the one employed in Expt. 5-11 where delay was generated in a similar manner. You are referred to it. We will not present a detailed analysis of that routine since it has been explained in Expt. 5-11. The delays are for providing time intervals between the sending of successive command buffers from master to slaves and for providing the on, off times of a machine controlled by the slave.

It should be stressed that a number of the key subroutines presented in the experiment are identical with those used in Expts. 8-3, 8-4, and 8-5. In particular, we suggest a review of the program in Expt. 8-5. Specifically, as with Expts. 8-3, 8-4, 8-5, this experiment uses the same PUT-CHR and GET-CHR routines. Further, the initializations of the serial port and Baud Rate are identical. Therefore, our analysis of those parts of the programs in this experiment will not be as detailed as in the previous experiments. This will again demonstrate a unity to this chapter, as more complex applications are built up from previously used subroutines.

We strongly urge you to carefully re-read the material on Mode 2, Mode 3, and Multiprocessor Communications on p. 2-18 of the Microcontroller Handbook (1985) (also reproduced on p. 25 of chapter 1). We also suggest that you re-read sections 3, 4, and 5 of part (B) of the introduction to this chapter. They, too, pertain to Modes 2 and 3 as well as to Multiprocessor Communications. We repeat the key points to keep in mind as they pertain to this experiment:

1. MODE 2: On transmit, a 9th data bit can be assigned the value 1 or 0 by setting or clearing TB8 in SP-CON. This bit is cleared on each transmission. ON RECEIVE, THE SERIAL PORT INTERRUPT IS NOT ACTIVATED UNLESS THE RECEIVED 9th DATA BIT IS 1.

2. MODE 3: A 9th data bit can be transmitted with the value of 1 or 0 as dictated by the value assigned to TB8 in SP-CON. ON RECEIVE, BIT 9 IS STORED IN SP-STAT.7 AND THE SERIAL PORT INTERRUPT IS ACTIVATED REGARDLESS OF ITS VALUE.

3. MULTIPROCESSOR COMMUNICATIONS: The slave is initially set to operate in Mode 2, the master in Mode 3. Remember, in Mode 2, if the received 9th data bit is not 1, the serial port interrupt is not activated. When the master wants to transmit a block of data to one of several slaves, it first sends out an address frame which identifies the target slave by its address. An address frame has its 9th bit = 1 (a data frame's is 0). Therefore, no slave in Mode 2 can be interrupted by a data frame. All slaves in Mode 2 will be interrupted by an address frame (9th bit = 1). In the slaves' serial interrupt ISRs, the interrupted slaves would compare the received byte (address) with their own addresses. If the comparison shows that a particular slave is being addressed, that slave switches to Mode 3 to receive the incoming DATA FRAMES (remember TB8, which was 1, clears on transmission so the next byte is a DATA frame). These data frames are in the nature of commands telling the slave to do what the master is dictating. The slaves not addressed remain in Mode 2 and continue their activity. The addressed slave, after receiving the commands from the master, will alter its activities accordingly, and then report back to the master as to the status of affairs at that slave.

   The nature of the data exchange is thus: a) transmission of a buffer of bytes from master to slave, the first byte being the address of a particular slave, the others being data (commands) for the addressed slave to act on; b) reception of the data commands by the addressed slave;

c) acting upon (processing) the received data commands by the slave; and d) reporting back by the slave to the master in the form of another buffer of data information transmitted from slave to master. This buffer will describe the status of activity at the slave after the commands from master were acted on. We often refer to the buffer of address/data being transmitted by the master to the slave as the TO BUFFER (or TBUF) and the buffer of data (status) transmitted back to master from slave as the FROM BUFFER (or FBUF).

FORMULATION

1. The Master 8096 sends out a 4-byte buffer every 6 sec. consisting of address/data to the slaves. The first byte is address and the other three are data (commands). We are not using those 3 data bytes for any useful purpose here, but they are there to be used in a more complex situation. They are included for that possibility. The master's port 1's LEDs toggle every 6 seconds to indicate a new TO BUFFER has been sent out. The master operates in serial Mode 3. The TO BUFFER is entered as a table at 5000 to 5003 at run-time.
2. The slave's duty will be to drive a machine (M0) on/off/on/off, etc. The machine is "stamping widgits". It is simulated by the LED at P1.6 of the slave's 8096 port 1. The slave operates in serial Mode 2.
3. A debounced switch is connected to the T2CLK source of timer T2 of the slave's 8096. Each press of this switch simulates another defective widgit caused by some malfunction in the stamping machine or incorrect placement of the widgit. The number of defectives at any time will be observed as the number represented by bits P1.4, P1.3, P1.2, P1.1, P1.0 at P1's LEDs on the slave's 8096.
4. Bit P1.5 at the slave's port 1 toggles every 6 seconds. Each TOGGLE indicates ANOTHER buffer of address/commands has been sent by the master and received by the slave.
5. If the number of actual defects reaches a programmed tolerable limit of defects, bit P1.7 of the slave's port 1 will go on to signify "FAULT". At that time the machine M0 at slave's P1.6 will go off and the "Buffer Received" LED at slave's P1.5 will stop toggling as no further address/data buffers from the master will be received (in our application). The situation at the slave's port 1 is thus: P1.7 = fault indicator; P1.6 = M0 (machine on/off); P1.5 = TO BUFFER received indicator; P1.4 to P1.0 = number of defects.
6. The addressed slave changes from mode 2 to mode 3 and stores the TO BUFFER address and DATA received from the

master in a table starting at 5000 in the slave's memory. It than monitors the defects in its event counter T2 and stores it in its memory location 5002. Thus the TO BUFFER has been processed to include the number of defects produced at the addressed slave. This processed buffer now becomes the FROM BUFFER and is sent back to the master. The master will now receive 4 bytes from the slave: the first is the address of the slave sending back information, the second is (in this application) a meaningless byte. The third is the number of defects at that slave, and the fourth byte is also (here) meaningless. We repeat, those "meaningless bytes" are there for you to modify the situation to include more process status information in the FROM BUFFER from the slave (or more commands from the master in the TO BUFFER). The FROM BUFFER from slave is stored by the master starting at 5010 in its memory.

7. Thus in this simple application, the TO BUFFER from master to slave has the address of the slave to be communicated with and 3 data (command) bytes for the slave (not utilized here). The FROM BUFFER back from addressed slave to master will also contain 4-bytes, the first its address and the third a report on the number of defects so far detected. The second and fourth bytes are, here, not used. We repeat that the 4-byte buffers allow for flexibility in the master-slave relationship so that a more complex and practical control and communication application between master and slave can be evolved from the programs given later. In a real application, the FBUF might be processed by the master's "other tasks" in its main program to prepare a NEW TBUF for the slave, based on the FBUF information it received from the slave (see problem 4, end of experiment), thus updating the control situation.

At this point it may be best to outline the experimental PROCEDURE before presenting and analyzing the program, as this will tie in with, and make clearer, the above formulation and give us a better feel for the program when we present and analyze it later. But first let us present the necessary connections on and between the two iSBE-96s used in the experiment.

CONNECTIONS

1. See Expt. 8-3, fourth paragraph in the introduction, for TXD, RXD connections on both master and slave.
2. The connection between the SBEs is made using a standard RS232C cable from J6 of one SBE to J6 of the other SBE. The cable should have its TXD and RXD (pins 2 and 3) reversed to allow the slave's TXD to be connected to the master's RXD and the slave's RXD to be connected to the

master's TXD. This cable is often referred to as a "Null Modem" type of cable.

3. Connect a debounced switch to T2CLK of the slave iSBE-96 to simulate production of defective widgits to be counted in T2.

PROCEDURE

1. AT THE SLAVE'S iSBE-96: enter BY 52 = 5. 5 is to represent the tolerable limit of defects produced by the slave's activity. 52 is the address of REG1 where this number is stored. Then enter BY 56 = 4. 4 in REG3 (56) will yield about 1/2 sec. on and 1/2 sec. off-times for the "widgit stamping" machine M0 (see Expt. 5-11). Then execute the slave's program (G FR 4500). Observe P1.6 (M0) at the slave go on/off at 1/2 sec. intervals.
2. AT THE MASTER'S iSBE-96: enter BY 56 = 30. 56 is the address of REG3 in master. 30 will yield about 6 sec. delay (see Expt. 5-11) between the sending of successive TO BUFFERs from master to slave (i.e. polling time interval). Then enter BY 5000 = 01, 0FF, 0FF, 0FF (TO BUFFER) and BY 5010 = 0FF, 0FF, 0FF, 0FF (a SIMULATED, INITIAL FROM BUFFER). The 01 at 5000 is the address of the slave selected for communication. All the other 0FF bytes are there to delineate initial values from changed values that will take place when the master's program executes and TO and FROM BUFFERs get transferred back and forth. Now execute the master's program from 4500.
3. We should observe at the slave's P1 LEDs the following: P1.7 = Fault LED = 0 (off); P1.6 = M0 machine LED flashing at 1/2 sec. intervals; P1.5 = TO BUFFER SENT LED = 0 (off); P1.4 - P1.0 = Defect Count LEDs = 00000 (no defects yet).
4. After about 6 seconds the TO BUFFER SENT LED at the slave (P1.5) will go on signifying that the first TO BUFFER was sent from the master to the slave(s) - slaves if more than one slave is being employed.
5. Enter the ESC key on the master.
6. Enter BY 5000 TO 5003 and BY 5010 to 5013 on the master to examine the TO BUFFER and the FROM BUFFER received back from slave.
7. We'll observe 5000: 01, 0FF, 0FF, 0FF and 5010: 01, 0FF, 00, 0FF. The TO BUFFER at 5000 is exactly the one entered at run time in the master in step 2 above. But now note that the "initialized" FROM BUFFER in the master at 5010 changes to indicate the addressed slave's address (01 at 5010) and the number of defects at that slave (00 so far at 5012). As mentioned earlier, in this application we are not using the other bytes in the TO BUFFER at 5001, 5002,

5003 or in the FROM BUFFER at 5011 and 5013, although they are included for a possible modification of the problem to include more actual commands from the master and more processed data back from the slave (see problems).

8. Depress the debounced switch at the slave's T2CLK to simulate one defective detected.
9. Observe the slave's LEDs at P1.4 - P1.0 display 00001, as expected.
10. Enter GO on the master to continue execution from where it left off when ESC was entered.
11. Observe the TO BUFFER SENT LED at P1.5 of slave go off before 6 seconds elapse. This signifies another TO BUFFER was sent.
12. Enter BY 5000 TO 5003 and BY 5010 TO 5013 both on the master.
13. Observe 5000: 01, OFF, OFF, OFF (TO BUFFER), and 5010: 01, OFF, 01, OFF (FROM BUFFER). One defect has been recorded at 5012 in the FROM BUFFER received back from the slave and the master now knows this.
14. At the master, enter BY 5000 = 02 (address of "another slave).
15. After about 6 seconds the TO BUFFER SENT LED at slave's P1.5 does NOT toggle this time. The 02 address did not match the slave's address 01, so that the slave 01 ignores the TO BUFFER address/data sent from the master and, as the program will show, does not send back any FROM BUFFER to the master. No further toggling at slave's P1.5 LED occurs.
16. Again depress the defect switch at slave's T2CLK. P1.4 - P1.0 at the slave will now show 00010 = 2 defects so far.
17. Enter BY 5010 TO 5013 at the master. Observe 5010: 01, OFF, 01, OFF (FROM BUFFER). What we're seeing here is the LAST FROM BUFFER returned from slave 01 when it was LAST addressed. Thus 5010 still shows address 01 and 5012 still shows the last defect count (01) when it was last addressed. The master has not been updated as far as the real defect count (2) since slave 01 was not now addressed.
18. Enter BY 5000 = 01 again at the master. We are going to address slave 01 again.
19. After about 6 sec. we'll see the TO BUFFER SENT LED toggle again (slave's P1.5). TO BUFFER from master is again being received by addressed slave 01.
20. Enter BY 5010 to 5013 at the master. Now we should observe 5010: 01, OFF, 02, OFF (FROM BUFFER). We do indeed now see the updated defect count (2) at 5012. The 01 slave was again addressed and reported back its latest defect count.
21. Depress the defect switches at T2CLK of the slave 3 more times for a total of 5 defects so far. The slave's P1.4 -

P1.0 bits will show 00101 = 5 defects. We have reached the tolerable limit 5 originally entered in the slave's REG1 (52) (see step 1 in Procedure). The slave will enter a halt state (see program later) and will turn off the machine M0 at P1.6 of the slave as well as turn on the FAULT LED at P1.7 of the slave to signify the process has been halted till tool-up or repairs are made. The TO BUFFER SENT LED at P1.5 of the slave stops toggling as no more TO BUFFERs from master are received. If we enter BY 5010 TO 5013 at the master, we'll now see 5010: 01, 0FF, 05, 0FF indicating the master has received the latest (limit) updated defective count from slave 01.

THE PROGRAMS

We'll first present the master's program and analyze it. After that we'll present the slave's program with its analysis.

The master's program at 4500 is shown below.

```
18 00        SP      EQU    18H
11 00        SP_CON  EQU    11H
11 00        SP_STAT EQU    11H
07 00        SBUF    EQU    07H
0E 00        BAUD    EQU    0EH
80 00        BAUD_HI EQU    80H
9B 00        BAUD_LO EQU    9BH            ;1200 BAUD
09 00        PINT    EQU    09H
08 00        MINT    EQU    08H
00 20        INVEC   EQU    2000H
0C 20        INVEC1  EQU    200CH
50 00        REG     EQU    50H
54 00        REG2    EQU    54H
56 00        REG3    EQU    56H
00 50        TBUF    EQU    5000H
60 00        TEMP    EQU    60H
A0 00        TEMP1   EQU    0A0H
16 00        IOC1    EQU    16H
70 00        CHAR_I  EQU    70H
90 00        CHAR_O  EQU    90H
0F 00        P1      EQU    0FH
```

```
4500                                  ORG    4500H
                            ;
4500   A1 C0 00 18                    LD     SP,#0C0H          ;Initialize SP.
4504   FA                             DI                       ;Disable interrutps.
4505   11 09                          CLRB   PINT              ;Clear any pending interrupts.
4507   B1 41 08                       LDB    MINT,#41H         ;Set mask bit 0 to enable timer
                                                               ;overflow interrupt source and
                                                               ;bit 6 to enable serial port interrupt.
450A   B1 24 16                       LDB    IOC1,#24H         ;Set bit 2 in IOC1 to enable Timer 1
                                                               ;overflow interrupt and bit 5 to
                                                               ;select TxD as function of P2.0.
450D   A1 86 45 A0                    LD     TEMP1,#T1OV       ;Load address of Timer 1 overflow
4511   C3 01 00 20 A0                 ST     TEMP1,INVEC[0]    ;interrupt service routine into INT
                                                               ;VECT table.
4516   A1 6A 45 A0                    LD     TEMP1,#SERINT     ;Load address of serial port
451A   C3 01 0C 20 A0                 ST     TEMP1,INVEC1[0]   ;interrupt service routine into INT
                                                               ;VECT table.
451F   B1 20 60                       LDB    TEMP,#20H         ;Initialize TEMP.
4522   B1 9B 0E                       LDB    BAUD,#BAUD_LO     ;Load low byte of baud rate into BAUD.
4525   B1 80 0E                       LDB    BAUD,#BAUD_HI     ;Load high byte of baud into BAUD reg.
4528   B1 0B 11                       LDB    SP_CON,#0BH       ;Initialize serial port: mode 3,
                                                               ;REN = 1, PEN = 0.
452B   A1 00 00 50                    LD     REG,#00H          ;Set character pointer to zero.
452F   B0 56 54                       LDB    REG2,REG3         ;Load time value into REG2.
4532   FB                             EI                       ;Enable interrupts.
4533   B1 00 0F                       LDB    P1,#00H           ;Turn LEDs off.
4536   27 FE                LOOP:     SJMP   LOOP              ;Loop here ("other tasks").

                            ;
                            ;         PUT_BUF - OUTPUTS TBUF TO SLAVES.
                            ;
4538   A1 00 00 50          PUT_BUF:LD       REG,#00H          ;Load character pointer with 0 to
                                                               ;point to slave address in buffer.
453C   B1 1B 11                       LDB    SP_CON,#1BH       ;Set TB8 (for address) transmission.
453F   B3 51 00 50 90 LOOP3:          LDB    CHAR_O,TBUF[REG];Get character from the buffer.
4544   EF 1A 00                       CALL   PUT_CHR           ;Output character to serial port.
4547   07 50                          INC    REG               ;Increment character pointer.
4549   89 04 00 50                    CMP    REG,#4H           ;Compare REG to 4.
454D   D7 F0                          JNE    LOOP3             ;If REG != 4, goto LOOP3.
454F   A1 00 00 50                    LD     REG,#00H          ;Reload character pointer.
4553   F0                             RET                      ;Else return to T1OV ISR.
                            ;
                            ;
                            ;         INPUT CHARACTER ROUTINE: GET_CHR
                            ;
4554   90 11 60             GET_CHR:ORB      TEMP,SP_STAT      ;Copy serial port status into TEMP.
4557   36 60 FA                       JBC    TEMP,6,GET_CHR    ;If RI = 0, goto GET_CHR.
455A   71 BF 60                       ANDB   TEMP,#0BFH        ;Else clear RI flag in TEMP.
455D   B0 07 70                       LDB    CHAR_I,SBUF       ;Read character from SBUF into CHAR_I.
4560   F0                             RET                      ;Return.
```

```
                        ;        OUTPUT CHARACTER ROUTINE: PUT_CHR
                        ;
4561  90 11 60          PUT_CHR:ORB    TEMP,SP_STAT    ;Copy serial port status into TEMP.
4564  35 60 FA                  JBC    TEMP,5,PUT_CHR  ;If TI = 0, goto PUT_CHR.
4567  B0 90 07                  LDB    SBUF,CHAR_O     ;Else load character from CHAR_O
                                                       ;into SBUF for transmission.
456A  71 DF 60                  ANDB   TEMP,#0DFH      ;Clear temp TI flag.
456D  F0                        RET                    ;Return.
                        ;
                        ;
                        ;
                        ;        SERIAL PORT INTERRUPT SERVICE ROUTINE:
                        ;              INPUTS FBUF FROM SLAVE.
                        ;
456E  F2                SERINT: PUSHF                  ;Save flags.
456F  90 11 60                  ORB    TEMP,SP_STAT    ;Copy serial port status into TEMP.
4572  36 60 13                  JBC    TEMP,6,NO_CHAR  ;If RI = 0, goto NO_CHAR.
4575  2F DD                     CALL   GET_CHR         ;Else call GET_CHAR to read character.
4577  C7 51 00 50 70            STB    CHAR_I,TBUF[REG] ;Store character in table and
457C  07 50                     INC    REG             ;increment character pointer.
457E  89 04 00 50               CMP    REG,#4H         ;Test if 4 characters received.
4582  D7 04                     JNE    NO_CHAR         ;If REG != 4, goto NO CHAR.
4584  A1 00 00 50               LD     REG,#00H        ;Initialize REG for the next FROM
                                                       ;BUFFFR.
4588  F3                NO_CHAR:POPF                   ;Restore flags.
4589  F0                        RET                    ;Return to main program.
                        ;
                        ;        TIMER 1 OVERFLOW INTERRUPT SERVICE ROUTINE
                        ;
458A  F2                T1OV:   PUSHF                  ;Save flags.
458B  E0 54 08                  DJNZ   REG2,RETURN     ;Decrement REG2, if != 0 time not
                                                       ;achieved, goto RETURN.
458E  B0 56 54                  LDB    REG2,REG3       ;Reload REG2 for another time delay.
4591  95 FF 0F                  XORB   P1,#0FFH        ;Toggle LED at P1.
4594  2F A2                     CALL   PUT_BUF         ;Send buffer.
4596  F3                RETURN: POPF                   ;Restore flags.
4597  F0                        RET                    ;Return to main program.
```

The main program first initializes the stack pointer and disables the interrupt system. Any pending interrupts are then cleared and 41 is loaded into MINT to enable the serial port interrupt and Timer 1 Overflow interrupts (we are using the latter to generate time delays as in Expt. 5-11). 24 is next loaded into IOC1. This sets IOC1.5 to 1, selecting P2.0 in its TXD operation, and it sets IOC1.2 to 1 to select the Timer 1 Overflow source for TOV interrupts. The address of the T1OV ISR is then entered into TEMP1 and stored in the vector interrupt table at 2000 (entry for TOV interrupts). Likewise the address of the SERINT ISR (serial interrupts) is entered into TEMP1 and stored in the vector interrupt table at 200C (entry for serial port interrupts). TEMP is then initialized to 20 for the same reason as in Expts. 8-3, 8-4, and 8-5 (to set TI flag in TEMP INITIALLY high). The Baud Rate is then set to 1200 Baud and SP-CON is loaded with 0BH. This selects Mode 3 for the master's serial operation and sets REN to 1 to enable receiver operation. PEN is set to 0 so that the 9th bit in the Mode 3 data will NOT be assigned a parity function. SO FAR we have not set TB8 to 1 in SP-CON. This comes LATER when we'll have the master interrupt all slaves in Mode 2 (that requires the 9th transmission bit from the master to be 1). REG (50) is then loaded with 00. REG will be an offset pointing to the TO BUFFER table of 4 bytes (entered at run-time) that will eventually be transmitted to each (in our case, one) slave. That table will have a base address of 5000 (TBUF EQU 5000). We next load REG2 (54) with the time value from REG3 (56) (entered at run-time). This will determine the time between successive outputting of the master buffer's 4 bytes to the slave (i.e. a polling of slaves every so often). The interrupt system is then enabled, P1's LEDs on the master are cleared, and "other tasks" are entered at SJMP LOOP.

And that's the way matters stand. Except that every 131 msec. T1 overflow interrupts dart in and out of the Timer 1 Overflow ISR at 458A. Each time it does, REG2 is decremented, and if not 0, a return to "other tasks" in the main program is made. Eventually REG2 will be 0. In that case REG2 is reloaded with REG3's contents, P1's LEDs on master are made to toggle, and a call to PUT-BUF is made, BEFORE the return, to send out the TO BUFFER to all slaves. The toggling of the LEDs at P1 on the master iSBE-96 is a convenient way of indicating to us that another TO BUFFER (entered at 5000 - 5003 at run-time) is about to be sent to the slave at each toggle. The entry into the T1OV ISR will occur the number of times given by the contents of REG3 (entered at run-time at register address 56). The time between toggles will thus be 0.131 sec. (time between T1OV interrupts) multiplied by (REG3). If the latter is 30H, delays between toggles (and transmission of the TO BUFFERs) will be about 6 sec.

We have just called PUT-BUF at 4538. The latter sends TO BUFFER from master's locations 5000 - 5003 to all slaves. Let's analyze PUT-BUF. First, the offset of the pointer into the TO BUFFER table is initialized to 0. And now, crucially, SP-CON is loaded with 1BH. This changes nothing in SP-CON EXCEPT that TB8 is now set to 1. Thus the 9th bit of the first 9-bit transmission from the master is programmed to be a 1. The consequences of this will be two-fold: the first character in TBUF about to be outputted from the serial port to the slaves will be an ADDRESS AND, as such, will INTERRUPT all slaves operating in Mode 2, precisely because the 9th bit received by each slave will be a 1. Don't forget, TB8 is CLEARED after transmission of that first byte so only the FIRST transmitted byte will be an ADDRESS and INTERRUPT all slaves in Mode 2 on reception.

Succeeding bytes in TBUF, now having bit 9 = 0, will NOT be able to activate serial interrupts in those slaves in Mode 2 on reception, but will again interrupt the ADDRESSED slave on reception IF THE LATTER HAS CHANGED TO MODE 3, which we'll arrange for on the slave side. Thus, the addressed slave, if now in Mode 3, will be able to receive those next TBUF data or command bytes with bit 9 = 0 because the RI and TI flags ARE affected by serial interrupts which are activated on reception in Mode 3, regardless of the value of the 9th bit. RI and TI would NOT be affected if bit 9 were 0 and the addressed slave were still in Mode 2. Remember, our GET-CHR and PUT-CHR routines depend on a polling of the RI and TI flags to receive or transmit characters. More on all this when we analyze the slave's program later.

The next instruction at 453F in PUT-BUF fetches the first character (slave's address) from 5000 (i.e. from TUBF [REG]) and loads it into register CHAR-0 (90H). A call is then made to PUT-CHR at 4561 where bit 5 in SP-STAT (TI) is polled. Since it is initially 1 in TEMP (see initialization at 451F in the main program), we fall through the JBC at 4564 and load CHAR-0 (slave's address at this point) into SBUF(TX) for transmission. The TI flag is then CLEARED for next time around (when the next character in the TO BUFFER is to be transmitted) and a return to 4547 in the PUT-BUF routine is executed. There, the offset, REG, is incremented to point to the next character in the 4-byte TBUF. A compare of REG is then made with 4. If they're not equal, JNE LOOP3 carries us back to 453F where the NEXT character in the 4-byte TBUF table is loaded into CHAR-0 for transmission. The call to PUT-CHR then polls TI at TEMP.5 till it goes high, indicating the PREVIOUS character from the table was transmitted out of SBUF(TX). The new character (NEXT table entry) is then loaded from CHAR-0 to SBUF(TX) for transmission. And so on. Eventually, the CMP REG, #4H at 4549 in PUT-BUF shows that 4 characters from TO BUFFER have been transmitted from master to slave. We fall through JNE LOOP3 at 454D to a RE-INITIALIZATION OF THE OFFSET POINTER, REG, to 00. We then return to 4596 of the T1OV ISR where the call to PUT-BUF was made. There, POPF and RET to the main program at SJMP LOOP are executed. The TO BUFFER has been transmitted from master to slave. "Other tasks" are continued by the master.

What next? After the addressed slave has received, and processed TBUF it will send back the information desired in the form of FBUF (FROM BUFFER) to the master. The master will receive it and store it at an FBUF block starting at 5010. Each such byte transmitted from slave to master will cause a serial I/O interrupt at the master when another complete byte from FBUF has been received in master's SBUF(RX). This causes a vector from SJMP LOOP to the serial port interrupt ISR at 456E (with RI high). We (master) are about to store the received information (the slave's transmitted FROM BUFFER characters).

After the PUSHF instruction at 456E in the SERINT ISR, RI at TEMP.6 is polled. IF it is 0, the interrupt must have been due to another completed TRANSMISSION of a byte out of TO BUFFER to slave. We ignore it by the JBC (at 4572) to NO-CHAR, where a POPF and RET to main program ("other tasks") are executed. (If RI was 0, TI must have been high, otherwise we'd not be in the SERINT ISR). When RI goes high (actually it is already high in this case), indicating a byte from the slave's FROM BUFFER was received by the master, we fall through the JBC at 4572 and call the GET-CHR routine at 4554 which is dedicated to reading the character received from the slave into CHAR-I (70H). To this end TEMP.6 (copy of RI flag) is polled till it goes high (in this case it is already high), signifying a complete character was received in SBUF(RX) from slave's FROM BUFFER. Fall-through JBC at 4557 then occurs where the RI flag in TEMP is cleared. The received character in SBUF(RX) is then loaded into CHAR-I and a return to 4577 in the SERINT ISR is made. There the received byte in CHAR-I is stored at 5010 on the master side i.e. FBUF [REG] = 5010 + 00 since REG was last re-initialized to 00 (see 454F in PUT-BUF). A FROM BUFFER table on the master side starting at 5010 is in the process of being formed. REG is then incremented to point to the next location in the FBUF receive table being formed. If REG is not equal to 4 (4 entries from FBUF not yet received), JNE NO-CHAR forces a return to the main program ("other tasks") after POPF. The next received character from slave's FROM BUFFER causes a repeat of the scenario i.e. a vector from SJMP LOOP ("other tasks") to SERINT ISR at 456E with RI = 1. Eventually, 4 FBUF characters from the slave will have been received and stored on the master side at 5010-5013. The CMP REG, #4H, JNE NO-CHAR instructions at 457E, 4582 then cause a fall-through to 4584 where the offset pointer, REG, is re-initialized to 0, to get ready for the NEXT FROM BUFFER that will be transmitted from slave to master. POPF and RET are then executed and we are back to SJMP LOOP ("other tasks") in the main program.

The master has now accomplished one TO BUFFER transmission to slave and received one FROM BUFFER from slave. After a delay

(6 sec. in our PROCEDURE description), another TO BUFFER will be transmitted to the slave and a receipt of a new FROM BUFFER from the slave will occur. The whole cycle of events will repeat every 6 sec. (or whatever, depending on the byte entered into REG3 (56H) at run-time). All the above descriptions and analysis apply each time a TBUF is transmitted and a FBUF is received. Thus a continual changing master-slave communications has been set up.

We are now ready for an analysis of the iSBE-96 slave's program. But before presenting the slave's program and its analysis, a few remarks are in order here. First, if we were dealing with N slaves, the PUT-BUF routine would be called N times with the first byte of each TO BUFFER changing from 1 to 2, ... to N (address of each slave). To optimize this operation, one additional facility should be implemented, namely the ability to specify other buffers' base addresses so that the data contained in the buffer to be sent can be different for each slave. This would then allow the "other tasks" in the main program to formulate the buffer data (TO BUFFERs) to be preloaded into each of the N buffers with specific data or commands for each slave as contrasted to entering tables at run-time. In conjunction with the above, the receive portion of the program would have to be modified to place each of the incoming FROM BUFFERs from the N slaves into an array of N buffer addresses. Again, "other tasks" would process each specific slave's returned data. We would not simply use one buffer location and have one slave's response overwriting another slave's response in the same buffer area. Since we are employing one 8096 slave, these remarks don't apply here (see problems at end of the experiment).

We are now ready to analyze the slave's program. It is presented below starting at 4500 on the slave side. The analysis is given immediately afterward.

```
18 00     SP      EQU   18H
11 00     SP_CON  EQU   11H
11 00     SP_STAT EQU   11H
07 00     SBUF    EQU   07H
0E 00     BAUD    EQU   0EH
80 00     BAUD_HI EQU   80H
9B 00     BAUD_LO EQU   9BH          ;1200 BAUD
09 00     PINT    EQU   09H
08 00     MINT    EQU   08H
00 20     INVEC   EQU   2000H
0C 20     INVEC1  EQU   200CH
40 00     DEF_LO  EQU   40H
40 00     DEFECTS EQU   40H
```

```
        50 00       REG       EQU     50H
        52 00       REG1      EQU     52H
        54 00       REG2      EQU     54H
        56 00       REG3      EQU     56H
        00 50       TBUF      EQU     5000H
        02 50       DEF_BYTE          EQU     5002H
        60 00       TEMP      EQU     60H
        A0 00       TEMP1     EQU     0A0H
        15 00       IOC0      EQU     15H
        16 00       IOC1      EQU     16H
        70 00       CHAR_I    EQU     70H
        0C 00       TIMER2    EQU     0CH
        90 00       CHAR_0    EQU     90H
        0F 00       P1        EQU     0FH
                    ;
                    ;
                    ;
                    ;
                    ;
                    ;
                    ;
                    ;
                    ;
                    ;
                    ;
                    ;
                    ;
                    ;
                    ;
```

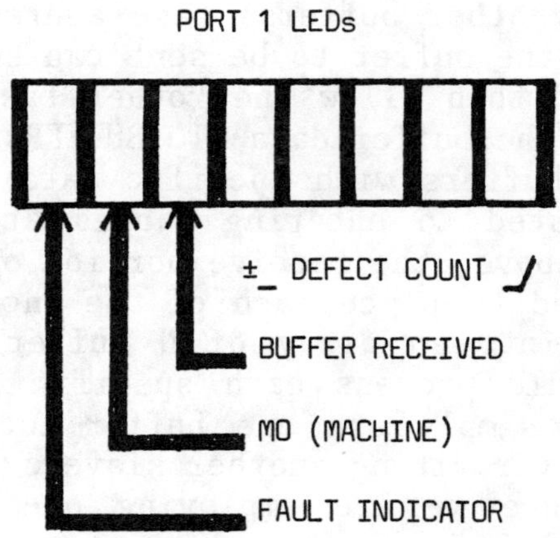


```
4500                        ORG     4500H
                    ;
4500  A1 C0 00 18           LD      SP,#0C0H          ;Initialize SP.
4504  FA                    DI                        ;Disable interrutps.
4505  11 09                 CLRB    PINT              ;Clear any pending interrupts.
4507  B1 41 08              LDB     MINT,#41H         ;Set mask bit 0 to enable timer
                                                      ;overflow interrupt source and bit 6
                                                      ;to enable serial port interrupt.
450A  B1 24 16              LDB     IOC1,#24H         ;Set bit 2 in IOC1 to enable Timer 1
                                                      ;overflow interrupt and bit 5 to
                                                      ;select TxD as function for P2.0.
450D  A1 C5 45 A0           LD      TEMP1,#T1OV       ;Load address of Timer 1 overflow
4511  C3 01 00 20 A0        ST      TEMP1,INVEC[0]    ;interrupt service routine into INT
                                                      ;VECT table.
4516  A1 88 45 A0           LD      TEMP1,#SERINT     ;Load address of serial port
451A  C3 01 0C 20 A0        ST      TEMP1,INVEC1[0]   ;interrupt service routine into INT
                                                      ;VECT table.
451F  B1 20 60              LDB     TEMP,#20H         ;Initialize TEMP.
```

```
4522  B1 9B 0E                 LDB   BAUD,#BAUD_LO     ;Load low byte of baud rate into BAUD.
4525  B1 80 0E                 LDB   BAUD,#BAUD_HI     ;Load high byte of baud into BAUD reg.
4528  B1 0A 11                 LDB   SP_CON,#0AH       ;Initialize serial port: mode 2,
                                                        ;REN = 1, PEN = 0.
452B  A1 00 00 50              LD    REG,#00H          ;Set character pointer to zero.
452F  B1 02 15       LOOP0:    LDB   IOC0,#02H         ;Load 02 into IOC0 to reset timer2
                                                        ;and select T2CLK pin as clock input.
4532  B0 56 54                 LDB   REG2,REG3         ;Load time value into REG2.
4535  FB                       EI                      ;Enable interrupts.
4536  B1 00 0F                 LDB   P1,#00H           ;Turn LEDs off.
4539  A0 0C 40       LOOP:     LD    DEFECTS,TIMER2    ;Load count from TIMER2 into
                                                        ;DEFECTS register.
453C  07 40                    INC   DEFECTS           ;Increment T2 counts.
453E  08 01 40                 SHR   DEFECTS,#1        ;Shift right to divide by two
                                                        ;for defects.
4541  71 E0 0F                 ANDB  P1,#0E0H          ;Clear lower 5 LEDs.
4544  74 40 0F                 ADDB  P1,DEF_LO         ;Add defect count to P1 for display.
4547  98 52 40                 CMPB  DEF_LO,REG1       ;Compare number of defects to limit.
454A  DF 02                    JE    FAULT             ;If num. defects = limit, goto FAULT.
454C  27 EB                    SJMP  LOOP              ;Else go back to LOOP.
454E  71 BF 0F       FAULT:    ANDB  P1,#0BFH          ;Clear M0 LED to turn process off.
4551  91 80 0F                 ORB   P1,#80H           ;Turn on fault LED.
4554  3F 0F FD       HALT:     JBS   P1,7,HALT         ;If fault LED = 1 loop on HALT.
4557  27 D6                    SJMP  LOOP0             ;Go back to LOOP0.
                     ;
                     ;         SPUTBUF - OUTPUTS FBUF TO MASTER.
                     ;
4559  A1 00 00 50    SPUTBUF:LD      REG,#00H          ;Load character pointer with 0 to
                                                        ;point to slave address in buffer.
455D  B3 51 00 50 90 LOOP3:    LDB   CHAR_O,TBUF[REG];Get character from the buffer.
4562  EF 16 00                 CALL  PUT_CHR           ;Output character to serial port.
4565  07 50                    INC   REG               ;Increment character pointer.
4567  89 04 00 50              CMP   REG,#4H           ;Compare REG to 4.
456B  D7 F0                    JNE   LOOP3             ;If REG != 4, goto LOOP3.
456D  F0                       RET                     ;Else return.
                     ;         INPUT CHARACTER ROUTINE: GET_CHR
                     ;
456E  90 11 60       GET_CHR:ORB     TEMP,SP_STAT      ;Copy serial port status into TEMP.
4571  36 60 FA                 JBC   TEMP,6,GET_CHR    ;If RI = 0, goto GET_CHR.
4574  71 BF 60                 ANDB  TEMP,#0BFH        ;Else clear RI flag in TEMP.
4577  B0 07 70                 LDB   CHAR_I,SBUF       ;Read character from SBUF into CHAR_I.
457A  F0                       RET                     ;Return.
                     ;         OUTPUT CHARACTER ROUTINE: PUT_CHR
                     ;
457B  90 11 60       PUT_CHR:ORB     TEMP,SP_STAT      ;Copy serial port status into TEMP.
457E  35 60 FA                 JBC   TEMP,5,PUT_CHR    ;If TI = 0, goto PUT_CHR.
4581  B0 90 07                 LDB   SBUF,CHAR_O       ;Else load character from CHAR_O
                                                        ;into SBUF for transmission.
```

```
4584  71 DF 60              ANDB   TEMP,#0DFH          ;Clear temp TI flag.
4587  F0                    RET                        ;Return.
                 ;
                 ;
                 ;
                 ;          SERIAL PORT INTERRUPT SERVICE ROUTINE
                 ;
4588  F2         SERINT:    PUSHF                      ;Save flags.
4589  90 11 60              ORB    TEMP,SP_STAT        ;Copy serial port status into TEMP.
458C  36 60 34              JBC    TEMP,6,NO_CHAR      ;If RI = 0, goto NO_CHAR.
458F  2F DD                 CALL   GET_CHR             ;Else call GET_CHAR to read character.
4591  99 01 70              CMPB   CHAR_I,#01H         ;Compare character to address 01.
4594  D7 2D                 JNE    NO_CHAR             ;If char != 01, goto NO_CHAR.
4596  B1 0B 11              LDB    SP_CON,#0BH         ;Change to mode 3 to receive rest of
                                                       ;buffer.
4599  A1 00 00 50           LD     REG,#00H            ;Initialize buffer character pointer.

459D  C7 51 00 50 70 SLOOP: STB    CHAR_I,TBUF[REG];Store character in buffer and
45A2  07 50                 INC    REG                 ;increment character pointer.
45A4  89 04 00 50           CMP    REG,#4H             ;Test if 4 characters received.
45A8  DF 04                 JE     PROBUF              ;If REG = 4, goto PROBUF
45AA  2F C2                 CALL   GET_CHR             ;Else call GET_CHR to read character.
45AC  27 EF                 SJMP   SLOOP               ;Loop back to SLOOP.

45AE  A0 0C 40      PROBUF: LD     DEFECTS,TIMER2      ;Load number of counts from TIMER2
                                                       ;into DEFECTS register.
45B1  07 40                 INC    DEFECTS             ;Increment T2 counts.
45B3  08 01 40              SHR    DEFECTS,#1          ;Shift right to divide by two
                                                       ;for defects.
45B6  C7 01 02 50 40        STB    DEF_LO,DEF_BYTE     ;Load number of defects into buffer.
45BB  2F 9C                 CALL   SPUTBUF             ;Call (slave) SPUTBUF.
45BD  95 20 0F              XORB   P1,#20H             ;Toggle buffer sent LED.
45C0  B1 0A 11              LDB    SP_CON,#0AH         ;Change serial port back to mode 2.
45C3  F3            NO_CHAR:POPF                       ;Restore flags.
45C4  F0                    RET                        ;Return to main program.

                 ;          TIMER 1 OVERFLOW INTERRUPT SERVICE ROUTINE:
                 ;                 (TOGGLES MO)
                 ;
                 ;
45C5  F2            T1OV:   PUSHF                      ;Save flags.
45C6  E0 54 09              DJNZ   REG2,RETURN         ;Decrement REG2, if != 0 time not
                                                       ;achieved, goto RETURN.
45C9  B0 56 54              LDB    REG2,REG3           ;Reload REG2 for another time delay.
45CC  3F 0F 03              JBS    P1,7,RETURN         ;If fault LED = 1, goto RETURN.
45CF  95 40 0F              XORB   P1,#40H             ;Toggle MO LED to signal process of
                                                       ;making widgets.
45D2  F3            RETURN: POPF                       ;Restore flags.
45D3  F0                    RET                        ;Return.
```

The main program for the slave starts with the exact same initializations at 4500 through 4536 as were performed in the master's main program, with two exceptions. First SP-CON is loaded with 0AH to select Mode 2 operation for the slave. If we had more than one slave, each would be programmed to operate in Mode 2. That will allow the master's first transmitted byte with its 9th bit set (TB8 = 1), representing a slave's address, to INTERRUPT all slaves so they can check to see if the address is theirs. That is crucial to multiprocessor communications. The slave whose address matches will change to Mode 3, the others will remain in Mode 2, as we'll see and describe later. Second, 02 has been loaded into IOC0 for the purpose of activating the T2CLK pin as event (defects) source for timer T2 and to reset T2 to 0. Note that the slave's port 1 is cleared. Remember, on the slave side P1.7 = fault indicator, P1.6 = M0 machine (on/off), P1.5 = TO BUFFER received indicator, and P1.4 through P1.0 will count defectives.

The main program continues at LOOP (4539). There T2, which holds the number of counts simulated by the debounced switch at T2CLK, is read into word register DEFECTS (40H) and adjusted so that one press and release of the switch yields just one more defect (event), not two (as T2 does). After clearing the lower 5 bits at P1, the low byte of the number of defects, held in DEF-LO (40H), is added to P1 so that the low 5 bits of P1 display the number of defects. A comparison is then made of the number of defects in DEF-LO with the tolerable limit stored in REG1 (52H), entered there at run-time. If the number of defects has reached the tolerable limit JE FAULT at 454A jumps to FAULT where the ANDB instruction turns off M0 at P1.6 and the ORB instruction turns on the FAULT LED at P1.7. The next instruction JBS P1, 7, HALT causes a halt condition to persist as long as P1.7 (fault indicator) is high. Should that fault indicator be cleared, fall-through JBS to SJMP LOOP0 will go back to LOOP0 to again read out number of defectives in a new start-up with T2 reset and LEDs off. (See problem 3 at end of the experiment). If the number of defects has not reached the limit, fall-through JE at 454A continues LOOP and widgits keep being stamped and defectives keep being recorded.

All during this monitoring of defectives in LOOP, T1OV interrupts are occurring every 0.131 sec. to the T1OV ISR at 45C5. There, after a PUSHF, we decrement REG2 (the time multiple) and if it's not yet 0 we jump around to POPF and RET to LOOP. Eventually, after (REG2) decrements, we fall through the DJNZ instruction at 45C6 to a re-load of REG2 from REG3 (REG3 is address 56H and is loaded at run-time to determine the on and off-times of machine M0). The next instruction JBS P1, 7, RETURN BYPASSES the toggling of M0 if the FAULT LED indicates a 1. In that case, we return to LOOP and eventually to HALT at 4554. If, however, P1.7 is 0 we fall through JBS at 45CC to the XORB P1, #40H instruction which toggles M0, the widgit stamping machine at P1.6. We then return to LOOP. Thus M0 is toggling with on and off times determined by (REG3) i.e. 0.131 sec. x (REG3) to be exact. Thus T1OV interrupts on a regular 131 msec. basis are being used to generate the M0 on/off times.

Now all during LOOP and T1OV interrupts, serial port interrupts will occur as the TO BUFFER's bytes from master are being received by the slave. In particular, TBUF's FIRST TRANSMITTED BYTE (address of slave), with 9th bit = 1, will interrupt all slaves, SINCE THE LATTER ARE IN MODE 2. When that byte is received, all slave's activities are interrupted by a serial port interrupt. This carries them to their SERINT ISRs (here at 4588 for our single slave). There a PUSHF is executed and SP-STAT is checked to see if RI is high. If it isn't, we must have had a serial interrupt due to the slave transmitting a byte back to master (more on that later). In that case, JBC at 458C jumps to NO-CHR and we return to LOOP or T1OV ISR. If RI is high, a byte has been received from the master with bit 9 = 1 i.e. an address has been received from the master and, because its 9th bit is 1, it was able to interrupt all slaves, (they are in Mode 2). We fall through JBC to a call of GET-CHR at 456E. This is the same GET-CHR routine used through-out the chapter. There we read out the received character from SBUF(RX) and load it into CHAR-I before returning to 4591. Remember, RI is high so we fall through 4571. At 4591 we compare the value (address) in CHAR-I with 01, the selected slave's address. If it's not 01, JNE NO-CHAR at 4594 jumps to NO-CHAR at 45C3 where a POPF and RET carry us back to either LOOP or the T1OV activity. The slave in that case ignores this address byte and the subsequent TBUF bytes (data/commands).

If, however, the received character in CHAR-I is 01 we fall through JNE to 4596 where 0B is loaded into SP-CON. THIS CHANGES THE SLAVE'S MODE TO 3. This is most important if we wish to receive the rest of the buffer. Remember, the rest of TBUF's bytes from the master do NOT have their 9th bits set (9th bit was cleared on transmission of the first address byte prior to which TB8 had been set to 1). Hence, if the addressed slave were still in Mode 2, those data bytes would NOT cause serial interrupts upon reception and the RI flag would not be set to 1. In that case the slave would not be able to read those subsequent buffer bytes, never being able to exit from the GET-CHR routine (called at 45AA) as RI would always be low. Remember, the GET-CHR routine reads the received character from SBUF(RX) into CHAR-I only after RI goes high. RI would not go high in Mode 2 if the 9th bit of the received character were 0.

Hence a reading of the rest of TBUF would not be possible. On the other hand, changing the addressed slave's mode to 3 ensures that ANY received byte, even with 9th bit 0, will cause a serial port interrupt at the addressed slave in Mode 3 so that RI will be 1. Then, when GET-CHR is called, fall-through 4571 will allow a reading of the masters data/command bytes in TBUF from SBUF(RX). All other slaves are allowed to remain in Mode 2 going about their dedicated slave activities. They are not interrupted by incoming data bytes whose 9th bits are 0.

An important observation must be made here. In Mode 3, the addressed slave, while in its GET-CHR routine finds RI going high TOGETHER with a serial interrupt to the SERINT ISR occurring, whenever it receives a data byte from master's TBUF. This serial interrupt becomes PENDING because of the PUSHF instruction in the SERINT ISR before the call at 45AA to GET-CHR (all interrupt mask bits were reset to 0). When we exit from GET-CHR upon reception of a character (RI went high), RI is cleared at 4574. We return to 45AC in SERINT and EVENTUALLY, after more calls of GET-CHR, end up at 45C3 where the POPF restores the interrupt mask bits. The RET to main program now allows the pending serial interrupt to be serviced. We re-enter SERINT WITH RI CLEARED. JBC at 458C now does an "end-around" to NO-CHAR since RI is 0. There a return to main program occurs. The pending interrupt has been "serviced" and its bit cleared in the process, with no visible effect on anything. Keep these remarks in mind as we continue our analysis at 4599.

We are now ready to store all received bytes from master in a slave table starting at 5000. To do that, we initialize the offset in the table pointer to 0. This is done at 4599. Then the first received character (address) is stored at 5000 (TBUF [REG]). The offset is then incremented and a check is made to see if 4 characters were received. If not, we fall through the JE PROBUF at 45A8 and again call GET-CHR at 456E to wait for the next received byte from master. When it arrives we return from GET-CHR (RI became 1 because of reception in Mode 3) to 45AC in SERINT ISR with the received character in CHAR-I. There SJMP SLOOP takes us back to 459D where the next received character is stored in the NEXT location in the table being formed. Eventually, REG will equal 4. Four characters from the TO BUFFER (including address) have been received and stored as a table by the slave. In that case, the JE instruction at 45A8 takes us to PROBUF at 45AE (Process Buffer).

The PROBUF routine starts by again reading the number of defects from T2 into the DEFECTS register (40H). We then store that value (from DEF-LO) into DEF-BYTE (5002 in the table). This PROCESSES the received TBUF from master to include information on the number of defects at the slave. The four bytes, including the modified one at 5002, form the FROM BUFFER which is now to be transmitted back to the master. The CALL SPUTBUF at 45BB does just that. SPUTBUF at 4559 is the slave's PUTBUF, and is identical to the master's PUTBUF routine at 4538 in the master's program, except that we do not now have the LDB SP-CON #1BH instruction which set TB8 (9th bit) to 1 for transmission of the first (address) byte out of the master. That is not necessary here, since we are sending a buffer back to the one MASTER, and the latter is in Mode 3 and will ALWAYS be interrupted on reception. It needs no address.

SPUTBUF at 4559 resets the offset (REG) to 0 to start transmission from the first table entry. LDB CHAR-0, TBUF [REG] fetches that byte into CHAR-0. A call is then made to PUT-CHR at 4578. Since TI was initially set (see 451F), we fall through JBC at 457E and load CHAR-0 into SBUF(TX) for transmission (same PUT-CHR routine we've been using through-out the chapter). We return from PUT-CHR to 4565 in SPUTBUF where the offset REG is incremented for transmission of the next table entry. If REG is not equal to 4 we jump back to LOOP3 (JNE LOOP3) at 455D till the whole processed FROM BUFFER is transmitted back to master. When that occurs, we fall through JNE at 456B to a return to 45BD in PROBUF. There we toggle P1.5, the TO BUFFER (or FROM BUFFER) indicator (both indicators occur at practically the same time, for all intents and purposes here). This indicates another FROM BUFFER was formed and sent back to the master. The next instruction loads SP-CON with 0AH again to insure that the slave is back in Mode 2 so that it can again be interrupted (with all other slaves) the next time the master sends out another TO BUFFER with its first byte an address (with 9th bit set). After that is done, POPF and RET carry us back to the main activity at LOOP and at T1OV ISR. When another TO BUFFER arrives from the master the whole SERINT ISR cycle of steps, just explained, repeats.

A last point to be made is a mention of where the RB8 bit in SP-STAT would be useful. If an addressed slave has just changed to Mode 3, it may happen that the master wants to readdress this slave (with 9th bit = 1) for it to receive new data/commands. Since the slave is in Mode 3, it won't know that this new received byte is an address (9th bit = 1) as it makes no distinction between 9 = 0 or 1, UNLESS it polls RB8 (SP-STAT.7) to determine whether it's high or not. If it is, then an appropriate jump to a new "address routine" would have to be made to receive new data/commands. Remember, in Mode 3 received characters with bit 9 = 0 or 1 have the same effect: they both cause interrupts so we can't separate address frames from data frames. A polling of RB8 settles the issue.

You are now ready to perform the experiment. Go back to the CONNECTIONS section and then the PROCEDURE section. Follow all the steps given in the PROCEDURE and confirm all our observations.

This experiment culminates this chapter and, hopefully, puts it all together. We have tried to build grandually and logically as we proceeded from experiment to experiment. Expt. 8-6 used all the techniques of the proceeding experiments and incorporated additional ones. A THOROUGH understanding of Expt. 8-6 is essential when working with serial I/O communications. We have covered all the 8096's serial port modes. Note how basic routines get used over and over even as the complexity of the experiment or application increases (GET-CHR, PUT-CHR, PUTBUF, etc.) This makes for a clearer structure to the programs and facilitates portability and flexibility in applying serial I/O to diverse applications. We also wish to point out that a COMPLETE interrupt-based serial communications approach could be taken without the need for GET-CHR and PUT-CHR polling routines (see PROBLEM 5 below). In Expts. 8-5, 8-6 we used a mixture of serial interrupt and RI/TI flag polling. For further comments on how you would implement a purely serial interrupt-based approach, without polling of any flags, read PROBLEM 5 below.

PROBLEMS

1. Enlarge the program to encompass 2 or 3 slaves with addresses 01, 02, 03.

2. In the experiment just done, assign meaningful data/commands to the second, third, and fourth bytes in the master's TO BUFFER. They're available, even though we did not use them in our simple application. Also assign other meaningful slave status data to the second and fourth bytes of the slave's FROM BUFFER. They're available even though we didn't use them. Thus we're asking to extend the scope of the application beyond the one discussed here. The structure is all there in the programs presented.

3. Expand the PROBUF routine to look at additional fields of the TO BUFFER. Select a field (byte) to be used to update the slave's defect LIMIT. Select a field to be used to cause the slave to leave the halt state (when detected defects reached the limit) and begin processing widgits again. In the latter case an alternative to the field would be to employ the EXTINT to get out of the halt state and return to SJMP LOOP0. LDB MINT, #0C1H and the appropriate EXTINT ISR are necessary.

4. Have "other tasks" on the master side process FBUF and arrange for the appropriate NEXT TBUF to be sent back to the slave, based on the data the master has just received from FBUF.

5. In Expt. 8-6, as we implemented it, the MAIN FUNCTION of the serial port interrupt on the slave side was to "wake up" all slaves so they could check to see if the first byte (address) sent out by the master was their address. This checking was done in each slave's Serial Interrupt ISR. After that, the non-addressed slaves returned to their main slave activities, remaining in Mode 2. The addressed slave remained in its ISR and then changed from Mode 2 to Mode 3. It then POLLED for the arrival of 3 bytes of data from the master in the GET-CHR loop routine. The RI flag was polled in that routine for reception of each successive byte. Likewise, when the whole TBUF was received by the slave, it was stored in a table, processed (for number of defects), and then transmitted back to the master as FBUF (based on a polling of the TI flag in the PUT-CHR loop routine). Thus reception and transmission at the slave was based on a polling of RI and TI flags. However, the WAKE-UP of slaves was based on a serial port interrupt of slaves in Mode 2 when an address character (bit 9 = 1) was forthcoming.
PROBLEM: We suggest that you modify the program SO THAT IT IS BASED ENTIRELY ON INTERRUPTS without the use of GET-CHR and PUT-CHR polling routines. Thus each individually received byte from the master will cause an interrupt, the addressed slave's ISR is to store the byte in a table by means of an appropriate receive pointer, and the ISR is to IMMEDIATELY return to the slave's main program. When another byte is received from the master, the slave's ISR is AGAIN entered (another interrupt occurs) and that character is to be stored in the NEXT location in the table. Again a return to the slave's main program should be executed. When 4 such bytes have been received, the ISR should process the table (so as to incorporate in it the number of widgit defects) and then start transmitting same, ONE BYTE AT A TIME, back to master. Thus, after EACH byte is fetched from the table for transmission, a return to the slave's MAIN PROGRAM is to take place. When another byte has been transmitted, an interrupt will be generated to cause another entry into the slave's ISR where the next byte from the processed table is to be loaded into SBUF for transmission, with subsequent return to slave's main program. When the whole FBUF table has been transmitted back to the master, the slave's transmit pointer is reset, the TBUF SENT LED is toggled, Mode 2 is re-programmed, and

a return to the slave's main program is to be executed. When a new TBUF from master is received by slave, all the above steps repeat.
This approach has its merits where minimal time interruptions of the slave's main program is an important consideration. No POLLING for received or transmitted characters is resorted to in that case. When characters are now received or transmitted, the associated interrupts to the SERINT ISR make it immediately known that characters were received or transmitted. The received character can be IMMEDIATELY read from SBUF(RX) while the character transmitted out of SBUF(TX) can be IMMEDIATELY replaced with the next character to be transmitted. More time is gained for the slave's other activities. Watch your changes from Mode 2 to Mode 3 and back to Mode 2 on the slave side. The first instruction in the slave's ISR should be a test of SP-STAT to decide if a receive or transmit was responsible for the ISR entry. Act accordingly on the result of the test.

CHAPTER 9

BROADER APPLICATIONS WITH THE 8096.

INTRODUCTION

Up to this point the book has concentrated on the fundamental and key capabilities of the 8096 and has provided a large number of applications illustrating those fundamentals. The emphasis on applications experiments was particularly strong in chapters 5, 6, and 8 and to some degree in chapter 4.

In this chapter we cover a broader range of hands-on applications not touched on before. These applications experiments, as in previous chapters, are meant to demonstrate to you the broad potential power, versatility and possibilities the 8096 posseses in many diverse applications areas. A glance at the listing of chatper 9's experiments in the table of contents will give you a good flavor of where you're headed and what you're about to experience in this chapter's experiments.

In addition to demonstrating the powerful features and facilities of the 8096, the experiments are designed to give you ideas for applications in your areas of interest. Naturally, the scope of this book does not permit addressing everyone's areas of interest (even if it were the scope, we couldn't fulfill that goal). Nor, do we attempt to present an experiment that's ready-made for your applications in your area of interest. The needs of your particular application will most likely require additional hardware and/or software considerations and the use of further development tools. But we hope the experiments will provide a good base to build on and give plenty of ideas. We hope, also, that the experiments will suggest areas of applications with the 8096 that may not have occurred to you otherwise. Therefore, we ask you to approach this chapter with the above thoughts in mind.

EXPERIMENT 9-1

A 1-250 KHz LINEAR FREQUENCY TO VOLTAGE CONVERTER.

INTRODUCTION

In the area of communications and instrumentation the need frequently arises for the linear conversion of frequency to voltage. Such conversion has important applications in: 1) frequency measurement where the size of the converted analog voltage is a measure of frequency, 2) frequency control where the converted voltage can be used, possibly in processed form, in a feedback loop to accurately control the output frequency of a voltage controlled oscillator (VCO), 3) in demodulation (detection) of a frequency-modulated (FM) carrier. In the latter case the swing in output voltage would be a measure of the degree of FM (modulation index) on the carrier frequency (the output voltage swing is easily displayed on a scope to indicate the degree of FM).

In this experiment, we'll demonstrate how the 8096 can be used in achieving frequency to voltage conversion. We'll use a variable 0 to 250 KHz pulse generator (set for 50% duty cycle and possessing TTL output levels of 0 and +5V on the pulses) to illustrate the method and approach. The ability of timer T2 to record 0 to 1 and 1 to 0 transitions separated in time by 2 usec. is instrumental in extending the frequency range coverage to 250 KHz. SEE IMPORTANT NOTE P. 464 on 1 KHz ERROR.

FORMULATION AND APPROACH

1. The output of the 0 to 250 KHz pulse generator will be input to the T2CLK (P2.3) source of timer T2.
2. A 1 msec. delay time in the program will separate successive readings of T2/2 (T2 always being cleared before the next reading of it). Thus a reading of T2/2 (remember T2 counts each 0 to 1 OR 1 to 0 transition on the pulse) will yield the frequency in KHz i.e. 200 KHz will read as 200 in T2/2.
3. The value of T2/2 is then output at port P1's LEDs so that P1 reads the frequency in KHz (albeit the HEX value).
4. This very same value of T2/2 is then loaded into the PWM SFR at 17H to drive the PWM output at P2.5. The filtered value at this output pin is then the analog voltage directly proportional to the value (duty cycle) in the PWM SFR, and that in turn is directly proportional to the frequency of the pulses since PWM was loaded with that frequency in KHz.

The program that implements the above is presented below at 2100. It is analyzed immediately afterward.

```
        18 00          SP       EQU     18H
        15 00          IOCO     EQU     15H
        16 00          IOC1     EQU     16H
        40 00          REG      EQU     40H
        50 00          REG1     EQU     50H
        0C 00          T2       EQU     0CH
        0F 00          P1       EQU     0FH
        17 00          PWM      EQU     17H
2100                            ORG     2100H
                       ;
2100    A1 C0 00 18             LD      SP,#00C0H     ;Initialize SP.
2104    B1 01 16                LDB     IOC1,#01H     ;Enable PWM at P2.5.
2107    B1 02 15       CLRT2:   LDB     IOCO,#02H     ;Select T2CLK as source for T2.
                                                      ;Reset T2 to 0.
210A    A1 4D 01 40             LD      REG,#014DH    ;Load REG for 1.0 msec. delay.
210E    05 40          DELAY:   DEC     REG           ;Decrement REG.
2110    D7 FC                   JNE     DELAY         ;If REG != 0, jump to DELAY.
2112    A0 0C 50                LD      REG1,T2       ;Else read T2 into REG1.
2115    07 50                   INC     REG1          ;Increment REG1.
2117    08 01 50                SHR     REG1,#01H     ;Divide result by 2 to give true #
                                                      ;of pulses recorded in T2 in 1 msec.
211A    B0 50 0F                LDB     P1,REG1       ;Display frequency in KHz at P1's LEDs.
211D    B0 50 17                LDB     PWM,REG1      ;Drive PWM to produce integrated
                                                      ;voltage at P2.5 proportional to
                                                      ;frequency.
2120    27 E5                   SJMP    CLRT2         ;Jump back to CLRT2 for new frequency
                                                      ;measurement.
2122                            END
```

After initializing the stack pointer, 01 is loaded into IOC1 to select the PWM function at P2.5. 02 is then loaded into IOC0 to reset T2 to 0 and to select T2CLK as the source of events for timer T2. A 1 msec. time delay is then executed by means of loading 014DH into REG and decrementing REG 333 times till it reaches 0 (DEC and JNE account for 12 state times = 3 usec. at 12 MHz, so 333 x 3 usec. = 1 msec. to within 0.1%). After that 1 msec. delay a reading of timer T2 is made, its contents being loaded into REG1. By incrementing REG1 and shifting right once (divide by 2) we convert the contents of T2 into the number of PULSES captured by T2 in 1 msec i.e. the frequency in KHz. That value is the low byte in REG1 (being less than or equal to 250 (dec) or FAH for our 0 to 250 KHz generator). That low byte in REG1 is then output to the LEDs at P1. They will display the frequency in HEX KHz. That same REG1 byte is next loaded into the PWM SFR to drive pin P2.5 with pulses of duty cycle proportional to the value in PWM (or to the frequency of the source pulse generator). The integrated value of the pulses at PWM pin P2.5 is then a voltage proportional to pulse generator frequency. Finally, SJMP CLRT2 ensures that T2 is reset to 0 before another 1 msec. window captures another sample of the frequency in KHz.

PROCEDURE

1. Connect the output of your TTL pulse generator (set for square waves) to T2CLK (P2.3). Have a VOM measure the filtered output voltage at P2.5 (PWM), using the same RC integrating circuit that we've been employing in the PWM experiments in this book.
2. Enter BY 09 = 00. Set the pulse generator to 0 KHz. Execute from 2100.
3. Measure the output (filtered) voltage at P2.5.
4. Set the input frequency at the pulse generator to the following values (in KHz): 10, 30, 50, 80, 120, 160, 200, and 250KHz. For each setting read the value on the LEDs at P1 and the voltage at P2.5.
5. Here were our results:

FREQUENCY IN	PWM = P1	VOLTAGE OUT
10 KHz	0B (11)	0.19V
30	1F (31)	0.55
50	33 (51)	0.89
80	52 (82)	1.56
120	7C (124)	2.28
160	A1 (161)	2.94
200	CC (204)	3.69
250	FB (251)	4.67

Note the good linearity re: V vs. f. Out settings for f on the pulse generator were made with its rotary dial. Its calibration was off somewhat.

REDUCING THE FREQUENCY RANGE AND FREQUENCIES TO ACHIEVE THE SAME OUTPUT VOLTAGE RANGE. SCALING.

In this experiment the results obtained in the last table indicate that a 0 to 250 KHz input frequency range produced a 0 to 4.67V output voltage range. That is the way we planned it, in that the time window of 1 msec. (#014DH at 210B, 210C in the delay loop), allowed exactly the frequency in KHz to be recorded in REG1 (from T2 counts), with the latter then directly loaded into the PWM to produce the proportional output voltage. If we wished to have a much smaller input frequency range produce the same output voltage (PWM) span, we merely have to change the time window to a larger value to capture the SAME number of pulses for loading the PWM from a smaller frequency. Thus, for example, suppose we wanted a 0 to 1250 Hz input frequency range to produce the same 0 to 4.67V output voltage range that 0 to 250 KHz just did. All we'd need is a 0.2 sec. delay window instead of the 1 msec. window just used. For then, 1250 Hz would produce 250 pulses in REG1 in 0.2 sec. just as 250 KHz produced in 1 msec. In either case, the PWM would receive the same value, 250 = FAH, from REG1 and thus produce the same output voltage 4.67V. As we know, 0.2 sec. delay will result if the value 014D at 210B, 210C is increased to FFFF (65,536 loops, each giving 3 usec. time). Then 250 Hz gives 50 pulses in 0.2 sec. just as 50 KHz did in 1 msec. In the same way, 500 Hz, 750 Hz, 1000 Hz, and 1250 Hz will now be equivalent (as far as PWM loading values) to the former 100 KHz, 150 KHz, 200 KHz, and 250 KHz, respectively. All we need do is enter BY 210B = 0FF, 0FF into the program. Do that, execute from 2100, observe P1 = PWM, and measure V at PWM's filtered output at P2.5. We found the following (expected) results:

FREQUENCY IN	PWM = P1	PWM VOUT
250 Hz	32H	0.89V
500	64H	1.76
750	96H	2.75
1000	C8H	3.71
1250	FAH	4.65

IMPORTANT NOTE ON 1 KHz ERROR.

Here, as in Expts. 9-3 and 9-4, we employed delay windows before capturing the count reading in T2 and converting it to number of pulses received. Thus, when we employ e.g. a 1 msec. delay window, a 1 KHz frequency becomes a reading of 1 at the display P1 and y KHz becomes a reading of y at P1, i.e. P1 gives frequency in KHz. Now that can easily lead to errors of as much as 1 KHz. Thus, if the frequency is e.g. 1 Hz and if its leading or trailing edge occurs DURING the 1 msec. window, then T2 will record 1 and P1 will display 1! This is all well if we are content to measure N KHz, with N = PRECISE INTEGERS. What happens in between? We remedy this shortcoming in Expt. 9-19.

EXPERIMENT 9-2

HSO PULSE GENERATOR WITH FREQUENCY CONTROLLED BY A VARIABLE VOLTAGE AT AN A/D INPUT CHANNEL (A VCO).

INTRODUCTION

An important device in communications and telecommuncations, be it for audio, video, intermediate, or radio frequency applications, is the VCO (Voltage Controlled Oscillator) in which the output frequency is controllable by a variable input voltage. As one example of the convenience such voltage control affords is the ease with which an FM modulated carrier can be implemented: a sinusoidal varying voltage of small amplitude about a fixed d.c. voltage will yield a sinusoidally varying output frequency about a fixed carrier frequency (assuming linearity between output frequency and input voltage for the VCO). The VCO is, therefore, the reverse aspect of the frequency to voltage converter treated in Expt. 9-1. The VCO is an example of "electronic tuning."

In this experiment, we use two of the 8096's powerful on-board features to implement a VCO. The output will be TTL pulses whose frequency is determined by the A/D input voltage. The two features we are referring to are the 8 input A/D channels available at port P0 and the ability of the independent HSO unit to generate pulses of any duty cycle and period on any one or more of six HSO output pins. While we shall produce output TTL pulses, there are methods for converting pulses to SINE WAVES to implement a VCO in the broader sense.

FORMULATION AND APPROACH

1. A 0 to 5 volt potentiometer will be connected to channel ACH.0 at P0.0. The output pulses will be generated at HSO.0. Their frequency will be controlled by the input voltage at the POT. The pulses will be observed on a scope.
2. We will arrange the program so that the output frequency will increase as input voltage increases. See (3) below.
3. The A/D converted word (actually 10 significant bits) (in REG1) will be subtracted from 7FFH and the result stored in a register (here REG3). REG3's VALUE will be doubled (but not REG3) and the result stored in another register (here REG2). (REG3) will then be made the on-time of the HSO-generated pulse. (REG3) will ALSO be the off-

time of the generated pulse i.e. the pulse will be made to go on "now" (at T1 + 0003), then to go off (REG3) from "now" [at T1 + (REG3)], and then to go back on (REG2) from "now" [at T1 + (REG2)], where (REG2) = 2 x (REG3). Thus we'll be generating square waves. The choise 7FF is arbitrary. It determines the frequency RANGE over 0 to 5V.

4. By making REG3 = 7FF minus the conversion value in REG1, we are ensuring that 0 input voltage will produce the largest on (REG3) and off (REG3) times i.e. 7FF x 2 usec., and hence the smallest square wave frequency, namely 1/(4094 x 2 usec) = about 122 Hz; and that the maximum input voltage (5V) i.e. 3FF, will produce the smallest on (REG3) and off (REG3) times i.e. 2.048 msec., or the largest (244 Hz) square wave frequencies. Thus frequency will increase with increasing voltage at ACH.0, but NOT linearly.
5. The main program will initiate the start of an A/D conversion on channel ACH.0 and will also call CAMLOAD where the three commands to generate one pulse are loaded into the CAM-FILE of the HSO unit. It will end in a self-loop simulating "other tasks". It is in this loop that A/D "conversion complete" interrupts will be made, as well as HSO interrupts at the end of each additionally generated pulse (although EITHER interrupt can certainly also occur while the OTHER'S ISR is being serviced. Things proceed smoothly either way, thanks to the RET instruction).
6. The HSO interrupt generated at the end of each pulse causes a vector to the HSO's ISR. There the CAMLOAD routine is again called to reload the CAM FILE with the 3 necessary commands to generate ANOTHER pulse.
7. The A/D "conversion complete" interrupt will vector us to the "A/D complete" ISR. There we read the 10 bit conversion result from the A/D Result Registers (HI and LO), subtract that result from 7FF (as explained in (3) and (4) above), and then store the result in REG3. That value is then doubled and stored in REG2, as explained in (3) above. Another A/D conversion is then initiated. These REG3, REG2 values are used by CAMLOAD...
8. The CAMLOAD routine loads T1 + (REG3) into HSOTIME to have (REG3) determine the on-time. It then loads (REG2) = 2 x (REG3) into HSOTIME to determine the off-time (= the on-time for a square wave). (It FIRST loads T1 + 0003 into HSOTIME to start a pulse "now").

The program at 2140 is given below. It is analyzed afterward.

```
      06 00          HSOCOM   EQU     06H    18 00      SP       EQU     18H
      04 00          HSOTIME  EQU     04H    08 00      MINT     EQU     08H
      0A 00          T1       EQU     0AH    09 00      PINT     EQU     09H
      40 00          TEMP     EQU     40H    02 00      ADCOM    EQU     02H
      50 00          REG1     EQU     50H    03 00      ADRESHI  EQU     03H
      51 00          REG1HI   EQU     51H    02 00      ADRESLO  EQU     02H
      50 00          REG1LO   EQU     50H
      60 00          REG2     EQU     60H
      70 00          REG3     EQU     70H
      06 20          INVEC1   EQU     2006H
      02 20          INVEC0   EQU     2002H

2140                          ORG     2140H
                     ;
2140  A1 C0 00 18             LD      SP,#00C0H          ;Initialize SP.
2144  FA                      DI                         ;Disable global interrupt.
2145  B1 0A 08                LDB     MINT,#0AH          ;Enable HSO and A/D Conv. Complete
                                                         ;interrupt sources.
2148  A1 80 21 40             LD      TEMP,#HSOINT       ;Load address of HSO ISR
214C  C3 01 06 20 40          ST      TEMP,INVEC1[0]     ;into location 2006 of VECT INT
                                                         ;table.
2151  A1 83 21 40             LD      TEMP,#ADCOMPL      ;Load address of A/D Conv. Complete
2155  C3 01 02 20 40          ST      TEMP,INVEC0[0]     ;into location 2002 of VECT INT
                                                         ;table.
215A  11 09                   CLRB    PINT               ;Clear any pendings.
215C  FB                      EI                         ;Enable global interrupt.
215D  B1 08 02                LDB     ADCOM,#08H         ;Start conversion on channel 0 now.
2160  EF 02 00                CALL    CAMLOAD            ;Loads CAM FILE with three commands
                                                         ;to produce a square pulse.
2163  27 FE          HERE:    SJMP    HERE               ;Loop ("busy tasks").
                     ;
                     ;
2165  B1 20 06       CAMLOAD:LDB      HSOCOM,#20H        ;HSO.0 to go on without generation
                                                         ;of HSO.0 interrupt.
2168  45 03 00 0A 04          ADD     HSOTIME,T1,#0003;HSO.0 to go on "now".
216D  FD                      NOP                        ;8 state times required.
216E  FD                      NOP                        ;
216F  B1 00 06                LDB     HSOCOM,#00H        ;HSO.0 is to go off without
                                                         ;generation of HSO.0 interrupt.
2172  44 70 0A 04             ADD     HSOTIME,T1,REG3    ;HSO.0 is to go off (REG3) from "now".
2176  FD                      NOP                        ;8 state times required.
2177  FD                      NOP                        ;
2178  B1 30 06                LDB     HSOCOM,#30H        ;HSO.0 is to go on with generation
                                                         ;of HSO.0 interrupt.
217B  44 60 0A 04             ADD     HSOTIME,T1,REG2    ;HSO.0 is to go back on at time
                                                         ;(REG2) = 2(REG3) from "now".
217F  F0                      RET                        ;Return to HERE in main program.
```

```
                    ;          HSO INTERRUPT SERVICE ROUTINE
                    ;
2180  2F E3         HSOINT: CALL  CAMLOAD          ;Another pulse was generated,reload
                                                   ;CAM FILE to generate another pulse.
2182  F0                    RET                    ;Return to where the HSO interrupt
                                                   ;was made.
                    ;
                    ;          A/D CONVERSION COMPLETE ISR
                    ;
2183  B0 03 51      ADCOMPL:LDB   REG1HI,ADRESHI   ;Store converted bits 9-2 into REG1HI.
2186  B0 02 50              LDB   REG1LO,ADRESLO   ;Store converted bits 1,0 int bits 7,6
                                                   ;of REG1LO.
2189  08 06 50              SHR   REG1,#06H        ;6 shifts right will put conversion
                                                   ;bits 7-0 into REG1LO and bits 9,8
                                                   ;into LSB bits of REG1HI, with bits
                                                   ;7-2 in REG1HI=0.
218C  A1 FF 07 70           LD    REG3,#07FFH      ;Load REG3 with 7FF.
2190  68 50 70              SUB   REG3,REG1        ;7FF - (REG1) is stored in REG3.
                                                   ;This will guarantee that high input
                                                   ;voltages will produce small periods
                                                   ;(high frequencies). See below and
                                                   ;CAMLOAD.
2193  44 70 70 60           ADD   REG2,REG3,REG3   ;2 X (REG3) is stored in REG2.
2197  B1 08 02              LDB   ADCOM,#08H       ;Start another conversion on CH.0.
219A  F0                    RET                    ;Return to where A/D Conv. Compl.
                                                   ;interrupt was made.
219B                        END
```

The main program starts by initializeing the Stack Pointer and disabling the interrupt system. 0A is then loaded into the interrupt mask register to unmask the HSO and "A/D conversion complete" interrupt sources. The address of the HOS ISR (#HSO INT = 2180H) is then loaded into the INT VECT table at 2006 (HSO location) and the address of the "A/D conversion complete" routine (#ADCOMPL = 2183) is loaded into the INT VECT table at 2002 (A/D complete location). Pendings are then cleared and the interrupt system is globally enabled. ADCOM is then loaded with 08 to start conversion on channel ACH.0 now. CAMLOAD at 2165 is then called to load CAM FILE with the commands necessary to generate the FIRST pulse out of the HOS unit. SJMP HERE then simulates "other tasks".

The CAMLOAD routine at 2165 first loads 20 into the Command Tag to turn HSO.0 on "now" (T1 + 0003) without the generation of any HSO interrupt. Two NOPs provide 8 state times to allow that command to enter the CAMFILE from the Holding Register. The next instruction loads 00 into HSOCOM to turn HSO.0 off without generation of any HSO interrupt. The next instruction places T1 + (REG3) into HSOTIME so that HSO.0 is to go off (REG3) from now. Thus (REG3) is to be the on-time. Again 8 state times are provided by the NOPs for that command to leave the Holding Register for the CAM FILE. The third command places 30 into HSOCOM to turn HSO.0 back on (completion of one pulse) with the generation of an HSO interrupt. T1 + (REG2) is then placed into HSOTIME ensuring that HSO.0 is to go on (REG2) from now. Since (REG2) = 2 x (REG3), the off-time will also equal (REG3) so that a square wave (50% duty cycle) is guaranteed. Finally a return to where the call of CAMLOAD was made is to be executed.

The HSO ISR at 2180 is simple. It is entered only at the end of the generation of another pulse, since an HSO interrupt was specified to occur ONLY after the third and last command (HSO.0 to go on) was entered into the CAM FILE. When entered, the CAM FILE is empty since the three previous commands were executed by this time. The HSO ISR reloads the CAM FILE with the same three commands by calling CAMLOAD. This will cause the generation of another pulse. The program then returns from the HSO ISR to the point where the HSO interrupt occurred.

The A/D "conversion complete" ISR at 2183 reads in the high byte (bits 9-2) of the 10-bit conversion result from ADRESHI into REG1HI, and the byte ad ADRESLO into REG1LO. Remember, bits 1 and 0 of the conversion result are located at bits 7 and 6, respectively, of ADRESLO. The WORD in REG1 is thus A/D9, ... A/D2, A/D1, A/D0, X, X, S, U, V, W where S is the status bit (0 here since the conversion is over) and U, V, W gives the A/D channel number (0 here i.e. U = V = W = 0 in our case). To have REG1 contain the proper 10-bit result (i.e. as the legitimate 10-bits of the word) clearly requires a shift right of the contents of REG1 6 times. Hence the SHR REG1, #06 instruction. The upper 6 bits in REG1 will be all 0s after the 6 shifts. For the reasons already discussed in sections (3) and (4) of the FORMULATION, this result is to be subtracted from 7FFH. That is accomplished by the loading of REG3 with 07FF and then subtracting of REG1 from REG3. This leaves 07FF - (REG1) remaining in REG3, which is what we wanted. Remember, REG3 becomes the on-time of the pulses generated at HSO.0 (see CAMLOAD routine at 2165). The 3-operand instruction ADD REG2, REG3, REG3 conveniently doubles REG3's value and deposits it in REG2 without affecting the contents of REG3. Remember, also, that REG2 is to be the time HSO.0 goes back on after having first gone on, then off. Since REG2 = 2 (REG3) this guarantees on = off times. Finally 08 is loaded into ADCOM to start another conversion on ACH.0 to update the 10-bit conversion. A return to where the A/D "conversion complete" interrupt occurred is then to be executed. NOTE THAT THE PERIOD WILL BE T = 2 x

(REG3) x 2 USEC. AND THE FREQUENCY WILL BE:
F = 1/T = 250 KHz/(REG3) = 250 KHz/(07FF-VAD) WHERE VAD IS THE CONVERTED INPUT VOLTAGE IN REG1.

PROCEDURE

1. Reset and enter BY 09 = 00. Connect a 0-5V POT to channel ACH.0 at P0.0. Set the POT to 0V. Connect the output from HSO.0 to your scope to observe the square waves generated by the HSO unit.
2. Enter WO 70 = (REG3) = 01FF and WO 60 (REG2) = 03FF. This ensures a definite initial frequency for the first pulse before the first A/D conversion is complete (42 usec). At that time the A/D "conversion complete" ISR will ITSELF load REG3 and REG2 on the basis of the 10-bit conversion result, as already discussed and explained. The initial loadings of 01FF and 03FF above specify 1022 usec. on and off-times or an initial transient frequency of about 500 Hz for the first pulse.
3. Execute from 2140. Observe the waveform on the scope. Measure its frequency.
4. Vary the POT position, measuring the voltage it generates into ACH.0 for each setting. Measure the corresponding frequency of the square waves observed on the scope. Frequency should go up as input voltage increases.
5. Here were our results: (excellent agreement with formula's predictions on 2nd line at top of this page):

POT VOLTAGE	SQUARE WAVE FREQUENCY (Hz)
0.00V	121 Hz
0.51	132
1.04	139
1.50	143
2.08	156
2.53	167
3.05	179
3.51	192
3.99	208
4.50	227
4.70	238

PROBLEM

The frequency response is not linear with respect to the input control voltage. The way we have programmed (REG3) causes the output frequency to be given by 250 KHz/(07FF - VAD), as already noted. This causes frequency to increase with voltage in a hyperbolic manner. Develop another algorithm that will cause the output frequency to increase linearly with voltage. Then modify the program accordingly. One approach might be to have on-time REG3 = 7FF/VAD with VAD restricted to 0 to 1.25 volts (00 to FF). This will involve a 16-bit by 8-bit divide with the 8 bit quotient residing in the low byte of REG3 and the remainder residing in the high byte of REG3. In this case you'd again first load REG3 with #07FF and then use the instruction DIVUB REG3, REG1LO. As noted, the quotient Q remains in REG3LO while the remainder R will be found in REG3HI. REG1, as before, holds the AD conversion WORD and REG1LO gives the 8 BIT conversion result in the range 0-1.25V. The trick will be to convert Q and R into PROPER FORM in REG3 for it to be properly treated by the HSO unit as a legitimate quantity in the ADD HSOTIME, T1, REG3 instruction in the CAMLOAD routine. Note that the period will be T = 2 x (REG3) x 2 usec. = 2 x (7FF/VAD) x 2 usec. so the frequency response will be linear with respect to V i.e. 1/T = 250 KHz x VAD/7FF.

NOTE

This experiment on VOLTAGE-TO-FREQUENCY CONVERSION has important application in "SENSOR TELEMETRY" where the temperature, or other, sensor's output voltage would be converted to frequency for transmission by telemetric methods over long distances. At the receiving end the frequency would be converted to a byte (or word) in e.g. timer T2 (SEE EXPT. 9-19: A FREQUENCY COUNTER USING T2). Thus, the size of the byte or word in T2 would represent frequency, which in turn represents voltage (e.g. table on p. 470), which in turn corresponds to the magnitude of temperature or other sensed parameter (e.g. see Expt. 9-13 on temperature sensing and control). Once the calibration relating the magnitude of the sensed parameter (pressure, temperature, etc.) to magnitude of received frequency (byte or word in T2) is made, look-up tables can be constructed at the receiver to fetch the magnitude of actual temperature or other sensed physical quantity corresponding to the magnitude of the frequency (byte or word) received in T2.

EXPERIMENT 9-3

A BANDPASS FREQUENCY DISCRIMINATOR IN THE RANGE 0 - 250 KHz.

INTRODUCTION

Another device useful in communications (be it audio, video, or higher frequencies) is the frequency DISCRIMINATOR. This passes certain desired frequencies as is, and blocks others. It is not to be confused with a FILTER (see later experiment in this chapter on a digital filter). The filter ATTENUATES certain frequencies MUCH LESS than other frequencies (giving rise to 3 db points, etc). In this experiment we'll have the 8096 pass ANY DESIRED BAND of frequencies input to it from a pulse generator (TTL levels), and completely block all frequencies outside this band. Timer T2 on the 8096 will be used to implement the discriminator. The fact that it can record 0 to 1 and 1 to 0 transitions separated in time by 2 usec. is responsible for range coverage from 1 to 250 KHz.

FORMULATION AND APPROACH

1. The output of a 0-250 KHz pulse generator (set for 50% duty cycle) is input to both the T2CLK source for timer T2 events and to one input of a 2-input AND gate (7408). The output line P2.7 will be the other input to the AND gate. The output of the AND gate is connected to a scope.
2. As the pulse generator's frequency is varied, port P1's LEDs will display that frequency and the scope will display the pulses, if the frequency is within the pass-band.
3. The desired lower and upper limits of the pass-band are entered outside the program code at run-time (at 5000 and 5002).
4. After the program is executed, the output pulses from the AND gate are observed on the scope. As the frequency of the pulse generator is varied, the scope will show no pulses as long as the frequency is outside the entered band limits. As soon as the input frequency at T2CLK enters the pass-band, that very frequency will be observed on the scope as pulses. As the input frequency varies upward from the lower limit of the pass-band we'll continue to observe the pulses from the gate on the scope, with the same frequency as that input to T2CLK from the pulse generator. The moment the input frequency exceeds the upper limit of the desired pass-band, the pulses on the scope will disappear.

5. The program will first generate a 2 MSEC. delay before reading T2 and divide it by 4 to get the true number of PULSES recorded in T2 in 1 MSEC. That value is the input frequency in KHz. The program then displays it (in HEX) at P1's LEDs. It next compares it with the low limit of the band-pass (entered at 5000 at run-time). If the frequency is less than or equal to the low limit of the band, port P2 (GATE) is ANDed with #7F. This makes P2.7 = 0, so no output pulses appear at the output of the AND gate. Similarly, a comparison of the input frequency is made with the upper limit of the desired band-pass (entered at 5002 at run-time). If the frequency is greater than that upper limit, GATE is again ANDed with 7F, so that P2.7 is still 0. Pulses are again blocked. If, however, the two comparisons fail, indicating that we are WITHIN the pass-band's limits, GATE is ORed with #80. This makes P2.7 = 1 and the AND gate passes the pulses to the scope.

The program at 21B0 is presented below and analyzed afterward.

```
        18 00           SP      EQU     18H
        15 00           IOCO    EQU     15H
        40 00           REG     EQU     40H
        50 00           REG1    EQU     50H
        0C 00           T2      EQU     0CH
        0E 00           P0      EQU     0EH
        0F 00           P1      EQU     0FH
        10 00           P2      EQU     10H
        10 00           GATE    EQU     P2

21B0                            ORG     21B0H
                        ;
21B0    A1 C0 00 18             LD      SP,#00C0H       ;Initialize SP.
21B4    71 7F 10        BLOCK:  ANDB    GATE,#7FH       ;And GATE with 7F to make P2.7=0.
21B7    B1 02 15        CLRT2:  LDB     IOCO,#02H       ;T2CLK chosen as source for T2.
                                                        ;T2 is reset.
21BA    A1 9B 02 40             LD      REG,#029BH      ;Load REG for 2 msec. delay.
21BE    05 40           DELAY:  DEC     REG             ;Decrement REG.
21C0    D7 FC                   JNE     DELAY           ;If REG != 0, jump to DELAY.
21C2    A0 0C 50                LD      REG1,T2         ;Else read value in T2 into REG1.
21C5    07 50                   INC     REG1            ;Increment REG1.
21C7    08 02 50                SHR     REG1,#02H       ;Divide by 4 to get true # of pulses
                                                        ;recorded in T2 in 1 msec.
21CA    B0 50 0F                LDB     P1,REG1         ;Display freq. in KHz at P1's LEDs.
21CD    8B 01 00 50 50          CMP     REG1,5000H[0]   ;Compare recorded freq. with low
                                                        ;limit freq. of bandpass.
```

```
21D2  D1 E0                     JNH   BLOCK          ;If recorded freq. <= low limit,
                                                     ;jump to BLOCK. (Pulses blocked).
21D4  8B 01 02 50 50            CMP   REG1,5002H[0]  ;Else compare recorded freq. with
                                                     ;high limit freq. of bandpass.
21D9  D9 D9                     JH    BLOCK          ;If recorded freq. > high limit
                                                     ;jump to BLOCK. (Pulses blocked).
21DB  91 80 10         PASS:    ORB   GATE,#80H      ;Else OR GATE with 80H to let
                                                     ;pulses through.
21DE  27 D7                     SJMP  CLRT2          ;Jump to take another recording
                                                     ;of freq., letting pulses through.
21E0                            END
```

The program loads the Stack Pointer with 00C0 and ANDs GATE with 7FH. IOC0 is loaded with 02 to select T2CLK as the source of T2 events and to reset T2. Remember, the input pulse generator is connected to both T2CLK and to one input of the AND gate. REG is next loaded with 029B to provide for a 2 msec. delay. The latter is generated by the loop consisting of DEC REG and JNE DELAY. The loop consumes 12 state times (3 usec.) and, with REG = 29BH = 667 (dec), 2 msec. will be generated at 12 MHz. After the loop is exited, T2's count is read into REG1 which is then incremented and divided by 4 to arrive at the true number of PULSES recorded in T2 in 1 msec. REG1 now gives the generator's frequency in KHz. It is outputted from the low byte of REG1 for display at P1's LEDs. Remember, we are restricting our frequencies to 0-250 KHz. The frequency (REG1) is next compared with the desired low limit of the band-pass stored at 5000H. If it is not higher than that low limit, the JNH BLOCK instruction carries us back to BLOCK where GATE is again ANDed with 7F (P2.7 still 0, pulses still blocked) and another 2 msec. delay window to record T2 is entered.

If the frequency is larger than (5000H), fall-through the JNH instruction at 21D2 occurs to a comparison of REG1 with the upper limit of the band-pass stored at 5002H. If (REG1) is higher than the desired upper limit of the band-pass, JH BLOCK carries us back to BLOCK where GATE is again ANDed with 7F, thereby continuing to keep P2.7 at 0 and blocking pulses. Another 2 msec. delay is entered before the updated T2 is again recorded (note that both JNH BLOCK and JH BLOCK not only keep P2.7 at 0, but reset T2 because of the next instruction after BLOCK at CLRT2. Thus a fresh reading of T2 can be made after each 2 msec. window).

If the frequency in REG1 is in the band-pass range between lower and upper limits, fall-through JH BLOCK to PASS will occur. There we ORB GATE with #80 and then jump back to CLRT2 where T2 is reset in preparation for the next reading of T2 after the NEXT 2 msec. delay. Now P2.7 is 1 and the AND gate passes pulses on to the scope. Continual JNH and JH tests every 2 msec. will respond to any input frequency changes to block or pass pulses as appropriate.

PROCEDURE

1. Connect the TTL level pulse generator (0 to 250 KHz) to T2CLK (P2.3) and to one input of the AND gate. Connect P2.7 to the other input of the AND gate and the output of the AND gate to the input of a scope. Set the pulse generator at its lowest frequency setting and for a 50% duty cycle.
2. Reset and enter BY 09 = 00.
3. Enter band limits as follows: WO 5000 = 20H and WO 5002 = 24H. This specifies the band-pass to be 32-36 KHz.
4. Execute from 21B0. Slowly vary the pulse generator's frequency. As you do, verify that P1 reads that frequency correctly in HEX KHz as it varies over the range 0 to 250 KHz.
5. Observe the scope. You should see 0 there as the frequency is varied until 32KHz is reached, at which point pulses appear on the scope. Verify that their measured frequency on the scope agrees with P1 and the pulse generator's reading i.e. 32 KHz.
6. As frequency proceeds on up from 32KHz to 36KHz pulses keep appearing on the scope. Notice how their frequency keeps increasing, always matching the frequency displayed at P1 and read on the pulse generator (measure a few frequencies on the scope to verify this). When the frequency reaches 36+ KHz the pulses should abruptly disappear from the scope. Verify this by reading P1 and the pulse generator setting. As frequency continues to increase beyond 36 KHz no further pulses are seen on the scope.
7. On-the-fly enter WO 5000 = 10 and WO 5002 = 12, specifying a band-pass from 16 KHz to 18 KHz. Set the pulse generator at its lowest frequency and repeat the procedure, noting how this time the scope displays pulses in the 16-18 KHz band, but not outside of it.
8. Repeat for other specified band-pass limits in the range 0 to 250 KHz.

EXPERIMENT 9-4

FREQUENCY TRACKING

INTRODUCTION

Another important problem in communications is "frequency tracking". Information usually rides on a "carrier frequency" as modulation (AM or FM). Detection of that information is best and most efficiently done at much lower frequencies than the carrier (one reason being that losses in received energy and noise in the receiver system will be much lower and, therefore, system sensitivity higher. Another reason is that circuitry is simpler and standard at the lower frequency). One way conversion of the carrier to the lower ("intermediate") frequency is accomplished is to "mix" the carrier frequency with a "local oscillator" which differs from the carrier frequency by just the desired value of the intermediate frequency. The mixing is usually done in a non-linear (crystal) mixer and this generates all kinds of sum and difference frequencies between carrier and L.O. (Local Oscillator), including a d.c. component. A band-pass filter or discriminator (see Expt. 9-3 and the digital filter experiment later in the chapter) is then used to pass only the DIFFERENCE (intermediate) frequency. Clearly, it is important that, as carrier frequency varies, the L.O. frequency should be made to track it so that the difference will always be the same, otherwise that difference will change and fall outside of the band-pass with resulting loss of information. This frequency tracking is related to the subject of "phase-locked loops".

Now in Expt. 9-1 we implemented a linear frequency to voltage converter and in Expt. 9-2 we implemented a voltage-controlled oscillator (voltage to frequency converter). This suggests that the carrier frequency should be input to T2CLK of ONE iSBE-96, with the converted voltage taken from the filtered PWM output at P2.5 of that SBE and input to ACH.0 of ANOTHER iSBE-96. The output at HSO.0 of the latter will then be square waves with frequency a function of the voltage input to ACH.0 (as in Expt. 9-2) which in turn is a function of the frequency input to the first SBE. Thus we should load the first iSBE-96 with the program of Expt. 9-1 and load the second iSBE-96 with the program of Expt. 9-2. The output frequency f2 of the second SBE will be our local oscillator frequency which will track the carrier frequency f1 input to the first SBE. However, because of the program and results in Expt. 9-2, we would not expect this tracking of f2 vs. f1 to be linear. If you can solve the problem posed at the end of Expt. 9-2, the tracking will be linear. We do the experiment even though we do not expect linear results. We want to open up possibilities.

To have a lower and smaller input frequency range control the output frequency range, we'll use a 0.2 sec. delay window in the program of Expt. 9-1 i.e. enter BY 210B = 0FF, 0FF there. As we saw on p. 464, this will give PWM output voltages at SBE #1 of 0.89V, 1.76V, 2.75V, 3.71V, and 4.65V for input frequencies f1 = 250 Hz, 500 Hz, 750 Hz, 1000 Hz, and 1250 Hz, respectively. From Expt. 9-2, p. 470, these voltages into the A/D of SBE #2 will produce HSO.0 output square wave frequencies (f2) there of abut 137 Hz to about 238 Hz as f1 ranges from 250 Hz to 1250 Hz.

PROCEDURE

1. Connect the output (f1) of a pulse generator (TTL square wave) to T2CLK (P2.3) of SBE #1. Connect the filtered output voltage at its PWM (P2.5) pin to ACH.0 of SBE #2. Connect the HSO.0 output (f2) of SBE #2 to a scope to measure frequencies f2.
2. Enter the program of Expt. 9-1 into SBE #1 and that of Expt. 9-2 into SBE #2. Enter BY 210B = 0FF, 0FF in SBE #1 for 0.2 sec. delay.
3. Reset each unit and enter BY 09 = 00 in each.
4. Execute SBE #1 from 2100 and SBE #2 from 2140.
5. Measure HSO.0's frequency, f2, on the scope as f1 at the pulse generator is made to vary. Record values.
6. Record also PWM (= P1) and voltage at P2.5 on SBE #1.
7. Here were our results for input vs. output (F1, F2) frequencies:

F1 (Hz)	PWM = P1	PWM VOUT	HSO.0, F2 (Hz)
250 Hz	32H	0.89V	132 Hz
500	62H	1.76V	156
750	98H	2.75V	167
1000	CBH	3.71V	200
1250	FAH	4.65V	238

Disregarding slight differences in the PWM column relative to the results on p. 464 (Expt. 9-1), the results show how nicely f1 controls f2. The relationship F2(f1) is certainly NOT linear. Refer back to the problem at the end of Expt. 9-2 re: the F2(V) linearity question. PROBLEM: What would you do with #7FF in Expt. 9-2 to change the f2 frequency range, and/or with the delay window at 210B, C in Expt. 9-1 to change the f1 frequency range (e.g. make it 1 sec.)?

EXPERIMENT 9-5

AN HSO-BASED SQUARE WAVE FREQUENCY SYNTHESIZER.

INTRODUCTION

In this experiment we'll have the HSO unit produce a square wave output at HSO.0, in which the frequency will be controlled at run-time (and thereafter on-the-fly) by the magnitude of the keyboard entry. To be more precise, entering WO 60 = 30 (REG = 60H) will produce a 30 Hz square wave; entering WO 60 = 60 will give 60 Hz; entering WO 60 = 120 will yield 120 Hz at HSO.0; WO 60 = 240 or WO 60 = 480 or WO 60 = 960 will produce 240 Hz or 480 Hz or 960 Hz, respectively. In other words, we shall implement a "frequency synthesizer".

We'll restrict the experiment to the above frequencies and keyboard inputs WITHOUT ANY LOSS IN GENERALITY. We wish to demonstrate the method. You should have no difficulty in producing frequencies well BEYOND the above-cited range and many frequencies IN BETWEEN those listed above, using the EXACT same program. That all depends on how large a look-up table you are prepared to use to store the necessary information that converts keyboard-inputted desired frequency to the required time word to be passed to the HSOTIME register. The latter, of course, controls the on/off times of the HSO-produced pulses. We are keeping things simple here with a short look-up table to illustrate the approach.

FORMULATION AND APPROACH.

To construct the look-up table, we proceed as follows: 30 Hz translates to about a 33 msec. period or to about 16 msec. on-off times. 16 msec. on-time will be produced if T1 + #2000H (approx.) is placed in HSOTIME after HSOCOM is loaded with the correct Command Tag. 2000H = 8192 (dec) which when multiplied by 2 usec. gives us about 16 msec. (we could be more exact by taking a 33.33 msec. period and a 16.67 msec. on/off time, and the precise necessary value to be added to T1). Similarly 60 Hz translates to about a 16 msec. period or to about 8 msec. on/off times. This will require T1 + #1000H be placed in HSOTIME after the correct Command Tag is loaded into HSOCOM. In the same way we can arrive at the required time words to produce 120 Hz, 240 Hz, 480 Hz, and 960 Hz. This leads to the following look-up table that must be accessed:

ADDRESS	INTERVAL FOR HSOTIME	FREQUENCY
5030	2000	30 Hz
5060	1000	60
5120	0800	120
5240	0400	240
5480	0200	480
5960	0100	960

In the CAML (Cam Load) routine in the program presented and analyzed below, you'll note what we do BEFORE any commands are entered in the CAM: we employ the instruction ADD REG1, REG, #5000H. This adds 5000 to REG (where REG is determined upon entering WO 60 = "value" at run-time or therafter on-the-fly), with the result stored in REG1. Thus if WO 60 is entered as 30, 60, 120, etc., 5030 or 5060 or 5120 or...5960 will be stored in REG1. REG1 then becomes the pointer into the above table so that a LD REG1, [REG1] instruction will fetch either 2000, or 1000, or 0800, etc. and store it in REG1. The ADD REG2, REG1, REG1 doubles any of those values and stores the result in REG2. REG1 will become the on-time when ADD HSOTIME, T1, REG1 is later executed and REG2 will become the period when ADD HSOTIME, T1, REG2 is then executed. This guarantees square wave output at HSO.0. This will be discussed in detail after the program is presented and analyzed below.

The program at 2200 is presented below. It is analyzed afterward.

```
        18 00        SP       EQU   18H
        06 20        INVEC    EQU   2006H
        04 00        HSOTIME  EQU   04H
        06 00        HSOCOM   EQU   06H
        40 00        TEMP     EQU   40H
        60 00        REG      EQU   60H
        70 00        REG1     EQU   70H
        80 00        REG2     EQU   80H
        08 00        MINT     EQU   08H
        09 00        PINT     EQU   09H
        0A 00        T1       EQU   0AH

2200                          ORG   2200H
                     ;
2200    A1 C0 00 18           LD    SP,#00C0H          ;Initialize SP.
2204    FA                    DI                       ;Disable interrupts.
2205    B1 08 08              LDB   MINT,#08H          ;Unmask HSO interrupt source.
2208    A1 40 22 40           LD    TEMP,#HSOINT       ;Load address of HSO ISR into
220C    C3 01 06 20 40        ST    TEMP,INVEC[0]      ;HSO VECT INT table location.
2211    11 09                 CLRB  PINT               ;Clear pendings.
```

```
2213  FB                        EI                       ;Enable interrupts.
2214  EF 02 00                  CALL   CAML              ;Call CAML to program HSO unit
                                                         ;for one pulse.
2217  27 FE           HERE:     SJMP   HERE              ;Loop ("busy tasks").
                      ;
                      ;
                      ;         CAM LOAD ROUTINE
                      ;
2219  45 00 50 60 70  CAML:     ADD    REG1,REG,#5000H   ;Add 5000 to (REG) and store in
                                                         ;REG1.  Becomes pointer to table
                                                         ;of necessary time words.
221E  A2 70 70                  LD     REG1,[REG1]       ;Fetch word at the location in the
                                                         ;table pointed to by (REG1) and
                                                         ;store in REG1.
2221  44 70 70 80               ADD    REG2,REG1,REG1    ;Add (REG1) to itself and store in
                                                         ;REG2.  Doubles REG1's value.
2225  B1 20 06                  LDB    HSOCOM,#20H       ;Load HSOCOM with command to turn
                                                         ;HSO.0 on (without HSO interrupt).
2228  45 03 00 0A 04            ADD    HSOTIME,T1,#0003H ;HSO.0 is to go on "now".
222D  FD                        NOP                      ;8 state times needed before next
222E  FD                        NOP                      ;entry into H.R. can be made.
222F  B1 00 06                  LDB    HSOCOM,#00H       ;Command to turn HSO.0 off (no HSO
                                                         ;intr.).
2232  44 70 0A 04               ADD    HSOTIME,T1,REG1   ;(REG1) + T1 loaded into HSOTIME
                                                         ;specifies that HSO.0 is to go off
                                                         ;(REG1) from "now".
2236  FD                        NOP                      ;8 state times needed.
2237  FD                        NOP                      ;
2238  B1 30 06                  LDB    HSOCOM,#30H       ;Command to turn HSO.0 on (with
                                                         ;HSO intr.).
223B  44 80 0A 04               ADD    HSOTIME,T1,REG2   ;HSO.0 is to go back on (REG2)
                                                         ;from now where (REG2) = 2(REG1)
                                                         ;i.e. square wave.
223F  F0                        RET                      ;Return.
                      ;
                      ;         HSO INTERRUPT SERVICE ROUTINE
                      ;
2240  2F D7           HSOINT:   CALL   CAML              ;A complete pulse (on,off,on) was
                                                         ;generated.  Program HSO unit for
                                                         ;generation of another pulse.
2242  F0                        RET                      ;Return.
2243                            END
```

After the stack pointer is initialized and the interrupt system disabled, the HSO interrupt source is unmasked. The address of the HSO ISR (#HSOINT) is then loaded into address 2006 in the interrupt vector location table. Pendings are cleared and the interrupt system enabled. The CAML (CAM Load) routine at 2219 is then called to generate one square pulse after which SJMP HERE simulates "other tasks".

The CAML Routine at 2219 adds 5000 to REG and stores the result in REG1. REG is to be entered at run-time or on-the-fly as WO 60 = 30, 60, 120, 240, 480, or 960. Thus REG1 = 5030, 5060, ... or 5960 and becomes the pointer into the table discussed and presented in the formulation. The next instruction in CAML fetches the word 2000, 1000, 0800, ... or 0100 stored at [REG1] in the table and loads it back into REG1. That word is then doubled in value by the 3-operand instruction ADD REG2, REG1, REG1 with REG2 holding that doubled value. The next two instructions specify that HSO.0 is to go on "now" without generation of any HSO interrupt. Two NOPs allow that command to enter the CAM from the Holding Register before another command is to be written into the H.R. That next command specifies that HSO.0 is to go off (REG1) from "now" (precisely the 2000 or 1000 or 0800 etc. fetched from the table previously). Again no HSO interrupt is to be generated. After another two NOPs, the third and final command for the CAM is written: HSO.0 is to go back on (REG2) = 2(REG1) from "now", WITH generation of an interrupt. This guarantees a square wave of the correct period to produce either 30 Hz, 60 Hz, ... or 960 Hz, as the case may be. Finally a return to the point where the call was made is to be executed. That return will be to HERE in the main program after the CALL at 2214 is executed.

During "busy tasks" at HERE the CAM's commands are being executed out of the CAM. When the first pulse is thereby generated at HSO.0, the HSO interrupt generated at the COMPLETION of that pulse causes a vector entry to the HSO ISR at 2240. There CAML is called to replenish the CAM with the same three commands as before to generate another pulse. The return from CAML is to the return at 2242 which takes us back to "busy tasks" at HERE. In that way continuous square wave pulse generation is assured with precisely the frequency given by the word entered into 60 (REG) at run-time or on-the-fly i.e. 30 Hz for WO 60 = 30, 60 Hz for WO 60 = 60, etc.

PROCEDURE

1. Reset and enter BY 09 = 00. Connect the HSO.0 output to a scope to observe and measure the frequency of the pulses.
2. Enter the look-up table discussed and presented in the FORMULATION section starting with WO 5030 = 2000 and ending with WO 5960 = 0100.
3. Enter WO 60 = 30 to ensure that when the program is first executed a 30 Hz square wave will be output at HSO.0.

4. Execute from 2200. Observe the pulse train on the scope. Measure its frequency. We found a 30.3 Hz square wave.
5. On-the-fly enter WO 60 = 60. Observe the scope. We found a square wave of frequency 60.9 Hz. Change WO 60 to 120, then to 240, then to 480, then to 960. In each case we observed 123 Hz, 245 Hz, 490 Hz and 981 Hz. The differences are accounted for by our taking the on-time for e.g. the 30 Hz pulse to be 2000H x 2 usec. = 16.4 msec. instead of 208FH which would give the exact 16.67 msec. required for a 30 Hz pulse train. The same considerations apply to the other table entries. A more accurate table would certainly give frequency outputs corresponding exactly to the frequency requested from the keyboard.

PROBLEM

Construct an algorithm that will allow you to convert any desired frequency inputted from the keyboard to the correct REG1, REG2 values to generate the pulse train at HSO.0 with the correct requested frequency. This would do away with table look up and the need for large memory storage to cover a wide frequency band with fine granularity.

NOTE

The two instructions at 2219, 221E could easily have been combined into the one instruction LD REG1, 5000H[REG].

EXPERIMENT 9-6

A "SQUARE LAW" DETECTOR IMPLEMENTED WITH THE 8096 TO MEASURE POWER.

INTRODUCTION

There are many situations in nature where the output from a device is a non-linear function of the input (current out of a crystal detector vs. input voltage, for example; or the "3/2" law found in many physical response situations). In the area of communications, one is mainly interested in received power, not voltage or electric field. Thus, for example, information imposed on a carrier wave in the form of a modulation can be retrieved at the receiver by first having some sort of filter block or ground the high frequency carrier leaving only the varying voltage envelope (if AM) for detection. Since it is power level that is of interest, the detection device (crystal, for example) should be "square law" i.e. output is to be proportional to the SQUARE of the voltage envelope at the input.

The arithmetic features of the 8096 make it well suited to implement non-linear relationships in software because of its multiply and divide capability. In that case the need for the square law crustal or other hardware would be obviated.

In this experiment, we'll input a voltage (0 to 5V) from a potentiometer into the A/D channel ACH.0. This voltage, Vin, SIMULATES the VOLTAGE level of the FILTERED carrier wave. We wish to detect and display the POWER in that signal. Thus we want Vout to be proportional to the square of Vin. The way we'll accomplish that is by using the multiply and divide instructions to square the NORMALIZED input (relative to 5 Volts max. -- or to the 3FF 10-bit conversion result corresponding to 5V max. input), and then having that squared value loaded into the PWM to produce the output voltage (integrated) at the PWM (P2.5) pin. Thus if UVWX is the 10-bit conversion of Vin at ACH.0 and 03FF is the 10-bit conversion that would result if 5V were at the input, we are asking that Vout be the following FRACTION of a FULL 5V output at the PWM pin: UVWX/03FF squared. Or Vout = [UVWX/03FF] EXP2 x 5V. Since 5V output at the PWM pin corresponds to FF in the PWM SFR, the required value needed for the PWM to produce the desired Vout is given by:

PWM BYTE VALUE = [UVWX/03FF] EXP2 x FF = [UVWX] EXP2/0FFF,

with Vout at P2.5 proportional to that PWM byte value. The square of UVWX will be implemented with a 3-operand 16-bit by 16-bit multiply i.e. UVWX by UVWX, giving a 32-bit result. The 32-bit result will then be divided by the 16-bit quantity 0FFF to give a 16-bit quotient and a 16-bit remainder. It is the quotient that we'll load into the PWM register. Since the maximum value obtained in the last formula will occur for UVWX = 3FF (5 volt input), we see that the formula in that case would give 256 = FF. Thus the quotient will be no higher than FF and hence it is the LOW BYTE of the "16-bit" quotient that is involved. That low-byte will be loaded into the PWM to produce the square law output Vout at P2.5 relative to the input Vin at ACH.0.

The program that implements this software square law detector is given below at 2280. It is analyzed at its conclusion.

```
      18 00          SP       EQU     18H
      16 00          IOC1     EQU     16H
      17 00          PWM      EQU     17H
      02 00          ADCOM    EQU     02H
      03 00          ADRESHI  EQU     03H
      02 00          ADRESLO  EQU     02H
      40 00          REG      EQU     40H
      41 00          REGHI    EQU     41H
      40 00          REGLO    EQU     40H
      50 00          REG1     EQU     50H
      60 00          REG2     EQU     60H
      50 00          IREG     EQU     50H

2280                          ORG     2280H
                     ;
2280  A1 C0 00 18             LD      SP,#00C0H         ;Initialize SP.
2284  B1 01 16                LDB     IOC1,#01H         ;Select P2.5 in PWM function.
2287  B1 08 02       CONVERT:LDB      ADCOM,#08H        ;Start conversion at ACH.0 now.
228A  FD                      NOP                       ;Need 8 state times.
228B  FD                      NOP                       ;
228C  3B 02 FD       BUSY:    JBS     ADRESLO,3,BUSY    ;Poll bit 3 of ADRESLO (S bit).
                                                        ;If hi, conversion not over.
                                                        ;Loop on BUSY.
228F  B0 03 41                LDB     REGHI,ADRESHI     ;Conversion over. Load bits 9-2
                                                        ;of result into REGHI.
2292  B0 02 40                LDB     REGLO,ADRESLO     ;Load ADRESLO into REGLO. Bits
                                                        ;1,0 of conversion result will be
                                                        ;in bits 7,6 of REGLO.
2295  08 06 40                SHR     REG,#06H          ;Shift right 6 times to form proper
                                                        ;word for the 10 bit conversion
                                                        ;result.
```

```
2298  4C 40 40 50         MULU  IREG,REG,REG   ;Square the conversion result and
                                               ;store 32 bit result in IREG.
229C  8D FF 0F 50         DIVU  IREG,#0FFFH    ;Divide result by 4095 to normalize.
                                               ;Stores quotient in low word of
                                               ;IREG and remainder in high word of
                                               ;IREG.
22A0  B0 50 17            LDB   PWM,REG1       ;Store low byte of quotient into
                                               ;PWM (high byte of quotient is 0).
22A3  B1 FF 60            LDB   REG2,#0FFH     ;Load time delay register.
22A6  E0 60 FD    DELAY:  DJNZ  REG2,DELAY     ;Decrement and test. If REG2 != 0
                                               ;goto to DELAY.
22A9  27 DC               SJMP  CONVERT        ;Else jump to CONVERT to start another
                                               ;conversion.
```

After SP is intitialized, 01 is loaded into IOC1 to select P2.5 in its PWM mode. 08 loaded into ADCOM starts conversion on channel 0. The two NOPs are needed for the 8 state times before conversion actually starts. JBS then polls the S bit of ADRES-LO. As long as it's high, conversion is not over and we remain in the BUSY loop. When conversion is over, S is low and we fall through the JBS instruction to the first of two LDB instructions. The first one loads bits 9-2 of the conversion result into REGHI, the second loads bits 1, 0 of the result into bits 7, 6 of REGLO. To produce a proper 10-bit result in a 16-bit register, SHR REG, #06 is employed. This shifts all the bits in REG (composed of the REGLO and REGHI 8-bit registers) to the right 6 times. The result will be that bits 7-0 of the conversion result will appear in REGLO and bits 9, 8 of the result will appear at bits 1 and 0 of REGHI with the other 6 bits in REGHI equal to 0. This gives us UVWX in REG.

Next, REG (= REGHI, REGLO) is multiplied by itself with the result [UVWX] EXP2 being stored in the 32-bit register IREG at 60 (low word in 50, 51; high word in 52, 53). The instruction is MULU IREG, REG, REG. That 32-bit result in IREG is then divided by 0FFF (DIVU IREG, #0FFFH), with the quotient (word) appearing in IREGLO (50, 51) and the remainder (word) appearing in IREGHI (52, 53). Remember, as was shown previously, the quotient will be an 8 bit result so it is the byte in byte register REG1 (50) that we want to load into PWM. This we do at 22A0 in the program. Remember from the experiments in chapter 5 and 6 involving the PWM that 64 usec. are needed before the PWM can be reloaded to possibly change its duty cycle (and filtered output voltage level) i.e. 64 usec. is the fixed PWM output period. We, therefore, program in a time delay at 22A3, 22A6. The time delay chosen is far more than needed i.e with FF in REG2 the delay will be 576 usec. (loading REG2 with 1DH would give about 65 usec). SJMP CONVERT then loops back to 2287 to start another conversion.

And that is how we've employed the 3-operand 16 x 16 bit multiply and the 32 by 16 bit divide to achieve square law detection, thanks to the 8096's arithmetic capabilities.

PROCEDURE

1. Connect a 0 to 5V potentiometer to the input at ACH.0. Measure filtered (integrated) d.c. output voltages at P2.5 (PWM) as well as the corresponding input voltages at the POT.
2. Reset. Enter BY 09 = 00.
3. Execute from 2280.
4. Set the POT for 1, 2, 3, and 4 volts in turn. Measure the corresponding voltages at the filtered PWM output. Confirm the square law characteristic i.e. each double of Vin should quadruple Vout; each triple of Vin should result in Vout going up by a factor of 9. A quadruple in Vin should result in Vout going up by a factor of 16, etc.
5. Our results were as follows:

VIN	VOUT MEASURED	VOUT EXPECTED
1.00V	0.290V	0.290V
2.00	1.14	1.16
3.00	2.50	2.61
4.00	4.60	4.64

   The results are quite good. Errors may be due to the PWM filter.
6. ESC. Replace REG1 (50) at 22A1 by REGHI (41) and place NOPs (0FD) at 2295-97. Re-run and measure Vout vs. Vin. The results should now be linear. Why?

PROBLEM

Think up other physical situations where Vout should be some other non-linear function of Vin. Implement them in software.

EXPERIMENT 9-7

USING THE HSI UNIT TO CALIBRATE ONE PULSE GENERATOR'S FREQUENCY (UNKNOWN) AGAINST ANOTHER'S (STANDARD).

INTRODUCTION

Frequency calibration is an important application in the field of instrumentation. In this experiment we shall employ two 0 to 500 KHz (50% duty cycle, TTL level) pulse generators to illustrate how the HSI unit can be employed to calibrate one frequency source (the unknown) against another frequency source (the standard). Frequency measurement errors and restrictions are discussed when employing the HSI unit.

FORMULATION AND APPROACH.

1. P.G.#1 (Pulse Generator 1) with variable known output frequency f1 (the "standard") is connected to input pin HSI.0 of the 8096.
2. P.G.#2 (Pulse Generator 2) with variable output frequency f2 (the "unknown") is connected to input pin HSI.1 of the 8096.
3. As f1 ("standard") is varied, with f2 set at a fixed, "unknown" value, a LED at P2.7 stays off as long as f2 and f1 are not equal. When f1 = f2, P2.7 goes on to indicate equality. The correct output frequency of the "unknown" P.G.#2 is then the KNOWN value of f1 read on the "standard" (P.G.#1).
4. Word REG2 (52H) will hold the changing period of the "standard" as f1 is varied. When f1 = f2, and P2.7 = 1, the reciprocal of that period is the frequency, f1, of the "standard", and that frequency in turn is the frequency of the "unknown", f2. Further, REG5 (62H) holds the period of the unknown.
5. The approach to the solution of the problem employing the HSI unit is as follows:
   a). The HSI interrupt source is unmasked and P2.7 is cleared.
   b). The mode is selected that allows only positive transitions on HSI.0 and HSI.1 to enter the HSI unit's FIFO.
   c). Initially, HSI.0 is enabled into the FIFO and HSI.1 is disabled.
   d). HSI interrupts are to occur only when the FIFO becomes full.

e). As positive transitions from f1 (the standard's frequency) enter the FIFO through HSI.0, an HSI interrupt will occur after the FIFO becomes full of those transitions. The HSI ISR is then entered.

f). The HSI ISR will disable HSI.0 and HSI.1 from the FIFO as it is being read out and cleared out. HSI STATUS is tested to confirm that it was NOT an event (s) on HSI.1 that occurred.

g). The times of the first two positive transitions on the standard (f1) are read into REG1 and REG2, respectively, and REG2 - REG1 will give the period of the standard f1. It, in turn, is stored in REG2.

h). Successive readings of HSITIME are made until the HSI Holding Register is finally empty (as indicated by bit IOS1.7 "HSI Holding Register Data Available" going low). The FIFO is then empty.

i). At that point HSI.1 is enabled into the FIFO with HSI.0 remaining disabled.

j). Return to the main program ("other tasks") is then made. Positive transitions on f2 (unknown) at HSI.1 are now recorded in the FIFO till it's again full when another interrupt to the HSI ISR occurs.

k). The ISR disables HSI.0 and HSI.1 from the FIFO and tests HSISTATUS to confirm that the event(s) occurred on HSI.1, not HSI.0.

l). The times of the first two positive transitions on the unknown (f2) are read into REG4 and REG5, respectively. REG5 - REG4 gives the period of the unknown f2. It is stored in REG5.

m). Successive readings of HSITIME are made until the HSI Holding Register is empty (IOS1.7 goes low). The FIFO is again empty.

n). The periods stored in REG2 (standard) and REG5 (unknown) are then compared. If they are unequal, P2.7 is kept at 0, HSI.0 is re-enabled, HSI.1 is kept disabled, and a return to the main program is made where positive transitions on f1 (standard) at HSI.0 are again recorded in the FIFO till it again becomes full and another HSI interrupt occurs. And so on, back and forth between alternate HSI.0 and HSI.1 FIFO recordings and alternate interrupts to the ISR.

o). If the comparison of REG2 with REG5 shows they are equal, P2.7 is set to 1 and HSI.0 is enabled, HSI.1 disabled and a return to the main program occurs where HSI.0 (f1) positive transitions are again recorded in the FIFO till it's full and another HSI interrupt occurs, whereupon alternate recordings of transitions into the FIFO from HSI.0 and HSI.1 are resumed.

THE PROGRAM

The program at 22C0 is shown below. In view of the detailed description of the approach to the program presented in 5(a) through 5(o) above, we will not analyze the program. The commentary in the program below, together with the discussion in section (5) of the FORMULATION AND APPROACH above, should make the program quite clear. Remember, however, several points: 1) Each reading of HSITIME empties the Holding Register and allows another FIFO entry to fall down into the H.R. to be read. Successive HSITIME readings will thus eventually clear the FIFO. 2) IOS1.7 going low is the indication that the FIFO is empty (no more "HSI Holding Register Data Available"). Hence the need to test IOS1.7 in the ISR routine. 3) readings of HSITIME should be separated by 8 state times since it may take that long after the first reading for the NEXT FIFO entry to fall into the H.R. before it, too, can successfully be read. Hence our use of two NOPs between readings of HSITIME into REG1 and then into REG2 (or into REG4 and then into REG5). The JBS IOS1, 7, EMPFIF (or CLRFIF) instruction consumes 9 state times before another reading of HSITIME is made (on the way to clearing the FIFO) - hence no problem there or the need to insert NOPs. 4) JBS HSISTAT, 2, HSI1 tests bit 2 of the HSISTATUS register. If that bit is 1, it's an indication that a transition (event) recorded in the FIFO was made on pin HSI.1 AT THE TIME RECORDED IN THE FIFO, and NOT on HSI.0 (since, if HSI.1 is enabled, HSI.0 is disabled and vice-versa). In that case the jump is to HSI1 where the period of f2 (unknown) (HSI.1 transitions) is determined. If, however, HSISTATUS.2 is 0, it has to mean that events occurred on HSI.0 (otherwise we'd not be in the HSI ISR due to the FIFO full interrupt). In that case fall-through the JBS instruction occurs and the period of f1 (standard) (HSI.0 transitions) is determined.

```
18 00        SP       EQU    18H
04 20        INVEC    EQU    2004H
15 00        IOS0     EQU    15H
16 00        IOC1     EQU    16H
16 00        IOS1     EQU    16H
10 00        P2       EQU    10H
03 00        HSIMODE  EQU    03H
06 00        HSISTAT  EQU    06H
04 00        HSITIME  EQU    04H
50 00        REG1     EQU    50H
52 00        REG2     EQU    52H
54 00        REG3     EQU    54H
60 00        REG4     EQU    60H
62 00        REG5     EQU    62H
40 00        TEMP     EQU    40H
08 00        MINT     EQU    08H
09 00        PINT     EQU    09H
```

```
22C0                              ORG     22C0H
                         ;
22C0   A1 C0 00 18                LD      SP,#00C0H         ;Initialize SP.
22C4   FA                         DI                        ;Disable interrupts.
22C5   71 7F 10                   ANDB    P2,#7FH           ;Clear P2.7 (frequency indicator).
22C8   B1 04 08                   LDB     MINT,#04H         ;Unmask HSI interrupt source.
22CB   B1 05 03                   LDB     HSIMODE,#05H      ;Only positive transitions on HSI.0,
                                                            ;HSI.1 lines will enter FIFO.
22CE   B1 01 15                   LDB     IOC0,#01H         ;Enable HSI.0 line, disable HSI.1
                                                            ;line into FIFO.
22D1   B1 80 16                   LDB     IOC1,#80H         ;HSI interrupt to occur only when
                                                            ;FIFO becomes full.
22D4   A1 E2 22 40                LD      TEMP,#HSIINT      ;Load address of HSI ISR into
22D8   C3 01 04 20 40             ST      TEMP,INVEC[0]     ;HSO VECT INT table location.
22DD   11 09                      CLRB    PINT              ;Clear pendings.
22DF   FB                         EI                        ;Enable interrupts.
22E0   27 FE             HERE:    SJMP    HERE              ;Loop here ("other tasks").
                         ;
                         ;
                         ;
                         ;        HSI INTERRUPT SERVICE ROUTINE
                         ;
22E2   F2                HSIINT:  PUSHF                     ;Save flags and mask all interrupts.
22E3   B1 00 15                   LDB     IOC0,#00H         ;Disable HSI.0 and HSI.1.
22E6   3A 06 19                   JBS     HSISTAT,2,HSI1    ;If transition occurred on HSI.1
                                                            ;jump to HSI1.
22E9   C0 50 04          HSI0:    ST      HSITIME,REG1      ;Else read time of first positive
                                                            ;transition on HSI.0 into REG1.
                                                            ;Next FIFO entry will soon enter
                                                            ;Holding Register.
22EC   FD                         NOP                       ;8 state times needed to allow
22ED   FD                         NOP                       ;next entry in FIFO to enter H.R.
22EE   C0 52 04                   ST      HSITIME,REG2      ;Read time of second positive
                                                            ;transition on HSI.0 into REG2.
22F1   68 50 52                   SUB     REG2,REG1         ;Store period of standard in REG2.
22F4   FD                         NOP                       ;Need 4 more state times.
22F5   C0 54 04          EMPFIF:  ST      HSITIME,REG3      ;Read rest of FIFO into dummy
                                                            ;register to clear it out.
22F8   3F 16 FA                   JBS     IOS1,7,EMPFIF     ;If Holding Register still loaded
                                                            ;continue reading out FIFO.
                                                            ;(JBS consumes 9 state times.)
22FB   B1 04 15                   LDB     IOC0,#04H         ;Else enable HSI.1 and disable
                                                            ;HSI.0 into FIFO. FIFO is empty of
                                                            ;HSI.0 transitions. It will now
                                                            ;only record HSI.1 transitions.
22FE   11 09                      CLRB    PINT              ;Clear any pendings.
2300   F3                         POPF                      ;Restore flags and INT mask.
2301   F0                         RET                       ;Return.
```

```
                     ;
2302   C0 60 04      HSI1:   ST     HSITIME,REG4    ;Read time of first positive
                                                    ;transition on HSI.1 into REG4.
                                                    ;Next FIFO entry will go to H.R.
2305   FD                    NOP                    ;8 state times needed.
2306   FD                    NOP                    ;
2307   C0 62 04              ST     HSITIME,REG5    ;Read time of second positive
                                                    ;transition on HSI.1 into REG5.
230A   68 60 62              SUB    REG5,REG4       ;Store period of unknown in REG5.
230D   FD                    NOP                    ;4 more state times needed before
                                                    ;next reading.
230E   C0 54 04      CLRFIF: ST     HSITIME,REG3    ;Read rest of FIFO into dummy
                                                    ;register to clear it out.
2311   3F 16 FA              JBS    IOS1,7,CLRFIF   ;If Holding Register still loaded
                                                    ;continue reading out FIFO.
2314   88 62 52              CMP    REG2,REG5       ;Else compare periods of standard
                                                    ;and unknown.  FIFO is now empty of
                                                    ;HSI.1 transitions.
2317   D7 05                 JNE    P27OFF          ;If they are not equal jump to P27OFF.
2319   91 80 10              ORB    P2,#80H         ;Else turn P2.7 on. Periods are equal.
231C   20 03                 SJMP   ENDIS           ;Jump to ENDIS.
231E   71 7F 10      P27OFF: ANDB   P2,#7FH         ;Turn P2.7 off. The periods are
                                                    ;unequal.
2321   B1 01 15      ENDIS:  LDB    IOC0,#01H       ;Enable HSI.0 and disable HSI.1 into
                                                    ;FIFO.
2324   11 09                 CLRB   PINT            ;Clear any pending interrupts.
2326   F3                    POPF                   ;Restore flags and INT mask.
2327   F0                    RET                    ;Return.
                     ;
2328                         END
```

PROCEDURE

1. Connect the "unknown" (f2) to HSI.1 and set it for a 1 KHz square wave. Connect the variable "standard" (f1) to HSI.0. Reset and enter BY 09 = 00. Have P2.7 drive a LED.
2. Execute from 22C0. Vary the frequency f1 of the "standard" till P2.7 goes on. The dial setting on the "standard" should indicate 1 KHz. Does it? It did for us.
3. Read WO 52 (REG2) when P2.7 = 1. It should read 1F4 (500 dec) which, when multiplied by 2 usec, will give 1000 usec. = 1 msec. = period of "standard" (or frequency = 1 KHz). We found WO 52 = 1F4. We also read WO 62 (REG5) and found 1F5 for the "unknown" period when P2.7 LED went on.

4. Change f2 at the "unknown" to 50 KHz. P2.7 should go off.
5. Vary the "standard"'s f1 till P2.7 goes on again. f1 should read 50 KHz on the "standard". Read WO 52. It should read 000A(10), which when multiplied by 2 usec. will give 20 usec. = 0.02 msec., corresponding to 50 KHz. Also read WO 62. Is it also 000A?

The experiment is but another applications showing the versatility of the High Speed Input unit. The ability to change the enable/disable status of any HSI pin into the FIFO on-the-fly is certainly a powerful attribute (just as Expt. 6-23 demonstrated the useful feature of being able to change HSI mode on-the-fly).

NOTE ON POSSIBLE FREQUENCY MEASUREMENT ERRORS AND RESTRICTIONS WHEN USING THE HSI UNIT.

In measuring the period with the HSI unit, as in this experiment, two readings of HSITIME are made: one for the time IN T1 at which the first transition occurred, and then for the time IN T1 at which the second transition occurred (both positive in our case). HSITIME records THE VALUES IN 16-BIT TIMER T1 when transitions on the HSI pins occur. The difference in these 16-bit T1 readings, when multiplied by 2 usec., gives the period because T1 is driven by a 2 usec. clock (at 12 MHz) i.e. each IMCREMENT in T1's WORD VALUE indicates another 2 USEC. TIME INTERVAL. Thus the period RECORDED AND READ will be EITHER 2 usec., 4 usec., 6 usec., ..., or 65,536 x 2 usec. i.e. integral multiplies of 2 usec. (even though the ACTUAL period may have been 2.5 usec., or 5.3. usec. or 7 usec., etc., the NEAREST time difference read from T1 would be 2 or 4 or 6 usec. etc., respectively). Thus frequencies INFERRED from period measurements with the HSI will be either 500 KHz or 250 KHz, or 166.67 KHz, ..., or 1 KHz, or 998 Hz, or 996 Hz, ... or 8 Hz. OUR METHOD IS, THEREFORE, ACCURATE ONLY FOR THOSE DISCRETE FREQUENCIES WHOSE ACTUAL PERIODS ARE INTEGRAL MULTIPLES OF 2 USEC. i.e. THOSE GIVEN ABOVE. To accurately measure ALL frequencies in the range 0 Hz to 250,000 Hz e.g. 49,536 Hz, 49,537 Hz, etc. REQUIRES THE USE OF THE T2 EVENT COUNTER. T2 can record ANY AND ALL 0 to 1 and 1 to 0 transitions, PROVIDED they are separated in time BY AT LEAST 2 USEC. Thus all transitions in a 4 usec. period square wave (250 KHz) and in ANY wave of period greater than 4 usec. (by ANY amount) can be recorded by T2. If a 1 sec. time base is used, T2/2 will give the frequency in Hz (due account being made of T2 overflows). SEE EXPT. 9-19. The restriction that periods be integral multiples of 2 usec. no longer holds when T2 is employed.

EXPERIMENT 9-8

A HIGH SPEED PROGRAMMABLE CONTROLLER.

INTRODUCTION

In this experiment we'll show how a fast programmable controller can be implemented with the HSO unit. The application will concern itself with discrete process control in a high speed sequential manufacturing or other control type operation. While the times we choose to illustrate the application are in the msec. range for purposes of visual demonstration, we, of course, know that the HSO unit is capable of creating on or off-times at its HSO pins as low as 2 usec. Our method can be extended to more general programmable controllers of broader scope.

DESCRIPTION OF THE PROBLEM

Pin HSO.0, when on, will cause the feeding of a part or object or material. HSO.1, when on, is to cause some action on the part or object (cutting, spraying, stamping, etc). Finally, HSO.2, when on, is to cause the ejection of the cut or sprayed object for further treatment or packaging, etc. down the assembly line. The process then repeats. The sequencing is:

HSO.2	HSO.1	HSO.0	COMMENT
0	0	1	Feed (16 msec. on)
0	1	0	Spray (33 msec. on)
1	0	0	Eject (82 msec. on)
0	0	1	Feed (16 msec. on)

etc.

Thus, HSO.0 is to go on for 16 msec., then go off just as HSO.1 goes on. The latter is to stay on for 33 msec. then go off just as HSO.2 goes on. The latter is to stay on 82 msec. then go off just as HSO.0 goes back on, etc. The sequencing repeats.

SOLUTION

The HSO unit will be employed to implement the solution. Six pairs of HSOCOM/HSOTIME byte/word commands are necessary. They are the following:

1. Load HSOCOM with 20H to turn HSO.0 on without the generation of an HSO interrupt. Load T1 + 0003 into HSOTIME to have HSO.0 go on "now".

2. Load HSOCOM with 00 to turn HSO.0 off without generation of HSO interrupt. Load T1 + 2000H into HSOTIME to have HSO.0 go off 2000H from "now". Thus its on-time will be 2000H x 2 usec. = about 16 msec. (16.384 to be exact).
3. Load HSOCOM with 21H to turn HSO.1 on without generation of HSO interrupt. Load T1 + 2003H into HSOTIME to have HSO.1 go on 2003 from "now" i.e. 16 msec. from "now" (just after HSO.0 went off).
4. Load HSOCOM with 01 to turn HSO.1 off without generation of HSO interrupt. Load T1 + 6000H into HSOTIME to have HSO.1 go off 6000 from "now" i.e. 6000 - 2000 = 4000 after it went on, for an on-time of 33 msec.
5. Load HSOCOM with 22H to turn HSO.2 on without generation of HSO interrupt. Load T1 + 6003H into HSOTIME to have HSO.2 go on 6003 from "now" i.e. just after HSO.1 went off.
6. Load HSOCOM with 12H to turn HSO.2 off WITH generation of HSO interrupt. Load T1 + 0FFFFH into HSOTIME to have HSO.2 go off FFFF from "now" i.e. FFFF - 6000 = A000 after it went on, for an on-time of 82 msec. So far one complete HSO.0, .1, .2 sequence has been specified for CAM loading and execution.
7. REPEAT the above loadings into HSOCOM/HSOTIME for the CAM in the HSO INTERRUPT SERVICE ROUTINE TO REPEAT THE SEQUENCING ALL OVER each time the CAM has been emptied and an HSO interrupt occurs.
8. We'll have the 6 loadings of HSOCOM/HSOTIME for the CAM implemented by FETCHING THE APPROPRIATE BYTES/WORDS FROM TWO TABLES ENTERED AT RUN-TIME: one table (the CMDTBL: Command Table) will have the command bytes 20, 00, 21, 01, 22, 12 (see above) entered at 5000-5005 for eventual loading into the HSOCOM part of the CAM FILE. The other table (the TMTBL: Time Table) will have the time words 0003, 2000, 2003, 6000, 6003, 0FFFF (see above) entered at 5100-510B for eventual loading into the HSOTIME part of the CAM FILE. These bytes/words are consistent with the values discussed in steps 1-6 above to produce the desired sequencing and on-times. REG1 will hold the table length (6).
9. The program itself will fetch the command bytes from the CMDTBL for the HSOCOM Command Tag register and the time words from the TMTBL for the HSOTIME time register. (See also program in Expt. 5-18 in chatper 5).
10. Flexibility is available by the ability to easily change the CMDTBL and/or TMTBL tables to achieve other kinds of sequencing patterns and/or other on/off times.

THE PROGRAM

We present the program at 2330, p. 495. It is analyzed afterward.

```
        18 00            SP      EQU     18H
        06 20            INVEC   EQU     2006H
        15 00            IOSO    EQU     15H
        04 00            HSOTIME EQU     04H
        06 00            HSOCOM  EQU     06H
        50 00            REG1    EQU     50H
        60 00            REG2    EQU     60H
        00 50            CMDTBL  EQU     5000H
        00 51            TMTBL   EQU     5100H
        70 00            OFFSET  EQU     70H
        40 00            TEMP    EQU     40H
        08 00            MINT    EQU     08H
        09 00            PINT    EQU     09H
        0A 00            T1      EQU     0AH

2330                             ORG     2330H
                         ;
2330    A1 C0 00 18              LD      SP,#00C0H        ;Initialize SP.
2334    FA                       DI                       ;Disable interrupts.
2335    B1 08 08                 LDB     MINT,#08H        ;Unmask HSO interrupt source.
2338    A1 53 23 40              LD      TEMP,#HSOINT     ;Load address of HSO ISR into
233C    C3 01 06 20 40           ST      TEMP,INVEC[0]    ;HSO VECT INT table location.
2341    11 09                    CLRB    PINT             ;Clear pendings.
2343    FB                       EI                       ;Enable interrupts.
2344    B0 50 60                 LDB     REG2,REG1        ;Load # CAM loads to be made into
                                                          ;counter.
2347    01 70                    CLR     OFFSET           ;Initialize OFFSET.
2349    EF 15 00         LOAD1:  CALL    SCAMLD           ;Call CAM load routine.
234C    07 70                    INC     OFFSET           ;Adjust OFFSET for next entry into
                                                          ;CAM.
234E    E0 60 F8                 DJNZ    REG2,LOAD1       ;If REG2 != 0, continue to load CAM
                                                          ;from tables.
2351    27 FE            HERE:   SJMP    HERE             ;Else loop ("busy tasks").
                         ;
                         ;
                         ;
                         ;       HSO INTERRUPT SERVICE ROUTINE
                         ;
2353    B0 50 60         HSOINT: LDB     REG2,REG1        ;Load # CAM loads to be made into
                                                          ;counter.
2356    01 70                    CLR     OFFSET           ;Initialize OFFSET.
2358    EF 06 00         LOAD2:  CALL    SCAMLD           ;Call CAM load routine.
235B    07 70                    INC     OFFSET           ;Adjust OFFSET for next entry into
                                                          ;CAM.

235D    E0 60 F8                 DJNZ    REG2,LOAD2       ;If REG2 != 0, continue to load CAM
                                                          ;from tables.
2360    F0                       RET                      ;Else return.
```

```
                    ;       CAM LOAD ROUTINE
                    ;
2361  3F 15 FD      SCAMLD: JBS   IOSO,7,SCAMLD               ;Test IOSO.7. If high, HSO's
                                                              ;H.R. is not empty. Wait.
2364  B3 71 00 50 06        LDB   HSOCOM,CMDTBL[OFFSET]       ;H.R. empty. Load HSOCOM with
                                                              ;Tag byte from command
                                                              ;table.
2369  09 01 70              SHL   OFFSET,#1                   ;Multiply OFFSET by 2 since
                                                              ;TIME is a word variable.
236C  47 71 00 51 0A        ADD   HSOTIME,T1,TMTBL[OFFSET];Load HSOTIME with word from
      04
                                                              ;TIME table.
2372  08 01 70              SHR   OFFSET,#1                   ;Divide to correct for word
                                                              ;access.
2375  F0                    RET                               ;Return.
```

The program begins with the familiar initializations: the stack pointer is set to 00C0, the interrupt system is disabled, the HSO interrupt source is unmasked and the address of the HSO ISR is loaded into address 2006 (HSO vector) in the VECT INT location table. Pendings are then cleared and the interrupt system is enabled. REG1 (50H) is then loaded into REG2. REG1 will be loaded at run-time with the number of table entries (i.e. # of bytes in CMDTBL or words in TMTBL) - in our case 6. The OFFSET (reg. 70H) into the tables is then cleared and a call to the CAM loading routine (SCAMLD) at 2361 is then made. There, the tag/times from the tables will be loaded into the CAM. At 2361 in that routine, we first test bit IOSO.7 ("HSO Holding Register is Full"). If the bit is 1, the HSO's H.R. is full and we should not attemt to load H.R. with the next HSO COM (Command Tag) and HSOTIME (time) commands. The JBS instruction at 2361 waits till IOSO.7 goes low, indicating an empty H.R. The next instruction at 2364 then loads HSOCOM with the BYTE from the CMDTBL at the OFFSET location in the table (base address is 5000). The OFFSET is multiplied by 2 to get ready to access the TMTBL which contains WORD variables. The word value from that table is fetched and added to T1 and the result placed in HSOTIME. Thus, the first complete (Tag/Time) command is placed in the H.R. and from there it enters the CAM. The next instruction divides OFFSET by 2 to correct for the WORD ACCESS so that we'll ALMOST be ready to access the NEXT BYTE from the CMDTBL. A return is then made to where the call was executed (in this case to 234C).

At 234C, the OFFSET is incremented. It IS now ready to access the next byte entry in the CMDTBL for HSOCOM. DJNZ REG2, LOAD1 decrements REG2 to reflect the fact that one CAM entry has been made. If REG2 is not 0, the DJNZ jumps back to LOAD1 where SCAMLD is called again, so that the second Tag/Time command from the CMDTBL and TMTBL tables can be fetched and placed in HSOCOM/ HSOTIME for the CAM. All repeats until REG2 is 0. The CAM is now loaded with 6 entries. We then fall through 234E to 2351 where SJMP HERE simulates "busy tasks".

While "busy tasks" are executing, the 6 entries in the CAM are being executed and pulled out, one after the other, thereby implementing the first HSO.0, HSO.1, HSO.2 sequence with the programmed on-times. When the 6th command is executed for HSO.2 to go off (after being on 82 msec.), an HSO interrupt is generated (since, as already discussed, the 6th entry into HSOCOM is 12 which turns HSO.2 off but with generation of an HSO interrupt). This interrupt takes us to the HSO ISR at 2353 where REG2 is re-loaded with the byte length of CMDTBL (or word length of TMTBL) from REG1. The OFFSET is then cleared in preparation for ANOTHER RELOADING OF THE CAM FROM THE TABLES TO GENERATE ANOTHER IDENTICAL SEQUENCE. SCAMLD is called and, as already analyzed, this loads HSOCOM and HSOTIME with the first byte/time command from the tables. Return from SCAMLD is this time to 235B. There, as in the main program, OFFSET is incremented and REG2 decremented to test whether all of each table has been loaded into the CAM. If it hasn't, DJNZ jumps back to LOAD2 to enter the next tag/time command from the tables into HSOCOM and HSOTIME. Eventually, each entire table has been accessed and the RET at 2360 carries us back to "busy tasks" at SJMP HERE. Another HSO.0,.1,.2 sequence will unfold with ultimate creation of another interrupt to the HSO ISR. All will repeat.

In this way a continual sequencing of HSO.0,.1,.2 will be sustained with the desired on-times as specified in the TMTBL table.

PROCEDURE

1. Reset and enter BY 09 = 00.
2. Connect LEDs to HSO.0, HSO.1, and HSO.2.
3. Enter BY 50 = 06 (REG1) to indicate there'll be 6 byte entries in CMDTBL and 6 word entries in TMTBL.
4. Enter BY 5000 = 20, 00, 21, 01, 22, 12 to establish the desired CMDTBL of tag bytes for HSOCOM which will produce the desired HSO.0,.1,.2 sequencing as indicated in the table given in the "Description of Problem" section earlier.
5. Enter WO 5100 = 0003, 2000, 2003, 6000, 6003, OFFFF to establish the desired TMTBL of time words for HSOTIME which will produce the desired on/off times (16 msec. on for HSO.0, 33 msec. on for HSO.1, and 82 msec. on for HSO.2).

6. Execute from 2330.
7. Observing the sequencing of the LEDs, fast to the eye, but qualitatively verifiable: on-time of HSO.0 is 1/2 that of HSO.1 and the latter is, in turn, less than the on-time of HSO.2.
8. Connect, in turn, HSO.0, then HSO.1, then HSO.2 to a scope to verify the on-times, off-times, and waveforms at each of those pins. We measured 16, 33, 82 msec, respectively, for the on-times of HSO.0,.1,.2, exactly as expected. Verify that each successive pin goes on just as the previous one turns off. If you can observe all three waveforms on the scope at one time, so much the better.
9. Enter another TMTBL table for different on-times and execute the program again.
10. Try other CMDTBL table entries for other sequencing patterns.
11. Remember, we have chosen on/off times in the msec. range for purposes of demonstration. On or off times down to 2 usec. are attainable with the HSO unit.

PROBLEM

Rewrite the SCAMLD (CAM LOAD) routine at 2361 using the "INDIRECT WITH AUTO-INCREMENT" addressing mode to load HSOCOM AND HSOTIME from the CMDTBL and TMTBL tables. We have accomplished the accessing of the tables here using "Long Indexed" addressing e.g. LDB HSOCOM, CMDTBL [OFFSET] in the program. The benefit of the "Indirect Auto-Increment" addressing mode is that an increment of 1 of the pointer into the table is automatically implemented if the table is a BYTE table, while the increment of the pointer is by 2 if the table is a WORD table e.g. LDB vs. ADD. A more compact program results. This is done in Expt. 9-9.

IMPORTANT NOTE

In a number of previous experiments dealing with HSO, we used in-line code to load SPECIFIC commands and times into the CAM. This is fine where the number of commands/times are small and fixed. It is awkward and rigid where a large number of commands/times are required, and where their values and number must be flexible to meet changing requirements. For that reason we loaded the CAM here from TABLES (as we'll do in subsequent HSO applications). Think of the tables as located in RAM and you can see the advantage of flexibility as well as more compact programs in ROM.

EXPERIMENT 9-9

A TWO-DIMENSIONAL HIGH SPEED FEED/CUTTING OPERATION IMPLEMENTED WITH THE HSO UNIT.

INTRODUCTION AND PROBLEM DESCRIPTION

In this experiment we will illustrate an application in which one or the other of two pairs of Tag/Time tables is invoked for loading into the HSOCOM/HSOTIME registers destined for the HSO unit's CAM. Which pair is accessed depends on the state of a sensor. If the sensor indicates low then one set of Tag/Time tables is fetched for loading into the HSO's CAM; if the sensor indicates high the other set of Tag/Time tables is accessed for loading into the CAM. Should the first set be invoked the HSO.1 and HSO.1 pins will go into alternate on-off sequencing with HSO.2 and HSO.3 off. If the second set is accessed, the HSO.2, HSO.3 pins will go into alternate on-off sequencing with HSO.0 and HSO.1 off. In the first case we are to think of each HSO.0 on-pulse as causing a quick, precise step or feed of a slab (wafer) in the X DIRECTION, while each HSO.1 on-pulse causes a precise VERTICAL slice (cut) of the slab or wafer to be made. With the sensor initially low, alternate step/slice/step/slice etc. operations occur in the x direction and will eventually cause the left end of the slab or wafer to clear the path of a light source. This will cause the sensor (e.g. photo-diode) to produce a high.

The sensor being high will cause the second Tag/Time table pair to be accessed for CAM loading, leading to HSO.0, HSO.1 going and staying off and HSO.2, HSO.3 going into on/off sequencing. This time each HSO.2 on-pulse cause a quick step of the slab or wafer in the Y DIRECTION while the subsequent HSO.3 on-pulse causes a HORIZONTAL slice or cut of the slab or wafer. Thus the slab or wafer is being cut into numerous small squares or rectangles. The size of these squares or rectangles can be made very fine because of the 2 usec. time intervals between successive x or y direction steps that can be programmed into the HSO unit. When the next slab or wafer arrives into position for cutting, the light source is again blocked and the sensor again goes low, invoking the first pair of Tag/Time tables for CAM loading. HSO.0, HSO.1 again team up to cause vertical cuts on the new slab as it is fed step by step in the x direction, until the sensor again goes high when HSO.2 and HSO.3 take over as a result of another access of the second pair of Tag/Time tables for CAM loading. And so on. This application would also fit under the aegis "Programmable Controller".

FORMULATION OF THE HSO.0, HSO.1 AND HSO.2, HSO.3 TAG/TIME TABLE PAIRS.

To arrive at the required table entries to implement the problem as described above, let us, for definitiveness, consider the following on/off sequencing times (again we choose msec. intervals for visual purposes. Much faster times are easily implemented by changing table entries):

1. With the sensor low, HSO.0 is to go on for 33 msec., then off, and HSO.1 is to go on for 99 msec. when HSO.0 goes off. HSO.0 is to go back on for 33 msec. when HSO.1 goes off, etc. These specifications require in the main program that: a) 20 be loaded into HSOCOM and T1 + 0003 be loaded into HSOTIME to turn HSO.0 on "now" without HSO interrupt; b) 00 and T1 + 4000 next be loaded into HSOCOM and HSOTIME to turn HSO.0 off 4000H x 2 usec. = 33 msec. from "now", without HSO interrupt; c) 21 and T1 + 4000 then be loaded into HSOCOM and HSOTIME to turn HSO.1 on at the time HSO.0 went off without HSO interrupt; d) 11 and T1 + 0FFFF be loaded into HSOCOM and HSOTIME to turn HSO.1 off FFFF - 4000 = C000 = 99 msec. after it went on WITH generation of HSO interrupt; e) a repeat of the above loadings IN THE HSO ISR ROUTINE AFTER EACH COMPLETE SEQUENCE IS DONE.
2. When the sensor indicates high, HSO.2 is to go on for 66 msec., then off, and HSO.3 is to go on for 66 msec. when HSO.2 goes off. HSO.2 is to go back on for 66 msec. when HSO.3 goes off, etc. These specifications require in the HSO ISR that: a) 22 and T1 + 0003 be loaded into HSOCOM/HSOTIME to turn HSO.2 on "now" without HSO interrupt; b) 02 and T1 + 8000 next be loaded into HSOCOM/HSOTIME to turn HSO.2 off 8000H x 2 usec. = 66 msec. from "now" without HSO interrupt; c) 23 and T1 + 8000 then be loaded into HSOCOM/HSOTIME to turn HSO.3 on at the time HSO.2 went off without HSO interrupt; d) 13 and T1 + 0FFFF be loaded into HSOCOM/HSOTIME to turn HSO.3 off FFFF - 8000 = 8000 = 66 msec. after it went on WITH generation of HSO interrupt; e) a repeat of the above in the HSO ISR routine after each complete sequence is done.
3. Thus, in this specific example, we are programming on-times of 33 msec. and 99 msec. for HSO.0, HSO.1, respectively, when they are in sequencing operation; and 66 msec. on-times for both HSO.2 and HSO.3 when they are in sequencing operation.
4. If we locate the HSO.0, HSO.1 (x-dimension) operation Tag/Time tables at 5000/5100, respectively, then the discussion in (1) above indicates that the first pair of tables should be as follows:

TAG (CMDTBL1)	TIME (TMTBL1)
5000 20 (HSO.0 on)	5100 0003 ("now")
5001 00 (HSO.0 off)	5102 4000 (33 msec. later)
5002 21 (HSO.1 on)	5104 4000 (33 msec. later)
5003 11 (HSO.1 off: INT)	5106 FFFF (131 msec. later)

5. If we locate the HSO.2, HSO.3 (y-dimension) operation Tag/Time tables at 5010/5110, respectively, then the discussion in (2) above indicates that the second pair of tables should be as follows:

TAG (CMDTBL2)	TIME (TMTBL2)
5010 22 (HSO.2 on)	5110 0003 ("now")
5011 02 (HSO.2 off)	5112 8000 (66 msec. later)
5012 23 (HSO.3 on)	5114 8000 (66 msec. later)
5013 13 (HSO.3 off: INT)	5116 FFFF (131 msec. later)

6. The times in the above tables can be changed to any other values desired (as can the tag for the sequencing pattern). (NOTE: "later" means relative to "now").
7. We refer to the first of the above tables as the CMDTBL1/TMTBL1 pair, and the second as CMDTBL2/TMTBL2 pair.
8. The length of the tables (4 here) will be entered in the appropriate register at run-time.

PROGRAM

The program that will access one or the other of the above table pairs for CAM loading, depending on sensor indication, is presented below at 2390 and discussed immediately thereafter. Note that the pointer to either CMDTBL is denoted by CPTR, while the pointer to either TMTBL is denoted by TPTR. In the former case CPTR will be loaded by the program with either 5000 or 5010 (base addresses), while in the latter case TPTR will be loaded by the program with either 5100 or 5110 (base addresses). Using these tables and accessing them with the indirect auto-increment addressing mode, as we do, achieves a large degree of program compactness.

```
18 00      SP       EQU   18H
06 20      INVEC    EQU   2006H
15 00      IOSO     EQU   15H
04 00      HSOTIME  EQU   04H
06 00      HSOCOM   EQU   06H
50 00      REG1     EQU   50H
60 00      REG2     EQU   60H
70 00      CPTR     EQU   70H
80 00      TPTR     EQU   80H
```

```
       00 50          CMDTBL1 EQU    5000H
       00 51          TMTBL1  EQU    5100H
       10 50          CMDTBL2 EQU    5010H
       10 51          TMTBL2  EQU    5110H
       40 00          TEMP    EQU    40H
       08 00          MINT    EQU    08H
       09 00          PINT    EQU    09H
       0E 00          P0      EQU    0EH
       0A 00          T1      EQU    0AH

2390                          ORG    2390H
                      ;
2390   A1 C0 00 18            LD     SP,#00C0H         ;Initialize SP.
2394   FA                     DI                       ;Disable interrupts.
2395   B1 08 08               LDB    MINT,#08H         ;Unmask HSO interrupt source.
2398   A1 B7 23 40            LD     TEMP,#HSOINT      ;Load address of HSO ISR into
239C   C3 01 06 20 40         ST     TEMP,INVEC[0]     ;HSO VECT INT table location.
23A1   11 09                  CLRB   PINT              ;Clear pendings.
23A3   FB                     EI                       ;Enable interrupts.
23A4   B0 50 60               LDB    REG2,REG1         ;Load # CAM loads to be made into
                                                       ;counter.
23A7   A1 00 50 70            LD     CPTR,#CMDTBL1     ;Load CMDTBL1 pointer with address
                                                       ;of CMDTBL1.
23AB   A1 00 51 80            LD     TPTR,#TMTBL1      ;Load TMTBL1 pointer with address
                                                       ;of TMTBL1.
23AF   EF 24 00       LOAD1:  CALL   CAMLD             ;Call CAM load routine for HSO.0,.1
                                                       ;operation.
23B2   E0 60 FA               DJNZ   REG2,LOAD1        ;If REG2 != 0, continue to load CAM
                                                       ;from tables.
23B5   27 FE          HERE:   SJMP   HERE              ;Else loop ("busy tasks").
                      ;
                      ;
                      ;
                      ;       HSO INTERRUPT SERVICE ROUTINE
23B7   30 0E 0A       HSOINT: JBC    P0,0,LD1          ;Test P0.0 (switch S0). If low
                                                       ;jump to LD1 to repeat HSO.0,HSO.1
                                                       ;operation.
23BA   A1 10 50 70            LD     CPTR,#CMDTBL2     ;Else load CMDTBL2 pointer with
                                                       ;address for HSO.2,.3 operation.
23BE   A1 10 51 80            LD     TPTR,#TMTBL2      ;Load TMTBL2 pointer with address.
23C2   20 08                  SJMP   CONT              ;Jump to CONT.
23C4   A1 00 50 70    LD1:    LD     CPTR,#CMDTBL1     ;Load CMDTBL1 pointer with address
                                                       ;for HSO.0,1 operation.
23C8   A1 00 51 80            LD     TPTR,#TMTBL1      ;Load TMTBL1 pointer with address.
23CC   B0 50 60       CONT:   LDB    REG2,REG1         ;Reload counter for tables.
23CF   EF 04 00       LOAD2:  CALL   CAMLD             ;Call CAM load routine.
23D2   E0 60 FA               DJNZ   REG2,LOAD2        ;If REG2 != 0, continue to load CAM
                                                       ;from tables.
23D5   F0                     RET                      ;Else return.
```

```
                          ;       CAM LOAD ROUTINE
                          ;
23D6   3F 15 FD           CAMLD:  JBS    IOSO,7,CAMLD      ;Test IOSO.7. If high, H.R.
                                                           ;not empty. Wait.
23D9   B2 71 06                   LDB    HSOCOM,[CPTR]+    ;H.R. empty. Load HSOCOM with
                                                           ;Tag command from command
                                                           ;table.
23DC   46 81 0A 04                ADD    HSOTIME,T1,[TPTR]+;Load HSOTIME with the time
                                                           ;interval from TIME table.
23E0   F0                         RET                      ;Return.
```

The main program's initializations between 2390 and 23A3 are quite clear. The LDB REG2, REG1 instruction then loads REG2 with the contents of REG1, the latter being loaded at run time with the value 04 (length of each table involved). 04 will represent, IN OUR CASE, the number of CAM loads to be made into the HSO unit. CPTR and TPTR are then loaded with 5000 and 5100, respectively, to point to the base addresses of CMD TBL1 and TMTBL1 (THE SENSOR IS ASSUMED LOW SO HSO.0, HSO.1 (X-DIMENSION) OPERATION IS CALLED FOR, AS A NEW SLAB JUST ARRIVED).

The CAMLD routine at 23D6 is then called. That routine simply waits till the HSO's H.R. is empty to accept a command (signified by bit IOSO.7 going low). The LDB instruction fetches (via [CPTR]+) the first byte command from CMDTBL1 for loading into HSOCOM. The pointer to that table, CPTR, is auto-incremented by 1 to get ready for the next byte command to be fetched from the CMDTBL1 later. The TPTR then accesses the first word from TMTBL1 via [TPTR]+. It is added to T1 and the result placed in HSOTIME. TPTR is auto-incremented by 2 (ADD is a word instruction) to get ready for the next time word to be fetched from TMTBL1 later. The return is made to 23B2. There the count length register REG2 is decremented and, if it's not 0, another fetch from the tables for HSOCOM/HSOTIME must be made. The complete sequencing of HSO.0, HSO.1 can not be implemented till the CAM is loaded with all four of the tables' entries. Thus the DJNZ carries us back to LOAD1 where another call of CAMLD is executed with the previously incremented pointers CPTR and TPTR ready to access the next byte and word entries in the CMDTBL1 and TMTBL1 tables, respectively. Eventually REG2 is decremented to 0 and fall-through to SJMP HERE ("busy tasks") ensues. The CAM is now loaded with the 4 tag/time entries from the CMDTBL1 and TMTBL1 tables to produce HSO.0, HSO.1 sequencing in x-dimension operation.

While "busy tasks" are being attended to, the 4 entries just made into the CAM are being executed out by the HSO unit. This will cause HSO.0 to go on for 33 msec., then off, followed by HSO.1 going on for 66 msec., then off. When HSO.1 goes off, the HSO unit generates an interrupt which vectors us to the HSO ISR at 23B7. There switch S0 at P0.0 (our "sensor") is tested. If it is still low, the JBC instruction causes a jump to LD1 where CPTR is RELOADED with the base address 5000 (CMDTBL1) and TPTR with the base address 5100 (TMTBL1). REG2 is RELOADED with the tables' count-length from REG1 (4) and CAMLD is called again to reload the CAM for ANOTHER HSO.0, HSO.1 sequencing cycle. The DJNZ REG2, LOAD2 instruction at 23D2 ensures that the CAM will again be loaded with the 4 HSOCOM/HSOTIME entries from CMDTBL1 and TMTBL1 for ANOTHER COMPLETE HSO.0,.1 SEQUENCING CYCLE. When that loading is finished, fall-through to RET back to "busy tasks" occurs. After another HSO.0,.1 sequencing cycle, another HSO interrupt causes a repeat of the series of events in the HSO ISR just described. Repeated x-dimension operations is occuring.

When the sensor S0 at P0.0 goes high, the entry into the HSO ISR finds the JBC test of S0 at 23B7 failing. Fall-through to 23BA occurs. There pointer CPTR is loaded with 5010 and pointer TPTR with 5110 to get ready to access the CMDTBL2 and TMTBL2 tables at 5010 and 5110, respectively. These tables will load the CAM with the 4 commands to produce HSO.2, HSO.3 sequencing (y-dimension operation). The SJMP CONT instruction skirts around LD1 (for obvious reasons) to 23CC where the count-length register is again loaded with 4 from REG1. The CAMLD routine is then called to load HSOCOM and HSOTIME with the 4 byte/word entries in the CMDTBL2 and TMTBL2 tables. The return from CAMLD to 23D2 finds the DJNZ instruction ensuring that the 4 byte/word entries in those tables do get into the CAM as HSOCOM, HSOTIME entries. The return at 23D5 is to "busy tasks". This time the HSO unit executes the four commands that puts HSO.2 on for 66 msec., then off, followed by HSO.3 going on for 66 msec., then off. When HSO.3 goes off the HSO unit generates an interrupt that vectors to the HSO ISR at 23B7. If S0 is still high the CAM is reloaded with the 4 byte/word entries from CMDTBL2 and TMTBL2. This will cause generation of another HSO.2, HSO.3 sequencing cycle (y-dimension operation is occurring).

Eventually the HSO interrupts generated by each successive HSO.2, .3 cycle will enter the HSO ISR only to find the sensor S0 low again (a new slab is in position). JBC will then jump to LD1 where the 4 CMDTBL1 and TMTBL1 table entries are loaded into the CAM for x-dimension (HSO.0, HSO.1 sequencing) operation again. And so it goes.

PROCEDURE

1. Reset and enter BY 09 = 00. Keep switch S0 at P0.0 low.
2. Enter WO 50 = 04 to indicate tables of length 4 each.
3. Enter the tables already discussed. CMDTBL1: BY 5000 = 20, 00, 21, 11. TMTBL1: WO 5100 = 0003, 4000, 4000, 0FFFF. CMDTBL2: BY 5010 = 22, 02, 23, 13. TMTBL2: WO 5110 = 0003, 8000, 8000, 0FFFF.
4. Connect LEDs to HSO.0,.1,.2, and .3 and use a scope to measure on-times.
5. Execute from 2390. Observe HSO.0 and HSO.1 blink on/off ... in turn. Measure their on-times on a scope. We found 33 msec. for HSO.0 and 99 msec. for HSO.1, as expected.
6. Throw switch S0 at P0.0 high. Observe HSO.0, HSO.1 go off immediately and HSO.2, HSO.3 start blinking on/off ... in turn. Measure their on-times on a scope. We found 66 msec. for HSO.2 and 66 msec. for HSO.3, as expected.
7. Throw S0 back low. Observe HSO.2, .3 go off at once and HSO.0, HSO.1 start theor on/off ... blinking sequence again.
8. ESC and enter new on times in the tables as follows: WO 5100 = 0003, 0C000, 0C000, 0FFFF. This should yield an on-time for HSO.0 of 99 msec. and an on-time for HSO.1 of FFFF - C000 = 4000 = 33 msec. Then enter WO 5110 = 0003, 4000, 4000, 0FFFF. This should yield on-times of 33 msec. for HSO.2 and 99 msec. for HSO.3. Execute from 2390 again with S0 low. Observe and measure the HSO.0,.1 on-times. Throw S0 high. Observe and measure the HSO.2,.3 on-times. Throw S0 low again and observe.
9. Now enter time words in the TMTBL1 and TMTBL2 tables that will produce real high speed feed/slice operations i.e. times in the usec. region. Execute and "observe" (measure times). Use a scope.
10. Formulate other applications involving new entries into the CMDTBL1, CMDTBL2 tables.

PROBLEM

3-dimensional cutting operation, anyone? (HSO.0,.1; HSO.2,.3; HSO.4,.5).

EXPERIMENT 9-10

A MATERIALS HANDLING APPLICATION: SORTING AND STORING OBJECTS BY SIZE. KEEPING TRACK OF THE SPECTRUM AND TOTALS.

INTRODUCTION

In this experiment we treat the application of sorting arriving objects (e.g. cartons) for storage in the proper bins according to their size; the tracking and recording of the number of objects of a given size stored in a given bin at any time; and the updating of the total number of objects of all sizes that have arrived to that point in time. As an object is detected, and its size determined by a sensor, the proper bin that stores ONLY objects of that size is to open to receive that object, then close. Correspondingly, the arrival and detection of an object of another size should activate the opening of another bin dedicated to holding objects only of THAT size, then close, etc. This application has assumed increasing importance in the automation of materials-handling in warehouses where received materials must be separated and stored, and an accurate record kept of the various materials, their characteristics (size, etc.), the number of objects stored with a given characteristic, and their various storage locations.

The following features of the 8096 will prove extremely useful in arriving at a compact solution to the problem: the existence of event counter T2 (to count objects as they arrive); of timer T1 (to record "size" of the arrived object in terms of the NUMBER of T1OV overflow interrupts (one every 131 msec.) recorded while the sensor (switch) is depressed by the object as it passes by); the 3-operand instructions; and the Shift instructions, e.g. SHLB breg, breg which shifts the contents of the destination register (first breg) as many times left as specified by the content of the source register (second breg above). The latter will prove most useful in arriving at an easy implementation of the opening of the correct bin to store a given size object.

FURTHER DESCRIPTION OF THE PROBLEM AND APPROACH TO A SOLUTION

1. A debounced switch S at T2CLK (P2.3) will be used, both to record the number of objects that pass by, and to record the "size" of each object in terms of the length of time (in units of 131 msec.) that it is depressed while a given

object passes over it before it is released.

2. Bin x at port 1 (x = 1, 2,....8) is to open to store objects of size x (x = 1, 2,....8) as the latter passes by.
3. As mentioned in (1) above, the size x of an object is proportional to the time that S is depressed as that object passes over it. That time will be recorded as the NUMBER OF T1OV OVERFLOWS that accrue from timer 1 DURING THE TIME S IS HIGH (DEPRESSED). Each T1OV overflow will cause another interrupt to a T1OV ISR where REG1 is incremented. REG1, therefore, will hold the object's size after it passes and releases S. That will inhibit any further T1OV interrupts (as we'll see). We are restricting ourselves, for simplicity, to sizes 1, 2,....8 (.131 sec up to about 1 sec in terms of times that S is depressed by an object).
4. Note that if REG1 = 3, for example, the size would really be between 3 and 4-, since the last T1OV INTERRUPT caused REG1 to be 3, but the object did not yet pass by. It will pass by, say, before the NEXT T1OV interrupt that WOULD HAVE made REG1 = 4. Thus bin 3 is really storing all objects whose size lies between 3 and 4. Fair enough.
5. REG0 will reveal the TOTAL number of objects of all sizes that passed and were detected.
6. Addresses 5001 - 5008 in memory, initialized to 0 at runtime, will keep a running record of the number of objects of sizes between 1 and 2-, 2 and 3-, 3 and 4-, ..., 8 and 9-, respectively, that passed by and are stored, respectively, in bins 1, 2, 3, ...8.
7. Thus at any given time the value stored in REG0 (total number of objects that passed by) should equal the sum of the CONTENTS of 500x with x running from 1 to 8 in the summation, where (500x) = number of objects of size between x and x + 1 that are stored in bin x up to the present time.
8. Port 1's LEDs simulate the 8 bins with bin 1 = P1.0 (for sizes 1 to 2-), bin 2 = P1.1 (sizes 2-3-), bin 3 = P1.2 (sizes 3-4-) .... bin 8 = P1.7 (sizes 8 to 9-). Please note that bin x (x = 1 to 8) corresponds to bit P1.(x-1) at port 1.

Before presenting and analyzing the program, it may be useful to first present the procedure, as this may help make the rationale behind the program clearer when we soon analyze it.

PROCEDURE

1. Reset and enter BY 09 = 00. Initialize memory locations 5001 - 5008 to 0: BY 5001 TO 5008 = 00. Enter BY 0F = 00 to close all bins at port 1. (Note that at any time on-the-fly we can open or close any bin(s) for whatever

purpose by simply entering BY 0F = XY, where XY is the appropriate byte for your purposes).

2. Connect a debounced switch S to T2CLK at P2.3.
3. Execute the program from 25A0.
4. Depress switch S anywhere from 10 to 40 (dec.) times with VARYING CONTACT TIMES. The latter should be no less than 0.131 sec. and no greater than 1 sec. to simulate sizes 1 (1 overflow of T1) to 8 (8 overflows of T1).
5. Each time S is depressed, note which bin at P1 opens. If bin 3 opened (LED P1.2 = 1), that would indicate size 3 passed (S was depressed about 0.4 sec). If bin 8 opened (LED P1.7 = 1), that would indicate size 8 passed (S was depressed about 1 sec). If bin 1 opened (LED P1.0 = 1), size 1 was detected (S was depressed around 0.131 sec), etc. Correlate the approximate times you keep S depressed with the size (which bin opened). Make a table of size x (bin x), x = 1, 2, ... 8, vs. # of times that bin x opened i.e. size x vs. FREQUENCY with which size x appeared during all those throws of S.
6. Enter BY 5001 TO BY 5008 to examine the contents of those memory locations. The value in 500x (x = 1, 2, ... 8) should exactly equal the number of times size x was recorded (i.e. that bin x opened) in the table you kept in (5) above.
7. Enter WO 50 = (REG0) to read the total number of objects of all sizes that passed by. That number should equal the total number of times you threw the switch in step (4) above, or alternatively the sum of the frequency column in the table you made in step (5) above, or still again the SUM of the contents read in memory locations 500x (x = 1, 2, ... 8).

PROGRAM

The program starting at 25A0 is presented below and analyzed afterward.

```
18 00        SP      EQU    18H
00 20        INVEC   EQU    2000H
16 00        IOC1    EQU    16H
15 00        IOC0    EQU    15H
0F 00        P1      EQU    0FH
10 00        P2      EQU    10H
40 00        TEMP    EQU    40H
08 00        MINT    EQU    08H
09 00        PINT    EQU    09H
50 00        REG0    EQU    50H
60 00        REG1    EQU    60H
70 00        REG2    EQU    70H
```

```
        80 00         REG3    EQU     80H
        90 00         REG4    EQU     90H
        0C 00         T2      EQU     0CH

25A0                          ORG     25A0H
                      ;
25A0    A1 C0 00 18           LD      SP,#00C0H        ;Initialize SP.
25A4    FA                    DI                       ;Disable interrupts.
25A5    B1 02 15              LDB     IOC0,#02H        ;Reset timer T2 and select T2CLK
                                                       ;as source for T2.
25A8    01 60                 CLR     REG1             ;Clear REG1 (size register).
25AA    B1 04 16              LDB     IOC1,#04H        ;Select T1 as source for timer
                                                       ;overflow interrupts.
25AD    B1 01 08              LDB     MINT,#01H        ;Unmask Timer Overflow interrupt
                                                       ;source.
25B0    A1 E4 25 40           LD      TEMP,#TOVINT     ;Load address of TOV ISR into
25B4    C3 01 00 20 40        ST      TEMP,INVEC[0]    ;TOV VECT INT table location.
25B9    33 10 FD      LOW:    JBC     P2,3,LOW         ;If switch at P2.3 is low, wait for
                                                       ;object.
25BC    11 09                 CLRB    PINT             ;Else clear pendings. Object arrived.
25BE    FB                    EI                       ;Enable interrupts.
25BF    3B 10 FD      HIGH:   JBS     P2,3,HIGH        ;Object size being measured. Wait
                                                       ;till it passes.
25C2    FA                    DI                       ;Else disable interrupt system.
                                                       ;Object passed. No more T1OV intrs.
25C3    A0 0C 50              LD      REG0,T2          ;Load value of T2 into REG0.
25C6    07 50                 INC     REG0             ;Increment REG0.
25C8    08 01 50              SHR     REG0,#01H        ;Divide it by 2 to count # of objects
                                                       ;that have passed.
25CB    45 00 50 60 70        ADD     REG2,REG1,#5000H;Add 5000 to # of overflows in REG1
                                                       ;(size) and store in REG2 (pointer
                                                       ;to table at 5000).

25D0    B2 70 80              LDB     REG3,[REG2]      ;Fetch count of # of objects of size
                                                       ;(REG1) that have passed so far.
25D3    07 80                 INC     REG3             ;Increment that count.
25D5    C6 70 80              STB     REG3,[REG2]      ;Store the incremented count back
                                                       ;in the table.
25D8    B1 01 0F              LDB     P1,#01H          ;Load port 1 (bins) with #01H.
25DB    05 60                 DEC     REG1             ;Decrement REG1 (size of object).
                                                       ;to adjust for correct # shifts
                                                       ;to open the proper bin.
25DD    19 60 0F              SHLB    P1,REG1          ;Shift each bit in P1 as many times
                                                       ;left as specified by value
                                                       ;in low byte of REG1. Thus bin x
                                                       ;will open for size x (x = 1,2,...8).
25E0    01 60                 CLR     REG1             ;Clear size register for next object.
25E2    27 D5                 SJMP    LOW              ;Jump to LOW to await arrival of
                                                       ;next object.
```

```
                   ;       T1 OVERFLOW ISR TO MEASURE SIZE
                   ;
25E4   07 60       TOVINT: INC     REG1          ;Increment size register by 1
                                                 ;for each T1 overflow ISR entry.
25E6   F0                  RET                   ;Return.
                   ;
25E7                       END
```

The program begins with the usual initialization of the stack pointer. The interrupt system is then disabled and 02 is loaded into IOC0 in order to select T2CLK as the source of T2 events and to reset T2. REG1 is cleared. It will count the number of T1 overflows as long as switch S at T2CLK is depressed simulating an object passing over it. As already discussed, the number of these overflows is an indication of size of the object (x overflows means size is between x and x + 1). Thus REG1 is the "size register". IOC1 is then loaded with 04 to select T1 as the source for timer overflow interrupts. Next, MINT is loaded with 01 to unmask the Timer Overflow interrupt source. #TOVINT (address 25E4 of the T1OV ISR) is loaded into TEMP and then stored at INVEC (2000H) in the VECT INT table, appropriate to Timer Overflow interrupts.

The state of switch S at T2CLK is next tested. Remember, T2CLK is at pin P2.3. If P2.3 is low, no object is present at the switch and we should wait. The JBC P2, 3, LOW instruction does just that at 25B9. When an object arrives, S is depressed and P2.3 goes high. We fall through to 25BC where any pending interrupts (e.g. Timer Overflow pendings) are cleared and the interrupt system is enabled. We want no T1OV pending interrupt to be serviced as this would give us a size, (REG1), one higher than it really is. JBS P2, 3, HIGH waits at 25BF as long as S is high (object over it). IT IS DURING THIS TIME THAT T1OV INTERRUPTS TO THE T1OV ISR AT 25E4 OCCUR EVERY 131 MSEC. REG1 IS INCREMENTED THERE EACH TIME THE ISR IS ENTERED. Hence size is being measured in REG1 as long as S is depressed and the object is moving over it. The moment the object passes by, S is released, P2.3 goes low, and we fall through 25BF to 25C2 WHERE THE INTERRUPT SYSTEM IS DISABLED. REG1 now holds the "final" size of the object (# of overflows of T1) and no more T1OV interrupts to the T1OV ISR will be serviced (they'll become pending). Hence REG1 stays "frozen" at its last overflow (size) value. Thus another object of size x has passed by and we now wish to update the total number of objects and the number of that size that have passed.

To record the total number of objects that passed over S we load T2 into REG0, increment REG0, and divide its value by 2 with the SHR REG0, #01 instruction. Remember, each press/release of S causes T2 to increase by 2, but that represents only one additional object that went by. Thus REG0 now contains the number of objects that passed to the present time.

To update the number of objects of a given size x that have passed, we shall construct and update a table of size x vs. the number of objects of that size that passed by. The table will start at 5001 in memory, where the number of size 1s will be stored, and end at 5008 in memory, where the number of size 8s that passed will be stored. Size 1s are stored in bin 1 (P1.0), ..., up to size 8s which are stored in bin 8 (P1.7). For that purpose, the 3-operand ADD instruction at 25CB adds 5000 to the contents of REG1 (size) and stores the result in REG2. Thus REG2 will hold 5001, 5002, ... or 5008 for size 1, size 2, ... or size 8. REG2 will now act as a pointer. The next instruction at 25D0 employs it in just that way: the number of objects of size x that passed and are stored at 500x (x = 1, 2, ...8) is fetched by indirect addressing ([REG2]). That number is stored in REG3, incremented, and then stored back in memory location 500x (again with [REG2] as the pointer). Remember that 500x (x = 1 to 8) will be initialized to 0 at run-time BEFORE any objects have arrived.

Having updated the total object count and the number of objects of size x that have been deteced and stored in bin x (i.e. the "spectrum", in the form of a table), we now have to actually open bin x to accept the object of size x that has just passed. This is done starting at 25D8 as follows: P1 is loaded with #01 and REG1 is then DECREMENTED by 1. The next instruction is crucial: SHLB P1, REG1 shifts P1 left by the number of times specified in REG1. Thus if the size were 1, REG1 would be 0 because of the decrement and #01 at P1 would be shifted left 0 times. Thus bin 1 (P1.0) would open as 01 would REMAIN at P1. If the size detected were 5, REG1 would be 4 because of the decrement and the byte at P1 (#01) would be shifted left 4 times. This would create 10 at P1 i.e. bin 5 (P1.4) would open. Similarly, if the size were 8, REG1 would be 7 after the decrement and P1 (#01) would be shifted left 7 times. This would create 80 at P1 i.e. bin 8 (P1.7) would open. You can see how useful the shift instructions are WHEN THE SHIFT COUNT IS SPECIFIED IN A REGISTER.

Finally, REG1 is cleared at 25E0 to get ready for the arrival of another object whose size in REG1 is to be measured all over in the T1OV ISR. SJMP LOW then carries us back to 25B9 where JBC P2, 3, LOW causes a wait for the arrival of another object.

Note that when it does arrive, and we fall through the JBC instruction to 25BC again, any T1OV pending interrupt that surely has been created during the wait at LOW (T1 overflowed time and again during that wait) is cleared by CLRB PINT. If we didn't include that instruction, we'd have a servicing of the pending interrupt after the ensuing EI instruction JUST AS THE NEW BODY ARRIVES. That would cause REG1 to already be 1 before the body hardly moved over switch S. Our sizes would all be in error by +1 (a too large indication).

The T1OV ISR at 25E4 to measure size, while S is depressed, is simple enough. Each time the ISR is entered, REG1 is incremented and a return is then made to the wait loop at 25BF (HIGH), where S may still be depressed as the body may not have cleared it. Thus REG1 is being incremented every 131 msec. till the body passes S and P2.3 goes low. DI at 25C2 then prevents further servicing to the ISR so that REG1 has attained its final value reflective of the object's size. Actual size would be given by (REG1) x 0.131 sec. x speed where "spped" would be the speed of the conveyor belt in e.g. cm/sec. or meters/sec. or feet/sec. etc. Remember, we are really measuring sizes between (REG1) and (REG1) + 1.

RESULTS

Following the procedure presented previously in the PROCEDURE section, we obtained the following sample results for two trial runs. In one run S was thrown 29 times and in the other run S was thrown 16 times (interim results were then checked) and S was then thrown an additional 10 times before final results were checked. In each run, we depressed S with arbitrary contact times before release, taking care not to have contact for more than 1 sec. or less than 0.131 sec. This assures that "sizes" are constrained to 1 through 8 only. Remember bin x is identified with bit P1.(x-1) at port 1. Resuts are on p. 513.

RUN #1: S THROWN 29 TIMES.

SIZE X (BIN X OPENED)	NO. OF TIMES BIN X OPENED FOR SIZE X	TOTAL NO. OF OBJECTS (REGO): WO 50	READING OF MEMORY SPECTRUM: WO 5001 TO 5008
1	2		5001: 02
2	2		5002: 02
3	5		5003: 05
4	7		5004: 07
5	6		5005: 06
6	3		5006: 03
7	3		5007: 03
8	1		5008: 01
	29	1DH	TOTAL: 29

RUN #2: S THROWN 16 TIMES, THEN AN ADDITIONAL 10 TIMES.

SIZE X (BIN X OPENED)	NO. OF TIMES BIN X OPENED FOR SIZE X	TOTAL NO. OF OBJECTS (REGO): WO 50	READING OF MEMORY SPECTRUM: WO 5001 TO 5008
1	1, (1)		5001: 01, (01)
2	2, (3)		5002: 02, (03)
3	3, (5)		5003: 03, (05)
4	1, (3)		5004: 01, (03)
5	6, (9)		5005: 06, (09)
6	2, (3)		5006: 02, (03)
7	0, (0)		5007: 00, (00)
8	1, (2)		5008: 01, (02)
	16, (26)	10H, (1A)	TOTAL: 16, (26)

In Run #2 there are 2 columns. The first column gives the results after S was thrown 16 times. At that point WO 50 and WO 5001 TO 5008 were read, with the interim results noted. The second column in ( ) gives the final results after an additional 10 throws of S were made, at which point WO 50 and WO 5001 TO 5008 were again read with the final results noted in ( ).

The results are perfectly consistent and substantiate the validity of the approach and the program.

EXPERIMENT 9-11

A "MOCK" POINT OF SALES TERMINAL

INTRODUCTION

An application of the microprocessor that is currently widespread is the "Point Of Sales Terminal". The POS is particularly useful where large inventories of many items are stocked, where sales are numerous and turnover is rapid, and where prices are subject to frequent change. This is the situation for example, in supermarkets. POSs are installed there at the check-out lines. In addition to scanning the bar code on each item to display its price, to arriving at the total price of all the items purchased, to calculating the change due the customer, and to printing out detailed receipts for the customer giving items purchased and individual and total prices, the POS serves other important functions: it keeps track of inventories as items are sold off; it can issue warning signals to indicate which, if any, items have reached critically low levels when replenishment of supplies is called for; it can print out or otherwise display the remaining inventories of all items at any given time. These are some of the important capabilities a POS should possess, among others.

This experiment will illustrate a "Mock POS" which actually is quite realistic as far as its intended scope. The 8096's 3-operand instructions, its indirect addressing mode (with and without auto increment) and its sign-extend instructions are most useful in the implementation of our solution to the problem.

FORMULATION

1. We'll assume an inventory of 4 items whose "bar codes" are 00, 01, 02, and 03. These codes will be simulated by employing our switch bank at Port 0. We refer to the items as 00, 01, 02, or 03 or simply 0, 1, 2, 3.
2. As each item is "passed through the scanner" (simulated by the pressing and releasing of a debounced switch at P2.7 from low to high to low), its price is to be displayed at the LEDs at Port 1. Prices of the items will be fetched from a price table at 5000 - 5003 (entered at run-time).
3. The original inventory of each item is stored (at run-time) in the inventory table at 5010 - 5013.
4. After any given item is sold (passed through the "scanner") the quantity remaining of that item is decremented by 1

and stored back in the inventory table. That table can be inspected at any time (BY 5010 TO 5013) to read out the remaining inventory.

5. If any item's inventory reaches a "critical level" of, say, 3, the LED at P2.6 is to go on and the code of that item is to be stored in another table in memory at 5020 - 5023. That table can be read out at any time (BY 5020 TO 5023) to see which items are in short supply. Thus if BY 5020 TO 5023 reads 01, 03, FF, FF, that would indicate that items 1 and 3 have reached critical low levels (that table is first initialized to FF, FF, FF, FF).
6. After each item has passed through the "scanner" and its price displayed, the press of a debounced switch connected to the EXTINT pin will cause the total bill to appear at P1's LEDs. The program then continues to execute from the main program where the interrupt occurred, waiting for the next customer and new items to be pushed through the scanner. The process and series of events described in (1) to (5) above repeats.
7. At run-time we'll enter the following data in memory initializing price/quantity (any other tables will do just as well, but for definitiveness you are referred to these tables to illustrate the points of the problem as they arise):

ITEM	ADDRESS	PRICE	ADDRESS	ORIGINAL QUANTITY
00	5000	26	5010	7
01	5001	32	5011	4
02	5002	07	5012	6
03	5003	15	5013	5

8. Those items that reach short supply (3 or less) will be recorded in memory locations 5020 and up. Thus locations 5020 to (arbitrarily) 5030 will be initialized to 0FF (BY 5020 TO 5030 = 0FF). They can be queried at any time to see which codes among 00, 01, 02, 03 appear there. Those that do indicate those items are in short supply.

THE PROGRAM

The program at 2520 is presented below and analyzed immediately thereafter.

```
18 00        SP      EQU     18H
0E 20        INVEC   EQU     200EH
16 00        IOC1    EQU     16H
0E 00        P0      EQU     0EH
0F 00        P1      EQU     0FH
```

```
        10 00           P2      EQU     10H
        50 00           TEMP    EQU     50H
        08 00           MINT    EQU     08H
        09 00           PINT    EQU     09H
        30 00           REG1    EQU     30H
        32 00           REG2    EQU     32H
        34 00           REG3    EQU     34H
        36 00           REG4    EQU     36H
        38 00           REG5    EQU     38H
        40 00           REG6    EQU     40H

2520                            ORG     2520H
                        ;
2520    A1 C0 00 18             LD      SP,#00C0H        ;Initialize SP.
2524    FA                      DI                       ;Disable interrupts.
2525    B1 80 08                LDB     MINT,#80H        ;Unmask EXTINT source.
2528    A1 73 25 50             LD      TEMP,#EXTINT     ;Load address of EXTINT ISR into
252C    C3 01 0E 20 50          ST      TEMP,INVEC[0]    ;EXTINT VECT INT table location.
2531    B1 00 16                LDB     IOC1,#00H        ;Select EXTINT as source instead of
                                                         ;ACH.7.
2534    A1 20 50 40             LD      REG6,#5020H      ;Load REG6 with 5020 (base of "low
                                                         ;inventory items" table).
2538    11 36                   CLRB    REG4             ;Clear "Price Totalizer" register.
253A    71 BF 10                ANDB    P2,#0BFH         ;Clear P2.6 (indicates item in
                                                         ;short supply when on).
253D    11 09                   CLRB    PINT             ;Clear any pending interrupts.
253F    FB                      EI                       ;Enable interrupt system.
2540    37 10 FD        HERE:   JBC     P2,7,HERE        ;If switch at P2.7 lo, wait.
2543    71 BF 10                ANDB    P2,#0BFH         ;Else clear P2.6 indicator. Item
                                                         ;scanned.
2546    B0 0E 30                LDB     REG1,P0          ;Read item's code into REG1 from
                                                         ;switch bank P0.
2549    16 30                   EXTB    REG1             ;Extend code to full word with
                                                         ;hi byte = 0.
254B    45 00 50 30 32          ADD     REG2,REG1,#5000H;5000 + code loaded into REG2
                                                         ;(pointer to price table).
2550    45 10 50 30 34          ADD     REG3,REG1,#5010H;5010 + code loaded into REG3
                                                         ;(pointer to inventory table).
2555    B2 32 0F                LDB     P1,[REG2]        ;Fetch price of item and display

                                                         ;it at P1.
2558    74 0F 36                ADDB    REG4,P1          ;Add P1 to REG4 and store in REG4
                                                         ;(total price so far).
255B    B2 34 38                LDB     REG5,[REG3]      ;Fetch inventory of item and store
                                                         ;in REG5.
255E    05 38                   DEC     REG5             ;Decrement REG5.
2560    C6 34 38                STB     REG5,[REG3]      ;Store updated inventory back in
                                                         ;[REG3] inventory table.
```

```
2563   99 03 38             CMPB   REG5,#03H      ;Compare decremented inventory with
                                                  ;03.
2566   D9 06                JH     WAIT           ;If REG5 is greater than 03 jump to
                                                  ;WAIT.
2568   91 40 10             ORB    P2,#40H        ;Else turn P2.6 indicator on.
                                                  ;Inventory of item is low.
256B   C6 41 0E             STB    P0,[REG6]+     ;Store code of itme in low supply
                                                  ;in table starting at 5020H.
256E   3F 10 FD   WAIT:     JBS    P2,7,WAIT      ;If P2.7 still high wait.
2571   27 CD                SJMP   HERE           ;Else jump to HERE to scan next item.
                  ;
                  ;         EXTINT ISR
                  ;
2573   B0 36 0F   EXTINT:   LDB    P1,REG4        ;Display total price in REG4 at P1's
                                                  ;LEDs.
2576   11 36                CLRB   REG4           ;Clear price totalizer for next
                                                  ;customer.
2578   71 BF 10             ANDB   P2,#0BFH       ;Clear P2.6 (low inventory indicator).
257B   F0                   RET                   ;Return.

257C                        END
```

The opening initializations involve the stack pointer and a disabling of the interrupt system. The EXTINT interrupt source is next unmasked and the address of the EXTINT ISR is stored at 200E (INVEC) in the VECT INT table (appropriate to EXTINT interrupts). 00 is then loaded into IOC1 to select EXTINT rather than ACH.7 as the external interrupt source. 5020 is then loaded into REG6 which establishes it as the pointer to the table of "low inventory items" that will be formed when the program executes. REG4 is then cleared. It will serve as the totalizer of price of all the items purchased by the customer. Next P2.6 is cleared (it will go on whenever an item's remaining quantity reaches 3 OR less). Any pending interrupts are then cleared and the interrupt system is enabled.

At 2540 the debounced switch at P2.7 is polled. As long as it is low, JBC keeps us in a wait loop at HERE. When it goes high, simulating an item going through the scanner, we fall through to 2543 where P2.6 (the "low inventory" indicator) is cleared. The next instruction reads the item's "bar code" from the switch bank at P0 (i.e. 00, 01, 02, or 03) and stores it in REG1. That code is sign extended into a full word, with high byte = 00 in our case. Thus REG1 will now contain the word 0000 or 0001 or 0002 or 0003. The 3-operand ADD at 254B adds that word code to 5000 and stores the result in REG2. This will allow REG2 to become the pointer to the price table at 5000 - 5003. Likewise 5010 is added to REG1 and the result stored in REG3.

This will allow REG3 to become the pointer to the inventory table at 5010 - 5013.

At 2555, the pointer REG2 fetches the price of the item from 5000 or 5001 or 5002 or 5003 and displays it at P1's LEDs. P1 is then added to the contents of REG4 (initially 0) so that REG4 will keep a running record of total price to that point. Next, the pointer REG3 fetches the current remaining inventory of the item from 5010 or 5011 or 5012 or 5013 and stores it in REG5. There that quantity is decremented and stored back in the table 5010 - 5013 by means of the STB instruction, again using REG3 as the pointer in indirect addressing. We now compare the decremented value of REG5 with #03 (critical low inventory level). If REG5 is higher than 03 a jump to WAIT at 256E is taken. There we wait as long as P2.7 is still high (remember the switch S at P2.7 was thrown high while in the loop at 2540 (HERE) and it takes some time before it is released. We do not yet want to go back to HERE to scan another item till S at P2.7 has been released, otherwise we'd have multiple passes through the path from HERE to 2571 with a false decrementing of inventory to 0). When S at P2.7 has been released we fall through to SJMP HERE at 2571. This carries us back to JBC P2, 7, HERE at 2540. There we wait for the next item to go through the "scanner". When it does, all repeats.

If, however, the CMPB at 2563 and JH at 2566 show that REG5 is not higher than 3 we fall through 2566 to the ORB instruction. This turns on the warning light at P2.6 to notify us that the item just purchased and scanned is now in short supply. Further, STB P0, [REG6]+ at 256B stores the code of that item (contents of switch bank at P0) that is now in short supply into the table starting at 5020. The auto-increment will allow REG6 to point to the next location in that table. This will cause storage of the Code of the item that might next be in short supply into the next location in that table. We then enter the wait loop at 256E till S at P2.7 goes low (for the same reasons given above). When it does, we jump to HERE to await the scan of the next item. Note that the "low inventory" indicator, P2.6, is on all this time, BUT GETS CLEARED AT 2543 WHEN THE NEXT ITEM PASSES THROUGH THE "SCANNER" AND FALL-THROUGH 2540 OCCURS.

Eventually, all the customer's items will have been scanned and it's time to ring up the total price. With the program counter in the wait loop at HERE, the creation of an EXTINT interrupt by means of a debounced switch connected to the EXTINT pin causes a vectoring to the EXTINT ISR at 2573. There the total accumulated price is retrieved from REG4 and displayed at P1's LEDs. REG4 is then cleared to prepare for the next customer and the new items. P2.6 is cleared in case it's been on and a return is made to the HERE loop in the main program where the EXTINT interrupt occurred. We await a new customer and new items. The series of events just described is repeated all over again.

PROCEDURE

Here is a sample run that we suggest. We have verified all the results indicated.

1. Enter BY 09 = 00. Connect debounced switches to P2.7 and to EXTINT.
2. Enter BY 5000 = 26, 32, 07, 15 (price table for items 00, 01, 02, 03, respectively).
3. Enter BY 5010 = 7, 4, 6, 5, (original inventory for items 00, 01, 02, 03, respectively).
4. Enter BY 5020 TO 5050 = 0FF to initialize the "low inventory" table. Any code(s) appearing later in that table will indicate that the item corresponding to that code is in short supply (a quantity of 3 or less remaining).
5. Execute from 2520.
6. Set the switches at P0 for item 2 (P0 = 02).
7. Throw S at P2.7 low/high/low and see 07 at P1's LEDs (price of item 2).
8. Set P0 to 00 (item 0). Throw P2.7 low/high/low and see 26 at P1 (price of item 0).
9. Throw P2.7 low/high/low again and see 26 again at P1 i.e. two of item 0 were purchased.
10. Set P0 to 01 (item 1). Throw P2.7 low/high/low and see 32 at P1 (price of item 1). Also see the LED at P2.6 go on because item 1's remaining inventory has just reached 3.
11. Set P0 to 03 (item 3). Throw P2.7 low/high/low and see 15 at P1 (price of item 3). At the same time see P2.6 go off.
12. Set P0 to 02 (item 2). Press and release P2.7. See 07 at P1 (price of item 2).
13. Set P0 to 03 (item 3). Throw and release P2.7. See 15 at P1 (price of item 3). See P2.6 go on again as item 3's remaining inventory has just reached 3.
14. Press and release the switch at the EXTINT pin creating an interrupt. See P2.6 go off and observe the total price displayed at P1. It should be 07 + 26 + 26 + 32 + 15 + 07 + 15 = B6. This we observed at P1.
15. Examine BY 5010 TO 5013 and see 5, 3, 4, 3 as the inventory REMAINING for items 00, 01, 02, and 03 respectively, as expected in view of steps (6) through (13) above.
16. Examine BY 5020 TO 5023 and see 01, 03, FF, FF, i.e. items 1 and 3 reached low inventory levels, in keeping with (15) above.

17. A new customer arrives. Set P0 = 02 and throw and release P2.7. See 07 at P1 (price of item 2) and P2.6 go on. Item 2's inventory has just reached critical level 3.
18. Set P0 = 00 and throw and release P2.7. See 26 at P1 (price of item 0). P2.6 goes off.
19. Set P0 = 01. Throw and release P2.7. See 32 (price of item 1) at P1. P2.6 goes on as item 1's inventory is now 2 (below citical level).
20. Throw and release the switch at EXTINT. See P2.6 go off and observe the total price displayed at P1: 07 + 26 + 32 = 5F. That is what we observed at P1.
21. Examine BY 5010 TO 5013 and observe 4, 2, 3, 3 as the remaining inventory of items 0, 1, 2, and 3, as expected in view of (15), (17), (18), and (19) above.
22. Examine BY 5020 TO 5030 and observe 01, 03, 02, 01, FF, FF, ... FF. This tells us that item 1 first reached critical inventory (3), then item 3 did, then item 2 did, then item 1 showed up again when its inventory went from 3 to 2 (below critical).

PROBLEMS

1. Modify the program to allow the CANCELLATION OF THE LAST ITEM THAT WAS SCANNED so that the price total in REG4 and the inventory count in memory locations 5010 - 5013 revert back to what they were before the item was scanned. Perhaps an HSI.0 external interrupt with its attendant ISR can be used to implement this feature.
2. Think up any and all modifications to make the POS terminal as realistic and as broad in scope as possible.
3. Add an interface and routine that will allow produce items to be weighed, with weight and price of the item being shown and added in to the total price. This would be the basis for a completely separate experiment. Weight could be sensed, for example, with a potentiometer whose output voltage is proportional to weight (spring displacement proportional to force). Inputting this voltage to one of the ACH channels will produce a 10-bit quantity proportional to weight. Price must then be fetched from the appropriate weight table (bananas vs. potatoes, etc).

EXPERIMENT 9-12

USING THE HIGH SPEED OUTPUT UNIT TO DRIVE STEPPER MOTORS.

INTRODUCTION

The stepper motor is an important electromechanical actuator device in "real world" interfacing where precise positioning is needed without feedback control. An axially oriented permanent magnet rotor placed in the magnetic field created by four independent current carrying coils will take up the precise position that results in minimum magnetic field energy (Earnshaw's Theorem). Further, if that position is one of stable equilibrium and if the energy is a "deep minimum" (both arranged by the proper coil/current arrangement), then any displacement of the rotor the LEAST bit away from the position of stable equilibrium (in any direction) will cause return forces that will restore the rotor to its original position of stable equilibrium. In a simple 4-coil arrangement, the rotor's south pole will align itself precisely between two coils that create north poles, and its north pole will align itself between the two coils that create south poles, as a result of the current flow directions imposed on the coils. When the currents in the various coils are changed, so that two other coils create north and south poles, the rotor will rotate into a new precise equilibrium ("midpoint") position. Thus, if we can arrange a distribution of two 1s for two coils (current flow) and two 0s for the two other coils (no current flow), and then sequence this distribution in the proper way, with any desired time delay between successive 1, 0 pattern distributions, we should succeed in having the rotor rotate from one precise equilibrium position to the next, separated by the desired time delay. The rotation will be in steps of precise amounts of rotation. Speed is given in steps/sec.

If the microprocessor is to drive the stepper, the requirement of the program is then simply to output the required 4-bit distribution and sequencing of 1s and 0s to a latched port where the bases of 4 transistors are connected to the pertinent 4 pins of the port. The 4 coils of the stepper are then connected to the collector circuits of the respective transistors, the emitters are grounded, and each coil is supplied with the proper d.c. voltage from a power source. The distribution of 1s, 0s output by the microprocessor to the bases of the transistors will then cause current flow through those coils that are connected to the transistors whose bases are 1 and no current flow through those coils that are connected to the transistors whose bases are 0. The sequencing of the 1, 0 pattern distribution at the port will cause the proper sequencing of currents among the stepper's four coils to induce precise rotor steps at a rate determined by the time delay between changes in pattern distribution. The step angle (the incrementation in degrees of rotor orientation between steps) is determined by the particular rotor /coil packaging in the unit provided by the manufacturer. This also determines number of steps per revolution.

Figure 9-1 on the next page shows the stepper/transistor drive circuitry and the required 1, 0 pattern distribution (and the sequencing thereof) needed to step a 4-coil unipolar stepper. The base of each transistor is driven by one of the 4 bits output by the microprocessor at the chosen latched I/O port. PLEASE NOTE IN FIG. 9-1 THAT OUR NOTATION FOR THE 4 COILS IS SHOWN AS Q4, Q3, Q2, Q1 AND ALSO AS Q3, Q2, Q1, Q0. THEY ARE EQUIVALENT. WE PREFER THE NOTATION Q3, Q2, Q1, Q0 AND WILL STICK TO THAT. NOTE ALSO IN FIG. 9-1 THAT WHERE YOU SEE 4,4' and 2,2' NOTED ON THE STEPPER CONNECTIONS, THE 4 and 4' SHOULD BE INTERCHANGED AND THE 2,2' SHOULD BE INTERCHANGED.

Now any microprocessor can control the movement and speed of most ordinary stepper motors (e.g. 2 or 3 msec. between steps, or slower), as the above discussion indicates. As stepper technology keeps moving ahead, extremely fast stepping motion well beyond the 2 or 3 msec. limits is becoming possible. The time between steps on some steppers is below 30 usec. It is for these ultra-fast steppers that the 8096's HSO unit is particularly well suited. It can drive its HSO pins with times between 0 to 1 and 1 to 0 transitions (or between 1 to 0 and 0 to 1 transistions) at those pins as low as 2 usec., as we've repeatedly pointed out. The HSO.0,.1,.2, and .3 pins, for example, can then be used to drive the Qj coils of the stepper.

This experiment employs the HSO unit to drive any 4-coil stepper, regardless of speed. The program is easily adapted to steppers of any speed by merely changing the word values in our time table from which HSOTIME is loaded. [The latter, together with the time tag in HSOCOM, becomes the command pair in the HSO CAM FILE that turns the specified HSO pin(s) on or off at the specified time(s)].

We used an Airpax K82201-P1 unipolar stepper (see Fig. 9-1 for connections) whose specifications are: 7.5 degree rotor rotation per step (48 steps per revolution), 475 RPM max. (about 8 RPS or about 2.7 msec. between steps), and 380 PPS max. (380 pulses per second, or about 2.7 msec. between PULSES which, of course, is equivalent to the 2.7 msec. between STEPS quoted

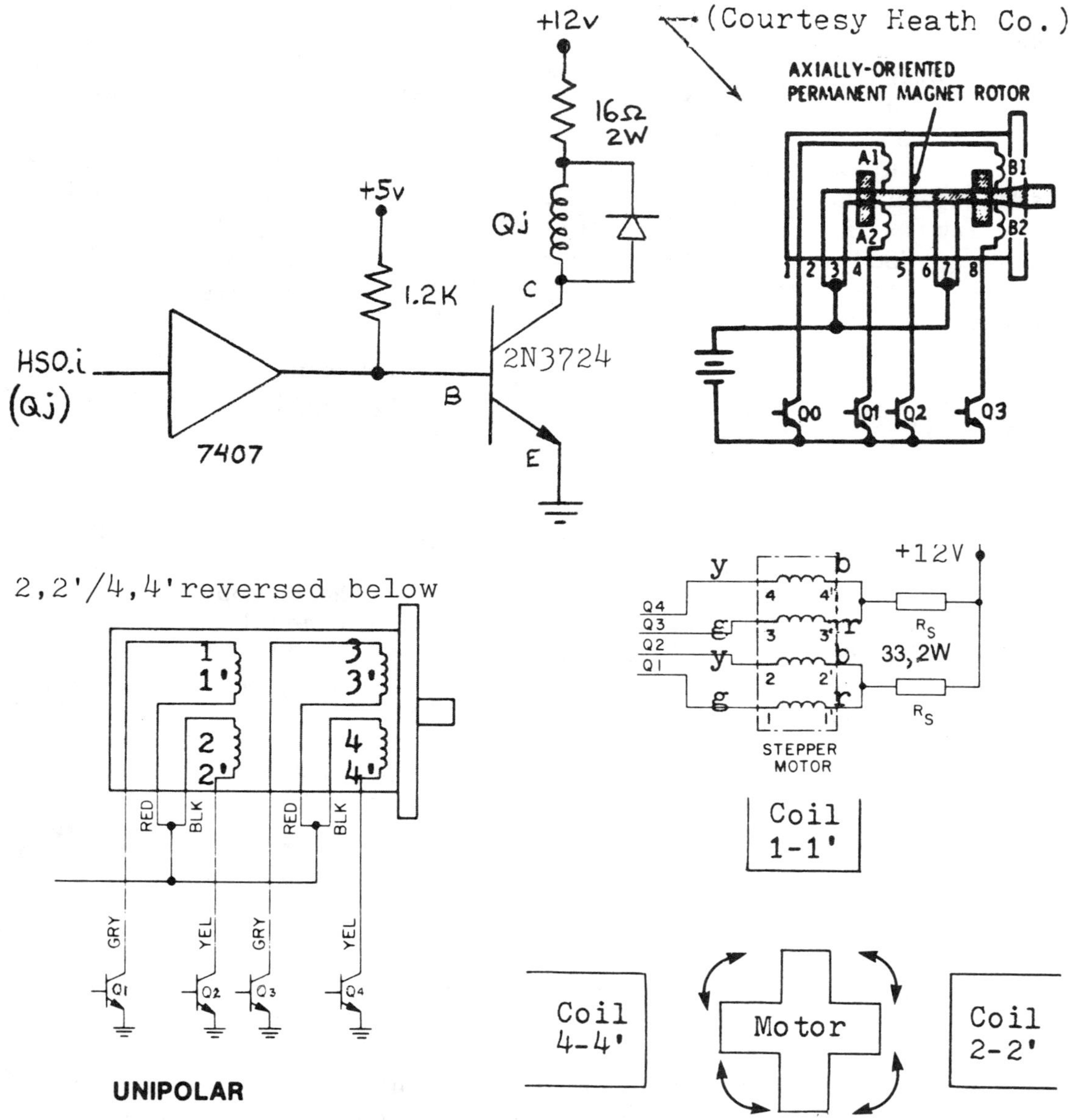

UNIPOLAR

CW ROTATION ↓

Step	Q_1	Q_2	Q_3	Q_4
1	ON	OFF	ON	OFF
2	ON	OFF	OFF	ON
3	OFF	ON	OFF	ON
4	OFF	ON	ON	OFF
1	ON	OFF	ON	OFF

CCW ROTATION ↑

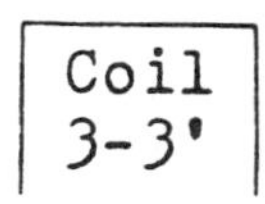

*R_S used to operate motors rated at 5 Volts.

FIGURE 9-1: Stepper connections for Expt. 9-12. The 1,0 pulse sequencing table is also shown. We used the Airpax K82201-P1 in the unipolar mode employing a normal 4-step sequence.

As the experiment and its results will show, we succeeded in driving the stepper with speeds as high as about 2 msec. between steps, which translates to about 100 msec. per revolution or 10 RPS (600 RPM), or equivalently 2 msec. between pulses, or 500 PPS. Anything lower than 2 msec. between pulses had no motional effect on the stepper - it "froze". We emphasize again that, while the stepper we employed was of the usual variety as far as speed specifications, the program employed and the HSO pin connections to the stepper are perfectly adaptable to the fastest of steppers, since the HSO unit can create transitions to within 2 usec. of each other.

THE HSO PIN CONNECTIONS AND THE SETTING UP OF THE HSO COMMAND TAG TABLE (CMDTBL) AND HSO TIME TABLE (TMTBL).

As we know, the HSO unit can drive individual HSO pins on or off and it can also drive pins HSO.0, HSO.1 on or off TOGETHER (ditto HSO.2, HSO.3). By connecting the HSO.i pins to the bases of the transistors driving coils Qj of the stepper in the following manner, we can take advantage of the above feature re: HSO.0/HSO.1 and HSO.2/HSO.3. This will allow the CMDTBL to be 8 bytes long rather than 10 bytes long, as we'll now see. From Fig. 9-1 the required table is:

STEP #	HSO.3 Q3	HSO.1 Q2	HSO.2 Q1	HSO.0 Q0
1	0	1	0	1
2	1	0	0	1
3	1	0	1	0
4	0	1	1	0
1	0	1	0	1

Sequencing the 4-bit pattern from top to bottom (steps 1-4 and repeat) produces CW rotation of the stepper, while sequencing the table from bottom (1) to top (2), via steps 4, 3 and then repeat, causes CCW rotation of the stepper.

The above table translates to the following required HSO.3, HSO.2, HSO.1, HSO.0 sequencing bit pattern:

STEP #	HSO.3 Q3	HSO.2 Q1	HSO.1 Q2	HSO.0 Q0	HSOCOM FOR CMDTBL AT 5000	HSOTIME INTERVALS FOR TMTBL AT 5100
1	0	0	1	1	26 then 07	4000 then 4000
2	1	0	0	1	01 then 23	8000 then 8000
3	1	1	0	0	06 then 27	C000 then C000
4	0	1	1	0	21 then 13	FFFF then FFFF
1	0	0	1	1	Repeat Steps 1 - 4.	

Again CW rotation involves a down reading of the table while CCW rotation involves upward reading. Note that, had you connected HSO.3,.2,.1,.0 directly to Q3, Q2, Q1, Q0 instead of to Q3, Q1, Q2, Q0, respectively, you would have needed 10 bytes for CMDTBL rather than the 8 bytes shown above (verify that -- see previous table). Step 1 above is achieved by loading 26 into HSOCOM from CMDTBL to turn BOTH HSO.0 and HSO.1 on and then loading 07 into HSOCOM from CMDTBL to turn both HSO.2 and HSO.3 off (both 4000, or 33 msec., from "now"). T1 + 4000 loaded into HSOTIME specifies that HSO.0 and HSO.1 are to go on 33 msec. from now. T1 + 4000 loaded AGAIN into HSOTIME specifies that HSO.2 and HSO.3 are to go off 33 msec. from now. Similar analyses hold for steps 2 and 3. Step 4 is achieved by loading 21 into HSOCOM to turn HSO.1 back on at FFFF (131 msec.) from "now", and then loading 13 into HSOCOM to turn HSO.3 back off (WITH HSO INTERRUPT TO BE GENERATED) also at FFFF from "now" (T1 + FFFF loaded into HSOTIME as the companion to 21 for HSOCOM and again into HSOTIME as the companion to 13 for HSOCOM specifies the 131 msec. from "now"). Going from step 3 to step 4 requires no change in HSO.0 and HSO.2. Note that in going from step 2 to step 3 we employ the byte for HSOCOM that turns HSO.0 and HSO.1 off TOGETHER and then the byte for HSOCOM that turns HSO.2 and HSO.3 on TOGETHER.

The 8 bytes for HSOCOM will be stored at run-time in CMDTBL starting at 5000. As indicated by the table, they are to be: 26, 07, 01, 23, 06, 27, 21, 13 (where only the LAST byte, 13, will have the HSO unit generate an interrupt so that the HSO ISR routine will be entered where the table will again be accessed to load the CAM for a repeat of steps 1-4 after the 4th step is made). Likewise, the 8 words for TMTBL will be stored at run-time starting at 5100. They are 4000, 4000, 8000, 8000, C000, C000, FFFF, FFFF. We are here choosing the time interval between steps to be, initially, 4000H, which translates to 16,384 x 2 usec. or about 33 msec. between steps (30 steps per sec). Later on, when the experiment is performed, we'll keep reducing the word value entries in TMTBL so that time intervals between steps of 2000H, then 1000H, then 0800H, then 0400H, then 0200H are tried on the stepper. We'll find that our stepper responds down to time intervals of 0400H = 1024 x 2 usec. = about 2 msec. between steps (or 500 PPS, or 96 msec. per rev (with 48 steps per rev. at 7.5 degrees rotation per setp), or 10 RPS, or 600 RPM). Anything less than 2 msec. time intervals between steps (pulses) will not draw a response from our stepper.

Finally, note that we'll need to enter the LENGTH (8) of the tables at run-time (that length corresponds to the number of CAM commands needed in our case). This we do by entering BY 40 = 08 where 40 is the address assigned to REG1, the table length counter. The loading of the tables into HSOCOM and HSOTIME will be accompanied by a constant decrementing of REG2 (loaded from REG1) till 0 in REG2 indicates completion of the loading of the 8 commands into the CAM FILE. Testing of bit IOS0.7 will hold up loading till the H.R. becomes available for another command entry.

THE PROGRAM

The program at 2420 is presented below and analyzed directly afterward.

```
     40 00      REG1     EQU   40H        18 00     SP       EQU   18H
     50 00      REG2     EQU   50H        06 20     INVEC    EQU   2006H
     00 50      CMDTBL   EQU   5000H      15 00     IOSO     EQU   15H
     00 51      TMTBL    EQU   5100H      04 00     HSOTIME  EQU   04H
     70 00      OFFSET   EQU   70H        06 00     HSOCOM   EQU   06H
     60 00      TEMP     EQU   60H
     08 00      MINT     EQU   08H
     09 00      PINT     EQU   09H
     0F 00      P1       EQU   0FH
     0A 00      T1       EQU   0AH

2420                     ORG   2420H
                ;
2420 A1 C0 00 18         LD    SP,#00C0H         ;Initialize SP.
2424 FA                  DI                      ;Disable interrupts.
2425 B1 08 08            LDB   MINT,#08H         ;Unmask HSO interrupt source.
2428 A1 45 24 60         LD    TEMP,#HSOINT      ;Load address of HSO ISR into
242C C3 01 06 20 60      ST    TEMP,INVEC[0]     ;HSO VECT INT table location.
2431 11 09               CLRB  PINT              ;Clear pendings.
2433 11 0F               CLRB  P1                ;Clear P1 LEDs. P1 will display count
                                                 ;of # steps/4.
2435 FB                  EI                      ;Enable interrupts.
2436 B0 40 50            LDB   REG2,REG1         ;Load # CAM loads to be made into
                                                 ;counter.
```

```
2439  01 70                     CLR    OFFSET               ;Initialize OFFSET.
243B  EF 17 00      LOAD:       CALL   SCAMLD               ;Call CAM load routine.
243E  07 70                     INC    OFFSET               ;Adjust OFFSET for next entry into
                                                            ;CAM.
2440  E0 50 F8                  DJNZ   REG2,LOAD            ;If REG2 != 0, continue to load CAM
                                                            ;from tables.
2443  27 FE         HERE:       SJMP   HERE                 ;Else loop ("busy tasks"). Four steps
                                                            ;specified.
                    ;
                    ;
                    ;
                    ;           HSO INTERRUPT SERVICE ROUTINE
                    ;
2445  17 0F         HSOINT:     INCB   P1                   ;Increment P1 to indicate that another
                                                            ;group of 4 steps were made.
2447  B0 40 50                  LDB    REG2,REG1            ;Load # CAM loads to be made into
                                                            ;counter.
244A  01 70                     CLR    OFFSET               ;Initialize OFFSET.
244C  EF 06 00      RELOAD:     CALL   SCAMLD               ;Call CAM load routine.
244F  07 70                     INC    OFFSET               ;Adjust OFFSET for next entry into
                                                            ;CAM.
2451  E0 50 F8                  DJNZ   REG2,RELOAD          ;If REG2 != 0, continue to load CAM
                                                            ;from tables.
2454  F0                        RET                         ;Else return.  Four more steps
                                                            ;specified.
                    ;
                    ;
                    ;
                    ;           CAM LOAD ROUTINE
                    ;
2455  3F 15 FD      SCAMLD:     JBS    IOS0,7,SCAMLD                ;Test IOS0.7. If high, H.R.
                                                                    ;not empty. Wait.
2458  B3 71 00 50 06            LDB    HSOCOM,CMDTBL[OFFSET]        ;H.R. empty. Load HSOCOM with
                                                                    ;step bits from command table.
245D  09 01 70                  SHL    OFFSET,#1                    ;Multiply OFFSET by 2 since
                                                                    ;TIME is a word variable.
2460  47 71 00 51 0A            ADD    HSOTIME,T1,TMTBL[OFFSET];Load HSOTIME from TIME table.
      04
2466  08 01 70                  SHR    OFFSET,#1                    ;Divide to correct for word
                                                                    ;access.
2469  F0                        RET                                 ;Return.
```

The main program starts by initializing the stack pointer and disabling the interrupt system. The HSO interrupt source is then unmasked and the HSO ISR address (#HSOINT = 2445H) is loaded into the INT VECT table at 2006H (INVEC) via the TEMP register. Any pending interrupts are then cleared as is port P1. P1 will display the count of the number of steps made by the stepper divided by 4. The interrupt system is then enabled.

The number of CAM loads to be made is next loaded into REG2 from REG1 (the latter will be loaded with the table length - here 8 - at run-time). An offset register OFFSET (word) is then cleared. It will be used as the offset part of a pointer into one or the other of the CMDTBL or TMTBL tables. The base of the pointer will be either 5000 (EQU CMDTBL) or 5100 (EQU TMTBL), respectively. Now the SCAMLD routine at 2455 is called (instruction at address 2438: "LOAD").

Let us analyze SCAMLD, the CAM LOAD routine at 2455. Bit IOS0.7 ("HSO Holding Register is Full") is tested at 2455. If it is 1, HR is full and we should not attempt to enter any command into it. The JBS instruction causes a wait till IOS0.7 goes low indicating H.R. is empty. Fall-through to 2458 occurs and there HSOCOM is loaded with the byte entry (Command Tag) from CMDTBL. The entry is fetched from address CMDTBL + OFFSET where CMDTBL = 5000H. OFFSET is then multiplied by 2 to get ready to access the appropriate word in TMTBL. The ADD instruction then places T1 + the word fetched from address TMTBL + OFFSET in TMTBL (where TMTBL = 5100) into HSOTIME. The SHR instruction divides OFFSET by 2 to get READY to access the CMD TBL table again for the NEXT byte in that table. The H.R. now has its first HSOCOM/HSOTIME command which, by this time, finds its way into the CAM (8 state times are needed after the ADD HSOTIME instruction for that to happen). The RET at 2469 in SCAMLD takes us back to 243E in the main program where OFFSET is incremented so that CMDTBL [OFFSET] will now point to the next byte to be fetched from CMDTBL for HSOCOM.

The DJNZ instruction at 2440 then decrements the table length register REG2. If the result is not 0, the table has not been exhausted and a jump back to LOAD is effected. There another call to SCAMLD is made in order to load HSOCOM and HSOTIME with another byte entry from CMDTBL and another word entry from TMTBL, respectively. This process continues until all the table entries have entered the CAM via HSOCOM/HSOTIME and the H.R. At that point REG2 is zero and the final return from SCAMLD results in a fall through 2440 to SJMP HERE at 2443 which simulates other tasks executing while the CAM is being loaded.

During this time the CAM commands are being executed by the HSO unit. The last HSO command is 13H which causes HSO.3 to turn off and the HSO unit to generate an interrupt. That will complete step 4. We are vectored to the HSO ISR at 2445. By now the CAM is empty as all 8 entries have been executed. The LEDs at P1 are incremented to indicate 4 steps have been made by the stepper. REG2 is then reloaded with the number of table entries from REG1. The OFFSET part of the pointer is cleared to get ready for another loading of the CMDTBL and TMTBL entries into the CAM via HSOCOM and HSOTIME. SCAMLD is then called and the return from it to 244F results in a replay of the events previously analyzed at 2436 - 2440 in the main program. Only, now, these events are associated with the instructions at 2447 - 2451 in the ISR. Return at 2454 in the ISR to "busy tasks" is made only after all table entries in CMDTBL and TMTBL have been fetched for loading into the CAM (indicated by REG2 being decremented to 0 at 2451). This reloading of the CAM with the 8 table entries will result in another 4 steps being made by the stepper, ALL THE WHILE "BUSY TASKS" ARE BEING PERFORMED. The completion of the 4th step again results in an HSO interrupt to the ISR where P1 is incremented once again (every 4 steps). The whole scenario repeats. "BUSY TASKS" AND STEPPER MOTION HUM ALONG, SIDE BY SIDE, TRANSPARENT TO EACH OTHER.

PROCEDURE

1. Connect HSO.0 to Q0, HSO.2 to Q1, HSO.1 to Q2, and HSO.3 to Q3 (coils of the stepper) as in Fig. 9-1. Actually, as shown there, HSO.i are connected to the bases of the respective transistors in whose collector circuits the coils Qj are connected. Follow the circuitry with respect to the resistors, the 7407 open collector buffer drivers, and the 12V d.c. power supply needed.
2. Reset and enter BY 09 = 00.
3. Enter BY 40 = 08 [8 CAM entries from the byte/word tables at 5000 (CMDTBL) and 5100 (TMTBL)].
4. Enter the CMDTBL: BY 5000 = 26, 07, 01, 23, 06, 27, 21, 13 to produce the correct bit sequence patterns at HSO.3, .2, .1, .0 that will result in a 4-step CW rotation.
5. Enter WO 5100 = 4000, 4000, 8000, 8000, 0C000, 0C000, 0FFFF, 0FFFF to set up the TMTBL to yield steps at 33 msec. intervals (30 steps/sec).
6. Execute from 2420. Observe the stepper rotate. After 3 revolutions of the stepper (as indicated by a pointed knob attached to its shaft) ESC. 48 x 3 steps should have been made. Therefore, P1 should read 36 dec. i.e. 48 x 3/4. We found 24H at P1, as it should be.
7. Reset, enter BY 09 = 00, execute again from 2420. Let the stepper rotate 5 times before pressing the ESC key. This time P1 should indicate 48 x 5/4 = 60 dec. = 3CH. We confirmed that at P1.
8. Reset, enter BY 09 = 00. Enter a new TMTBL: WO 5100 = 2000, 2000, 4000, 4000, 6000, 6000, 8000, 8000. The time interval between steps will now be 2000H x 2 usec. = about 16 msec. or about 62 steps per sec.

9. Execute from 2420. Observe a doubling in stepper speed. After 3 revolutions of the stepper ESC. There are 48 steps per revolution. P1 should thus display 48 x 3/4 = 36 dec. = 24H. This was observed. Reset and enter BY 09 = 00 again. Execute from 2420 and allow 8 revolutions of the stepper before pressing the ESC key. P1 should now indicate 48 x 8/4 = 96 dec. = 60H. We observed 61H (pressing the ESC key at "precisely" the time that a specified number of revolutions have been completed will result in a margin of error). Redo allowing 13 revolutions before pressing the ESC key. P1 should display 48 x 13/4 = 156 dec. = 9CH. We observed 9DH.
10. Reset and enter BY 09 = 00. Set up a new TMTBL: WO 5100 = 1000, 1000, 2000, 2000, 3000, 3000, 4000, 4000. Now 1000H x 2 usec. = about 8 msec. between steps, or about 125 steps per sec. Execute from 2420. The speed of the stepper doubled again. ESC after 10 revolutions of the stepper. P1 should read 48 x 10/4 = 120 dec. = 78H. We observed 6E. Our eye could not accurately follow the fast rotating stepper so we could only estimate when the 10th revolution was approaching. Hence the 6EH vs. 78H discrepancy.
11. Reset and enter BY 09 = 00. Set up another TMTBL: WO 5100 = 0800, 0800, 1000, 1000, 1800, 1800, 2000, 2000. This will result in 800H x 2 usec. = about 4 msec. between steps or about 250 steps per sec. Execute from 2420 and observe the extremely fast rotational speed of the stepper. We could not accurately count the revolutions.
12. Reset and enter BY 09 = 00. Try another TMTBL: WO 5100 = 0400, 0400, 0800, 0800, 0C00, 0C00, 1000, 1000. This should result in 0400H x 2 usec. = about 2 msec. between steps, or 500 steps per sec. Execute from 2420. We observed exceedingly fast rotation of the stepper - much faster than in (11) above and again too fast for us to count revolutions.
13. Reset and enter BY 09 = 00. Now try the following entries in TMTBL: 0300, 0300, 0600, 0600, 0900, 0900, 0C00, 0C00. Execute from 2420. This time the stepper did not respond - the time interval between steps being specified (0300H x 2 usec. = about 1.5 msec.) is too fast for our stepper.

CONCLUSION

We achieved a maximum speed of about 2 msec. between steps which translates to 500 steps per sec. (or 500 PPS) or 48 x 2 = 96 msec. per revolution (or about 10 RPS = 600 RPM). This exceeded the specification of the Airpax K82201-P1 stepper (475 RPM max. and 380 PPS max). The HSO unit should easily match the fastest steppers available today or in the forseeable future: 2 usec. time intervals between steps are available from the HSO!

PROBLEMS

1. Modify the HSO ISR after the INCB P1 instruction so that the stepper will stop after having made a prescribed number of steps (divisible by 4). In this case, when the prescribed number of steps is reached, your test in the HSO ISR, if met, should cause a jump around the CALL SCAMLD instruction and a return to HERE in the main program. In that way no more steps or HSO interrupts will occur.
2. How would you modify the program so that P1 will display the actual number of steps AS THEY OCCUR AND NOT JUST AFTER EVERY 4th STEP? Hint: Perhaps an HSO interrupt should be specified when EACH new step is implemented. The ISR routine will have to change. Make that change.
3. Modify the HSOCOM CMDTBL so that the stepper rotates in a CCW direction. See the 2nd table in the section "THE HSO PIN CONNECTIONS ...." and read it from bottom (step 4) to top (step 1) to construct the proper CMDTBL of HSOCOM bytes. This time you'll find that 10 bytes are needed for the CMDTBL and 10 words for the TMTBL. We are assuming that the HSO.i connections to the coils Qj are still HSO.3 to Q3, HSO.2 to Q1, HSO.1 to Q2, and HSO.0 to Q0.
4. Incorporate your solutions to Problems (1), (2), and (3) above into the program of this experiment to have the stepper rotate a finite number of steps CW, stop for a specified amount of time, rotate back CCW the same number of steps, stop for another specified amount of time, rotate back CW, etc., etc. This, in itself, is an important application in fluid, pressure, etc. control in which stepper controlled valves are employed, or in XY table motion for accurate cutting, drilling, spraying, surface depositions, or in positioning of any kind.

EXPERIMENT 9-13

A TEMPERATURE CONTROLLER USING A SENSOR AND THE 8096's ACH INPUT CHANNEL (ADC).

INTRODUCTION AND DESCRIPTION OF PROBLEM

In this experiment we shall demonstrate the use of the 8096 in implementing one type of temperature controller. Upper and lower bounds of a temperature range are established. If the actual temperature lies between these limits no effort is made to change it. If, however, the temperature exceeds the upper limit, a blower or cooler is turned on to drive the temperature down to within the desired range. The cooler is turned off as soon as the temperature reaches the specified upper limit on the way down. Should the temperature drop to or below the specified lower limit, a heater is to be turned on to drive the temperature back up. The heater will then go off the moment the temperature exceeds the specified lower limit on the way up. Thus a stability region with respect to temperature is established. A sensor converts temperature to analog voltage for input to ACH.0. Digital vs. analog output control is distinguished.

IMPLEMENTATION OF THE SOLUTION

1. The voltage output of a temperature sensor (we used the National Semiconductor LM 135H) is input to one of the ACH ADC channels of the 8096 (we used channel ACH.0). We shall use 8 bits (9-2) of the 10-bit conversion result as the byte proportional to temperature. Thus we are treating the ADC as an 8-bit converter. Clearly we are losing granularity since bits 1 and 0 of the 10-bit result are being discarded (i.e. as temperature, for example, increases, the increase will not manifest itself in bits 9-2 UNTIL bits 1 and 0 go through ANOTHER 00, 01, 10, 11 sequence). We are taking this approach for purposes of simplifying the solution -- in particular from the viewpoint of the compactness of the look-up table that we shall construct, in which actual temperature will be fetched from an address which is determined by the SIZE OF THE CONVERTED BYTE. Thus, if the 8-bit conversion byte corresponding to the input temperature/output voltage at the sensor is e.g. 9C and if it corresponds to a room temperature of 24 degrees C, then the table entry would be e.g. 509C 24. Since the 8-bit conversion value (bits 9-2) goes up by 1 as temperature increases, the next table entry would be 509D XY, where XY would be the temperature that produced 9D as its

conversion byte. We are missing those temperatures that affect only bits 1,0 till spillover to bits 9-2 occurs. Clearly, if we wanted greater accuracy, we'd need to use the full 10-bit AD conversion result. In that case, with the 10-bit conversion result spanning 000 to 3FF as temperature increases, we'd need a table in which addresses ranged from e.g. 5000 to 5001, to 5002, ... to 50FF, to 5100, to 5101, ... to 51FF, to 5200, ... to 53FF, with corresponding temperatures XY placed at each address in the table. In that case we'd have a 10-bit accuracy but a table of length 1024 for a given FULL temperature range (0 to 5V). In our 8-bit approach we are clearly losing accuracy, as we are missing temperatures that cause the first two bits to increment from 00 to 11 before spillover to bits 9-2 occurs, when we first see the effect of the temperature rise. But the table would now be only 256 bytes long for the FULL temperature range 0 to 5V. Granularity will now be 4 times coarser. But the implementation of the problem would be simpler. Clearly, no loss in generality results from our 8-bit approach. We are interested in demonstrating the method. You can easily implement the solution using the full 10-bit capability of the 8096's ADC (see Problem at end of the experiment). That's one of the nice features of the 8096's ADC facility.

2. Figure 9-2 p. 534 shows the temperature sensor and the circuit connections needed to produce the sensor's output voltage which is to be input, in our case, to ACH.0 of the 8096 for conversion. Also shown are the output voltages vs. temperature in the 0 to 100 degree C range for the LM 135H, as specified by National Semiconductor. Thus at ice point (0 degrees C) the output voltage 2.73V must lead to a 10-bit conversion result given by (2.73/5) x 1024 or 560 dec. = 230H. Bits 9-2 of this result would be given by 8CH. At the boiling point of water, the output voltage 3.73V would lead to a 10-bit conversion result given by (3.73/5) x 1024 = 765 dec. = 2FDH. Bits 9-2 of this result would be given by BFH. Room temperature (2.98V sensor output @ 25 degrees C) would lead to 615 dec. = 267H as the 10-bit conversion result, or to 99H for bits 9-2. Thus we'd EXPECT A/D results in ADRESHI (high byte of A/D Result Register - address 03) ranging from 8CH at ice point to 99H at room temperature (25 degrees C) to BFH at the boiling point of water. WE'LL CORRELATE THE ACTUAL 8-BIT CONVERSION RESULT AT BITS 9-2 IN ADRESHI WITH INPUT TEMPERATURE before constructing our look-up table of conversion byte vs. actual temperature. This is discussed in (3) below.

3. To calibrate the temperature sensor i.e. conversion bits 9-2 vs. input temperature, we'll input the sensor's output

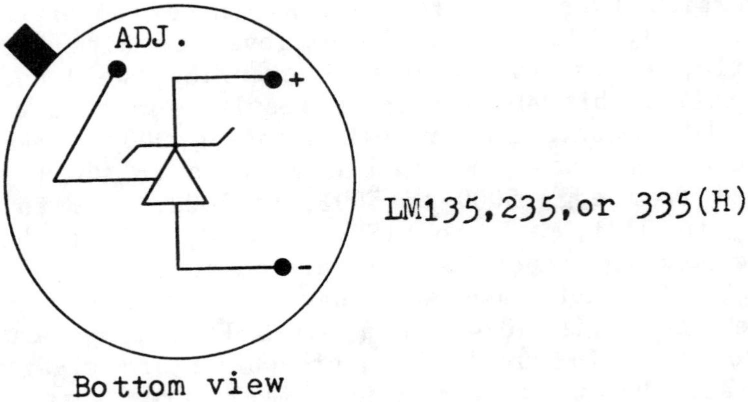

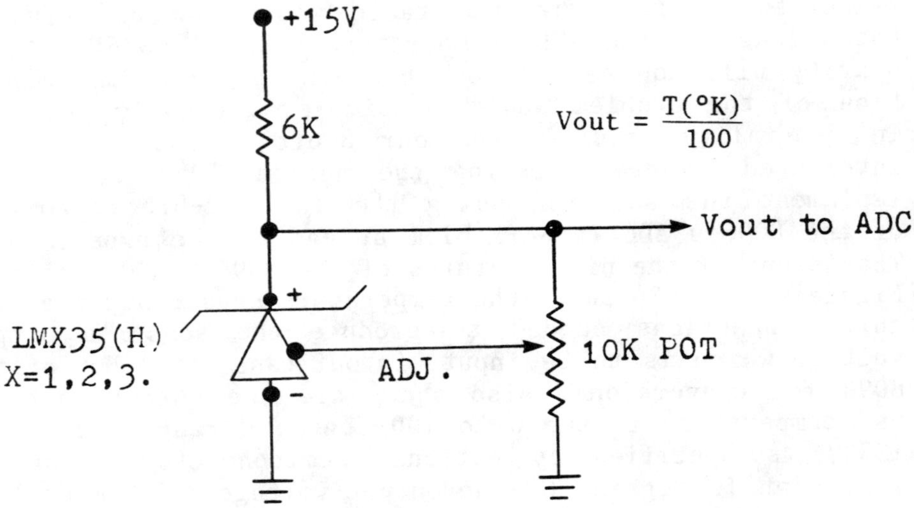

SPECS FOR LMX35(H)(X=1,2,or 3) TEMP. SENSOR (NATL. SEMI.):

Temp °C, °K	Vout (Volts) (analog in)	ADC HEX Output-Byte (based on 0 to 5V input analog swing)
0°C,273.2°K	2.73V	8A
*25°C,298.2°K	2.98V*	96
50°C,323.2°K	3.23V	A4
75°C,348.2°K	3.48V	B2
100°C,373.2°K	3.73V	BE

(*Room Temp.)

FIGURE 9-2: LM135(H) temperature sensor connections and circuitry used in Expt. 9-13. Output voltage vs. temperature specifications.

to ACH.0 and write a simple calibration program that will display the 8-bit conversion byte at P1's LEDs. As the input temperature is varied a short table will first be constructed showing the converted byte vs. measured temperature for a few temperatures from ice point to room temperature to the ambient near a light bulb in the light fixture. This table will then be interpolated on a linear basis (the temperature sensor's Vout vs. Tin characteristic is supposed to be linear) to construct a look-up table in which the AD conversion byte is listed in 1 bit increments of the byte 9-2 vs. actual temperature. Further, the actual table will start at 508C (ice point) and then proceed on up covering addresses 508D, 508E, etc. with corresponding interpolated temperatures listed in BCD form. Here 508C supposes that ice point will lead to ADRESHI = 8C as discussed in (2) above. Actually, we may find it to be slightly otherwise when we carry out the actual calibration discussed above. If ice point turns out to give the byte 89H (as we found) then the table will start at 5089 and go up in 1 bit increments of bits 9-2. Thus, for example, BCD 00 would be entered at 5089 and, if we found (as we did) 9C as the converted byte at our room temperature (24 degrees C), then we'd enter BCD 24 at 509C, with linear interpolated insertions for temperature between 5089 and 509C in the table i.e. from 00 to 24. The table will, of course, go beyond 509C 24 to cover temperatures above room temperature i.e. to the temperature and conversion byte corresponding to light bulb ambient.

4. The actual temperature controller program, as distinct from the calibration program in (3) above, will address itself to initializing P2.7 (heater) and P2.6 (blower or cooler) to the off state and then starting conversion at ACH.0 (where the sensor's output voltage is input). The converted 8-bit result in ADRESHI (bits 9-2) is extended into a word in REG1 with high byte = 0 and low byte = bits 9-2 of the conversion. This word is then added to #5000 and stored in a register (REG2) which becomes the POINTER into the temperature table. Thus if 91H were the result in ADRESHI, REG2 would hold 5091 and an instruction LDB P1, [REG2] would fetch the actual temperature (BCD degrees C) from the table constructed in (3) above and display it at P1. Thus, actual temperature would always be observed at P1. We'd next want to compare that temperature with the lower acceptable limit (entered at run-time in REG3) and then with the upper acceptable limit (entered at run-time in REG4). If the first of the two comparisons shows the temperature to be equal to or below the lower limit, a jump to LOW in the program will turn the cooler off (if it was on) and turn the heater on. If that was not

the case then a fall-through to the other comparison will occur. If that shows the temperature is above the upper limit, a jump to HIGH in the program will turn the heater off (if it was on) and turn the cooler on. If neither was the case, fall-through to a jump to "OK" keeps (or turns) both heater and cooler off, since we are between the upper and lower temperature limits and nothing needs to be done. Another conversion at ACH.0 is started and the above steps in the program are repeated. This approach to output control is digital. See PROBLEM 3 for analog output control.

THE PROGRAMS

This time we'll analyze the programs first and present them afterwards. The first program at 2490 below is the calibration program needed before a look-up table of conversion byte (8 bits) vs. actual temperature can be constructed. It simply starts conversion at channel 0, waits 8 state times for conversion to start, tests status bit S in the ADRESULT(LO) register to determine when conversion is over, at which time outputs the 8-bit result to the LEDs at P1 and then starts another conversion. Thus as temperature is varied we can read the conversion byte at each temperature. That data will then be used to construct our address vs. temperature look-up table in which the conversion byte becomes a pointer into the table. The table will be constructed so that address 50XY will contain the BCD byte UV, where XY is the conversion byte and UV is the temperature in degrees C that produced that byte (bits 9-2).

The next program at 24B0 below is the main program that implements the temperature controller. It initializes P2.7 and P2.6 to 0 (heater and cooler, respectively), starts conversion of input temperature at ACH.0, waits 8 state times for conversion to start, gathers in the high XY byte (bits 9-2) from ADRESHI into REG1 when S indicates conversion is over (S goes low), and clears the high byte of REG1, so that REG1 contains the word 00XY. REG1 is then added to #5000 to create the pointer 50XY in REG2. This will point to address 50XY in the table (see above) where the actual temperature in degrees C can be found. The instruction LDB P1, [REG2] fetches the actual temperature from the table (BCD degrees C) and outputs it to the display at P1 so that temperature is continually monitored and displayed. CMPB P1, REG3 then compares the actual temperature vs. the specified lower limit on temperature (entered into REG3 at run-time). If it is less than or equal to this lower limit, a jump is made to LOW where P2.6 is set to 0 (cooler) and P2.7 is turned on (heater). In that case the SJMP ANOTHER instruction initiates another conversion of the temperature input by the sensor and all repeats. If, however, the comparison shows that the temperature is above the lower limit, fall-through to

24D1 occurs. There the temperature is compared with the acceptable upper limit (entered into REG4 at run-time). If it is higher than that limit, a jump is made to HIGH where the heater (P2.7) is turned off and the cooler (P2.6) is turned on. The SJMP ANOTHER instruction then causes another conversion of temperature. Again all repeats.

Should the test at 24D4 fail, the indication is that the temperature lies between the specified limits. Fall-through 24D4 to 24D6 results in a jump to OK where heater and cooler are turned off (should either have been on). After OK we start another conversion and all repeats.

The programs are presented below.

```
         18 00          SP       EQU    18H
         02 00          ADCOM    EQU    02H
         03 00          ADRESHI  EQU    03H
         02 00          ADRESLO  EQU    02H
         50 00          REG1     EQU    50H
         51 00          REG1HI   EQU    51H
         50 00          REG1LO   EQU    50H
         60 00          REG2     EQU    60H
         70 00          REG3     EQU    70H
         80 00          REG4     EQU    80H
         0F 00          P1       EQU    0FH
         10 00          P2       EQU    10H

                        ;
                        ;        CALIBRATION ROUTINE FOR EXPT. 9-13
                        ;

2490                             ORG    2490H
                        ;
2490     A1 C0 00 18             LD     SP,#00C0H          ;Initialize SP.
2494     B1 08 02       THERE:   LDB    ADCOM,#08H         ;Start a conversion at ACH.0 now.
                                                           ;(temp. sensor input).
2497     FD                      NOP                       ;8 state times needed.
2498     FD                      NOP                       ;
2499     3B 02 FD       HERE1:   JBS    ADRESLO,3,HERE1    ;Poll A/D status bit S. Wait until
                                                           ;S bit is cleared.
249C     B0 03 0F                LDB    P1,ADRESHI         ;Conversion complete. Output bits
                                                           ;9 - 2 of result to P1 LEDs.
249F     27 F3                   SJMP   THERE              ;Loop to THERE to start another
                                                           ;conversion.
```

```
                        ;       MAIN PROGRAM OF EXPERIMENT 9-13
                        ;
24B0                            ORG     24B0H
                        ;
24B0   A1 C0 00 18              LD      SP,#00C0H         ;Initialize SP.
24B4   71 3F 10         OK:     ANDB    P2,#3FH           ;Initialize P2.7 = P2.6 = 0. Temp OK.
24B7   B1 08 02         ANOTHER:LDB     ADCOM,#08H        ;Start conversion on channel 0 now.
24BA   FD                       NOP                       ;8 state times needed
24BB   FD                       NOP                       ;
24BC   3B 02 FD         HERE2:  JBS     ADRESLO,3,HERE2   ;Poll A/D S bit. If high, wait.
24BF   B0 03 50                 LDB     REG1,ADRESHI      ;Else conversion over, read bits
                                                          ;9 - 2 into REG1.
24C2   11 51                    CLRB    REG1HI            ;Clear high byte of word REG1.

24C4   45 00 50 50 60           ADD     REG2,REG1,#5000H;Add 5000H to word in REG1 and store
                                                          ;in REG2 (table ptr.).
24C9   B2 60 0F                 LDB     P1,[REG2]         ;Fetch actual temp. (degrees C as BCD
                                                          ;number) from table location [REG2] and
                                                          ;display at P1 LEDs.
24CC   98 70 0F                 CMPB    P1,REG3           ;Compare actual temp. T with lower limi
                                                          ;T1 stored in REG3.
24CF   D1 07                    JNH     LOW               ;If T is not higher than T1, jump to
                                                          ;LOW.
24D1   98 80 0F                 CMPB    P1,REG4           ;Else compare T with upper limit T2
                                                          ;stored in REG4.
24D4   D9 0A                    JH      HIGH              ;If T is higher than T2, jump to HIGH.
24D6   27 DC                    SJMP    OK                ;Else jump to OK. Keep P2.7 and P2.6
                                                          ;off since T is between the desired
                                                          ;limits.
24D8   71 BF 10         LOW:    ANDB    P2,#0BFH          ;Temp. is too low. Turn cooler (P2.6)
24DB   91 80 10                 ORB     P2,#80H           ;off and heater (P2.7) on.
24DE   27 D7                    SJMP    ANOTHER           ;Loop back to do another conversion.
24E0   71 7F 10         HIGH:   ANDB    P2,#7FH           ;Temp is too high. Turn heater (P2.7)
24E3   91 40 10                 ORB     P2,#40H           ;off and cooler (P2.6) on.

24E6   27 CF                    SJMP    ANOTHER           ;Loop back to do another conversion.


24E8                            END
```

PROCEDURE

1. Reset and enter BY 09 = 00. Connect the output of the LM 135H temperature sensor to A/D input channel ACH.0. See Fig. 9-2. We are using a 15V d.c. bias and voltage divider at the sensor's terminals. The ADJUST at the 10K POT in Fig. 9-2 allows for adjustment of Vout to make sure that room temperature will result in a conversion byte in the neighborhood of 99H at a room temperature of 25 degrees C.

2. Execute the "static" (calibration) program from 2490. Vary the temperature at the sensor, measuring it in degrees C. Read out the A/D conversion byte (bits 9-2) at P1's LEDs as a function of temperature. Also measure the output analog voltage at the sensor with a VOM. Here are the results we found at three different temperatures (24°C was our room temperature):

TEMP	Vout = Vin TO ADC	CONVERTED BYTE AT P1
0°C	2.62V	89H
24°C	2.98V	9CH
64°C	3.29V	ACH

3. On the basis of the above results, we constructed the temperature look-up table tiven below. Note that we have 20 points between 89H and 9CH (0 to 24 degrees) inclusive, and another 16 points between 9DH and ACH (25 to 64 degrees) inclusive. It is clear that there is a good degree of non-linearity. Also, because we won't represent 10ths of degrees, we'll have to fit in e.g. 20 points to cover 0 to 24 degrees and 16 points to cover 25 to 64 degrees. With that in mind, we constructed the following (somewhat arbitrary) coarse table, not with accuracy in mind, obviously, but to facilitate demonstrating the method. In other words we've attempted a very rough fit to the 3 points 89H, 0; 9CH, 24; ACH, 64.

ADDRESS 50XY. XY = CONVERTED BYTE.	TEMPERATURE, DEGREES C. BCD.
5089	00
508A	02
508B	04
508C	06
508D	08
508E	10
508F	11
5090	12
5091	13
5092	14
5093	15
5094	16
5095	17
5096	18
5097	19
5098	20
5099	21

509A	22
509B	23
509C	24
509D	25
509E	26
509F	27
50A0	28
50A1	30
50A2	33
50A3	36
50A4	39
50A5	42
50A6	45
50A7	48
50A8	51
50A9	54
50AA	57
50AB	60
50AC	64

4. Reset and enter BY 09 = 00. Enter the above table as follows: BY 5089 = 00, 02, 04, ... 64.
5. Enter the lower and upper limits of the desired temperature band. Take 20 degrees C and 30 degrees C, initially, as the lower and upper limits: BY 70 = 20, BY 80 = 30.
6. Execute the "dynamic" (temperature control) program from 24B0 with the temperature sensor at room temperature. You should see 24 at P1 (if that's your room temperature) and P2.7 = P2.6 = 0 (heater and cooler off). Enter BY 70 and then BY 80 and observe 20 and then 30 on the screen of your terminal.
7. Now vary the input temperature using ice and the nearest electric bulb as the means for varying the temperature at the sensor. Note that as soon as T reaches 20 degrees, the heater (P2.7) goes on and stays on as T decreases below 20. P2.6 remains off. This is verified by reading the LEDs at P1 the moment P2.7 goes on. P1 should read 20 (BCD).
8. As T goes back up (use your finger to make body contact with the sensor), P2.7 goes off as soon as T goes above 20 degrees C (verified by reading P1). As T keeps increasing (use proximity to a light bult), P2.6 (cooler) goes on the moment T goes above 30 degrees C (verified by reading P1). Now lower T at the sensor and observe the cooler P2.6 go off the moment T reaches 30 degrees on the way down (verified at P1).
9. Note in both (7) and (8), P1 reads temperature in BCD as T varies below the band, through the band, and above the band. P1 is thus our thermometer read-out.

10. Enter new temperature limits on-the-fly e.g. BY 70 = 16 and BY 80 = 36 for an acceptable temperature range of 16 to 36 degrees C. Starting at room temperature, gradually lower T at the sensor. Observe the heater P2.7 now go on the moment T reaches 16 degrees on the way down (as observed at P1). It goes back off when T goes back above 16 degrees and stays off as T increases further. When T first goes above 36 degrees, the cooler P2.6 goes on (read P1) and stays on as T is increased further. As T is now made to go back down, the cooler will go off the moment T reaches 36 degrees (read P1). It stays off as T decreases further. Query BY 70 and BY 80. Observe 16 and 36.

PROBLEMS

1. Implement a temperature controller using the full 10 bits of the A/D converter. This needs a table length of 2FDH - 230H to cover the range 100°C to 0°C (3.73V to 2.73V). The table length would thus be 204 bytes compared to an 8-bit conversion table length of BFH - 8CH = 51 bytes for the same temperature and voltage range (the expected 4 to 1 ratio). In that case you can construct a temperature look-up table at 1/2°C intervals from one address to the next, compared to our average interval of 2°C for our table that was based on an 8-bit conversion.
2. Write a program to calculate °C EXACTLY from the formula (Fig 9-2): °C = 100 x Vout - 273.2, where Vout = (UVW/3FF) x 5V, and UVW = 10-bit A/D conversion word. Use no tables, do by ARITHMETIC. The 8096 is well suited for this.
3. As an alternative to the "cooler/heater" approach to temperature control, one could implement such control by having an analog voltage created by the microcomputer whose magnitude, if input to the temperature controller, will force the temperature to go up if the actual temperature is below the acceptable band or to go down if the actual temperature is above the acceptable band. This will necessitate a knowledge of the input voltage/output temperature characteristic of the temperature controller. In that case the necessary analog voltage to implement temperature control could be generated using the PWM unit with a d.c. smoothing filter at the output of the PWM pin (P2.5). Actual temperature, of course, would still be monitored by means of the sensor and A/D conversion at ACH.0. The size of the conversion byte would reveal which temperature region we're in and thus decide the necessary analog voltage to be output to the temperature controller to get us back in the acceptable band. Try to implement such a temperature controller using the PWM unit. Analog output control thus replaces digital output control.

EXPERIMENTS 9-14(A),(B)

REMOTE CONTROL OF 8096 - DRIVEN I/Os FROM A LOCAL "DUMB TERMINAL" VIA SERIAL LINK.

A. SELECTION OF PARAMETERS FOR I/Os AT REMOTE 8096 MADE FROM LOCAL TERMINAL: THE I/O NUMBER, THE NUMBER OF ON/OFF CYCLES, AND THE ON/OFF TIMES. REMOTE CONTROL OF REP-RATE ON-THE-FLY.

B. REMOTE TERMINAL CONTROL OF MOTOR SPEED, OR TEMPERATURE, OR PRESSURE, ETC. VIA SERIAL LOADING OF THE PWM. ASCII-TO-HEX CONVERSION ROUTINE.

INTRODUCTION

Up to now, parameter set-up and/or parameter control on-the-fly have been accomplished by using the SBE commands e.g. BY REG = XY (or WO REG = UVXY) AT RUN-TIME, and/or BY REG = X'Y' (or WO REG = U'V'W'X') DURING EXECUTION OF THE PROGRAM. Here, XY or (UVWX) are the parameter values being set up and X'Y' (or U'V' W'X') are the NEW parameter values being imposed on-the-fly AFTER set-up. The iSBE-96 monitor did the function of reading the data entered at the KBRD and placing it into memory at the specified address. By using this facility, we didn't have to concern ourselves with writing our own program to "read the keyboard" for those parameters. See, for example, Expts. 6-13, 6-16, 6-17 and many, many others through-out the book.

Now we'd like to become independent of any monitor or operating system in this regard. We'd like to include OUR OWN ROUTINES which will allow us to interact with a user via a terminal and accept data from it for parameter set-up or for changing their values on-the-fly. This can be accomplished by connecting a serial I/O device (e.g. a terminal or another microcomputer) to the serial port of our 8096. The TXD output line of the terminal (or other microcomputer) would be connected to the RXD input line of our microcomputer and the RXD of the terminal (or other microcomputer) would be connected to our TXD. Then, as in chapter 8, a calling of the "GET-CHR" routine in our microcomputer (which polls the RI flag) will pass any character received in its SBUF(RX) from the terminal or other microcomputer into a register when RI goes high (indicating SBUF(RX) has received a COMPLETE byte serially from the terminal or other microcomputer). The character received would be transmitted back to the terminal or other microcomputer to allow a visual echo for the user. GET-CHR can be called as many times as there are parameters to SET UP. On the other hand, a vectoring to a SERIAL INTERRUPT ISR can be arranged when a key is pressed DURING PROGRAM EXECUTION and a fully received byte has been stored in SBUF(RX) of our microcomputer via its RXD line. The serial interrupt generated will be SERVICED if the global interrupt is enabled and the serial port's interrupt line is unmasked. The servicing would merely consist of the ISR reading the newly received character in SBUF(RX) into the parameter register, thus changing that parameter and some aspect of the I/O control or performance ON-THE-FLY. A new change can be imposed each and every time that a new key is pressed. In the previous parameter set-up stage, we can, if we wish, read in the characters from the keyboard (GET-CHR) without necessarily servicing the attendant serial port interrupt (e.g. it can be masked - see Expt. 8-3).

In this experiment we'll write our own routines, based on serial I/O, which will allow us to "READ THE KEYBOARD" at run-time and return with a parameter(s) stored in a register(s) for parameter set-up; or which will allow us to update those parameters from the keyboard as the program is executing. The approach is based on the material covered in chapter 8 on Serial I/O. We'll use the technique in two different applications that are of important interest in their own right (see title to this experiment) where remote control of microcomputer driven I/Os (either via RS232 or fiber optics or modems) must be implemented.

THE IMPORTANCE OF REMOTE CONTROL (OR COMMUNICATIONS) VIA SERIAL I/O IN REAL WORLD APPLICATIONS CAN NOT BE OVEREMPHASIZED. THE LINK CAN BE RS232, MODEM, OR FIBER OPTICS - OUR PROGRAMS APPLY EQUALLY WELL.

EXPERIMENT 9-14(A).

SELECTION OF PARAMETERS FOR I/Os AT REMOTE 8096 MADE FROM LOCAL TERMINAL: THE I/O NUMBER, THE NUMBER OF ON/OFF CYCLES, AND THE ON/OFF TIMES. REMOTE CONTROL OF REP-RATE ON-THE-FLY.

DESCRIPTION OF THE PROBLEM

The application we'll solve can be described as follows:

1. A "dumb terminal" (ASCII keyboard with CRT display and

RS232 serial I/O facility) is serially linked to an iSBE-96 board via the TXD, RXD lines at both devices. See Expt. 8-3, 4th paragraph in the introduction section p. 419, for the necessary RS232 connections to implement the serial link between the terminal and the SBE-96.

2. After execution of the program is initiated, key 0, 1, 2, ..., or 7 is entered from the terminal's keyboard to select I/O P1.0, P1.1, P1.2, ... or P1.7 for on/off action at the SBE-96. An echo back from the 8096 displays the I/O # on the CRT.
3. Key 1, 2, ... or 9 is then entered to specify the number of on/off cycles at the selected I/O P1.x. That number also is displayed at the CRT.
4. Key 1, 2, ... or 9 is next entered to specify the on/off times of the selected I/O (in multiples of 0.2 sec). That multiple is also to be echoed back to the CRT.
5. Any key is then pressed to start the I/O cycles (it, too, is displayed).
6. At ANY TIME during either the parameter set-up, or while the on/off cycles are occurring, you can create an EXTINT interrupt (a debounced switch S is used at EXTINT) to abort the cycles at P1, or nullify the entered parameters. You can then enter new parameters for new cycles. S is to be considered located at the local terminal and is connected to EXTINT at the remote 8096 to create the abort interrupt.
7. DURING EXECUTION OF THE ON/OFF CYCLES, any number from 1 to 9 can be entered from the keyboard to "instantly" change the on/off times on-the-fly before all the cycles are done. In fact, we'll be able to change those times more than once by further presses among keys 1 to 9 before the cycles are completed. "Instantly" will mean "to within 0.2 sec". (See Problem 3).
8. When all cycles are completed (or after an abort via switch S at EXTINT is accomplished) a NEW SET of parameters can be entered to define a new on/off operation (number of cycles and on/off times) of another (or the same) I/O from among P1.x (x = 0 to 7).

Let us now present and discuss the program that will implement the above features of the problem.

THE PROGRAM

The program at 2600 is presented below and analyzed afterward.

```
            18 00          SP       EQU   18H
            11 00          SP_CON   EQU   11H
            11 00          SP_STAT  EQU   11H
            07 00          SBUF     EQU   07H
            0E 00          BAUD     EQU   0EH
            80 00          BAUD_HI  EQU   80H
            9B 00          BAUD_LO  EQU   9BH         ;1200 BAUD
            09 00          PINT     EQU   09H
            08 00          MINT     EQU   08H
            0E 20          INVEC0   EQU   200EH
            0C 20          INVEC1   EQU   200CH
            20 00          TEMP1    EQU   20H
            30 00          TEMP     EQU   30H
            40 00          OFFSET   EQU   40H
            50 00          REG0     EQU   50H
            51 00          REG1     EQU   51H
            52 00          REG2     EQU   52H
            53 00          REG3     EQU   53H
            80 00          REG4     EQU   80H
            16 00          IOC1     EQU   16H
            70 00          CHAR_I   EQU   70H
            60 00          CHAR_O   EQU   60H
            0F 00          P1       EQU   0FH
                           ;
                           ;
2600                                ORG   2600H
                           ;
2600        A1 C0 00 18             LD    SP,#0C0H         ;Initialize SP.
2604        FA                      DI                     ;Disable interrutps.
2605        11 0F                   CLRB  P1               ;Initialize P1 LEDs to 00.
2607        B1 20 16                LDB   IOC1,#20H        ;Select EXTINT, not ACH.7 interrupt
                                                           ;source and enable TxD.
260A        B1 80 08                LDB   MINT,#80H        ;Unmask EXTINT interrupt source.
260D        A1 AB 26 30             LD    TEMP,#EXTINT     ;Load TEMP with EXTINT ISR address
2611        C3 01 0E 20 30          ST    TEMP,INVEC0[0]   ;and store in VECT INT table at
                                                           ;200EH.
2616        A1 92 26 30             LD    TEMP,#SERINT     ;Load address of serial port
261A        C3 01 0C 20 30          ST    TEMP,INVEC1[0]   ;interrupt service routine into INT
                                                           ;VECT table at 200CH.
261F        B1 20 30                LDB   TEMP,#20H        ;Initialize TEMP with 20 (RI and TI).
2622        B1 9B 0E                LDB   BAUD,#BAUD_LO    ;Load low byte of baud rate into BAUD.
2625        B1 80 0E                LDB   BAUD,#BAUD_HI    ;Load high byte of baud into BAUD reg.
2628        B1 09 11                LDB   SP_CON,#09H      ;Initialize serial port: mode 1,
                                                           ;REN = 1, PEN = 0.
```

```
262B  11 09                    CLRB   PINT               ;Clear any pending interrupts.
262D  FB                       EI                        ;Enable interrupts.
262E  A1 00 00 40    NEWSET:   LD     OFFSET,#00H        ;Initialize register table pointer
                                                         ;offset.
2632  EF 32 00       PARAMS:   CALL   GET_CHR            ;Call GET_CHR ("Read Keyboard")
                                                         ;routine.  Waits for key to
                                                         ;be pressed.
2635  B0 70 60                 LDB    CHAR_O,CHAR_I      ;Copy input key to CHAR_O for echo.
2638  EF 39 00                 CALL   PUT_CHR            ;Echo key to terminal.
263B  71 0F 70                 ANDB   CHAR_I,#0FH        ;Mask out upper nibble. Parameter
                                                         ;value (0 to 9) now in CHAR_I.
263E  C7 40 50 70              STB    CHAR_I,REG0[OFFSET] ;Load parameter into register
2642  07 40                    INC    OFFSET             ;table and increment OFFSET.
2644  99 04 40                 CMPB   OFFSET,#04H        ;Compare OFFSET to 4.
2647  D7 E9                    JNE    PARAMS             ;If OFFSET != 4, four keys have not
                                                         ;been entered, goto PARAMS for more.
2649  11 09                    CLRB   PINT               ;Clear any pending interrupts.
264B  B1 C0 08                 LDB    MINT,#0C0H         ;Unmask serial port interrupt source.
264E  B1 01 20       CYCLE:    LDB    TEMP1,#01H         ;Load TEMP1 with 01.
2651  19 50 20                 SHLB   TEMP1,REG0         ;Shift left # times specified by
                                                         ;I/O number in register at table
                                                         ;location 0 (REG0).
                                                         ;This will turn on P1.X where X
                                                         ;is 0,1,2,... or 7.
2654  B0 20 0F                 LDB    P1,TEMP1           ;Copy TEMP1 to P1 LEDs.
2657  EF 27 00                 CALL   TIME               ;Keep P1.X on for time determined
                                                         ;by REG2 (third key entered).
265A  11 0F                    CLRB   P1                 ;Clear P1.X
265C  EF 22 00                 CALL   TIME               ;Call time delay for off time (REG2).
265F  E0 51 EC                 DJNZ   REG1,CYCLE         ;Decrement REG1 contents. If != 0,
                                                         ;jump to CYCLE to do another cycle.
2662  B1 80 08                 LDB    MINT,#80H          ;Else mask serial port interrupt
                                                         ;source again.
2665  27 C7                    SJMP   NEWSET             ;Specified # of cycles complete.
                                                         ;Jump to NEWSET to read in new
                                                         ;parameters for I/O, # cycles, and
                                                         ;on/off time.
                     ;
                     ;
                     ;
                     ;         INPUT CHARACTER ROUTINE: GET_CHR
                     ;
2667  90 11 30       GET_CHR:ORB      TEMP,SP_STAT       ;Copy serial port status into TEMP.
266A  36 30 FA                 JBC    TEMP,6,GET_CHR     ;If RI = 0, goto GET_CHR.
266D  71 BF 30                 ANDB   TEMP,#0BFH         ;Else clear RI flag in TEMP.
2670  B0 07 70                 LDB    CHAR_I,SBUF        ;Read character from SBUF into CHAR_I.
2673  F0                       RET                       ;Return.
```

```
                              ;       OUTPUT CHARACTER ROUTINE: PUT_CHR
                              ;
2674    90 11 30        PUT_CHR:ORB     TEMP,SP_STAT     ;Copy serial port status into TEMP.
2677    35 30 FA                JBC     TEMP,5,PUT_CHR   ;If TI = 0, goto PUT_CHR.
267A    B0 60 07                LDB     SBUF,CHAR_O      ;Else load character from CHAR_O
                                                         ;into SBUF for transmission.
267D    71 DF 30                ANDB    TEMP,#0DFH       ;Clear temp TI flag.

2680    F0                      RET                      ;Return.
                              ;
                              ;
2681    B0 52 53        TIME:   LDB     REG3,REG2        ;Pass multiples from REG2 to
                                                         ;REG3 (i.e. # outer loops).
2684    A1 FF FF 80     LOAD:   LD      REG4,#0FFFFH     ;Load REG4 with FFFF for 0.2 sec.
                                                         ;(# inner loops).
2688    05 80           AGAIN:  DEC     REG4             ;Decrement inner loop counter (REG4).
268A    D7 FC                   JNE     AGAIN            ;If REG4 != 0, jump to AGAIN.
268C    E0 53 F5                DJNZ    REG3,LOAD        ;Else decrement outer loop counter
                                                         ;and jump to LOAD if != 0.
268F    F0                      RET                      ;Outer loop counter = 0, return.

                              ;
                              ;       SERIAL PORT INTERRUPT SERVICE ROUTINE:
                              ;
2690    F2              SERINT: PUSHF                    ;Save flags.
2691    90 11 30                ORB     TEMP,SP_STAT     ;Read SP_STAT for RI, TI test.
2694    36 30 10                JBC     TEMP,6,NO_CHAR   ;If RI = 0, jump to NO_CHAR.
2697    2F CE                   CALL    GET_CHR          ;Get character just entered (RI is
                                                         ;high).
2699    B0 70 60                LDB     CHAR_O,CHAR_I    ;Copy character received into CHAR_O
                                                         ;register for echo.
269C    2F D6                   CALL    PUT_CHR          ;Call PUT_CHR to echo back CHAR_O.
269E    B0 70 52                LDB     REG2,CHAR_I      ;Load character from CHAR_I into REG2.
26A1    71 0F 52                ANDB    REG2,#0FH        ;Mask upper nibble.
26A4    B0 52 53                LDB     REG3,REG2        ;Copy REG2 into REG3.
26A7    F3              NO_CHAR:POPF                     ;Restore flags.
26A8    F0                      RET                      ;Return to main program.
                              ;
                              ;       EXTERNAL INTERRUPT SERVICE ROUTINE
                              ;
26A9    11 0F           EXTINT: CLRB    P1               ;Clear P1 LEDs. P1.X on/off activity
                                                         ;ceases.
26AB    A1 C0 00 18             LD      SP,#00C0H        ;Reinitialize SP.
26AF    B1 80 08                LDB     MINT,#80H        ;Disable serial port interrupts.
26B2    E7 79 FF                LJMP    NEWSET           ;Jump to NEWSET to accept new
                                                         ;parameters.
                              ;
                              ;
26B5                            END
```

The main program starts by initializing SP, disabling the interrupt system, and resetting all I/Os at P1 (P1.x, x = 0 to 7). IOC1 is then loaded with 20H to both select the EXTINT source (rather than ACH.7) and to enable the TXD line at P2.0 of the 8096 (for echo back to the CRT). The EXTINT interrupt source is next unmasked (the serial port interrupt source is kept masked at this point). The addresses of the EXTINT and Serial Interrupt ISRs are then loaded into the INT VECT table at 200E and 200C, respectively (the SERINT ISR will be used when MINT.6 is LATER set to 1). 20 is then loaded into TEMP to set our TI flag indicator to 1 and to clear the RI flag indicator (TEMP.5 and .6, respectively). WE WANT TO MAKE CERTAIN, WHEN WE HAVE THE FIRST KBRD CHARACTER WHICH WE WISH TO TRANSMIT BACK TO THE CRT, THAT WE'LL GET OUT OF THE TI POLLING LOOP IN PUT-CHR SO THAT WE CAN LOAD SBUF(TX) WITH THE FIRST RECEIVED CHARACTER FOR TRANSMISSION BACK TO THE CRT. OTHERWISE WE'D BE HUNG UP IN THAT LOOP FOREVER. This only applies to the FIRST received character. For subsequent received characters, TI will go high when the PREVIOUS character loaded into SBUF(TX) has been transmitted out. We'll then be able to fall through the TI polling to load SBUF(TX) with the NEXT received character to be echoed back on the CRT. (This matter was also taken up and discussed in Expts. 8-3, 8-4, 8-5, and 8-6 where the same situation arose).

The initializations continue with a loading of BAUD to specify a baud rate of 1200, the loading of 09 in SPCON to seLect mode 1 operation for the serial port and to enable its receiver [RXD to SBUF(RX)] facility, the clearing of any pending interrupts, and the enabling of the interrupt system (to service any EXTINT interrupts - NOT serial I/O interrupts YET).

We are now at the point of analyzing the part of the program dealing with parameter set-up (and echoing of same). Three registers REG0 (50), REG1 (51), and REG2 (52) are assigned to store the values of I/O number selected, number of cycles desired, and on/off time required, respectively. With REG0 (0050) serving as a BASE ADDRESS to the parameter table to be formed at 0050, 0051, and 0052, and OFFSET (0040) serving as the offset from REG0 (0050) into this table to be constructed, we should initialize OFFSET to 0. This we do at NEWSET (at 262E). NEWSET indicates a new set of parameters is about to be entered and stored in REG0, REG1, REG2 at 0050, 51, 52 in the table, respectively. We now call the GET-CHR routine (located at 2667) to await the reception of the first character from the terminal's keyboard (which will then be processed to become the first parameter i.e. I/O # selected). GET-CHR simply waits till RI in the TEMP flag register goes high (as read from SP-STAT). This will occur when a complete byte from the terminal is received in SBUF(RX) in the 8096. Fall-through at 266A then occurs.

The RI flag in TEMP is cleared and the received byte in SBUF(RX) is loaded into CHAR-I for subsequent transmission (echo back to the CRT). Return to 2635 in the main program then results in CHAR-I being loaded into register CHAR-O. A call to PUT-CHR is then made where (with TI flag being high as a result of the prior initialization of TEMP) fall-through the test of the TI flag at 2677 results in the loading of CHAR-O (first received character) into SBUF(TX) for transmission and echo back at the CRT. The TI flag in TEMP is then cleared. It will go high again as soon as the CHAR-O byte just loaded into SBUF(TX) is fully transmitted out. Return to 263B in the main program then results in a masking out of the upper nibble in the character received from the terminal. Thus ASCII codes 30, 31,....or 39 (corresponding to presses of keys 0, 1,....or 9) become 00, 01, 02,....or 09, respectively: they'll serve as our PARAMETERS for I/O # (0 thru 7), or # cycles (1 thru 9), or on/off time multiples of 0.2 usec. (1 thru 9). That parameter is then stored in the table at REGO [OFFSET], which at this point is at 0050. The OFFSET is then incremented to get ready to point to 0051 in the parameter table being constructed.

We shall be entering 3 parameters associated with the I/O control in this application, as already explained. They'll be stored at REGO, REG1, and REG2 at 0051, 52, 53 as previously indicated. The first (I/O #) has just been stored in REGO at 0050. A FOURTH key (any key) will ALSO be pressed merely for the purpose of initiating the I/O process AFTER 3 keys have been entered and stored as parameters. Its storage in REG3 at 0053 will be superfluous and ignored. To test when 4 keys have been entered, the CMPB OFFSET, #04H instruction at 2644 and the JNE PARAMS instruction at 2647 have been inserted. If 4 keys have not been entered, the JNE instruction takes us back to PARAMS where another call of GET-CHR takes us to 2667 to await the entry of another key. When that occurs, RI in TEMP goes high again (it was cleared after the last character from the terminal was received) and CHAR-I is loaded with the newly received character in SBUF(RX). Again a return to 2635 occurs (with RI in TEMP cleared). There PUT-CHR is again called and entered. It is MOST IMPORTANT to realize that when we enter PUT-CHR AGAIN, the TI flag in TEMP is high again (or will shortly become high) as a result of the LAST byte previously loaded into SBUF(TX) having been transmitted out by this time (or being transmitted out shortly). This results (or will result) in fall-through at 2677 and a loading of the newly received character into SBUF(TX) for subsequent transmission. Again, the TI flag is cleared in TEMP. BUT, NOTE: AFTER THE 4th (LAST) KEY IS PRESSED AND TRANSMITTED BACK IN PUT-CHR, THE TI FLAG WILL AGAIN GO, AND REMAIN, HIGH WHEN THE KEY'S CHARACTER IS FULLY TRANSMITTED OUT OF SBUF(TX). THIS IS VERY IMPORTANT FOR LATER WHEN THE SERIAL AND EXTINT ISRS ARE ANALYZED.

The above events repeat until 4 key presses have been made (I/O #, # cycles, on/off time, and ANY KEY to initiate the process). At that point fall-through JNE at 2647 occurs. PINT is cleared of any pending interrupts. Remember that the characters received in SBUF(RX) from the terminal, as well as characters transmitted back to the terminal from SBUF(TX), will generate serial port interrupts which become PENDING because MINT contains 80. We now clear those pendings. We don't want SERINT interrupts to be serviced (yet). MINT is then loaded with C0H TO NOW UNMASK THE SERIAL I/O INTERRUPT SOURCE, keeping EXTINT unmasked. Our purpose here is to GET READY for vectoring to the SERINT ISR during the I/O on/off cycles about to unfold SHOULD key presses during THOSE CYCLES be made FOR THE PURPOSE OF CHANGING THE TIME PARAMETER IN REG2 ON-THE-FLY. Any such key press will cause a byte to be serially transmitted to the 8096 from the terminal and stored in SBUF(RX) there. The serial I/O interrupt generated when the FULL BYTE is received in SBUF(RX) will THIS TIME be serviced since we'll then vector to the SERINT ISR. There, that byte (with upper nibble unmasked) can be loaded into REG2 (time parameter register) to update the on/off time on-the-fly. More on that aspect later. After the loading of MINT at 264B, the I/O cycles unfold.

In order to turn P1.x on (x = 0, 1,....or 7), TEMP1 is loaded with 01 AND THEN SHIFTED LEFT THE NUMBER OF TIMES INDICATED IN REG0 (I/O #). THIS WILL RESULT IN TEMP1.X BEING SET WITH ALL OTHER BITS IN TEMP1 CLEARED. LDB P1, TEMP1 then turns P1.x on. Time is then called (located at 2661) to keep P1.x on for the desired time (the parameter stored in REG2 determines that time). Note that TIME retrieves the time multiple of 0.2 sec. from REG2 and loads it into REG3. (REG3 is available to us even though previously used to store "any key", as we have no further need for "any key"). REG4 is then loaded with FFFF so that a 0.2 sec. inner loop delay (the loop at AGAIN at 2688) results. The DJNZ REG3, LOAD insures that precisely (REG2) such loops will be made before the exit at 268F takes us back to 265A in the main program where P1.x is turned off and TIME is again called to produce an off-time of the same amount as the previous on-time. Returning from TIME now takes us to 265F where the cycle-count register, REG1, is decremented to see whether all the I/O cycles specified by the parameter in REG1 (at 0051) have been completed. If not the jump taken by DJNZ is back to CYCLE where all repeats to implement another I/O cycle. When the specified number of cycles are done the program falls through 265F and we re-load MINT with 80H to mask the serial I/O interrupt source again, as we are about to enter new parameters and we are not now concerned with changing the on/off time on-the-fly. We do not want serial interrupts in GET-CHR or PUT-CHR to be honored during this phase. The SJMP NEWSET instruction then carries us back to 262E where a new set of 3 parameters for I/O #, # cycles, and on/off time are to be entered. IT IS MOST IMPORTANT TO REALIZE THAT WHEN WE ARE CARRIED BACK TO NEWSET, WE ARRIVE THERE WITH TEMP.5 (TI FLAG) HIGH AGAIN BECAUSE THE 4TH AND FINAL KEY ("ANY KEY") PREVIOUSLY LOADED INTO SBUF(TX) IN PUT-CHR HAS, BY THIS TIME, BEEN TRANSMITTED OUT CAUSING THE TI FLAG, PREVIOUSLY CLEARED IN PUT-CHR, TO GO HIGH AGAIN. THIS IS EXTREMELY IMPORTANT, OTHERWISE WHEN THE FIRST OF 4 NEW KEYS IS ENTERED, FOR A NEW PARAMETER SET-UP AND PUT-CHR IS AGAIN CALLED AFTER A RETURN FROM GET-CHR, WE'D NEVER GET OUT OF THE PUT-CHR LOOP TESTING TI. WE'D NEVER BE ABLE TO LOAD SBUF(TX) WITH THE FIRST OF THE 4 NEW PARAMETERS JUST ENTERED AT THE KEYBOARD.

What happens, either during parameter set-up or during the I/O on-off cycles, if an EXTINT interrupt is made with our debounced switch S? In either case, we are simply vectored to the EXTINT ISR at EXTINT (26A9) where the I/O, P1.x, is turned off (if it was on), SP is re-initialized to 00C0 and MINT is reloaded with 80. The latter is done in case the interrupt was made in that part of the program where the contents of MINT are C0 i.e. during the I/O's on or off times. 80 in MINT again assures that, when a jump to NEWSET is made, (the last instruction in the EXTINT ISR), we'll arrive there with the serial interrupt source MASKED, as we'll then be ready for a NEW parameter set-up. We don't want any serial I/O interrupts to be serviced while new parameters are entered from the terminal. Remember that the serial I/O interrupt is to be serviced in its ISR ONLY when entering keys DURING THE ON OR OFF TIMES OF P1.X IN ORDER TO CHANGE THOSE TIMES ON-THE-FLY. Note, also, that the EXTINT ISR ends in a jump to NEWSET, at 262E, where we now want to be. Normally, a more conventional RET would be used, but that would take us back to the point where the EXTINT was made, and would not lead to the ABORT situation we are trying to implement with EXTINT. In following this approach, we make certain that SP is back to 00C0 before undertaking the LJMP instruction. Remember, the stack pointer has moved up as TWO return addresses have been saved on the top of the stack (one from CALL TIME and the other from the EXTINT interrupt), and so it is imperative, using our approach, that SP be brought back to its original value before the CALL and EXTINT were made. (See Problem 4).

On the other hand, if the EXTINT interrupt was made between PARAMS and CYCLE, during parameter set-up, and before the latter was completed, then 80 was in MINT all along and no harm is done by a re-loading of 80 into it in the EXTINT ISR. This time, the interrupt would have been made somewhere in GET-CHR or PUT-CHR (most likely in GET-CHR, where we'd be waiting to receive the next parameter entry from the terminal when we decide to abort and enter new parameters to replace the others previously entered). Again, the EXTINT ISR will carry us back to NEWSET (LJMP NEWSET) with 80 in MINT, ready for a new set of parameters to be entered. (There'll be no servicing of any serial I/O interrupts to the SERINT ISR when RECEIVE COMPLETE or TRANSMIT COMPLETE serial I/O interrupts are generated as parameter entries are made from the terminal's keyboard). IN EITHER CASE, THE ARRIVAL AT NEWSET AFTER EXTINT FINDS US WITH TI FLAG HIGH AS A RESULT OF THE LAST KEY ENTRY'S CHARACTER HAVING BEEN TRANSMITTED OUT OF SBUF(TX) SOME TIME BACK. THIS IS IMPORTANT BECAUSE IT GUARANTEES THAT WE'LL GET OUT OF THE PUT-CHR LOOP TO TRANSMIT NEW KBRD CHARACTERS.

Finally, an analysis must be made of the serial port ISR (SERINT) at 2690. This ISR is ONLY entered when a key is pressed at the terminal's keyboard DURING ANY I/O ON OR OFF/TIME as I/O cycles are unfolding (remember, MINT is loaded with C0 only during those times). That causes a byte to be received in the 8096's SBUF(RX) from the terminal. The subsequent serial port interrupt is generated (and RI goes high) at the time the COMPLETE BYTE IS RECEIVED in SBUF(RX). The SERINT ISR's purpose is to gather in and echo the received character and store it in the time registers REG2 and REG3 (upper nibble masked). The subsequent return to TIME, where the serial port interrupt was made, will result in an immediate change in the current time delay (a glance at TIME shows that this change in on or off time will be made WITHIN 0.2 USEC. i.e. at the END of the INNER loop at AGAIN when the DJNZ REG3, LOAD instruction is encountered). In that way, the ORIGINAL time delay parameter in REG2 is replaced, on-the-fly, by the update entered at the terminal's keyboard during the on/off cycles.

The details of the SERINT ISR at 2690 follow. The PSW (flags and MINT) is pushed on the stack leaving the interrupt system disabled (PUSHF leaves 0 in the PSW). The RI flag in TEMP (TEMP.6) is polled after SPSTAT is written into TEMP (RI = SPSTAT.6). Since RI is high because a byte HAS been received in SBUF(RX) from the terminal (otherwise we wouldn't find ourselves in this ISR to begin with), we IMMEDIATELY fall through the JBC instruction at 2694 to the CALL of GET-CHR (why, then, the polling of TEMP.6? Read on). GET-CHR at 2667 also polls the RI flag in TEMP and, for the same reason as above, immediately falls through to 266D where the RI flag in TEMP is cleared and the character received in SBUF(RX) is loaded into CHAR-I. The return at 2673 is to 2699 in the SERINT ISR. There, the byte just received is loaded into CHAR-O for transmission (echo) back to the terminal. That is accomplished by a CALL at 269C of PUT-CHR at 2674. In PUT-CHR TEMP.5 is polled. This flag is high from the time the 4th key was entered in the PARAMS set-up and then echoed back to the terminal. The subsequent complete transmission out of SBUF(TX) AT THAT TIME (see PUT-CHR) left TI high ever since. Hence, when we now call PUT-CHR at 269C in the SERINT ISR, we immediately fall through the JBC instruction at 2677 and load the PRESENT received character (in CHAR-0) into SBUF(TX) for transmission back to the terminal. The TI flag in TEMP is then cleared (it will go high again just as soon as the present transmission out of SBUF(TX) is completed). A return is then made to the LDB REG2, CHAR-I instruction in the ISR at 269E. (Please note that the present TRANSMISSION out of SBUF (TX) will ALSO create a serial port interrupt. It becomes PENDING because the PSW has 0 all during this ISR till POPF at the end. We'll shortly see what becomes of this pending interrupt). The LDB instruction mentioned above loads REG2 with the character entered at the terminal. The upper nibble in REG2 is masked so that REG2 now containes the newly updated, on-the-fly, value of time multiples. This value is also placed in REG3 so that time will change NO LATER than 0.2 usec. after the new key was pressed (see TIME routine). The POPF insturction restores flags, MINT, and PSW.9 (global bit). A return at 26A8 is then made to the location in TIME where the serial port interrupt was created. The effect on the on/off times there will be "immediate" (to within 0.2 sec). (See Problem 3).

But we are not yet "off the hook". The very last statement made in the last paragraph is true but is not yet in order. Remember, there is a pending serial port interrupt to be serviced due to TRANSMISSION COMPLETE out of SBUF(TX) that occurs after the present entered key has been echoed back to the terminal in PUT-CHR. This pending is now serviced because of POPF at the end of the SERINT ISR. With the TI flag high (because of TRANSMISSION COMPLETE) and RI low (as a result of its clearing in the GET-CHR routine called from the SERINT ISR), the entry into the SERINT ISR does a jump around at 2694 (JBC TEMP, 6, NO-CHAR) to POPF and RET. We are out of the ISR, with no effect on anything, and back to TIME. The last statement in the last paragraph now applies. Therein lies the need for polling TEMP at the beginning of the SERINT ISR.

PROCEDURE

1. Connect a "local" debounced switch S to the EXTINT interrupt line on the remote 8096. Interface RXD/TXD of a CRT terminal with an ASCII keyboard to TXD/RXD of the remote SBE-96 by means of an RS232 cable as in Expt. 8-3 (see p. 419, paragraph 4 in the introduction to that experiment).
2. Reset and enter BY 09 = 00.
3. Execute from 2600. Enter parameters: key 5 to select I/O P1.5, key 7 to specify 7 on/off cycles by P1.5, key 1 to

specify 0.2 sec. on and off times. Then press any key to initiate the cycles. Observe the echoes 5, 7, 1, x on the terminal (x being "any key") as you enter the keys. See P1.5 go on/off 7 times with 0.2 sec. on/off times after "any key" is pressed.

4. Enter new parameters: 7, 9, 9, then any key. See the echoes. Observe P1.7 go on/off 9 times with 9 x 0.2 = 1.8 sec. on/off times.
5. Enter the same parameters again: 7, 9, 9, any key, with echoes. Before the 9 cycles are done, and during an on-time, abort by throwing S lo/hi/lo at EXTINT. Observe P1.7 clear. No further cycles are observed. Re-enter the same parameters (see echoes) and throw S during one of the off cycles. Observe.
6. Enter new parameters: 3, 2, 1. Then abort with switch S at EXTINT before pressing any key. Enter 3, 4, 9, any key. See P1.3 go on/off 4 times with 1.8 sec. on and off-times. In each case observe the key press echoes on the CRT.
7. Enter parameters 0, 6, 7, any key. Observe the echoes on the terminal. See P1.0 go on/off after "any key" is pressed. The on/off times are each 1.4 sec. Abort before the 5 cycles requested are done (EXTINT).
8. Re-enter 0, 6. Create another EXTINT abort. Nothing happens. Enter 6, 4, 2, any key. See P1.6 go on/off 4 times with 0.4 sec. on/off times.
9. Enter 2, 9, 9, any key. Observe P1.2 go on/off with 1.8 sec. on and off times. After two such cycles, enter key "4". See the on/off times change to 0.8 sec. (almost immediately, to the eye). After 3 more cycles key in "1". The on/off times change to 0.2 sec. Four more cycles finish up.
10. Enter 4, 0, 1, any key (0 cycles really means 256 cycles because of DJNZ at 265F). Observe P1.4 go on/off with 0.2 sec. on and off-times. Gradually enter keys 2, 3, 4, 5, 6, 7, 8, 9 in turn, and observe the oscillations at P1.4 proceed with slower and slower on/off times (0.4 sec, 0.6 sec.,...1.8 sec). Then enter keys 8, 7, 6, 5, 4, 3, 2, 1 and observe the on/off times speed up again (1.6 sec., then 1.4 sec.,....and finally 0.2 sec). Continue pressing various keys from among 1 through 9 until the cycles finish up. Shades of a pinao KBRD? (See Problem 1).

PROBLEMS

1. What changes must be made in the program to implement a piano keyboard played from the terminal? For a piano keyboard, frequencies of the on-off cycles must be in the audio range and controlled on-the-fly from the keyboard.

2. Modify the program to allow for entry of different on vs. off-time parameters during set-up. How would you arrange for changing BOTH these parameters, independently, on-the-fly?
3. Modify the SERINT ISR so that a full WORD UVWX can be created by key presses on-the-fly. Have that word passed to REG4 (the other time parameter in TIME). In that way you'll have just about INSTANTANEOUS time response to keyboard entry on-the-fly. Remember, REG4 is being decremented in the very tight loop at 2688-268B. Further, you'll have much better time delay granularity. The way we've approached TIME, we've assured MULTIPLES of 0.2 sec., in which the REG2 parameter is the multiple (1, 2, ...9). In this new approach, REG2 is fixed and REG4 can be changed by minimal amounts corresponding to 1 part in 65, 536, or 3 usec. (DEC and JNE produce another 12 state times for each additional loop specified by REG4).
4. Emplement the EXTINT ISR so that you end it on a RET to get back to NEWSET. The SP should be back to 00C0 when you arrive at NEWSET.

EXPERIMENT 9-14(B)

REMOTE KBRD CONTROL OF MOTOR SPEED, OR PRESSURE, OR TEMPERATURE, ETC. VIA SERIAL LOADING OF THE PWM. ASCII TO HEX CONVERSION ROUTINE.

DESCRIPTION OF THE PROBLEM

1. The physical set-up between local CRT terminal and remote SBE-96 via a RS232 link is exactly as in Expt. 9-14(A) just concluded (see also p. 419, Expt. 8-3). Debounced switch S is again used to create an abort. S is situated at the local terminal and is connected to EXTINT at the remote 8096 to create the abort interrupt.
2. After the program below is executed, two keys from among 0, 1, 2,....9, A, B, C, D, E, F will be entered at the local terminal to create a full HEX byte, XY (00 to FF). It is stored in a register (and then in the PWM) of the remotely located 8096 via the RS232 serial link. We include an ASCII-to-HEX routine in the program (ASCHEX) since the CRT terminal has a standard ASCII keyboard. ASCII codes 30, 31, 32,....39, 41, 42, 43, 44, 45, 46 for the keys 0, 1,....F must be converted to HEX codes 00, 01,.... 09, 0A, 0B,....0F. The two HEX codes (after 4 shifts left on the first HEX code) are added to form the HEX byte XY

(= 00, 01,....,FE, or FF). (Our ASCHEX routine actually works a little differently, as we'll see).

3. The two keys entered at the terminal are echoed on the CRT AS THEY ARE KEYED IN and the HEX byte XY formed in ASCHEX is loaded into the 8096's PWM (and is also displayed at LEDs at the 8096's port P1 AFTER the two keys are entered).
4. The loading of XY in the PWM (above) results in a d.c. level voltage proportional to XY at the output of the R-C filter we've been employing at the PWM pin P2.5. THIS VOLTAGE CAN THEN BE USED TO CONTROL MOTOR SPEED, TEMPERATURE AT A TEMPERATURE CONTROLLER, PRESSURE AT A PRESSURE CONTROLLER, ETC. (The voltage or current output may need to be amplified or otherwise conditioned).
5. At any time, two new keys can be entered at the terminal to change the XY value in the PWM so as to achieve instantaneously a new control voltage at the filter's output at P2.5. The 2 keys are again individually echoed on the CRT and together at P1 on the 8096 as the new HEX byte X'Y'.
6. Abort can be achieved by throwing switch S at EXTINT from low to high to low. In that case the PWM is cleared and the d.c. output voltage at P2.5 drops to 0. New X,Y keys can again be entered to produce a new voltage at P2.5. They are again echoed on the CRT and at P1's LEDs.
7. There is no SERINT interrupt or ISR in this experiment. It is not needed, since changing XY on-the-fly is easily implemented: after any entry of keys X,Y occurs to produce the parameter XY, the program jumps back to the point where another X',Y' parameter set-up is awaited. When such new entry occurs, the PWM value is INSTANTLY changed and a new voltage IMMEDIATELY produced.

PROGRAM

The program at 2700 is presented below. It, too, is based on the GET-CHR and PUT-CHR serial I/O routines we've been using to have the 8096 receive, and echo, bytes from, and to, the remote terminal. We analyze the program after it is presented. The main new point in the analysis will be the ASCII to HEX routine, ASCHEX, to allow a HEX byte XY to be formed from the entry of two ASCII keys X,Y. Parameter set-up, utilizing the GET-CHR and PUT-CHR routines, follows along the same lines as discussed in the analysis of the program of Expt. 9-14(A). The resulting HEX byte XY is then simply loaded into the PWM and displayed at P1.

```
        18 00         SP      EQU    18H
        11 00         SP_CON  EQU    11H
        11 00         SP_STAT EQU    11H
        07 00         SBUF    EQU    07H
        0E 00         BAUD    EQU    0EH
        80 00         BAUD_HI EQU    80H
        9B 00         BAUD_LO EQU    9BH               ;1200 BAUD
        09 00         PINT    EQU    09H
        08 00         MINT    EQU    08H
        0E 20         INVECO  EQU    200EH
        30 00         TEMP    EQU    30H
        40 00         OFFSET  EQU    40H
        50 00         REGO    EQU    50H
        51 00         REG1    EQU    51H
        16 00         IOC1    EQU    16H
        70 00         CHAR_I  EQU    70H
        60 00         CHAR_O  EQU    60H
        80 00         ASC_H   EQU    80H
        81 00         ASC_L   EQU    81H
        82 00         HEX     EQU    82H
        17 00         PWM     EQU    17H
        0F 00         P1      EQU    0FH
                      ;
                      ;
2700                          ORG    2700H
                      ;
2700    A1 C0 00 18           LD     SP,#0C0H          ;Initialize SP.
2704    FA                    DI                       ;Disable interrutps.
2705    11 17                 CLRB   PWM               ;Initialize PWM to 00.
2707    B1 21 16              LDB    IOC1,#21H         ;Select EXTINT, not ACH.7 interrupt
                                                       ;source and enable TxD and PWM.
270A    B1 80 08              LDB    MINT,#80H         ;Unmask EXTINT interrupt source.
270D    A1 66 27 30           LD     TEMP,#EXTINT      ;Load TEMP with EXTINT ISR address
2711    C3 01 0E 20 30        ST     TEMP,INVECO[0]    ;and store in VECT INT table at
                                                       ;200EH.
2716    B1 20 30              LDB    TEMP,#20H         ;Initialize TEMP with 20 (RI and TI).
2719    B1 9B 0E              LDB    BAUD,#BAUD_LO     ;Load low byte of baud rate into BAUD.
271C    B1 80 0E              LDB    BAUD,#BAUD_HI     ;Load high byte of baud into BAUD reg.
271F    B1 09 11              LDB    SP_CON,#09H       ;Initialize serial port: mode 1,
                                                       ;REN = 1, PEN = 0.
2722    FB                    EI                       ;Enable interrupt system.
2723    A1 00 00 40   NEWSET: LD     OFFSET,#00H       ;Initialize register table pointer
                                                       ;offset.
2727    EF 22 00      PARAMS: CALL   GET_CHR           ;Call GET_CHR ("Read Keyboard")
```

```
                                                        ;routine.  Waits for key 0-F to
                                                        ;be pressed.
272A    B0 70 60                LDB     CHAR_O,CHAR_I   ;Copy input key to CHAR_O for echo.
272D    EF 29 00                CALL    PUT_CHR         ;Echo key to terminal.
2730    C7 40 50 70             STB     CHAR_I,REGO[OFFSET] ;Load key into register table and
2734    07 40                   INC     OFFSET          ;Increment OFFSET.
2736    99 02 40                CMPB    OFFSET,#02H     ;Compare OFFSET to 2.
2739    D7 EC                   JNE     PARAMS          ;If OFFSET != 2, two keys have not
                                                        ;been entered, goto PARAMS for more.
273B    B0 50 80                LDB     ASC_H,REGO      ;Load first character entered into
                                                        ;ASC_H (for high nibble).
273E    B0 51 81                LDB     ASC_L,REG1      ;Load second character entered into
                                                        ;ASC_L (for lower nibble).
2741    EF 2B 00                CALL    ASCHEX          ;Call ASCII to HEX conversion routine.
2744    B0 82 17                LDB     PWM,HEX         ;Load HEX byte result into PWM.
2747    B0 82 0F                LDB     P1,HEX          ;Output HEX result to P1 LEDs.
274A    27 D7                   SJMP    NEWSET          ;Jump to NEWSET.
                        ;
                        ;
                        ;
                        ;       INPUT CHARACTER ROUTINE: GET_CHR
                        ;
274C    90 11 30        GET_CHR:ORB     TEMP,SP_STAT    ;Copy serial port status into TEMP.
274F    36 30 FA                JBC     TEMP,6,GET_CHR  ;If RI = 0, goto GET_CHR.
2752    71 BF 30                ANDB    TEMP,#0BFH      ;Else clear RI flag in TEMP.
2755    B0 07 70                LDB     CHAR_I,SBUF     ;Read character from SBUF into CHAR_I.
2758    F0                      RET                     ;Return.

                        ;
                        ;
                        ;       OUTPUT CHARACTER ROUTINE: PUT_CHR
                        ;
2759    90 11 30        PUT_CHR:ORB     TEMP,SP_STAT    ;Copy serial port status into TEMP.
275C    35 30 FA                JBC     TEMP,5,PUT_CHR  ;If TI = 0, goto PUT_CHR.
275F    B0 60 07                LDB     SBUF,CHAR_O     ;Else load character from CHAR_O
                                                        ;into SBUF for transmission.
2762    71 DF 30                ANDB    TEMP,#0DFH      ;Clear temp TI flag.
2765    F0                      RET                     ;Return.
                        ;
                        ;
                        ;
                        ;       EXTERNAL INTERRUPT SERVICE ROUTINE
                        ;
2766    11 17           EXTINT: CLRB    PWM             ;Clear PWM to stop motor.
2768    A1 C0 00 18             LD      SP,#00C0H       ;Reinitialize SP.
276C    E7 B4 FF                LJMP    NEWSET          ;Jump to NEWSET to accept new
                                                        ;parameters.
```

```
                            ;
276F   F2                   ASCHEX: PUSHF                          ;Save flags.
2770   36 80 03                     JBC     ASC_H,6,DIGIT1         ;If bit 6 = 0, jump to DIGIT1.
2773   75 09 80                     ADDB    ASC_H,#09H             ;Else add 9 to form binary nibble.
2776   19 04 80             DIGIT1: SHLB    ASC_H,#04H             ;Shift 4 bits to the left to move
                                                                   ;binary result into high nibble.
2779   36 81 03                     JBC     ASC_L,6,DIGIT2         ;If bit 6 = 0, jump to DIGIT2.
277C   75 09 81                     ADDB    ASC_L,#09H             ;Add 9 to form binary nibble.
277F   71 0F 81             DIGIT2: ANDB    ASC_L,#0FH             ;Mask out upper nibble.

2782   54 80 81 82                  ADDB    HEX,ASC_L,ASC_H        ;Add low and high nibbles and
                                                                   ;store result in HEX.
2786   F3                           POPF                           ;Restore flags.
2787   F0                           RET                            ;Return.
                            ;
2788                                END
```

The main program starts by initializing SP and disabling interrupts. The PWM register in the remote 8096 is cleared. 21 is loaded into IOC1 to select EXTINT, not ACH.7, as the external interrupt source, and to select pin P2.5 in its PWM role and pin 2.0 in its TXD role (for echo). 80 loaded into MINT unmasks the EXTINT interrupt source. The address of the EXTINT ISR is then stored in the VECT INT table at 200E via the TEMP register. 20 is then loaded into TEMP to initially clear the RI flag copy and set the TI flag copy. (TEMP is the register that holds copies of those flags from SP-STAT). Baud rate is then set to 1200. SP-CON is loaded with 09 to select Mode 1 serial port operation and to enable serial reception from RXD into SBUF(RX). OFFSET is initialized to 0 and GET-CHR is then called at PARAMS to await the arrival of a key character (parameter) from the terminal. GET-CHR is the same routine we have been using through-out and needs no analysis. It is located at 274C. We return from GET-CHR with the ASCII code of the key, read from SBUF(RX), in CHAR-I. The latter is loaded into CHAR-O (at 272A) for echo back to the terminal. That feature is implemented by the call of PUT-CHR at 272D in the main program. Again, PUT-CHR is the same routine we have been using through-out and should be familiar. It is located at 2759. We return from PUT-CHR with the key character to be echoed in SBUF(TX). Transmission (echo) occurs out of SBUF(TX). We now find ourselves at 2730 where the first ASCII character entered from the keyboard at the terminal is stored in the table at REG0 (50H) i.e. at REG0 [OFFSET]. OFFSET is then incremented. If it is not equal to 2 (2 keys not yet entered) a jump back to PARAMS is made (JNE at 2739) to await entry of the second key. When that key is entered, a repeat of the above events occurs. The second ASCII code is now stored at REG0 [OFFSET], which by now is 51 i.e. in REG1. The CMPB, JNE instructions at 2736, 2739 fall through to 273B since

OFFSET is now 2 due to the increment at 2734. At 273B and 273E the ASCII codes of the first key in REG0 and of the second key in REG1 are loaded into byte registers ASC-H and ASC-L, respectively.

At this point a call to ASCHEX (at 276F) is made in the program (2741). This routine will convert the ASCII codes into a compact HEX byte. Thus if keys A,B were pressed, ASC-H will contain 41 and ASC-L will contain 42. At the end of ASCHEX, we'll return with AB (HEX) in the byte register HEX. This comes about as follows: the PUSHF instruction in ASCHEX saves flags and disables the interrupt system. If bit 6 in the FIRST ASCII code (ASC-H) is low (key was BELOW A i.e. one of the numbers 0 to 9) a jump to DIGIT1 is made by the JBC instruction at 2770. There the code ASC-H is shifted left 4 times so ASC-H now contains 00, or 10, or 20,....,or 90. Then bit 6 of the SECOND ASCII code (ASC-L) is tested. If it is also low (another number key was pressed) a jump to DIGIT2 at 277F is made. There the upper nibble of ASC-L is masked out so ASC-L also now contains 00, 01, 02,....or 09. The three-operand instruction at 2782 (there it is again!) adds the processed ASC-L byte to the processed ASCH-H byte and stores the result in register HEX. The latter will, therefore, contain the HEX byte XY with X,Y = 0, 1, 2,....,or 9. After the POPF instruction return is made to 2744 where this HEX byte is loaded into the PWM and also displayed at P1. At P2.5, after the R-C filter, we should sense a d.c. voltage proportional to XY. The SJMP NEWSET instruction jumps back to re-initialize OFFSET and await new keyboard entries (if any) to produce another voltage. Reader: trace what happens if bit 6 in the SECOND ASCII code were high.

If, however, bit 6 in the FIRST ASCII code (ASC-H) were high (key A or greater was pressed) fall-through JBC at 2770 would occur and 09 would be added to that code. Thus 41 (for A) + 09 = 4A, or 42 (for B) + 09 = 4B. The SHLB instruction at 2776 converts 4A or 4B, etc., to A0 or B0, etc. The JBC instruction at 2779 tests bit 6 of the SECOND ASCII code (ASC-L). If it was low (i.e. a number key), the 3 in the code 3N is masked at DIGIT2 to give 0N. The 3-operand ADD will then yield HEX bytes AN or BN, etc., where N = 0, 1, 2,....or 9. If bit 6 in the SECOND ASCII code (ASC-L) were high (letter key) fall-through to the ADDB instruction at 277C occurs where 09 is added to ASC-L. This converts e.g. A or B's ASCII codes from 41 or 42, etc., to 4A or 4B, etc. The following ANDB instruction at 277F masks out the upper nibble so we are left with 0A or 0B, etc. in ASC-L. When this is added to the code (A0, B0, etc.) in ASC-H at 27B2, we are left with XY in HEX, where X and Y are LETTER keys.

Thus in every case we return from ASCHEX 2744 with the true

HEX byte XY in register HEX where X,Y = 0, 1, 2,....,9, A, B, ...or F. PWM is loaded with XY and P1 is made to display that byte. A jump to NEWSET then re-initializes OFFSET and awaits new keyboard entries, if any, to produce another voltage at P2.5. Early on, PUT-CHR echoed X, then Y at the terminal.

The EXTINT ISR at 2766 merely clears PWM (driving the output voltage back to 0 at P2.5), reloads the SP with its initial value 00C0, and jumps to NEWSET to re-initialize OFFSET and wait for two new keys to produce another voltage.

PROCEDURE

1. Reset and enter BY 09 = 00. The terminal-to-SBE-96 serial link is exactly as in Expt. 9-14(A). The abort switch S is located at the terminal and is connected to EXTINT of the remote 8096.
2. Execute from 2700. Since PWM was initialized to 0 in the program, the voltage at P2.5 should be 0. We measured 0.2 mv. (offset).
3. Enter keys 3,A to form HEX byte 3A. We observed 3, then A, appear one after the other on the CRT. The byte 3A appeared at P1 after the second key (A) was entered. We measured the voltage at the output of the R-C filter at P2.5 to be 1.13V.
4. Enter two new keys 8,0 to form the byte 80 for the PWM. We observed 8 then 0 on the CRT and 80 at P1's LEDs. The voltage at P2.5 immediately changed to 2.28V.
5. When keys F,F were entered we observed FF on the CRT, FF at P1. The voltage at P2.5 jumped to 4.67V.
6. When keys 0,0 were entered, we saw 00 on the CRT, 00 at P1, the voltage at P2.5 immediately dropped to 0.2mv.
7. Enter keys C,0. We observed C0 on the CRT, C0 at P1,. The voltage increased to 3.47 volts.
8. Create an EXTINT interrupt with switch S. The voltage at P2.5 immediately dropped to 0.2mv.
9. Enter two new keys 6,0. See 60 on the CRT and at P1. We found the voltage at P2.5 increase to 1.69 volts.
10. Throw S lo/hi/lo again and observe the voltage immediately decrease to 0.2mv. again.
11. Etc.

CONCLUSION

The importance of serial I/O in implementing remote control through parameter set-up and parameter changes on-the-fly from a local CRT terminal to a distant microcontroller should be apparent from the two experiments just concluded. In the next experiment (9-15) we have a local microcontroller (another SBE-

96) direct the control of a remotely situated 8096 microcontroller in a manner different than the master-slave approach taken in Expt. 8-6. We come back to the "dumb CRT terminal" and remote microcontroller again in Expt. 9-16 where a number of keys on the terminal are assigned "special tasks". Pressing one such key initiates one of a set of tasks, pressing another at any time initiates another task, etc.

EXPERIMENT 9-15

LOCAL MICROCONTROLLER (8096) DIRECTS A REMOTE SENSOR/ACTUATOR CONTROLLER (8096) VIA SERIAL LINK. CLOSED LOOP CONTROL.

INTRODUCTION

In this experiment a local (master) microcontroller (SBE-96) is employed to direct a remote sensor/actuator controller (SBE-96). Thus we'll have the "dumb terminal" of Expt. 9-14 replaced by another (master) iSBE-96 with the TXD, RXD lines of master controller connected to the RXD, TXD lines of the remote controller via a RS232 serial link (same connections as described on pp. 438, 439 of Expt. 8-6).

In this application, we'll have the remote microcontroller sense pressure, temperature, speed, flow etc. and report back serially the constantly monitored results to the local master microcontroller. The latter will decide what to do to maintain the remote temperature, pressure, etc. within a specified band. It will accomplish this by transmitting back to the remote microcontroller the necessary I/O control action via the serial link. THIS IS AN IMPORTANT APPLICATION THAT FREQUENTLY ARISES IN THE SMART ACTUATOR CONTROL BUSINESS.

The approach we'll take is a more straight-forward implementation of the solution than the broader master-slave approach taken in Expt. 8-6. The application treated in the present experiment could certainly be brought under the broad umbrella of the master-slave solution presented in Expt. 8-6 where the 4-parameter fields in TBUF (from master to slave) and FBUF (from slave to master) could easily encompass the requirements of the problem here. However, we feel it is instructive to treat the present application in another, if more specialized, manner. To make clear the distinction between the two approaches, we refer to the application here as the "master-remote" problem, as opposed to the broader "master-slave" problem of Expt. 8-6. The connections in the two experiments are the same (see pp. 438, 439 of Expt. 8-6).

FORMULATION (DIGITAL OUTPUT IN THE CONTROL LOOP)

1. A potentiometer at ACH.0 on the remote 8096 will simulate the voltage input to the remote 8096 from any one of several kinds of sensors: temperature, pressure, flow, speed, etc. The relevant parameter is to be kept within specified

limits (set points). The connections between master and remote are as in Expt. 8-6 (pp. 438, 439).

2. The remote microcontroller converts the sensed voltage into a 10-bit A/D digital value and then transmits (in our case) bits 9-2 of the result back to the master controller via the serial link.
3. The master controller polls the RI flag for a received byte of sensor information from the remote controller. When one is received, its value is compared with specified upper and lower limits. If the received value falls between these limits, the master outputs 00 serially to the remote controller. If the received value is higher than the specified upper limit, the master outputs 01 serially to the remote controller. If the received value is less than or equal to the specified lower limit, the master outputs 02 serially to the remote controller. In each of these cases the master then goes back to polling the RI flag for another received sensor byte from the remote controller. As usual, reception at the master of remote sensor information and transmission back of controller action (bytes 00, 01, 02) rely on the GET-CHR and PUT-CHR RI and TI flag polling routines we've been using through-out.
4. The remote controller, after sending the sensed A/D value to the master, now polls RI for a serially received byte from the master which will direct the control action at the actuators. When a byte is received (00 or 01 or 02, depending on the sensed value's magnitude relative to the specified limits) it is output to port P1 (the actuators) of the remote controller. There, either P1.0 and P1.1 are made to go (or stay) off, or P1.0 goes on with P1.1 off, or P1.1 goes on with P1.0 off. P1.1 and P1.0 are to be thought of as driving one or the other of two actuators (valves, motors, steppers, solenoids, relays, etc.) That will control temperature, pressure, flow, speed, etc. by means of any of a number of devices - heaters, coolers, pumps, etc. They will force the sensed parameter to increase or decrease to lie within the specified band, depending on whether P1.0 or P1.1 goes on, or to stay within the band if neither goes on. See, for example, Expt. 9-13 on temperature control. The remote controller than goes back to converting the sensed parameter again before sending its updated value back to the master for new (or same) control directives. As with the master, the transmission of sensed information to master and the reception of control directives from master rely on the use of the PUT-CHR and GET-CHR polling routines (the TI and RI flags) in the remote controller's program. (See p. 570 for analog output control).
5. We'll not employ serial or external interrupt facilities or ISRs. They are not needed in this experiment.

THE PROGRAMS

The remote controller's program resides at 2800, as does the local master's program in its memory space. We first present the remote controller's program with its analysis, then the master's program with its analysis.

The remote controller's program at 2800 in its memory space is presented below and analyzed afterward.

```
        18 00          SP       EQU    18H
        11 00          SP_CON   EQU    11H
        11 00          SP_STAT  EQU    11H
        07 00          SBUF     EQU    07H
        02 00          ADCOM    EQU    02H
        03 00          ADRESHI  EQU    03H
        02 00          ADRESLO  EQU    02H
        0E 00          BAUD     EQU    0EH
        80 00          BAUD_HI  EQU    80H
        9B 00          BAUD_LO  EQU    9BH             ;1200 BAUD
        30 00          TEMP     EQU    30H
        16 00          IOC1     EQU    16H
        70 00          CHAR_I   EQU    70H
        60 00          CHAR_O   EQU    60H
        0F 00          P1       EQU    0FH
                       ;
                       ;
2800                            ORG    2800H
                       ;
2800    A1 C0 00 18             LD     SP,#0C0H        ;Initialize SP.
2804    FA                      DI                     ;Disable interrutps.
2805    11 0F                   CLRB   P1              ;Initialize P1 LEDs to 00.
2807    B1 20 16                LDB    IOC1,#20H       ;Load IOC1 to select TxD function.
280A    B1 20 30                LDB    TEMP,#20H       ;Initialize TEMP with 20 (RI and TI).
280D    B1 9B 0E                LDB    BAUD,#BAUD_LO   ;Load low byte of baud rate into BAUD.
2810    B1 80 0E                LDB    BAUD,#BAUD_HI   ;Load high byte of baud into BAUD reg.
2813    B1 09 11                LDB    SP_CON,#09H     ;Initialize serial port: mode 1,
                                                       ;REN = 1, PEN = 0.
2816    B1 08 02       CONVERT:LDB     ADCOM,#08H      ;Start A/D Conversion on channel 0.
2819    FD                      NOP                    ;8 state times needed.
281A    FD                      NOP                    ;
281B    3B 02 FD       HERE:    JBS    ADRESLO,3,HERE  ;Wait until conversion is complete.
                                                       ;If status bit S = 1, loop on HERE.
```

```
281E   B0 03 60          LDB    CHAR_O,ADRESHI  ;Else read ADRESHI into CHAR_O for
                                                ;transmission.
2821   EF 15 00          CALL   PUT_CHR         ;Call PUT_CHR to send A/D value to
                                                ;master.
2824   EF 05 00          CALL   GET_CHR         ;Call GET_CHR which waits for byte
                                                ;to be received from master.
2827   B0 70 0F          LDB    P1,CHAR_I       ;Output received byte to P1 LEDs
                                                ;(actuators).
282A   27 EA             SJMP   CONVERT         ;Loop back to CONVERT.
                 ;       INPUT CHARACTER ROUTINE: GET_CHR
                 ;
282C   90 11 30  GET_CHR:ORB    TEMP,SP_STAT    ;Copy serial port status into TEMP.
282F   36 30 FA          JBC    TEMP,6,GET_CHR  ;If RI = 0, goto GET_CHR.
2832   71 BF 30          ANDB   TEMP,#0BFH      ;Else clear RI flag in TEMP.
2835   B0 07 70          LDB    CHAR_I,SBUF     ;Read byte from SBUF into CHAR_I.
2838   F0                RET                    ;Return.

                 ;
                 ;
                 ;       OUTPUT CHARACTER ROUTINE: PUT_CHR
                 ;
2839   90 11 30  PUT_CHR:ORB    TEMP,SP_STAT    ;Copy serial port status into TEMP.
283C   35 30 FA          JBC    TEMP,5,PUT_CHR  ;If TI = 0, goto PUT_CHR.
283F   B0 60 07          LDB    SBUF,CHAR_O     ;Else load byte from CHAR_O
                                                ;into SBUF for transmission.
2842   71 DF 30          ANDB   TEMP,#0DFH      ;Clear temp TI flag.
2845   F0                RET                    ;Return.
                 ;
2846                     END
```

After initializations that sets SP, disables interrupts, and clears P1 (actuators), 20 is loaded into IOC1 to select the TXD function for pin P2.0 at the remote controller. 20 is also loaded into TEMP to set bits RI (6) and TI (5) in the SP-STAT copy register to 0 and 1, respectively. The baud rate is then set to 1200 and Mode 1 (with REN = 1) is specified when 09 is loaded into SP-CON. Conversion of the sensor's analog voltage input to ACH.0 at the remote controller is then started at 2816. After 8 state times are allowed to elapse, the S bit in ADRESLO is tested for "conversion complete". This is indicated when S goes low. When it does, fall-through to 281E takes place. There A/D conversion bits 9-2 in ADRESHI are read into CHAR-O and PUT-CHR (at 2839) is called. The latter loads CHAR-O into SBUF(TX) for transmission of the A/D sensor conversion byte (upper 8 bits) back to the master. After the TI flag in TEMP is cleared, return is made to 2824 where GET-CHR (at 282C) is called. That routine polls the RI flag for an indication as to when a character (directive) from the master is received. When it is received (RI high), the received byte in SBUF(RX) is read into CHAR-I after the RI flag in TEMP is first cleared. Return is then made to 2827 where CHAR-I (directive from master) is output to the actuators at P1. The SJMP CONVERT instruction jumps back to start another conversion of the sensor input. The events described above repeat.

We next present, and then analyze, the master's program at 2800 in its space.

```
      18 00        SP      EQU    18H
      11 00        SP_CON  EQU    11H
      11 00        SP_STAT EQU    11H
      07 00        SBUF    EQU    07H
      0E 00        BAUD    EQU    0EH
      80 00        BAUD_HI EQU    80H
      9B 00        BAUD_LO EQU    9BH              ;1200 BAUD
      30 00        TEMP    EQU    30H
      40 00        REG     EQU    40H
      16 00        IOC1    EQU    16H
      70 00        CHAR_I  EQU    70H
      60 00        CHAR_O  EQU    60H
                   ;
                   ;
2800                       ORG    2800H
                   ;
2800  A1 C0 00 18          LD     SP,#0C0H         ;Initialize SP.
2804  FA                   DI                      ;Disable interrutps.
2805  B1 20 16             LDB    IOC1,#20H        ;Load IOC1 to select TxD function.
2808  B1 20 30             LDB    TEMP,#20H        ;Initialize TEMP with 20 (RI and TI).
280B  B1 9B 0E             LDB    BAUD,#BAUD_LO    ;Load low byte of baud rate into BAUD.
280E  B1 80 0E             LDB    BAUD,#BAUD_HI    ;Load high byte of baud into BAUD reg.
2811  B1 09 11             LDB    SP_CON,#09H      ;Initialize serial port: mode 1,
                                                   ;REN = 1, PEN = 0.
2814  EF 1F 00     POLL:   CALL   GET_CHR          ;Call GET_CHR which waits for character
                                                   ;to be received from remote controller.
2817  B0 70 40             LDB    REG,CHAR_I       ;Copy byte received from remote
                                                   ;into REG.
281A  99 90 40             CMPB   REG,#90H         ;Compare remote  temp., pressure, etc.
                                                   ;with specified upper limit (90H).
281D  D9 0A                JH     HIGH             ;If it exceeds upper limit jump to
                                                   ;HIGH to transmit byte to remote to
                                                   ;cause action to decrease. (Turn
                                                   ;e.g. blower on.)
```

```
281F   99 70 40              CMPB   REG,#70H         ;Else compare remote value (temp.
                                                     ;pressure, etc.) with specified lower
                                                     ;limit.
2822   D1 0A                 JNH    LOW              ;If it is less than lower limit jump
                                                     ;to LOW to transmit byte to remote
                                                     ;to cause increase. (Turn e.g. heater
                                                     ;on).
2824   B1 00 60              LDB    CHAR_O,#00H      ;Else load 00 byte into CHAR_O for

                                                     ;transmission. (keep e.g. blower and
                                                     ;heater off at remote location.)
2827   20 08                 SJMP   SEND             ;Jump to transmit byte.
2829   B1 01 60     HIGH:    LDB    CHAR_O,#01       ;Load byte to turn blower on at remote
                                                     ;location.
282C   20 03                 SJMP   SEND             ;Jump to transmit byte.
282E   B1 02 60     LOW:     LDB    CHAR_O,#02       ;Load byte 02 to turn heater on at
                                                     ;remote location.
2831   EF 0F 00     SEND:    CALL   PUT_CHR          ;Send byte to remote location.
2834   27 DE                 SJMP   POLL             ;Jump back to POLL and wait for byte
                                                     ;from remote.
                    ;
                    ;
                    ;
                    ;        INPUT CHARACTER ROUTINE: GET_CHR
                    ;
2836   90 11 30     GET_CHR:ORB     TEMP,SP_STAT     ;Copy serial port status into TEMP.
2839   36 30 FA              JBC    TEMP,6,GET_CHR   ;If RI = 0, goto GET_CHR.
283C   71 BF 30              ANDB   TEMP,#0BFH       ;Else clear RI flag in TEMP.
283F   B0 07 70              LDB    CHAR_I,SBUF      ;Read byte from SBUF into CHAR_I.
2842   F0                    RET                     ;Return.

                    ;
                    ;
                    ;        OUTPUT CHARACTER ROUTINE: PUT_CHR
                    ;
2843   90 11 30     PUT_CHR:ORB     TEMP,SP_STAT     ;Copy serial port status into TEMP.
2846   35 30 FA              JBC    TEMP,5,PUT_CHR   ;If TI = 0, goto PUT_CHR.
2849   B0 60 07              LDB    SBUF,CHAR_O      ;Else load byte from CHAR_O
                                                     ;into SBUF for transmission.
284C   71 DF 30              ANDB   TEMP,#0DFH       ;Clear temp TI flag.
284F   F0                    RET                     ;Return.
```

The initializations at the master from 2800 to 2813 are exactly the same as for the remote controller in the previous program (except for the CLRB P1 instruction, which is not needed at the master). The GET-CHR routine (at 2836) is then called at 2814. It waits for an A/D converted byte from the remote sensor to be transmitted back to the master. When one is received (RI goes high) it is gathered in from SBUF(RX) to CHAR-I (after the RI flag in TEMP was first cleared). Return from GET-CHR to 2817 is then made. There CHAR-I is loaded into REG and a comparison of REG with the (arbitrary) upper limit 90H is made (remember, the conversion byte sent from remote controller are the bits 9-2 = 00 to FF). This upper limit can represent the upper limit to temperature, or pressure, etc. that we are specifying. (It can be changed at 281B to another value, if we wish). If the A/D sensor conversion byte is larger than 90, a jump (JH) to HIGH is taken where 01 is loaded into CHAR-O. If not, fall-through to 281F occurs. There comparison of the sensed conversion byte in REG with an arbitrary lower limit (here 70H) is made. (That limit can also be changed at 2820, if we wish). If the sensed value is 70 or lower a jump (JNH) to LOW is taken where 02 is loaded into CHAR-O. If the sensed value lies between the limits 70 and 90 fall-through to 2824 occurs where CHAR-O is loaded with 00.

In each of the above three cases, after CHAR-O is loaded with the appropriate byte, we end up at the label SEND (2831) where the PUT-CHR routine (at 2843) is called. There, the byte in CHAR-O is loaded into SBUF(TX) for transmission to the remote controller. A return to 2834 is then made where the SJMP POLL instruction takes us back to 2814 for another call of GET-CHR to await new sensed data from the remote controller. The above sequence of events then repeats.

PROCEDURE

1. Reset and enter BY 09 = 00 on both local and remote iSBE-96s. Connect RXD and TXD on master and remote controllers for serial I/O as in Expt. 8-6 (pp. 438, 439).
2. Connect a potentiometer (0 to 5V) at ACH.0 of the remote 8096. Set it at the low end of the 0 to 5V scale.
3. Execute the master 8096 from 2800, THEN the remote 8096 from 2800.
4. You should observe P1.1 on at the remote, as the converted byte is less than 70H.
5. Slowly increase the POT setting at ACH.0 on the remote till P1.1 goes off (P1 = 00). Check the A/D conversion byte by reading ADRESHI (i.e. BY 03) on the remote SBE-96. It should read 71H when P1.1 just went off. We found BY 03 = 73H (hard to precisely control the turning of the POT).
6. Continue to increase the voltage at the output of the POT till P1.0 goes on alone at the remote 8096. This should occure when the sensor's conversion byte just goes above 90 to 91H. Check the A/D conversion byte by reading BY 03. We found BY 03 = 94H.

7. Continue to increase the POT setting till 5V is reached. P1.0 remains on.
8. Now decrease the POT setting from 5V back to 0V. We found that P1.0 went off when BY 03 read 8FH and P1.1 went on when BY 03 read 6FH (again, precise settings on the POT were hard to maintain with release of the turning mechanism). The results are in excellent agreement with what is expected.
9. ESC on both SBEs and enter BY 281B = 50 and BY 2820 = 30 at the master for new upper and lower limits on the sensed parameter. Execute the master from 2800 and then the remote from 2800 again. Vary the POT from 0 to 5V and then back down from 5V to 0V. Observe P1.1 and P1.0. On the way up we found P1.1 stayed on till BY 03 read 33H when it went off. Then P1.0 went on when BY 03 read 51H. On the way down P1.0 went back off when BY 03 read 50H and P1.1 went back on when BY 03 read 2FH. Excellent results.

PROBLEM

Modify the program in the master so that the upper and lower limits on the parameter being controlled are no longer fixed values in the program (at 281B and 2820 in the master), but can be entered from the local master at run-time and changed any time on-the-fly. We suggest you review Expt. 9-14(B), since the set-up of the HEX X1Y1 (upper) and X2Y2 (lower) bounds will require the GET-CHR and PUT-CHR (for echo) routines as shown there, as well as the ASCHEX ASCII to HEX conversion routine used there. You may, or may not, want to use the EXTINT interrupt for the purpose of entering new limits at any time, after an abort.

PROBLEM: ANALOG OUTPUT IN THE CONTROL LOOP.

The approach taken in the experiment was closed-loop in which the output part of the loop involved pure digital control i.e. outputting of bits 0,0 or 0,1 or 1,0 to actuators at P1.0 and P1.1. The input part of the loop involved analog sensing and the ADC facility. If e.g. the temperature transducer functions in ANALOG fashion i.e. Tout = f(Vin), then the master should be outputting digital correction bytes to the remote's PWM unit, with the latter's ANALOG FILTERED OUTPUT applied to the input at the temperature transducer. Modify the program to implement this analog output control approach. At 2827 in the remote controller's program, replace LDB P1, CHAR-I (digital approach with actuators) by LDB PWM, CHAR-I (analog approach using PWM's output). All now depends on what you do in the master's program at 2829 (HIGH), 282E (LOW), and 2824. There you must come up with the correct control bytes for CHAR-O to be sent at 2831 (SEND) to the remote's PWM.

EXPERIMENT 9-16

TERMINAL INTERFACE FOR TASK EXECUTION (FUNCTION KEYS).

INTRODUCTION

In many cases the user is interested in a package of applications software in which any one of several applications, utilities, or routines can be selected and executed by the press of a specific key. The user would also like the flexibility of selecting and executing any other of the applications or routines by the mere press of another dedicated key, even as the previous task or application is executing. And, of course, to make the package even more useful, it should be written so that, when used at a remote controller where the application is taking place, the latter can accept the dedicated key assignments from a local terminal via a serial communications set-up. By "remote" we mean any application that requires serial I/O for the communications, be it short distance (RS232) or longer paths (modem or optics). This experiment illustrates how the above objectives are accomplished using a local "dumb terminal" and a remote 8096 controller whose serial port is activated. The physical set-up and connections are as in Expt. 8-3, 9-14(A), and 9-14(B).

FORMULATION

1. After the program in the remote controller is executed, P1 displays 00. Any one of the keys at the local terminal is then to be keyed in. We'll assign function keys 1, 2, ... 8 to the dedicated tasks 1, 2, ...8, respectively.
2. Entering any key x from among 1, 2, ...8 will result in P1 at the remote controller displaying the byte xx (Task x: x = 1, 2, ...8). After task x displays xx at P1, it goes into a loop on itself. This loop SIMULATES the actual task application BEYOND the mere display of xx (which display simply identifies for us that it is task x that's executing).
3. Pressing any other key in the range 1, 2, ...8 will IMMEDIATELY result in yy being displayed at P1 (y = 1, 2, ... 8) indicating that ANOTHER task (y) is now executing.
4. Entering any key OUTSIDE the range 1, 2, ...8 will result in 00 being shown on the display at P1 (no task is then executing) i.e. an "abort" of the previous task activity.
5. Pressing any key from among 1, 2, ...8 again will result in the execution of the task corresponding to that key num-

ber. P1 will again display zz where z = 1, 2, ...or 8, indicating task z is executing.

6. Etc.

APPROACH TO THE SOLUTION

1. The program will set up the remote 8096 to receive characters (ASCII key codes) from the local terminal. This will entail the usual serial port and baud rate initializations. Port P1 is cleared. The serial port interrupt source is temporarily masked.
2. The GET-CHR routine will then be entered to wait for a received character from the terminal.
3. When a character is received it will be passed to register CHAR-0 for echo back at the terminal.
4. The PUT-CHR routine is then entered to transmit the character back for display at the terminal.
5. Comparisons are then made between the received code and 30H and 38H (the key codes for keys 0 and 8, respectively). If the key entered was not among 1, 2, ...8, the comparisons cause jumps back to the clearing of P1. The program then awaits a new character entry in GET-CHR until another key is entered representing a valid task number x (1, 2, ...8).
6. Should the key represent a valid task number, then the upper nibble of its code is masked, leaving 01, 02, ...or 08 in the byte register REG1 that holds the received character's code. A shift left (by one) and an EXTB instruction, both on REG1, then leaves either 0002, or 0004, ... or 0010 in the WORD register EXTENSION of the BYTE register (REG1).
7. This word value is added to #5000 to yield 5002, 5004, ... or 5010, which is then stored in another register, REG2. 5002, 5004, ...5010 are to be word addresses in a table where the starting addresses of each task will be stored. [REG2] then fetches the starting address of task x (x = 1, 2, ...8) from that table and stores it in REG3. We'll assign the following task x starting addresses: 2A00, 2A05, 2A0A, ...2A23: 8 addresses in all. The table is entered at run-time i.e. WO 5002 = 2A00, 2A05, ...2A23. (The program itself will execute from 2900).
8. An indirect branch is then made to [REG3] i.e. to either 2A00, or 2A05, ...or 2A23 to execute the task x specified by the key entry.
9. During execution of task x, another key from among 1, 2, ...8 (or outside that range if we wish to abort) may be entered to select another task on-the-fly. If one is entered, a serial I/O interrupt is created upon reception of the new character in SBUF(RX). By this time, as we'll see,

we will have UNMASKED the serial port interrupt line so the entry of a new character, while task x is executing, will, when received, cause a vectoring to the SERINT ISR. There, a TEST is made as to whether the RI flag is high (due to entry of a NEW key) or whether the TI flag is high (due to transmission/echo back to the terminal of the PREVIOUS key entered). If the interrupt was due to the completion of TRANSMISSION of the previous key entered (TI high), the ISR forces a RETURN TO TASK X (LOOP at HEREX) TO CONTINUE EXECUTION OF TASK X AS IF NOTHING HAPPENED. If, however, the interrupt was the result of the entry of ANOTHER key to select ANOTHER task (leading to RECEPTION of a new character in SBUF(RX) i.e. RI high) then the ISR will force a return to the MAIN PROGRAM where GET-CHR and PUT-CHR are AGAIN called and the address of the NEW TASK REQUIESTED is fetched from the table and branched to. If the key just entered is outside the range 1, 2, ...8 then the return to the main program and the GET-CHR, PUT-CHR routines will subsequently result in the abort of the previous task: P1 will display 00 till a legitimate task key is entered.

10. The above description of our approach will be filled in with other details (particularly those relating to the serial interrupt aspects of the problem) when the program is presented and analyzed (below).

THE PROGRAM

The program at 2900 is shown below and analyzed afterward.

```
18 00        SP       EQU    18H
11 00        SP_CON   EQU    11H
11 00        SP_STAT  EQU    11H
07 00        SBUF     EQU    07H
0E 00        BAUD     EQU    0EH
80 00        BAUD_HI  EQU    80H
9B 00        BAUD_LO  EQU    9BH           ;1200 BAUD
09 00        PINT     EQU    09H
08 00        MINT     EQU    08H
0C 20        INVEC    EQU    200CH
30 00        TEMP     EQU    30H
40 00        REG1     EQU    40H
50 00        REG2     EQU    50H
60 00        REG3     EQU    60H
16 00        IOC1     EQU    16H
70 00        CHAR_I   EQU    70H
80 00        CHAR_O   EQU    80H
0F 00        P1       EQU    0FH
```

```
2900                         ORG     2900H
                      ;
2900  A1 C0 00 18            LD      SP,#0C0H          ;Initialize SP.
2904  FA                     DI                        ;Disable interrutps.
2905  B1 20 16               LDB     IOC1,#20H         ;Enable TxD function at P2.0.
2908  B1 00 08               LDB     MINT,#00H         ;Mask all interrupt sources.
290B  A1 6C 29 30            LD      TEMP,#SERINT      ;Load address of serial port
290F  C3 01 0C 20 30         ST      TEMP,INVEC[0]     ;interrupt service routine into INT
                                                       ;VECT table at 200CH.
2914  B1 20 30               LDB     TEMP,#20H         ;Initialize TEMP with 20 (RI and TI).
2917  B1 9B 0E               LDB     BAUD,#BAUD_LO     ;Load low byte of baud rate into BAUD.
291A  B1 80 0E               LDB     BAUD,#BAUD_HI     ;Load high byte of baud into BAUD reg.
291D  B1 09 11               LDB     SP_CON,#09H       ;Initialize serial port: mode 1,
                                                       ;REN = 1, PEN = 0.
2920  11 09                  CLRB    PINT              ;Clear any pending interrupts.
2922  FB                     EI                        ;Enable interrupts.
2923  11 0F         CLRP1:   CLRB    P1                ;Clear LEDs at P1.
2925  EF 2A 00      POLLKEY:CALL     GET_CHR           ;Call GET_CHR to wait for keyboard
                                                       ;entry.
2928  B0 70 80               LDB     CHAR_O,CHAR_I     ;Load key entered into CHAR_O for
                                                       ;echo.
292B  EF 31 00      ECHO:    CALL    PUT_CHR           ;Call PUT_CHR to echo the key to the
                                                       ;terminal.
292E  99 30 70               CMPB    CHAR_I,#30H       ;Compare key to '0' ('1' is lowest

                                                       ;valid key).
2931  D1 F0                  JNH     CLRP1             ;If key is not higher jump to CLRP1.
2933  99 38 70               CMPB    CHAR_I,#38H       ;Else compare key to '8' (highest valid
                                                       ;key).
2936  D9 EB                  JH      CLRP1             ;If key is higher jump to CLRP1.
2938  B0 70 40               LDB     REG1,CHAR_I       ;Else load key into REG1 for
                                                       ;modification.
293B  71 0F 40               ANDB    REG1,#0FH         ;Mask upper nibble of key in REG1.
293E  19 01 40               SHLB    REG1,#01H         ;Multiply key by 2 to adjust for word
                                                       ;entries in address table.
2941  16 40                  EXTB    REG1              ;Extend REG1 to word table
                                                       ;offset.
2943  45 00 50 40 50         ADD     REG2,REG1,#5000H;Add offset to 5000H and store result
                                                       ;in REG2.
2948  A2 50 60               LD      REG3,[REG2]       ;Fetch address from table and load it
                                                       ;into REG3.
294B  11 09                  CLRB    PINT              ;Clear any pending interrupts.
294D  B1 40 08               LDB     MINT,#40H         ;Enable serial port interrupt.
2950  E3 60                  BR      [REG3]            ;Branch to routine whose address was
                                                       ;fetched from table.
```

```
                        ;       INPUT CHARACTER ROUTINE: GET_CHR
                        ;
2952    90 11 30        GET_CHR:ORB     TEMP,SP_STAT      ;Copy serial port status into TEMP.
2955    36 30 FA                JBC     TEMP,6,GET_CHR    ;If RI = 0, goto GET_CHR.
2958    71 BF 30                ANDB    TEMP,#0BFH        ;Else clear RI flag in TEMP.
295B    B0 07 70                LDB     CHAR_I,SBUF       ;Read character from SBUF into CHAR_I.
295E    F0                      RET                       ;Return.

                        ;
                        ;
                        ;       OUTPUT CHARACTER ROUTINE: PUT_CHR
                        ;
295F    90 11 30        PUT_CHR:ORB     TEMP,SP_STAT      ;Copy serial port status into TEMP.
2962    35 30 FA                JBC     TEMP,5,PUT_CHR    ;If TI = 0, goto PUT_CHR.
2965    B0 80 07                LDB     SBUF,CHAR_O       ;Else load character from CHAR_O
                                                          ;into SBUF for transmission.
2968    71 DF 30                ANDB    TEMP,#0DFH        ;Clear temp TI flag.
296B    F0                      RET                       ;Return.
                        ;
                        ;
                        ;
                        ;       SERIAL PORT INTERRUPT SERVICE ROUTINE:
                        ;
296C    90 11 30        SERINT: ORB     TEMP,SP_STAT      ;Read SP_STAT for RI test.
296F    36 30 10                JBC     TEMP,6,NO_CHR     ;If RI = 0 goto NO_CHR(was echo).
2972    A1 23 29 40             LD      REG1,#CLRP1       ;Else load REG1 with address of CLRP1
                                                          ;(was function key).
2976    A1 BE 00 18             LD      SP,#00BEH         ;Load SP with initial value - 2.
297A    C2 18 40                ST      REG1,[SP]         ;Put address onto stack.
297D    11 09                   CLRB    PINT              ;Clear any pending interrupts
297F    B1 00 08                LDB     MINT,#00H         ;Mask out all interrupt sources.
2982    F0              NO_CHR: RET                       ;Return.

                        ;       ROUTINES
2A00                            ORG     2A00H
                        ;
2A00    B1 11 0F        KEY1:   LDB     P1,#11H           ;Load KEY1 routine LED value into P1.
2A03    27 FE           HERE1:  SJMP    HERE1             ;Loop here "routine's operation".
                                                          ;
2A05    B1 22 0F        KEY2:   LDB     P1,#22H           ;Load KEY2 routine LED value into P1.
2A08    27 FE           HERE2:  SJMP    HERE2             ;Loop here "routine's operation".
                                                          ;
2A0A    B1 33 0F        KEY3:   LDB     P1,#33H           ;Load KEY3 routine LED value into P1.
2A0D    27 FE           HERE3:  SJMP    HERE3             ;Loop here "routine's operation".
                                                          ;
2A0F    B1 44 0F        KEY4:   LDB     P1,#44H           ;Load KEY4 routine LED value into P1.
2A12    27 FE           HERE4:  SJMP    HERE4             ;Loop here "routine's operation".
```

```
2A14   B1 55 0F     KEY5:   LDB    P1,#55H       ;Load KEY5 routine LED value into P1.
2A17   27 FE        HERE5:  SJMP   HERE5         ;Loop here "routine's operation".
                                                 ;
2A19   B1 66 0F     KEY6:   LDB    P1,#66H       ;Load KEY6 routine LED value into P1.
2A1C   27 FE        HERE6:  SJMP   HERE6         ;Loop here "routine's operation".
                                                 ;
2A1E   B1 77 0F     KEY7:   LDB    P1,#77H       ;Load KEY7 routine LED value into P1.
2A21   27 FE        HERE7:  SJMP   HERE7         ;Loop here "routine's operation".
                                                 ;
2A23   B1 88 0F     KEY8:   LDB    P1,#88H       ;Load KEY8 routine LED value into P1.
2A26   27 FE        HERE8:  SJMP   HERE8         ;Loop here "routine's operation".
                    ;
2A28                        END
```

The main part of the program starts by initializing SP to 00C0 and disabling all interrupts. 20H is loaded into IOC1 to enable the TXD function at P2.0 (for purposes of echoing back from 8096 to terminal). All interrupt sources are then masked in MINT. The address of the serial interrupt (#SERINT = 296C here) is then stored in the VECT INT table at 200C. TEMP (which will hold a copy of SP-STAT's RI,TI flags) is initialized to 20H for reasons we've explained in a number of experiments dealing with serial I/O. The baud rate between terminal and 8096 is set to 1200 and the serial port operating mode is selected to be Mode 1 with receiver (RXD to SBUF(RX) buffer) enabled. All pending interrupts are cleared and the interrupt system is enabled, even though the interrupt sources are all masked at this point.

Port P1 is now cleared. Task identification xx will be displayed there once key x is entered. The GET-CHR routine is next called. It is located at 2952. When entered, the RI flag in SP-STAT is copied into TEMP. As long as it's low the polling of TEMP.6 continues. When it's high (character received in SBUF (RX) of 8096 from local terminal), fall-through 2955 occurs. TEMP.6 is cleared and the received character is loaded into CHAR-I. A return to 2928 then occurs where the received character is loaded into CHAR-O and the PUT-CHR routine at 295F is called. There TEMP.5 is tested after the TI flag from SP-STAT.5 is copied into TEMP.5. Since it is high (see address 2914) we fall through 2962 and load the received character from CHAR-O into SBUF(TX) for transmission. TEMP.5 is then cleared. (Remember SP-STAT.5 will again go high when the character is fully TRANSMITTED out of SBUF(TX), and so TEMP.5 will eventually be set high after the COPY at 295F is again performed next time we call PUT-CHR or GET-CHR).

The return to 292E from the PUT-CHR routine is followed by two compare instructions in which the ASCII code of the received character is compared, first with 30H (key 0), then with 38H (key 8). Should the key entered have been anything below key 1 or above key 8 a jump back to CLRP1 results. P1 is kept at 00. No task is selected. The JNH and JH instructions accomplish this. If the key entered was one of the task keys 1, 2, ...or 8, fall-through to 2938 occurs. There the received key code is loaded into REG1, its upper nibble is masked out, the resulting byte is shifted left one bit, and that byte result in turn is sign-extended into a word. REG1 will, therefore, now contain the word 0002, 0004, ...or 0010 corresponding to the case where either key 1, key 2, ...or key 8, respectively, was entered.

At 2943, 5000 is added to one of the word values just mentioned and the result 5002, ..., or 5010 is stored in REG2. The instruction at 2948 then fetches the specified task's starting address from the table whose entries are made at 5002, 5004, ...5010 and are themselves the addresses of the 8 tasks corresponding to key 1, key 2, ..., or key 8. The task's address is loaded into REG3. These addresses are to be 2A00, 2A05, ... 2A23.

UP TO NOW THE SERIAL PORT'S INTERRUPT SOURCE HAS BEEN MASKED. Now, the previous reception of a character into SBUF(RX), and the subsequent transmission of that character out of SBUF(TX), certainly created serial interrupts. Because MINT.6 was 0 up to now, those interrupts became PENDING. They caused no vectoring to the SERINT ISR that we've written at 296C. Since we are about to branch to the selected task's routine, WHERE WE WANT THE POSSIBILITY OF CHOOSING ANOTHER TASK WHEN ANOTHER KEY IS ENTERED AT THE TERMINAL, we should now unmask the serial port's interrupt source. Then the entry of another key during execution of task x, to select another task y, WOULD, this time, create a serial interrupt that would IMMEDIATELY vector to the SERINT ISR where we can set the stage for the execution of the new task. With that in mind we clear the serial pending interrupts that were previously created and then load 40 into MINT to unmask the serial interrupt source. The BR [REG3] indirect branch instruction at 2950 simply executes a jump to [REG3] i.e. to the starting address of task x.

The starting addresses of tasks x (x = 1, 2, ...8) are 2A00, 2A05, 2A0A, 2A0F, 2A14, 2A19, 2A1E and 2A23. In each, we first simply output xx to P1's display (x = 1, 2, ...or 8) to identify the task as that belonging to key x. EACH TASK'S MAIN FUNCTION IS THEN SIMULATED BY THE SJMP HEREx INSTRUCTION, WHERE

THE LABEL HEREx (x = 1, 2, ...8) IS SITUATED TO THE LEFT OF SJMP. AT THIS POINT, TWO POSSIBILITIES EXIST: 1) either we enter another key y (with attendant serial interrupt on reception) to select another task, in which case we'd expect to see yy at P1; or 2) we don't enter another key, but a serial interrupt is caused by the ultimate transmission out of SBUF(TX) of the LAST character received from the terminal which was PREVIOUSLY placed in SBUF(TX) for transmission back to the terminal. Remember, at 1200 baud, transmission out of SBUF(TX) will take some 7 or so msec. before the serial interrupt will manifest itself, whereas the execution time of the program from 292E after PUT-CHR to 2950 will only take about 20 or so usec. In the latter case, the program is vectored from the looping in task x to the SERINT ISR at 296C with TI flag high and RI flag low (it was last cleared in GET-CHR). There the test of TEMP.6 at 296C indicates RI = 0 (no received character, as no key was pressed). The JBC instruction jumps to NO-CHR because RI is 0. At NO-CHR a simple return to the task x loop is made and TASK X CONTINUES EXECUTING. The delayed serial interrupt caused no problem for us.

Eventually, while we're in the SJMP HEREx task loop, we'll enter another key y to select another task y. When we do, the SUBSEQUENT COMPLETELY RECEIVED KEY CODE in SBUF(RX) will cause a serial interrupt to SERINT. This time RI = 1 and the test at 296C,6F falls through to 2972. There we load the address #CLRP1 (i.e. 2923) into REG1 and set SP to 00BEH. (REG1) is then stored at [SP] i.e. the address of CLRP1 is stored at the address pointed to by SP, namely at 00BE and 00BF (word on even boundary). Pending interrupts are cleared (unlikely that any exist) and MINT is loaded with 00, MASKING THE SERIAL INTERRUPT SOURCE AGAIN. Now the return instruction at 2982 pops the return address off the top of the stack (i.e. #CLRP1 = 2923 from 00BE, 00BF) into the PC AND LEAVES SP AT 00C0 WHERE THE SP WAS AT 2923. The return to 2923 (CLRP1) clears P1 and immediately calls the GET-CHR routine again. Since RI at TEMP.6 is still high (although cleared in SP-STAT after the reading of the latter at 296C), the test in GET-CHR at 2952 falls right through and loads CHAR-I with the newly received key code from SBUF(RX). The return is to 2928 in the main program. The analysis now repeats verbatum. If the key entered during task x was not 1, 2, ...or 8, the JNH and JH instructions at 2931, 2936 keep P1 cleared ("abort" resulted) and another key y (1, 2, ...or 8) can now be entered to select another task. If the key entered during task x was from among 1, 2, ...8, we fall through both the JNH and JH instructions and, as before, branch to the newly specified task's starting address. We'll observe yy at P1. All repeats as before i.e. another key inside or outside the range 1, 2, ...8 can be entered to replace task y by an abort or by another task z. Remember, after the ISR, the serial interrupt source is again masked between addresses 2923 and 294B till it is again unmasked at 294D to allow ISR servicing during execution of any new task subsequently being executed.

PROCEDURE

1. The set-up and connections are as in Expt. 8-3 or 9-14(A), 9-14(B).
2. Reset and enter BY 09 = 00.
3. Enter the table of branch addresses i.e. the starting addresses of the various tasks: WO 5002 = 2A00, 2A05, 2A0A, 2A0F, 2A14, 2A19, 2A1E, 2A23.
4. Execute from 2900. Observe 00 at P1.
5. Enter key 8 (task 8). Observe 88 at P1.
6. Enter key 6 (task 6). Observe 66 at P1.
7. Enter key A. Observe 00 at P1 (abort). Enter key 0. 00 is still displayed at P1. Enter the space bar. P1 does not change.
8. Enter key 3 (task 3). Observe 33 at P1.
9. Enter key Z. See 00 at P1.
10. Enter keys 4 and 7 in succession and observe 44, then 77, at P1 (tasks 4 and 7).
11. Strike key B. P1 changes to 00 (abort).
12. Enter key 1 and observe 11 at P1 (task 1).
13. Etc.

EXPERIMENT 9-17

A DIGITAL FILTER. SAMPLING.

The introductory material on digital filter theory below is reproduced from the book "The 8085 Microprocessor, Vol. 2: 54 Hands-On Control Experiments", by Howard Boyet, MTI Publications, 1982, pp. 703-707. This material is pertinent and relevant to the 8096-based digital filter we shall implement in this experiment. (The first 3 lines of the last paragraph on p. 581 have been changed to indicate that the experiment is centered around the 8096).

INTRODUCTION

In this Digital Signal Processing (DSP) application to electrical filtering, the aim is to remove certain frequency components from an incoming signal or waveform. In the experiment we shall create a microprocessor-based low pass filter whose function is to pass frequency components below a certain cut-off frequency, fc, and attenuate frequency components above fc (3 db. attenuation at fc). If, then, a wave or signal is input, and contains many frequency components in varying degrees of amplitude (described by its "frequency spectrum"), the result at the output will be a waveform in time which is different in shape than the input signal, precisely because certain frequency components have been removed. We say that the input signal has been "processed" (altered) to yield a different waveform at the output. If a microcomputer and its software are to do this signal processing, then clearly there must be an A to D converter to transform the input (analog) signal to digital for microprocessor processing or alteration, and then a D to A converter to transform the processed (digital) signal back to an analog output signal vs. time. The actual digital signal processing will usually contain multiply and add and subtract routines as well as a routine involving the accumulator holding previous values of the arithmetic operations in preparation for the next stage of the signal processing (i.e. an iterative type or recursive type of routine in which a sampling delay time enters).

The techniques of DSP have a wide range of applications: filtering as explained above; speech synthesis in which white noise (all frequency components equally present) is filtered on a selective frequency basis so that a signal results which is an audio type signal; speech recognition in which the frequency components of the incoming signal are selectively passed through a filter(s) and the output strengths or amplitudes measured (the resulting FREQUENCY SPECTRUM is then the speech's "signature"); signal analysis in which the amplitudes of the various frequency components are identified by the digital filter thus identifying the time nature of the signal (pulse, ramp, or whatever). Our DSP application in this experiment will be to filtering.

The advantages of microprocessor-based DSP to realize a filter are the same that appear time and again in microprocessor-based control applications in general: 1) absence of hardware and discrete R,L,C components, which in communication systems can amount to lots of "real estate" and components; 2) size; 3) tolerance (no R,L,C drift induced by changing temperature, humidity and other environmental parameters which can change cut-off frequency and filter response); 4) flexibility and versatility whereby a simple change of a couple of bytes in the program changes the cut-off frequency and filter response, as contrasted to a hardware approach in which a circuit re-design would be necessary to effect a new filter; 5) easier to manufacture; 6) multiplexed filtering capability in which many channels can be filtered by the same microprocessor and its software, given the necessary microprocessor speed, obviating the need for many hardware filters, one for each channel; 6) better performance with smaller size; 7) multiple filters can be realized from a single DSP by cascading various basic DSP units. In short, it is the old story that has appeared in every experiment in this book and in Volume 1: AN INPUT (EXCITATION) IS TRANSFORMED TO AN OUTPUT (RESPONSE), NOT BY A HARDWARE-BASED TRANSFER FUNCTION, T, BUT BY A SOFTWARE-BASED T, WITH ALL THE ADVANTAGES OF FLEXIBILITY, VERSATILITY, ADAPTABILITY, SIZE, COST, RELIABILITY, ETC. THAT WE HAVE CONSTANTLY STRESSED.

The microprocessor is the element which gave DSP its impetus and popularity: the availability of a small, fast, low cost computer is the key. As microprocessor speed has been increasing, allowing higher signal sampling rates (giving a more faithful output waveform, relative to what is desired), the DSP applications grew rapidly into many areas, some of which were noted above. One such example of a very specialized DSP device is Intel's powerful 2920 signal processing microprocessor. It is a chip expressly devoted to DSP. The advent of fast mutliply instructions for signal processing and of 16 bit microprocessors have been more recent forces behind the DSP surge. Faster A to D (signal-in) and D to A (signal-out) converters with larger bit sizes have also been important factors. They result in more accuracy and resolution in signal processing applications where needed.

Our experiment is the implementation of a low-pass digital filter in which the 8096, its ACH.0 A/D converter, and an external D/A converter (AD558) are used. The signal to be filtered is input via the A/D on a regular sampled interrupt basis, then digitally processed (altered) by the software routine, and output back in analog form via the DAC. There are two methods of designing a digital filter: the DIRECT method and the TRANS-

FORMATION method. The latter entails designing a continuous or analog filter and then using one of the many transformation techniques to realize the filter using DSP. The transform method takes advantage of the enormous amount of experience, tools, and methods available to design analog filters. We shall pursue the transform method in designing our digital filter. We will be giving only the basic theory needed for the design, in our case, of a simple LOW PASS FILTER. Details on DSP, digital filters, and filters generally can be obtained in many references, two of which are listed here:

1. Digital Signal Processing: Theory, Design, and Implementation - by A. Peled and Bede-Liu. (John Wiley).

2. Continuous and Discrete Signal and System Analysis - by McGillem and Cooper. (Holt, Rinehart, and Winston).

A simple circuit for a low pass filter is shown below:

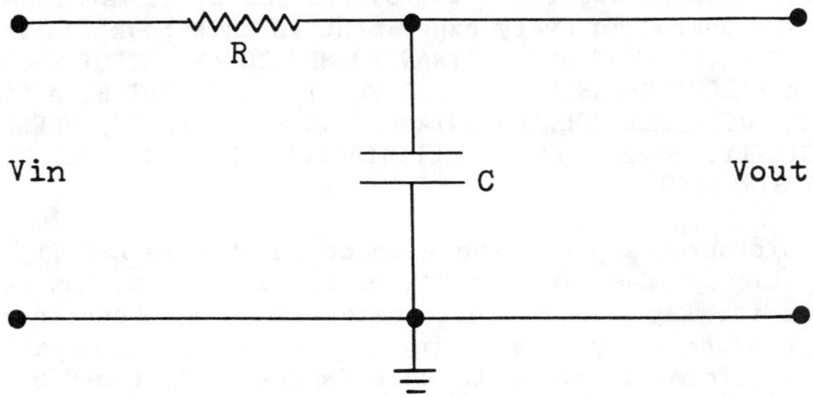

For large sinusoidal frequencies, the impedance of C is low, and so input currents at those frequencies are shorted to ground and do not appear at the output. For low frequencies, C's impedance is high and so input currents at those frequencies are blocked from ground and appear at the output. Hence a "low pass" filter. At some frequency, called the cut-off frequency, the output power is cut in half relative to the input power (3 db point). The cut-off frequency for the above low pass filter is given by:

(1): $$fc = \frac{1}{2\pi RC}$$

This can be shown by a "sinor" or "phasor" analysis in which Vout (sinor) is a fraction of Vin, the fraction being the ratio of C's impedance to R+ C's impedance (voltage-divider circuit in above diagram).

Using Laplace Transforms, applicable to any type of signals, not just sinusoids, the impedance-voltage divider relationship becomes:

(2): $$\frac{Vout\ (s)}{Vin\ (s)} = \frac{1/Cs}{R+1/Cs} = \frac{a}{s+a},$$

where $a = 1/RC = 2\pi\ fc$.

The Z Transform is needed for digital implementation or realization of the filter. It is defined as

(3): $$Z = \frac{1}{1 - sT},$$

where T is the sampling period. 1/T would be the sampling rate i.e. the rate at which Vin is sampled. The above gives:

(4): $$s = \frac{1 - 1/Z}{T}$$

(4) into (2) gives:

(5): $$\frac{Vout\ (Z)}{Vin\ (Z)} = \frac{aT}{1+aT-1/Z}$$

(5) above can be re-structured to yield:

(6): $$Vout\ (Z) = K\ Vin\ (Z) + M\ Vout\ (Z) \times 1/Z.$$

where:

(7): $$K = \frac{aT}{1+aT},\ M = \frac{1}{1+aT}$$

1/Z represents a DELAY of one T sample (period). Note also that

(8): $$K/M = aT = (1/RC) \times T = 2\pi\ fc \times T$$

The parameter procedure in our design approach is then the following:

a) Choose a cut-off frequency, fc, desired for your LP filter. This determines a=1/RC from equation (1).

b) Choose a sampling rate, 1/T, as high as possible and still allow each sample to be processed and output. The sample rate chosen thus determines T.

c) With a and T now known, K and M from equation (7) are determined from the product aT.

d) With K and M known, the output signal can be calculated for a given input signal from eq. (6). Eq. (6) merely says that the input (ADC) SAMPLE, Vin, is to be multiplied by K and added to M times the PREVIOUS (delayed) output Vout x (1/Z). The result, Vout, is output to the DAC. It should differ from Vin by the absence (or attenuation) of frequency components above fc. Our software routines must, therefore, contain one that implements the fractional multiply and addition comprising equation (6).

Note, in the above, that there are no references whatsoever to ACTUAL, REALIZED lumped elements R and C. They SIMPLY DO NOT EXIST. An A to D input signal is sampled, processed (eq. 6) for a desired sampling rate 1/T and cut-off frequency fc, and then output through a DAC. The R.C. CONCEPT is used only as an INTERMEDIATE stage in the transform method.

One implementation of eq. (6) above is the following:

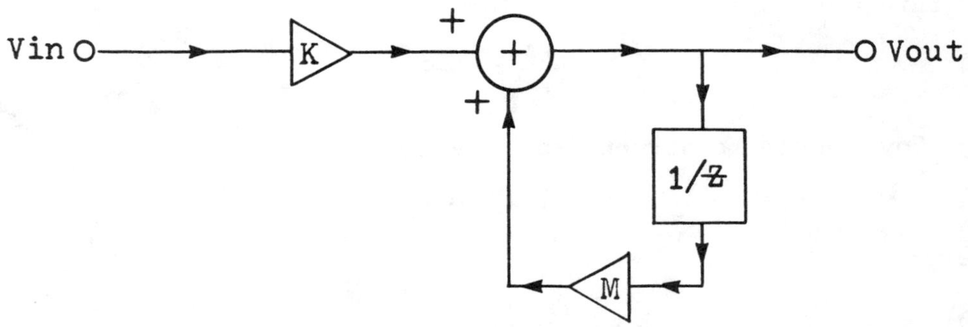

where 1/Z is a DELAY (next sample occurs T secs. later), and its reciprocal represents SAMPLING RATE.

HARDWARE SET-UP AND FURTHER COMMENTS

1. The set-up consists of a low frequency (0-10,000 Hz) sine wave signal generator as the source Vin for ACH.0 A/D conversion. Port P1's output pins P1.0 to P1.7 are tied to an external 8-bit DAC (see sections 2, 3 below). A switch at P0.7 is used to select the filtered (processed) output wave form (if high) or the unfiltered, straight-through signal (if low). The DAC's output, Vout, will show either of these on a scope. (P1 also has 8 LEDs).
2. The reason we shall be using an EXTERNAL DAC (here the AD 558), rather than the PWM unit with its pulse train output

at P2.5, is simply to avoid the hardware implementation of a BROAD-BAND integrating filter at the output of the PWM. That would be necessary to have faithful true D/A output waveforms over the broad audio range we intend to operate our digital filter.

3. The pin-out for the AD558 DAC, as we used it, is shown below. Pins 1-8 (DB0-DB7) are driven by the 8 output lines P1.0-P1.7 at port 1. What we output at P1, if switch P0.7 is high, is the A/D sampled (input) conversion byte after software processing (filtering). The filtered analog waveform is then available at the DAC's output. If switch P0.7 is low, we simply copy the A/D sampled conversion byte straight out to P1 (the unfiltered input analog waveform is, in that case, also available at the DAC's output). This is convenient for visually demonstrating the effect of filtering (sampling and processing) vs. no filtering.

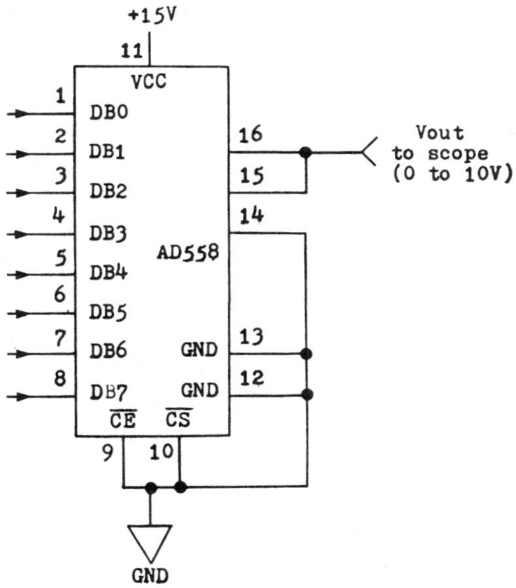

4. Note that, since the AD558 is an 8-bit DAC, we shall be using only bits 9-2 of the 10-bit A/D conversion result (with bits 9-2 rounded up if bit 1 of the neglected bits 1,0 is a 1). Clearly, we can synthesize more accurate, smoother filtered output waveforms if we employed all 10-bits of the 8096's A/D conversion capability in conjunction with a matching 10-bit output DAC. In that regard the PWM output of the 8096 would not suffice. Hence, our program, with slight modifications, is easily adapted to the case of 10-bit accuracy if we are willing to use an EXTERNAL 10-bit DAC. With 8-bit A/D and D/A, our processing consists,

among other things, of an 8 by 8 bit, three-operand multiply. If 10-bit A/D and D/A were involved we'd need to employ 16 by 16-bit multiply with the 8096.

5. In calculating the HEX values to be associated with the fractions K and M, which are crucial parameters in the fractional multiply method and in the program (see addresses 2B45 and 2B49 in the program), we would proceed as follows: if we took fc to be 1000 Hz and a sampling period of 126 usec. (sampling rate = about 7900 Hz) then K and M would turn out to be the fractions 0.4419 and 0.5581, respectively (see Eq. 7). Multiplying these fractions by 255(FF) gives, respectively, 113 and 142 (dec) which become 71H and 8EH. These would be the values used in the fractional multiply part of our program which implements Eq. 6 to give the output waveform. Similar procedure would hold for other cut-off frequencies and sampling periods fc and T. (For more on fractional multiply, see Expt. 8-5, p. 376, in the book "The 8051: 81 Hands-On Experiments" by the authors, MTI Publications).
6. Aside from the accuracy considerations (10-bit vs. 8-bit) discussed in (4) above, the basic condition to be satisfied, above all else, is SHANNON'S SAMPLING THEOREM. This states that the frequency of sampling must be at least twice the frequency of the wave being sampled, otherwise information and accuracy will be lost. We are sampling at 7900 Hz and our input signals varied from 100 to 2000 Hz.
7. The sampling PERIOD should be NO LESS than the sum of a) the time for A/D conversion, PLUS b) the time it takes to process that digitally converted sample into filtered form before a new sample should be taken in. In reality, that period should be comfortably larger than this sum in case multiple filter units (higher order filters with better overall response) are to be implemented. In that case, repeated fractional multiplications are involved, leading to larger overall processing time. In our simple one-unit software filter, the processing time in our program between 2B2E and 2B58 (see program below) is a fast 35 usec. (as a result of the speed of execution of the 8096's 3-operand multiply and add instructions), and the A/D conversion time on our 8096 was 42 usec. Thus a total time of about 80 usec. is needed between samplings. Our 126 usec. sampling period (sampling rate = 7900 Hz) more than covers this. With the latest 8096, A/D conversion times of 22 usec. are specified. In that case we could use sampling periods as low as 35 usec + 22 usec. = about 60 usec. (for a one-unit filter), or sampling rates as high as about 17,000 Hz. The filter band-pass could then cover input frequencies up to over 8000 Hz (Sampling Theorem). The fast MUL and ADD instructions of the 8096 make it well suited for digital filtering and all other kinds of DSP.

THE METHOD AND THE PROGRAM

1. Refer to the hardware set-up in section (1) above.
2. Refer to the pin-out and set-up of the AD558 DAC shown in section (3) above.
3. The processing (filtering) part of our program is essentially a software solution of equations (6) and (7) in the Introduction section above, in which fractional multiply and add are involved (in 3-operand forms) for which the 8096 is so well-suited.
4. The method behind our program will be brought out as we analyze it. The program (at 2B00) is shown below.

```
18 00      SP       EQU   18H       60 00    PROD    EQU   60H
08 00      MINT     EQU   08H       61 00    PROD_1  EQU   61H
09 00      PINT     EQU   09H       70 00    PP      EQU   70H
02 20      INVECO   EQU   2002H     71 00    PP_1    EQU   71H
0A 20      INVEC1   EQU   200AH     80 00    TEMP    EQU   80H
06 00      HSOCOM   EQU   06H       0A 00    T1      EQU   0AH
04 00      HSOTIME  EQU   04H       0E 00    P0      EQU   0EH
02 00      ADCOM    EQU   02H       0F 00    P1      EQU   0FH
02 00      ADRESLO  EQU   02H       8E 00    M       EQU   8EH
03 00      ADRESHI  EQU   03H       71 00    K       EQU   71H
40 00      INPUT    EQU   40H

2B00                         ORG    2B00H
                    ;
2B00  A1 C0 00 18   START:   LD     SP,#0C0H          ;Initialize SP.
2B04  B1 00 0F               LDB    P1,#00H           ;Initialize D/A Converter.
2B07  FA                     DI                       ;Disable interrupts.
2B08  B1 22 08               LDB    MINT,#22H         ;Enable HSO Software Timer intr.
                                                      ;and A/D Completion interrupt.
2B0B  11 09                  CLRB   PINT              ;Clear any pending interrupts.
2B0D  A1 2E 2B 80            LD     TEMP,#ADCPLT      ;Load address of A/D complete
2B11  C3 01 02 20 80         ST     TEMP,INVECO[0]    ;ISR into INT VECT table.
2B16  A1 59 2B 80            LD     TEMP,#SOFTINT     ;Load address of SOFTINT ISR
2B1A  C3 01 0A 20 80         ST     TEMP,INVEC1[0]    ;into INT VECT table.
2B1F  EF 03 00               CALL   HSOTAG            ;Call HSO command routine.
2B22  FB                     EI                       ;Enable interrupts.
2B23  27 FE         HERE:    SJMP   HERE              ;Loop HERE. ("BUSY").
                    ;
                    ;
2B25  B1 38 06      HSOTAG:  LDB    HSOCOM,#38H       ;Load HSO command tag for
                                                      ;software timer to generate
                                                      ;an interrupt.
2B28  45 40 00 0A 04         ADD    HSOTIME,T1,#0040H ;Program time of HSO command to
                                                      ;be 126 microseconds from "now".
2B2D  F0                     RET                      ;Return.
```

```
                        ;        A/D CONVERSION COMPLETE ISR
                        ;
2B2E    F2              ADCPLT: PUSHF                       ;Save flags.
2B2F    3B 02 FD        ADBUSY: JBS    ADRESLO,3,ADBUSY;If A/D not complete loop.
2B32    B0 03 40                LDB    INPUT,ADRESHI        ;Load high byte (BITS 9-2)
                                                            ;of A/D result into INPUT.
2B35    37 02 07                JBC    ADRESLO,7,NO_RND;If AD_LO.7 = 0, jump to NO_RND.
2B38    99 FF 40                CMPB   INPUT,#0FFH          ;Else compare INPUT with 0FFH.
2B3B    DF 02                   JE     NO_RND               ;If INPUT = 0FFH, jump to NO_RND.
2B3D    17 40                   INCB   INPUT                ;Else add 1 to input (round-up).
2B3F    EF 02 00        NO_RND: CALL   FILTER               ;Call filter processing routine.
2B42    F3                      POPF                        ;Restore flags.
2B43    F0                      RET                         ;Return.
                        ;
                        ; FRACTIONAL MULTIPLY ROUTINE
                        ;
2B44    5D 71 40 60     FILTER: MULUB  PROD,INPUT,#K        ;Multiply (8 bit) input by constant
                                                            ; 'K'.
2B48    5D 8E 0F 70             MULUB  PP,P1,#M             ;Multiply output from previous
                                                            ;sample (P1) by constant M and
                                                            ;store result in PP (Partial Product).
2B4C    3F 0E 05                JBS    P0,7,FIL             ;If P0.7 = 1, jump to FIL.
2B4F    B0 40 0F                LDB    P1,INPUT             ;Else simply copy INPUT to P1.
2B52    20 04                   SJMP   RETURN               ;Jump to RETURN.
2B54    54 71 61 0F     FIL:    ADDB   P1,PROD_1,PP_1       ;Add K*INPUT to (M*VOUT)* 1/Z
                                                            ;(output delayed by one sample time).
                                                            ;The result is the new output and
                                                            ;is loaded into P1 for D/A Converter
                                                            ;and LEDs.
2B58    F0              RETURN: RET                         ;Return.
                        ;
                        ;
                        ;        SOFTINT ISR
                        ;
2B59    F2              SOFTINT:PUSHF                       ;Save flags.
2B5A    B1 08 02                LDB    ADCOM,#08H           ;Start A/D Conversion on channel 0
                                                            ;now.
2B5D    2F C6                   CALL   HSOTAG               ;Call HSOTAG to reload the HSO
                                                            ;command.
2B5F    F3                      POPF                        ;Restore flaqs.
2B60    F0                      RET                         ;Return.
```

Behind the program are three main points: 1) Software Timer 0 (ST0) is programmed at 2B25 to create an interrupt 126 usec. from "now". 126 usec. is to be our sampling period. 2) At the time the interrupt occurs, the SOFTINT ISR at 2B58 programs the IMMEDIATE start of A/D conversion on channel 0, where the analog waveform to be filtered is input. 3) An "A/D Conversion Complete" interrupt, generated when conversion is over, vectors to the "A/D Complete" ISR at 2B2E where the filter processing is implemented in software. The sequence of events repeats after the SOFTINT ISR programs STO for another interrupt 126 usec. later. These three points will now be amplified. Also keep in mind that the main program ends on SJMP HERE at 2B23. That loop is to represent other "busy tasks" which will be interrupted by the STO and A/D Complete interrupts on a regular basis. Hence, again, the 8096's ability to carry out various tasks and tasks within tasks.

The main part of the program initializes SP to 003C and the DAC output to 0. Interrupts are disabled and the Software Timer and A/D Complete interrupt sources are unmasked. Pending interrupts, if any, are cleared. The addresses of the A/D Complete and Software Timer Interrupt routines are then loaded into the interrupt vector table at 2002 and 200A, respectively. At 2B1F HSOTAG (at 2B25) is called. There HSOCOM and HSOTIME are programmed to have STO generate a Software Timer interrupt 126 usec. from "now". (Remember, T1 + 0040H loaded into HSOTIME corresponds to 64 (dec) or 128 usec. from "now"; but it takes 2 usec. for the ADD HSOTIME command to get into the CAM FILE, so "now" is really 2 usec. not 0 usec. -- hence the 126 usec. value for the sampling period). The return from HSOTAG to 2B22 results in the enabling of global interrupts. "Busy tasks" (the loop at 2B23) is then entered.

When the STO interrupt is created at the end of 126 usec., the SOFTINT ISR at 2B59 is entered. There flags and interrupt mask are pushed on the stack (the system is disabled) and conversion of the analog signal at ACH.0 is immediately started. STO is again programmed for an interrupt another 126 usec. later (see the call of HSOTAG at 2B5D). Flags and interrupt mask are then restored and the RET instruction causes a return to the point at which the STO interrupt occurred in the program flow. When A/D conversion is complete, the "A/D Complete Interrupt" generated vectors the program to the A/D Complete ISR at 2B2E. There, the heart of the digital filter signal processing (fractional multiply) takes place. Flags and mask are pushed. The JBS ADRESLO, 3, ADBUSY instruction polls the status bit S to make sure conversion is indeed complete. It is a backup, precautionary measure not absolutely necessary. Bits 9-2 of the valid conversion result in register ADRESHI are then loaded into register INPUT. Next, bit 1 of the 10-bit result is tested (it is represented by bit 7 in ADRESLO). If ADRESLO.7 is 0 no rounding up of INPUT is needed and the JBC instruction jumps directly to NO-RND where the filter processing routine at FILTER is called. If, however, that bit is high, fall-through to the CMPB instruction occurs. We want to make sure, before INPUT is incremented by 1 to effect rounding up, that ADRESHI was not FF, otherwise the rounding up will give 00 in INPUT.

If the CMPB INPUT, #0FFH instruction shows INPUT to be FF, the JE instruction also jumps to NO-RND where the filter processing routine at FILTER is called. If INPUT is not equal to FF then it is rounded up by 1 (INCB INPUT) and FILTER (at 2B44) is called from 2B3F.

Let us now analyze the FILTER routine at 2B44. The K value (calculated before-hand from Eq. 7 for a specified cut-off frequency fc and sampling period T) is then multiplied by INPUT (the latter represents the rounded 8-bit cnversion byte at the input i.e. Vin in Eq. 6) and the result is stored in the PROD word register at 60H. The 8-bit by 8-bit MULUB instruction in 3-operand form is used. This 16-bit result is thus stored in registers 60H (lo byte) and 61H (hi byte). Next, the M value corresponding to fc and T from Eq. 7 is multiplied by the PREVOUS OUTPUT BYTE Vout at P1 (one sample time ago i.e. the term Vout x 1/Z in Eq. 6) and the result is stored in the PP (Partial Product) word register at 70H. Again, the 3-operand MULUB instruction is used so 70H contains the low byte and 71H the high byte of this new 16-bit result. Please note that the Equates in the program show K = 71H and M = 8EH. They are the values Eq. 7 gives (after multiplying by 255 and converting to HEX) for the case of a 1000 Hz fc cut-off frequency and a sampling period, T, of 126 usec. Thus, so far, PROD contains K x Vin and PP contains M x Vout x 1/Z in Eq. (6).

The instruction JBS P0, 7, FIL at 2B4C tests the switch at P0.7. If its status is low, fall-through to the LDB P1, INPUT instruction causes an exact duplication at the output of the DAC of the input waveform at ACH.0. We have that option. The SJMP to RETURN then returns to 2B42 where POPF and return to the main program are executed. If, however, P0.7 is high, then the jump to FIL at 2954 is taken. There the high BYTE quantities in PP-1 (at 71H) and PROD-1 (at 61H) are added and the 8-bit result is stored in P1 to drive the output DAC and produce the new filtered output Vout = K x Vin + M x Vout x 1/Z, in conformity with Eq. (6). The RET instruction at 2B58 causes a return to 2B42 where POPF and then RET are executed. Program flow returns to the main program to "busy tasks". Another ST0 sampling interrupt, when created, will cause a repeat of the whole series of events analyzed above.

Please note that the crucial ADDB instruction at 2B54 adds the HIGH BYTES of PROD and of PP to each other, not the 16-bit values. We do the addition that way so that we end up with the most significant 8-bit result for outputting to P1 to drive the 8-bit DAC. Effectively, each 16-bit result in PROD and PP has been divided by 255 to leave an 8-bit result (the values in high byte registers PROD-1 and PP-1).

PROCEDURE

1. Connect the output of a low frequency, level sine wave generator to ACH.0.
2. Connect output port P1 to an 8-bit DAC (see diagram in section (3) of Hardware Set-Up where a AD558 DAC is shown). Connect the output of the DAC to a scope. The amplitude of the input to ACH.0 should not exceed 5V.
3. Connect a switch S to bit P0.7. Keep it low.
4. Reset and enter BY 09 = 00.
5. Execute from 2B00. The declared values of M and K in the program, as is, are 8EH and 71H, i.e. fc = 1000 Hz and a sampling period 126 usec. (7900 Hz rate) [see Eq. (7)].
6. Set the generator to 100 Hz and observe its waveshape on the scope (remember S = P0.7 is low so we observe the straight-through sampled, but unfiltered signal at the DAC's output). Measure the peak to peak voltage of the input on the scope (absolute or in terms of boxes). Now flip S high and observe the filtered output waveform on the scope. Measure its peak to peak voltage. Record results. Note the steps because of the finite number of samples.
7. Repeat (6) for frequencies of 500 Hz and 1000 Hz, recording input amplitude vs. output amplitude at each frequency (simply throw S from low to high in each case). Observe the filtered wave shape and notice the step-wise effects of the sampling on accuracy. See Expt. 9-21 for smoothing. Naturally, the input amplitude will not vary with frequency if you're employing a level generator. The output amplitude variation with frequency gives the filter response. We found the filtered output had amplitudes of 5.0 boxes, 4.4 boxes, 3.5 boxes at 100, 500, and 1000 Hz, respectively. The POWER RATIO of the amplitudes at 100 and 1000 Hz is thus (5 x 5)/(3.5 x 3.5) = 2.04. It should be exactly 2 i.e. 3 db down at fc. Agreement is excellent.
8. Repeat the experiment for a cut-off frequency of 2000 Hz and the same sampling period 126 usec. Eq. (7) now gives K = 9CH and M = 63H. ESC and enter 9C at 2B45 for the new K and 63 at 2B49 for the new M. Execute. Flipping S from low to high, observe the unfiltered and then filtered output waves on the scope as you vary frequency from 100 Hz to 2000 Hz. We found the output filtered wave amplitudes at 100, 500, 1000, 1500, and 2000 Hz to be 5.0, 4.9, 4.2, 3.7, and 3.5 boxes, respectively. Again, we find the ratio of the powers at 100 Hz to that at fc = 2000 Hz to be 2.04, almost exactly as it should be. Observe in close detail the output filtered waveforms and the steps due to the finite sampling rate.
9. Observe the output waveforms in the last case as you go beyond fc = 2000 Hz and as you then go beyond 4000 Hz (exceeding 1/2 the sampling rate). Explain your observations.
10. PROBLEM: Add filters (cascade fractional multiplies).

EXPERIMENT 9-18

A MATERIALS HANDLING PROBLEM IMPLEMENTED USING EVENT COUNTER T2 AS THE REFERENCE FOR THE HSO UNIT.

INTRODUCTION AND FORMULATION

In Expt. 9-10 we treated a materials handling problem in which objects were sorted by size, and counts of total number of objects, as well as number of objects of any given size, were tracked. Varous bins to accommodate the various sizes detected were opened and closed at the proper times. In that experiment, we used real-time timer T1 to "measure" size and event counter T2 to record numbers of objects. The HSO unit and its HSO pins were NOT used to open and close the bins (they were located at port P1 in the approach we took there i.e. bin x = P1.x, x = 0, 1, 2, ...7). As written, the program in Expt. 9-10 was dedicated to that task. "Other tasks" did not enter the picture.

This experiment will treat a different materials handling problem. T2 and the HSO unit are employed. The first n0 objects are to pass to bin 0, the next n1 objects are to pass to bin 1, the next n2 objects are to pass to bin 2, etc., where now bin 0, bin 1, bin 2, etc. are opened or closed by positive or negative transitions at HSO pins HSO.0, HSO.1, HSO.2, etc., respectively. The "bins" may not even be bins; HSO.i may simply open or close doors or cartons where the objects n0, or n1, or n2 are to be packaged or crated separately in individual GROUPS no, n1, n2, etc.

Now, in the many experiments in this book employing the HSO unit, we have, with two exceptions, always used real time timer T1 as the reference for the HSO unit, so that events (transitions) at any pin(s) HSO.i were to occur at specified REAL TIMES relative to time in free-running 16-bit timer T1 (2 usec. increments). Remember, bit6 (T) in the HSO Command Tag Register (06H) can specify the reference to be T1 OR EVENT COUNTER T2 (T = 0 or 1, respectively). The only two experiments where T2 was chosen as the reference for the HSO unit were Expt. 5-15 and 6-6. In each of those experiments we used the HSO unit only to reset T2 by software. That involved the two instructions LDB HSOCOM, #4EH (or #6EH) and ADD HSOTIME, T2, #0000H. The first of the above instructions specifies that T2 is to be reset AT THE MOMENT THAT T2 (REFERENCE SPECIFIED AS T2) REACHES A CERTAIN VALUE. The second one specifies the value reached in T2 when T2 is to be reset. As written, T2 will reset when its value equals T2 + 0000 i.e. for the PRESENT VALUE in T2, not one count later. T2 + 0004 would specify that reset is to occur when T2 has incremented by 4. We could also have written LDB HSOCOM, #0EH (or #2EH) and ADD HSOTIME, T1, 0003. This selects T1 as the REFERENCE and specifies that T2 is to be RESET (0E or 2E in HSOCOM specifies that action) "NOW" i.e. when T1 = T1 + 0003 in REAL TIME. Aside from those two experiments, T1 was always used as the reference for real time events occurring at HSO.i. So far in the book's experiments, events (transitions) at HSO.i have never been tied to counts in T2 reaching certain values.

We shall now be employing EVENT COUNTER T2 as the REFERENCE for events (openings and closings) which we want to occur at HSO.i. Thus we may want to specify that HSO.0 is to open when T2 reaches a certain value and close when T2 reaches a certain higher value; that HSO.1 is to be 1 when T2 reaches a certain value and that it go to 0 when T2 reaches a specified higher value, etc. That is just what we want to, and will, do to implement the materials handling problem described above. Events will enter T2 through T2CLK at P2.3. Employing the HSO unit has the added advantage of greater through-put: "other tasks" can be attended to while the HSO unit attends to its business.

APPROACH

All we need do is use, as is, the program in one of the HSO unit experiments where the CAM file was loaded with the HSO Command Tag bytes and the HSOTIME words from the two tables CMDTBL (HSO COM Command table bytes) and TMTBL (HSOTIME word Timer values). Those tables, as appropriate to the application, were loaded at run-time. The flexibility and convenience in having the program written around loading the CAM from such tables will now be apparent. All we need do is load the tables at run-time with command bytes and time words appropriate to having event counter T2 as the reference for the problem at hand. We'll use the program as written in Expt. 9-8 at address 2330 ("A High Speed Programmable Controller"). BUT, T1 (0A) AT ADDRESS 2370 THERE SHOULD NOW BE REPLACED WITH T2(0C). Note "busy tasks" at 2351 in that program (multitasking).

Let us analyze the approach taken to arrive at the bytes/words needed for the CMDTBL/TMTBL tables for this problem (refer to the HSOCOM Command Tag register format p. 31). Remember, T2 will count events from a debounced switch input at T2CLK.

1. To reset T2 using the HSO unit, all we need execute are the HSO instructions LDB HSOCOM, #4EH and ADD HSOTIME, T2, #0000H. This selects T2 as the reference and specifies

that T2 is to be reset "now" i.e. when T2 = T2 + 0000, whatever the value that T2 may presently have. Channel E in HSOCOM specifies that a reset of T2 is wanted. Thus, so far, the byte/word combination is 4E, 0000.

2. We want bin 0 (HSO.0) to open (HSO.0 = 1) when the first object arrives. This can be achieved with the instructions LDB HSOCOM, #60H and ADD HSOTIME, T2, #0001H. The first specifies that T2 is the reference timer and that HSO.0 is to be set. The second specifies that HSO.0 is to be set when T2 = T2 + 0001 (on arrival of first object). The next byte/word for the table is thus to be 60, 0001.
3. We want bin 0 to close (HSO.0 = 0) when the count in T2 reaches a definite value. Thus, if this definite value is specified as 0008 (corresponding to n0 = 4 objects passing T2CLK i.e. one lo/hi/lo throw of the switch corresponds to one object but 2 counts in T2), then the appropriate HSO instructions would be LDB HSOCOM, #40H and ADD HSOTIME, T2, #0008H. These specify T2 as the reference (40) and that HSO.0 is to be cleared when T2 reaches the value 0008 (4 objects passed into bin 0). Thus the next byte/word for our tables is to be 40, 0008.
4. We want bin 1 to open (HSO.1 = 1) on arrival of the 5th object. Thus the HSO instructions should be LDB HSOCOM, #61H and ADD HSOTIME, T2, #0009H. 61 selects T2 as the reference and specifies that HSO.1 is to be set. The ADD instruction specifies this is to happen when T2 reaches 0009 (arrival of the 5th object). Thus the next byte/word in the table is to be 61, 0009.
5. Bin 1 is to close (HSO.1 = 0) when the count in T2 reaches another definite value, say 0018 (= 24 dec). This would correspond to a TOTAL of 12 objects being recorded by T2 so far, with the 13th about to arrive. In terms of n, this would correspond to n0 = 4 being let into bin 0 and n1 = 8 being let into bin 1. The appropriate HSO instructions should thus be LDB HSOCOM, #41H and ADD HSOTIME, T2, #0018H. The next byte/word pair for the table is thus to be 41, 0018.
6. Bin 2 is to open (HSO.2 = 1) on arrival of the 13th object. This requires LDB HSOCOM, #62 and ADD HSOTIME, T2, 0019H. Again, this specifies T2 as the reference timer. Next byte/word = 62, 0019.
7. Bin 2 is to close (HSO.2 = 0) when the count in T2 reaches another definite value, say 002C (= 44 dec). This would correspond to a total of 22 objects being recorded by T2 so far, with the 23rd to arrive later. In terms of n, this would correspond to n0 = 4 in bin 0, n1 = 8 in bin 1, and n2 = 10 in bin 2. The HSO instructions should thus be LDB HSOCOM, #52H, ADD HSOTIME, T2, #002CH. WE HAVE CHOSEN 52H FOR HSOCOM TO ASSURE, NOT ONLY THAT HSO.2 IS CLEARED

WHEN T2 REACHES 44 DEC., BUT ALSO THAT AN HSO INTERRUPT IS GENERATED TO THE HSO ISR AT 2353 IN EXPT. 9-8 (FOR A RE-LOAD OF THE CAM). The last byte/word in the table is thus to be 52, 002C.

8. The HSO interrupt specified in (7) above will cause a re-loading of the CAM in the HSO ISR (address 2353 in Expt. 9-8) for a repeat of the "packaging sequence": 4, 8, 10 to bins 0, 1, 2, respectively (or at the times the TOTALS 4, 12, 22 (objects) are detected by T2).
9. The table values in TMTBL could be changed at any time to specify new n0, n1, n2 values for the bins 0, 1, 2, (at HSO.0,.1,.2).
10. Thus the tables we'll enter at 5000 and 5100 will be BY 5000 = 4E, 60, 40, 61, 41, 62, 52 and WO 5100 = 0000, 0001, 0008, 0009, 0018, 0019, 002C. The number of entries is thus 7 and we'll have to enter that at run-time i.e. BY 50 = 07. The above table specifying n0, n1, n2 can be changed during execution time to specify other bin loading conditions.

PROCEDURE

1. Connect a debounced switch S to T2CLK (P2.3). Use LEDs at HSO.0,.1,.2.
2. Change the byte 0A at 2370 in Expt. 9-8's program to the byte 0C (that changes T1 to T2 in the ADD HSOTIME command in the CAM LOAD routine there. Remember, event timer T2 is now to be the reference for the HSO unit instead of real-time timer T1).
3. Reset and enter BY 09 = 00.
4. Enter the CMDTBL and TMTBL tables as follows: BY 5000 = 4E, 60, 40, 61, 41, 62, 52 and WO 5100 = 0000, 0001, 0008, 0009, 0018, 0019, 002C.
5. Enter the table length: BY 50 = 07.
6. Enter BY 15 = 02. This loads 02 into IOC0 to select T2CLK as the source of T2 events (it also resets T2 to 0 - not necesary since the first table entry will do that when executed in the CAM).
7. Execute the program as given in Expt. 9-8 from 2330 (with the T1 to T2 change noted in (2) above).
8. Throw the debounced switch S at T2CLK and observe HSO.0 go on at the FIRST THROW HIGH OF S. Throw S high 3 more times and observe HSO.0 go off after the RELEASE of S on the fourth throw. 4 objects are now in bin 0.
9. Continue to depress and release S. HSO.1 goes high on the 5th throw of S high. HSO.1 wll go off after the release of S on the 12th throw. 8 objects are now in bin 1.
10. Continue to depress and release S. HSO.2 goes on at the 13th throw of S high. HSO.2 will go off after release of S

on the 22nd throw. 10 objects are now in bin 2. HSO.0, .1, .2 are now all off.

11. Continue throwing S to simulate arrival of the next batch of 22 objects. You should observe only HSO.0 on during arrival of the first 4 objects; then only HSO.1 on during arrival of objects 5 through 12; and then only HSO.2 on during arrval of objects 13 through 22, after which HSO.0, .1,.2 remain off till the next batch of objects starts arriving.
12. While the program is executing, but with no throws of S occurring, change the TMTBL as follows: enter WO 5100 = 0000, 0001, 0004, 0005, 000A, 000B, 0012. Now resume throwing S. You should observe 2 objects enter bin 0, 3 enter bin 1, and 4 enter bin 2. Why?
13. Enter WO 5100 = 0000, 0001, 0006, 0007, 000C, 000D, 0016. Continue to press and release S. What do you observe?
14. Why, when you enter a new T2 TMTBL after the previous batch goes through, does the next batch follow the PREVIOUS n0, n1, n2 specifications ONE MORE TIME AROUND before the new n0, n1, n2 values are implemented?

PROBLEM

Introduce the HSI unit into the program to measure time between press and release of each throw of S. This will give the "size" of each object. Then have bin x open at either port P1 or at the HSO pins to receive size x. How would you have the HSI unit operate on each GROUP n0 (for bin 0), n1 (for bin 1) and n2 (for bin 2) (with bin x driven by HSO.x) so that each GROUP is sorted by size? Thus T2 is still to be the reference for HSO (to divide the objects into groups of n0, n1, and n2), but HSI is to add another dimension to the problem (sorting each group by size).

PROBLEM

Correct the situation in (14) above so that the new specified n0, n1, n2 values are obeyed for the very next batch.

EXPERIMENT 9-19

A FREQUENCY COUNTER USING THE T2 EVENT COUNTER (1 HZ RESOLUTION TO 250 KHZ).

INTRODUCTION AND APPROACH

In Expt. 9-7 frequencies were measured using the HSI unit. Actually, an unknown frequency was calibrated against a standard by varying the standard until the PERIODS of unknown and standard, as measured by the HSI unit, were equal. The reciprocal of the standard's period at the point of equality (indicated by the turning on of a LED) gave the frequency of the unknown. It was then pointed out on p. 492 that, since periods could only be inferred to the nearest integral multiple of 2 usec. [the resultion of time increments in timer T1 (which is the basis of time in the HSITIME register of the HSI unit)], the calculated frequency could be in error; and further, that only those DISCRETE frequencies whose periods were INTEGRAL MULTIPLES of 2 usec. would be accurately indicated by the HSI unit.

It was then stated there that the only accurate way of measuring frequency (ALL frequencies in the range 0 - 250,000 Hz for EVERY Hz) would be by means of event counter T2, PROVIDED THE MAXIMUM FREQUENCY OF THE SQUARE WAVE TO BE MEASURED DID NOT EXCEED 250,000 Hz, since T2 can not count transitions (0 to 1, 1 to 0) that are separated in time by an amount less than 2 usec. With that restriction met, there is no reason that T2 can't measure ANY frequency LESS than 250,000 Hz (in steps of 1 Hz if desired). For then, the time between transitions in square waves will be greater than 2 usec., by WHATEVER amount. To accomplish this frequency measurement with T2, all we need do is set up a time base of 1 sec. (a delay loop) and allow 0 to 1 and 1 to 0 transitions from the square waves (input to the T2CLK (or HSI.1) clock source of T2) to be counted by T2. Clearly T2/2 (T2 = transition count) at the end of 1 sec. will give the number of PULSES recorded in 1 sec. i.e. the frequency. The only thing to remember is that any FREQUENCIES LARGER than 32,768 Hz will cause the COUNT in T2 to reach 65,536 and then OVERFLOW before 1 sec. elapses. By counting the number of T2 overflows, multiplying it by 32,768, and adding the result to the value T2/2 (where T2 is the count ACCUMULATED in T2 after the LAST T2 overflow), we'll arrive at the frequency of the square wave. The overflows from T2 are easily recorded in a T2OV ISR, provided T2 is enabled as the source of Timer Overflow interrupts (set bit 3 to 1 in IOC1 and bit 0 to 1 in MINT). We'll not only increment a register (REG2) every time the T2OV ISR is entered, but also output that overflow count to the LEDs at P1. The following program gives the details.

PROGRAM

The program at 2D00 is presented below. It is analyzed afterward.

```
      18 00        SP      EQU    18H
      00 20        INVEC   EQU    2000H
      16 00        IOC1    EQU    16H
      15 00        IOC0    EQU    15H
      0F 00        P1      EQU    0FH
      0E 00        P0      EQU    0EH
      40 00        TEMP    EQU    40H
      08 00        MINT    EQU    08H
      09 00        PINT    EQU    09H
      60 00        REG1    EQU    60H
      70 00        REG2    EQU    70H
      80 00        REG3    EQU    80H
      90 00        REG4    EQU    90H
      0C 00        T2      EQU    0CH

2D00                       ORG    2D00H
                   ;
2D00  A1 C0 00 18          LD     SP,#00C0H      ;Initialize SP.
2D04  FA                   DI                    ;Disable interrupts.
2D05  B1 01 08             LDB    MINT,#01H      ;Unmask Timer Overflow interrupt
                                                 ;source.
2D08  B1 08 16             LDB    IOC1,#08H      ;Select T2 as source for timer
                                                 ;overflow interrupts.
2D0B  A1 3E 2D 40          LD     TEMP,#T2OVFL   ;Load address of T2OVFL ISR into
2D0F  C3 01 00 20 40       ST     TEMP,INVEC[0]  ;T2OVFL VECT INT table location.
2D14  01 70        CLROV:  CLR    REG2           ;Clear REG2.
2D16  11 0F                CLRB   P1             ;Clear LEDs at P1.
2D18  B1 02 15             LDB    IOC0,#02H      ;Reset timer T2 and select T2CLK
                                                 ;as source for T2.
2D1B  11 09                CLRB   PINT           ;Clear pending interrupts.
2D1D  FB                   EI                    ;Enable interrupt system.
2D1E  EF 0E 00             CALL   TIME           ;Call TIME for 1 second delay.
2D21  FA                   DI                    ;Disable interrupt system.
2D22  A0 0C 60             LD     REG1,T2        ;Load REG1 with count in T2.
2D25  07 60                INC    REG1           ;Increment REG1 for adjustment.
2D27  08 01 60             SHR    REG1,#01H      ;Divide by 2 to complete adjustment.
2D2A  30 0E FD     HERE:   JBC    P0,0,HERE      ;Test switch 0 at P0. If P0.0 = 0,
                                                 ;jump to HERE.
```

```
2D2D   27 E5                SJMP    CLROV          ;Else jump to CLROV to measure
                                                   ;frequency again.
                  ;
                  ;
2D2F   B1 05 80   TIME:     LDB     REG3,#05H      ;Load outer loop REG3.
2D32   A1 FF FF 90 LOAD:    LD      REG4,#0FFFFH   ;Load inner loop REG4.

2D36   05 90      MORE:     DEC     REG4           ;Decrement inner loop.
2D38   D7 FC                JNE     MORE           ;If REG4 != 0, jump to MORE.
2D3A   E0 80 F5             DJNZ    REG3,LOAD      ;Else decrement outer loop, if
                                                   ;REG3 != 0, jump to LOAD.
2D3D   F0                   RET                    ;Else return.
                  ;
                  ;         T2 OVERFLOW ISR
                  ;
2D3E   07 70      T2OVFL:   INC     REG2           ;Increment REG2 (no. of overflows).
2D40   B0 70 0F             LDB     P1,REG2        ;Output REG2 to LEDs at P1.
2D43   F0                   RET                    ;Return.
                  ;
2D44                        END
```

The main program starts by initializing the SP, disabling the interrupt system, unmasking the timer overflow interrupt source, and unmasking the timer overflow interrupt source, and selecting T2 overflows as the source of timer overflow interrupts. The address of the T2OV interrupt ISR (#T2OVFL = 2D3E) is then loaded into TEMP before storing it in the VECT INT table at INVEC[0] = 2000 appropriate to timer overflow interrupts. REG2 is cleared. It will serve as the counter of the number of T2 overflows that might occur during the 1 sec. sampling of 0 to 1 and 1 to 0 transitions in T2 originating from the square waves input at T2CLK. P1 is cleared and 02 is loaded into IOC0 for the purpose of selecting T2CLK as the input source for T2 transition counts and to reset T2 to 0. Any pending interrupts are then cleared and the interrupt system is enabled.

A 1 second delay is then called (located at 2D2F). It is during this time that the 0 to 1 and 1 to 0 transitions on the square wave are counted by T2. Should any overflow(s) during this time occur in T2 (which will happen if the frequency being measured is greater than 32,768 Hz), then an interrupt(s) to the T2OV ISR at 2D3E will occur where REG2 is incremented to record the number of T2OV interrupts (T2 overflows) each time one occurs. That number is displayed at P1 and a return to the time delay then takes place. At the end of 1 sec. a return from TIME back to 2D21 transpires. There the interrupt system is disabled (no further T2OV interrupts will be serviced, should they occur, during the JBC wait instruction at 2D2A). The number of 0 to 1 and 1 to 0 TRANSITIONS recorded in T2 (after the last T2OV overflow occurred - if any did occur) is read into REG1. The latter is incremented and then divided by 2, so that REG1 now contains the number of PULSES that entered T2 (after the last T2 overflow, if any, occurred).

At this point we poll the status of a debounced switch S at P0.0. If it's low we loop on the label HERE. It is during this wait loop that we can read out the word value in REG1 (WO 60) to give the "remainder" number of PULSES in T2 that occurred after the last T2 overflow. Frequency (in Hz) is then given by (P1) x 32,768 + (REG1), where (P1) is the number of T2 overflows that occurred in 1 sec. as seen on the P1 display, and (REG1) is read from WO 60 and converted to decimal. After that determination, the frequency at the 0 - 250,000 Hz pulse generator can be changed prior to undertaking another frequency measurement. The latter is accomplished by throwing S high and quickly releasing it (in less than 1 sec). Fall-through 2D2A to the instruction SJMP CLROV loops back to CLROV at 2D14. There REG2 and P1 are cleared, T2 is reset, interrupts from T2OV pendings (developed during the JBC wait loop when T2 may have overflowed) are cleared and the interrupt system is re-enabled. Another measurement in T2 is made during another 1 sec. window (called again at 2D1E) and all repeats as before. At the end of that 1 sec. P1 is observed and WO 60 is read again in order to calculate the new frequency, which is again given by f = (P1) x 32,768 + (REG1) with (REG1) = WO 60 (and converted to decimal).

The time delay at TIME (2D2F) is the usual one based on loops: REG3 is loaded with 5 so that 5 outer loops will be made. The inner loop consists of 65,536 decrements of REG4 (initialized to FFFF). Because the DEC and JNE instructions comprising the inner loop (MORE) consume 12 state times (3 usec), the inner loop will create 196.61 msec. delay which, when multiplied by 5, WILL CAUSE A TOTAL DELAY OF 0.938 SEC. (2% ERROR). Keep this error in mind as you analyze the results given below in the Procedure section. PROBLEM: Choose the loading word for REG4 and the loading byte for REG3 so that the total time delay will come out AS CLOSE TO 1.000 SECONDS AS POSSIBLE.

PROCEDURE

1. Connect the output of a 0 - 250,000 Hz pulse generator (TTL level square waves) to the T2CLK (P2.3) source of T2 transitions.
2. Connect a debounced switch S to P0.0.
3. Reset and enter BY 09 = 00.

4. Set the pulse generator to 100,000 Hz, if possible.
5. Execute from 2D00. Read (P1) and WO 60 = (REG1). Calculate f = (P1) x 32,768 + WO 60 (the latter converted to decimal). Compare with 100,000 Hz. We found P1 = 3, REG1 = 001A = 26 dec., giving f = 98,330 Hz. Remember that our "1 sec." time base is really 0.983 sec. The agreement is, therefore, excellent.
6. Change the setting on the pulse generator to 150,000 Hz, if possible. Throw S at P0.0 high and quickly release. Calculate the new frequency from your new (P1) and WO 60 readings. Compare with 150,000 Hz. We found P1 = 4, REG1 = 484CH = 18,508 dec., f = 149,580 Hz.
7. Change the setting on the pulse generator to 50,000 Hz, if possible. Throw S high/low again. Calculate the new frequency from your new (P1) and WO 60 readings. We found P1 = 1, REG1 = 42A7H = 17,063 dec., f = 49,831 Hz.
8. With a setting of 25,000 Hz on the generator, throwing S hi/low again resulted in P1 = 0, REG1 = 60B4H = 24,756 dec., f = 24,756 Hz.

In all cases we measured the pulse generator's output frequency on a scope. This may have introduced errors that account for differences more or less than the 2% error in the time base i.e. 1.000 sec. vs. 0.983 sec.

NOTE ON FREQUENCY MEASUREMENT OF ANY PERIODIC WAVEFORM.

In this experiment we used input square waves and measured their frequency with the T2 event counter. The input need not be restricted to only pulses or square waves. Any periodic waveform can be converted to pulses (or square waves in the case of symmetric periodic waveforms) of the same frequency by various hardware techniques (e.g. clamping). The method employed in this experiment is then directly applicable, and the pulse or square wave frequency measured represents the frequency of the original periodic waveform. Hence a true frequency counter.

EXPERIMENT 9-20

AN ULTRASONIC RANGE-FINDER MADE INTELLIGENT: CLASSIC VS. HSI APPROACHES WITH THE 8096.

INTRODUCTION

The accurate measurement of distance by means of a sensor(s) is important in many areas of controls. Examples: monitoring and control of distance to objects in robotics; or of liquid levels in tanks or other vessels in the areas of manufacturing and packaging, in heating and cooling systems, in nuclear generation, and the chemical industry; in "smart" focusing, etc.

The determination of distances is useful and necessary but, of itself, would be of limited value in controls without the added intelligence that a microcomputer can provide. That intelligence is essential if control decisions are to be implemented based on the results of the distance measurement. For example, if distance to an object becomes less than a critical value, the robot is to recoil (human too close), or if greater than that value, robot is to approach till the object (part) is reached. Or, if distance from sensor to fluid level exceeds critical (nuclear generation application) emergency control measures (more fluid, alarms, shut-down, etc.) are to be taken

In this experiment, we have added intelligence to distance sensing by interfacing the 8096 to an ultrasonic ranging system and incorporating the appropriate software. The sensor employed was Polaroid's "Ultrasonic Ranging System (Designer's Kit)". By accessing and inputting the appropriate signals from that range-finder system into the 8096, we shall have the 8096 itself measure and display distance (in addition to it being displayed on the Polaroid system's board). Our program will then allow the 8096 to indicate when distance to object or fluid level exceeds a specified critical value and then implement a simple control function. A problem at the end of the experiment then suggests the implementation of feedback in the form of digital or analog signals output from 8096 back to mechanism(s) which could control the object's distance or the fluid level in response to the received distance data. In that way control of distance to within certain limits, if desired, could be achieved.

The experiment implements the intelligent range-finder with the 8096 in two ways: A) a classic approach in which the EXTINT, HSI.0 (interrupt), and T2CLK inputs to the 8096 are employed, and B) an approach based on the use of the HSI unit of the 8096. The interfacing and part of the program are different for the two cases.

BRIEF DESCRIPTION OF THE POLAROID ULTRASONIC RANGING SYSTEM.

An excellent article on the Polaroid Ultrasonic Ranging System and Designer's Kit giving the theory, board circuitry, and other details regarding that ranging system can be found in the Nov. 1980 issue of Byte Magazine ("An Ultrasonic Ranging System" by Steve Ciarcia). We now describe some of the salient features of that ultrasonic sensor as they pertain to our application.

The kit contains two electrostatic ultrasonic transducers, an ultrasonic transceiver circuit board (patterned after the SX-70 Sonar One-Step Land Camera's automatic focusing system), a demonstrator display board (EDB), and Polapulse 6V batteries. The ranging unit's main components are the electrostatic ultrasonic transducer and the ultrasonic transceiver board. They can detect the presence and distance of objects within a range of about 0.9 feet to 35 feet. When operating, an ultrasonic pulse is transmitted and the echo from the target is detected. The time interval from initiation of transmission to detection of echo can be measured by counting the number N of clock pulses of definite period (178 usec. period clock in the Polaroid ranging unit) emitted and recorded during that time interval. From this time value, the ROUND-TRIP DISTANCE from transmit transducer to target and back can be calculated, since the speed of sound is known (1125 ft./sec. at normal pressure and temperature). Thus, if N clock pulses were counted, each with period 178 usec., the ONE-WAY DISTANCE from source to object would be given by d = 1/2 (1125 x 12"/sec. x N x 0.178 msec.), or:

(1)... $$d = N \times 1.20''$$

where N is the number of 178 usec. period clock pulses recorded in the time between initiation of transmission and reception of echo from target.

It is clear from the above equation that distance to objects can not be resolved with accuracy better than 1.2" i.e. to the nearest 0.1 ft. with a 178 usec. clock. To achieve greater accuracy requires a clock source whose period is less than 178 usec. Free-running timer T1 in the 8096 would be perfect for such an application. Its period is 2 usec. and it is the time base in the HSITIME SFR which, with the HSISTATUS SFR, is the basis of time-event measurement in the HSI unit and its FIFO. Thus if N1 is the word value of HSITIME when transmission is initiated and N2 is its value when the relevant echo is received, then the time interval would be (N2 - N1) x 2 usec. = N' x 2 usec. (where N' = N2 - N1). The one-way distance from source to object would thus be given by d = 1/2 (1125 x 12"/sec. x N' x 2 usec.), or:

(2)... d = N' x 0.0135"

indicating a resolution of about 0.014" or about 0.001 ft. In Eq. (2), N' is the word value INCREMENT in HSITIME between transmission and echo reception i.e. N' = HSITIME(ECHO) - HSITIME (TRANSMIT).

In this experiment we'll employ two approaches: one using the 178 usec. period clock available on the Polaroid range-finder system with Eq. (1) above being relevant, and the other using the 2 usec. T1 clock available with the HSI unit on the 8096, for which Eq. (2) above is relevant. The 90-fold greater accuracy that can be achieved using the HSI unit is apparent. Whereas the EDB board or our classic approach gives distances to only 0.1 ft., the HSI-based method will measure distances to 0.001 ft.

The ultrasonic transducer acts as a "speaker" when transmitting and as a "microphone" when receiving echoes from a target. It measures 1.5" in diameter and has a gold plated foil 0.003" thick stretched over aluminum plate. The metallic backplate and the foil form a capacitor in which the foil is the moving element that converts varying a.c. electrical energy (and, therefore, electrostatic force on the foil) into sound waves of the same frequency for transmission, and then converts the sound energy in the echo from target back to electrical (a.c.) energy. THE ROUND-TRIP TIME IS MEASURED FROM THE TIME AN ELECTRICAL PULSE TRIGGERS THE TRANSMITTED SOUND TO THE TIME THE SOUND ECHO RECEIVED FROM TARGET TRIGGERS A RECEIVED ELECTRICAL PULSE. Round-trip distance is this time multiplied by the speed of sound. Actually, the transmission consists of bursts of four different ultrasonic frequencies (60 KHz, 57 KHz, 53 KHz, and 50 KHz) so as to accommodate possible different reflectivities that might be associated with various parts of an object's surface i.e. to overcome possible frequency absorption selectivity.

The Experimental Demonstration Board (EDB) that comes with the Polaroid Ranging System converts the transmit/receive time interval discussed above into a figure indicating distance in feet. It is presented on a 3-digit LED display (e.g. 14.6 feet), in increments of 0.1 ft. (i.e. 1.2" resolution using their clock).

The next section describes which signals we accessed from the Polaroid Ultrasonic Ranging System for inputting to the 8096 in order to have the latter itself monitor and display distance and in order to program intelligence into the sensor for control purposes. Part (A) below pertains to the "classic" approach with the 8096 and Part (B) below relates to using the 8096's HSI unit.

INTERFACING THE 8096 TO THE ULTRASONIC RANGING SYSTEM TO ACCESS THE NECESSARY SIGNALS.

METHOD (A) INTERFACING: USING EXTINT, HSI.0 INT, AND T2CLK (CLASSICAL).

The beginning of each burst of ultrasonic sound transmission on the Polaroid board is initiated in conjunction with a signal (XLG) going high. That signal is avalable at input pin 3 of the MC14044 R-S flip-flop on the Polaroid EDB board. This signal is needed to establish time t = 0 as the start of time interval measurement from source to target back to source. We tied this signal to the EXTINT pin of the 8096 in this classic approach.

The detection of an echo on the Polaroid board causes the creation of a pulse, FLG, whose leading (0 to 1) edge occurs at the time the echo is detected. This pulse is needed to establish the time t = T of arrival of an echo back, thus allowing determination of the relevant time interval to establish 2-way distance. FLG is available at input pin 11 of another MC14044 R-S flip-flop on the EDB board. We connected this signal to the HSI.0 pin of the 8096 (to be used as a SECOND EXTERNAL INTERRUPT SOURCE IN ADDITION TO EXTINT).

Finally, the 178 usec. period clock source (A7CLK) was accessed at output pin 4 (A7) of the MC14040 12-stage binary ripple counter on the EDB board. WE INPUT THIS CLOCK SIGNAL TO THE T2CLK CLOCK SOURCE OF EVENT COUNTER T2 ON THE 8096. T2 will be used to count the number, N, of 178 usec. wide clock pulses IN THE TIME INTERVAL BETWEEN TRANSMISSION (EXTINT INTERRUPT) AND RECEPTION OF ECHO (HSI.0 INTERRUPT) IN ORDER TO CALCULATE TIME INTERVAL AND DISTANCE (see Eq. (1) above where distance is given in terms of N).

Notice that the chips on the EDB board referred to above are CMOS. We had to do a bit of cleaning of the associated and relevant signals to get good 0 to 5V TTL levels for input to the 8096. This was accomplished by inputting the EDB signals to 74LS14 Schmitt-Trigger Inverters and using their outputs as the inputs to the 8096.

METHOD (B) INTERFACING: USING THE 8096'S HSI UNIT.

In the method employing the HSI unit, the XLG pulse generated on the EDB board upon transmission (see above) is tied to the HSI.0 pin of the 8096 WHERE NOW THE HSI.0 INPUT TO THE HSI UNIT'S FIFO WILL BE ENABLED. Thus, the start of transmission will create a 0 to 1 transition (event) at HSI.0, and the FIFO will record event/time data for this transition in the HSISTATUS and HSITIME registers in said FIFO.

Further, the FLG pulse generated when the echo is received is now tied to the HSI.1 pin of the 8096. IT, TOO, WILL BE ENABLED INTO THE HSI'S FIFO. Reception of echo will, therefore, create a 0 to 1 transition event at HSI.1 and the FIFO will record this transition's event/time data in its HSISTATUS and HSITIME registers.

Subsequent successive readings of HSITIME out of the FIFO will establish the incremented word value N' = HSITIME(ECHO) - HSITIME(TRANSMIT). The distance to target in terms of N' is then given by Eq. (2) above.

Note that the A7 CLK 178 usec. clock from the EDB board is now disconnected from the 8096's T2CLK input - it is not now used as far as the 8096 is concerned. Note, also, that distances determined by the 8096 can be compared with the corresponding distance read-out on the 3-digit display on the Polaroid EDB board which is operative while the 8096 is functioning [this applies for both Methods (A) and (B)].

SOFTWARE APPROACH IN CALCULATING AND DISPLAYING DISTANCE, AND IN ESTABLISHING CONTROL OF TARGET DISTANCE. METHOD (A) VS. METHOD (B).

The main programs in both approaches are almost identical. Their differences lie in establishment of different ISR addresses corresponding to the employment of different interrupt vectors in Methods (A) and (B), and in different initializations of the same or different SFRs. These differences will be brought out later when analyzing the programs associated with the two approaches. At this point we'll analyze the approach taken in that part of the main programs which are identical in the classic and HSI approaches.

In both approaches a switch S (at P0.7), initially set low, is polled. During the time it is low, the target is placed at a distance from the transducer that is to represent "critical distance". A register COUNT counts the number N or N' of clocks [in Method (A) or Method (B)] that transpire between transmission and reception of echo. This count, proportional to distance, is established in one or the other of the interrupt ISRs appropriate to the method employed. Further discussion of this aspect is presented below. In Method (A) the value of N is displayed at P1's LEDs, in Method (B) the high byte of N' is displayed there. The critical distance can then be calculated from Eq. (1) or Eq. (2), as appropriate, and compared with the read-out on the Polaroid EDB board. All this time switch S is maintained low. So far, critical distance has been established in COUNT.

Switch S is then thrown high. In response, the software in both approaches loads the N or N' value in COUNT into register LIMIT (which now holds the limit or critical source-to-target distance). At the same time an "alarm" at P2.7 (or other warning mechanism) is turned off (it will signal target distance greater than critical when, and if, it goes on). Another wait loop is created, as long as S is high. During this time target distance to source may change in keeping with the realities of the application (fluid level descends, etc). The interrupt ISRs in each approach are constantly updating N or N' in COUNT, (as we'll see) and displaying same at P1. Thus any change in actual distance will be reflected at P1 and the new distance can be calculated from Eqs. (1) or (2) and compared with the read-out on the EDB board.

When switch S is thrown low, the software responds with an instruction that compares the value in LIMIT with that in COUNT i.e. critical distance vs. PRESENT ACTUAL distance (in terms of N or N'). As long as COUNT does not exceed LIMIT (present distance less than or equal to critical) the program loops back on the compare instruction. Whenever the actual distance exceeds critical (e.g. water level in tank too low) COUNT becomes larger than LIMIT and a fall-through occurs. Here, in each approach, we turn on the alarm at P2.7. It is precisely here that more realistic and elaborate control can be undertaken by e.g. causing digital or analog signals to be output to the control mechanism(s) at the target (or source), to cause actual distance to recede back to critical or less (e.g. allow more water into the tank, etc). The programs then both jump back to the original loop where a wait is imposed as long as S is low. The WHOLE SITUATION CAN BE REPEATED with establishment of a NEW CRITICAL DISTANCE, just as before, so long as S is low.

As stated, the above main program features are identical in the two approaches--only the initializations and ISR addresses and interrupt sources differ.

The only software question remaining is how each approach records N or N' in COUNT in the relevant interrupt routines. In Method (A), where EXTINT, HSI.0 INT, and T2CLK are employed, the software approach consists of 1) the EXTINT ISR, whenever entered, resetting T2CLK to 0, and 2) the HSI.0 INT ISR, whenever entered (i.e. on reception of each echo) reading the number of transitions counts in T2 (from range-finder's A7CLK) and converting same to number of clock pulses, N, that transpired between initiation of transmission and reception of echo. That number, N, is then loaded into COUNT and displayed at P1's LEDs. In that way, constant updating of COUNT (distance to target) on an interrupt basis is realized.

In Method (B), where HSI.0 and HSI.1 inputs to the HSI's FIFO are employed, the software approach consists of 1) having a "FIFO BECOMES FULL" interrupt generated whenever the FIFO becomes full with HSI.0 (start of transmission) and HSI.1 (reception of echo) events (transitions), 2) reading the times of the first two HSITIME entries, 3) subtracting those values to establish the distance (or time) value N' in COUNT, 4) outputting hi-byte of N' to P1, and 5) clearing out the FIFO so a new update of transmission/echo transitions can be entered. Again COUNT is updated on a constant interrupt (here FIFO BECOMES FULL) basis. Of course, the FULL word, N', can be read from the COUNT register (which we'll do) for COMPLETE ACCURACY.

PROGRAM. METHOD (A): CLASSIC WAY

The program at 2E00 to display distance in terms of N and to implement control action is shown below. This program is the software implementation of the classic approach--Method (A).

```
      18 00       SP      EQU    18H         60 00       LIMIT  EQU   60H
      08 00       MINT    EQU    08H         0C 00       T2     EQU   0CH
      09 00       PINT    EQU    09H         16 00       IOC1   EQU   16H
      0E 20       INVEC0  EQU    200EH       15 00       IOC0   EQU   15H
      08 20       INVEC1  EQU    2008H       0E 00       P0     EQU   0EH
      40 00       TEMP    EQU    40H         0F 00       P1     EQU   0FH
      50 00       COUNT   EQU    50H         10 00       P2     EQU   10H
      50 00       COUNT0  EQU    50H
2E00                      ORG    2E00H
                  ;
2E00  A1 C0 00 18 START:  LD     SP,#0C0H        ;Initialize SP.
2E04  B1 00 0F            LDB    P1,#00H         ;Initialize LEDs at P1.
2E07  71 7F 10            ANDB   P2,#7FH         ;Clear error LED at P2.7.
2E0A  FA                  DI                     ;Disable interrupts.
2E0B  B1 90 08            LDB    MINT,#90H       ;Enable EXTINT and HSI.0 interrupts.
2E0E  B1 00 16            LDB    IOC1,#00H       ;Clear IOC1.1 to select EXTINT.
```

```
2E11   B1 02 15                    LDB    IOCO,#02H         ;Clear IOCO.7 to select T2CLK
                                                            ;and set IOCO.1 to reset T2.
2E14   A1 4D 2E 40                 LD     TEMP,#EXINT       ;Load address of EXTINT intr.
2E18   C3 01 0E 20 40              ST     TEMP,INVECO[0]    ;ISR into INT VECT table.
2E1D   A1 3F 2E 40                 LD     TEMP,#HSIOINT     ;Load address of HSI.0 intr.
2E21   C3 01 08 20 40              ST     TEMP,INVEC1[0]    ;ISR into INT VECT table.
2E26   11 09                       CLRB   PINT              ;Clear any pending interrupts.
2E28   FB                          EI                       ;Enable interrupts.
2E29   37 0E FD          HERE1:    JBC    P0,7,HERE1        ;If P0.7 = 0, jump to HERE1.
                                                            ;Set critical distance.
2E2C   A0 50 60                    LD     LIMIT,COUNT       ;Else load critical distance into
                                                            ;LIMIT.
2E2F   71 7F 10                    ANDB   P2,#7FH           ;Clear error LED at P2.7.
2E32   3F 0E FD          HERE2:    JBS    P0,7,HERE2        ;If P0.7 = 1, jump to HERE2.
                                                            ;Change distance.
2E35   88 60 50          TEST:     CMP    COUNT,LIMIT       ;Else compare COUNT (present distance)
                                                            ;to LIMIT.
2E38   D1 FB                       JNH    TEST              ;If COUNT <= LIMIT, jump to TEST.
2E3A   91 80 10          ERROR:    ORB    P2,#80H           ;Else turn on error LED. Critical
                                                            ;distance reached.
2E3D   27 EA                       SJMP   HERE1             ;Jump to HERE1 to record new
                                                            ;LIMIT.

                         ;         HSI.0 ISR
                         ;
2E3F   F2                HSIOINT:PUSHF                      ;Save flags and disable interrupts.
2E40   A0 0C 50                    LD     COUNT,T2          ;Load value of T2 into COUNT.
2E43   07 50                       INC    COUNT             ;Increment to adjust COUNT.
2E45   08 01 50                    SHR    COUNT,#01H        ;Divide COUNT by to provide
                                                            ;number of pulses.
2E48   B0 50 0F                    LDB    P1,COUNTO         ;Output low byte of COUNT(N) to LEDs.
2E4B   F3                          POPF                     ;Restore flags.
2E4C   F0                          RET                      ;Return.
                         ;
                         ;         EXTINT ISR
                         ;
2E4D   F2                EXINT:    PUSHF                    ;Save flags.
2E4E   B1 02 15                    LDB    IOCO,#02H         ;Reset T2 for next cycle.
2E51   F3                          POPF                     ;Restore flags.
2E52   F0                          RET                      ;Return.
```

The initializations between addresses 2E00 and 2E28 need very little explanation. P2.7 is reset to 0 (alarm). At 2E29 the status of switch S is tested. As long as it is low, the program waits in a loop. It is during this time that the critical distance to the object is set and calibrated. Fall-through 2E29 occurs when S is thrown high. The critical N value in COUNT (recorded in the HSI.0 ISR) is loaded into register LIMIT and the alarm at P2.7 is reset (in case it was turned on in response to a previous violation of the critical distance limit). The JBS instruction at 2E32 results in another wait loop. Here distance may be changing. When S is thrown low again, fall-through the JBS instruction occurs and the present N value in COUNT (actual object distance by now has changed) is compared to the critical N value established in LIMIT. If COUNT is less than or equal to LIMIT, the JNH instruction at 2E38 jumps back to TEST for another comparison. This continues until such time as the actual distance (in terms of N) becomes greater than the critical value established during the calibration procedure. Fall-through the JNH instruction at 2E38 then occurs and the alarm P2.7 is turned on at ERROR (2E3A). (See Problem for more realistic control suggestions to be implemented at 2E3A). The SJMP HERE1 instruction then jumps back to 2E29 where the program again waits, as S is still low. A new critical value of distance to object is set (if desired) and the switch S is again thrown high. It is then thrown low and the whole series of events described above repeats.

The critical and actual values of N in COUNT are established in the HSI.0 ISR after the EXTINT ISR resets the count in T2 to 0. Thus, initiation of ultrasonic transmission causes a vector to EXINT at 2E4D where T2 is reset to 0 and a return to main program is executed. The next interrupt is associated with reception of the echo from the target and causes vectoring to HSI0INT at 2E3F. There, the number of 0 to 1 and 1 to 0 transitions recorded in T2 from the range-finder's 178 usec. period clock, which is input to T2CLK, is loaded into COUNT. The latter is then adjusted to convert that number to the number of clock pulses, N, received during the transmit to echo time interval. The number N is then displayed at P1's LEDs. Distance d = N x 1.2" is now known.

PROCEDURE. METHOD (A): CLASSIC WAY

1. Follow the interfacing procedure described in the section on Interfacing the 8096 to the Range-Finder [Method (A)].
2. Reset and enter BY 09 = 00. Keep switch S at P0.7 low.
3. Execute the program from 2E00. Observe that the error LED at P2.7 is off.
4. Set the object at some critical distance from the range-finder's transducer. Read N at P1's LEDs. We found P1 = 14H = 20 dec. corresponding to d (critical) = 20 x 1.2" = 2.0 ft. This agreed with the 3-digit reading on the Polaroid EDB board.
5. Throw S at P0.7 high and bring the object closer to the transducer. Throw S back low. We observed P1's reading change to 12H = 18 dec. giving d = 18 x 1.2" = 1.8 ft.,

again in agreement with the range-finder's reading on its EDB board. P1 continues to decrease as the object is brought closer to the transducer.

6. Slowly cause the object to recede. Observe N's value at P1 increase. P2.7's LED went on ("error") when P1 reached 15H = 21 dec. or for d = 21 x 1.2" = 2.1 ft. (same reading as on EDB board). 2.1 ft. is larger than d (critical) = 2.0 ft.
7. Set the object at some new, smaller critical distance and read N at P1. This time we read P1 = 12H = 18 dec. or d (critical) = 1.8 ft. Throw S high. P2.7 goes off. Decrease the object's distance from the transducer. Throw S low. Observe P1's display decrease in value to, in our case, N = 10H = 16 dec., or d = 16 x 1.2" = 1.6 ft. (also read on the EDB board). Move the object still closer to source. P1 decreases further.
8. Now increase the object's distance from the transducer. P2.7 went on when P1 reached a value 13H = 19 dec. or d = 19 x 1.2" = 1.9 ft. which is larger than d (critical) = 1.8 ft.

PROBLEM

1. At 2E3A (ERROR), call a routine that not only puts on the alarm at P2.7 but also outputs the correct digital or analog signals to a mechanism that can control forward or backward motion of the object, or that can control height of water (or other fluid) level. The former case might simply involve reversing current flow in the motor that drives the object forward or back a definite amount. The latter case could involve controlling valves or solenoids that allow more liquid to flow into the tank to cause liquid height to always be a definite amount greater than critical (or transducer distance to liquid surface to be less than critical).

PROGRAM. METHOD (B): HSI WAY

The program at 2E70 below gives the APPROXIMATE distance in terms of the HIGH BYTE of N' at P1 and the EXACT DISTANCE by reading the FULL WORD VALUE of N' in register COUNT (WO 50) at any time. This program is the implementation of Method (B): the HSI approach. As Eqs. (1) and (2) show, our classic approach, based on using the EDB's 178 usec. clock as the source of T2CLK transitions, will lead to measured distances good to every 0.1 ft. (same as the EDB's distance read-out accuracy), while our HSI-based approach will give measured distances valid to 0.001 ft. - a considerable improvement in accuracy of almost 100-fold (178 usec. clock vs. 2 usec. clock on the HSI). Remember, we are now connecting XLG to HSI.0 and FLG to HSI.1 inputs to the HSI's FIFO in order to measure their time difference.

```
18 00          SP       EQU   18H            51 00          COUNTHI EQU   51H
08 00          MINT     EQU   08H            60 00          LIMIT   EQU   60H
09 00          PINT     EQU   09H            70 00          REG1    EQU   70H
04 20          INVEC    EQU   2004H          80 00          REG2    EQU   80H
06 00          HSISTAT  EQU   06H            16 00          IOS1    EQU   16H
04 00          HSITIME  EQU   04H            16 00          IOC1    EQU   16H
03 00          HSIMODE  EQU   03H            15 00          IOCO    EQU   15H
30 00          REG      EQU   30H            0E 00          P0      EQU   0EH
40 00          TEMP     EQU   40H            0F 00          P1      EQU   0FH
50 00          COUNT    EQU   50H            10 00          P2      EQU   10H
2E70                            ORG     2E70H
                       ;
2E70   A1 C0 00 18     START:   LD      SP,#0C0H          ;Initialize SP.
2E74   71 7F 10                 ANDB    P2,#7FH           ;Clear error LED at P2.7.
2E77   FA                       DI                        ;Disable interrupts.
2E78   B1 04 08                 LDB     MINT,#04H         ;Unmask HSI interrupt source.
2E7B   B1 05 03                 LDB     HSIMODE,#05H      ;Set HSI mode for 0 to 1 transitions
                                                          ;on HSI.0 and HSI.1 pins.
2E7E   B1 05 15                 LDB     IOC0,#05H         ;Enable HSI.0 and HSI.1 transitions
                                                          ;into HSI FIFO.
2E81   B1 80 16                 LDB     IOC1,#80H         ;Specify HSI interrupt when FIFO
                                                          ;becomes full.
2E84   A1 A6 2E 40              LD      TEMP,#HSIINT      ;Load address of HSIINT
2E88   C3 01 04 20 40           ST      TEMP,INVEC[0]     ;ISR into INT VECT table.
2E8D   11 09                    CLRB    PINT              ;Clear any pending interrupts.
2E8F   FB                       EI                        ;Enable interrupts.
2E90   37 0E FD        HERE1:   JBC     P0,7,HERE1        ;If P0.7 = 0, jump to HERE1. Set
                                                          ;critical distance.
2E93   A0 50 60                 LD      LIMIT,COUNT       ;Else load critical distance into
                                                          ;LIMIT.
2E96   71 7F 10                 ANDB    P2,#7FH           ;Clear error LED at P2.7.
2E99   3F 0E FD        HERE2:   JBS     P0,7,HERE2        ;If P0.7 = 1, jump to HERE2. Change
                                                          ;distance.
2E9C   88 60 50        TEST:    CMP     COUNT,LIMIT       ;Else compare COUNT (present distance)
                                                          ;to LIMIT.
2E9F   D1 FB                    JNH     TEST              ;If COUNT <= LIMIT, jump to TEST.
2EA1   91 80 10        ERROR:   ORB     P2,#80H           ;Else turn on error LED. Critical
                                                          ;distance reached.
2EA4   27 EA                    SJMP    HERE1             ;Jump to HERE1 to record new
                                                          ;LIMIT.
                       ;
                       ;        HSI FIFO FULL ISR
                       ;
2EA6   F2              HSIINT:  PUSHF                     ;Save flags and disable interrupts.
2EA7   B1 00 15                 LDB     IOC0,#00H         ;Disable HSI.0 and HSI.1 into FIFO.
2EAA   38 06 05                 JBS     HSISTAT,0,HSI0    ;If transmission transition ocurred
                                                          ;on HSI.0, jump to HSI0.
2EAD   C0 30 04                 ST      HSITIME,REG       ;Else read time of echo into dummy
                                                          ;register REG. Discard.
```

```
2EB0   FD                   NOP                       ;8 state times needed between reads.
2EB1   FD                   NOP                       ;
2EB2   C0 70 04    HSI0:    ST     HSITIME,REG1       ;Read time of occurrence of
                                                      ;transmission.
2EB5   FD                   NOP                       ;8 state times needed between reads.
2EB6   FD                   NOP                       ;
2EB7   C0 80 04    HSI1:    ST     HSITIME,REG2       ;Read time of occurrence of echo.
2EBA   48 70 80 50          SUB    COUNT,REG2,REG1    ;Subtract REG1 from REG2 and store
                                                      ;difference(N') in COUNT.
2EBE   B0 51 0F             LDB    P1,COUNTHI         ;Display high byte of COUNT at P1's
                                                      ;LEDs.
2EC1   C0 30 04    EMPFIFO:ST      HSITIME,REG        ;Read next FIFO time entry into
                                                      ;dummy register.
2EC4   3F 16 FA             JBS    IOS1,7,EMPFIFO     ;Poll IOS1.7 and loop on EMPFIFO if
                                                      ;high.
2EC7   B1 05 15             LDB    IOC0,#05H          ;Else re-enable HSI.0 and HSI.1
                                                      ;transitions into FIFO. FIFO is
                                                      ;empty.
2ECA   11 09                CLRB   PINT               ;Clear pending interrupts.
2ECC   F3                   POPF                      ;Restore flags.
2ECD   F0                   RET                       ;Return.
```

The main program for Method (B) above is, with slight differences, the same as for Method (A). The differences lie in the new initializations. Since the HSI unit will be employed in this method we need to: 1) unmask the HSI interrupt source by setting MINT to 04, 2) set HSIMODE to 05 to have the FIFO record only 0 to 1 transitions at HSI.0 and HSI.1, 3) set IOC0 to 05 to enable the HSI.0, HSI.1 input lines to the HSI, 4) set IOC1 to 80 to have an HSI interrupt generated when the FIFO BECOMES FULL, 5) set up the address of the HSIINT ISR (2EA6) in the Interrupt Vector Table. All this is done as the program indicates. After that the main program is the same as for Method (A).

The HSI FIFO FULL ISR at 2EA6 is now analyzed. We have programmed for an HSI interrupt when the FIFO becomes full with alternate HSI.0 (transmit: XLG) and HSI.1 (echo: FLG) 0 to 1 transitions (event/times). When this occurs, the main program is vectored to 2EA6. There we want to ascertain the number (N') of T1 counts between the first (transmission) FIFO entry and the next (echo) entry. Flags and mask are pushed and the HSI.0, .1 lines are disabled from the FIFO. Bit 0 of HSISTAT is tested with the JBS instruction at 2EAA. If it is set, an event (transition) occurred on the HSI.0 line (transmission started) and a jump to HSI0 is taken (where a reading of the time of transmission into REG1 will be executed). If it is not set, the event must have been on the HSI.1 line (echo received) and fall-through the JBS instruction occurs. The ST HSITIME, REG instruction at 2EAD simply DISCARDS the time reading of this first echo in the FIFO (we want to START by reading the first transmission time). REG is a "dummy register". 8 state times (2 NOPs) are needed before the next event/time drops from FIFO to Holding Register for accessing availabilty. At HSI0 (2EB2) the time of the first transmission recorded in the FIFO (HSITIME) is read into REG1. Again 2 NOPs provide the required 8 state times before the next entry in the FIFO can be accessed. At HSI1, HSITIME of the next entry is read into REG2 to provide the time of occurrence of the first echo after the last transmission occurred. The 3-operand SUB instruction stores the value N' = REG2 - REG1 in COUNT, where N' = number of T1 clocks between transmit and echo. The high byte of N' is then output at P1 to get "an idea" of the size of N' (its exact value can be read from WO 50, where 50 is COUNT's address, and this we'll do). We must now empty the FIFO of the rest of its transmit/echo recordings before we can fill it up again for the next COUNT = N' determination. This we do in the EMPFIFO loop where the other FIFO entries are read into the dummy register REG and IOS1.7 is polled until it reveals 0 (indicating HSI Holding Register has no more data available, i.e. FIFO has been emptied). Fall-through 2EC4 then occurs and the HSI.0,.1 inputs to the FIFO are re-enabled so that future transmit/echo transitions can be recorded. Pending interrupts are cleared, flags and interrupt mask are restored and the program returns to the main program with the distance from transducer to target stored (as N') in register COUNT (and hi-byte of N' showing at P1). Remember, d = N' x 0.0135" = (about) N' x .0011 feet. Distance is thus known with 0.001 accuracy.

PROCEDURE. METHOD (B): HSI WAY

1. Connect XLG on the EDB board to HSI.0 and FLG to HSI.1.
2. Reset and enter BY 09 = 00. Keep switch S at P0.7 low.
3. Execute the program from 2E70. Note error LED at P2.7 is off.
4. Set the object at some critical distance from the transducer. Read N' at P1 and in register 50. We observed P1 = 04 and WO 50 = 04A6 = 1190 (dec). This corresponds to a critical d = 1190 x 0.0011 ft. = 1.309 ft. The EDB readout was 1.3 ft. (note the resolutions).
5. Throw S high and bring the target closer to the transducer. We now observed P1 = 03, WO 50 = 03CF = 975 (dec) giving d = 975 x 0.0011 ft. = 1.073 ft. vs. the EDB read-out of 1.1 ft.
6. Throw S low. Slowly move the target away from the transducer. Observe P1 increase. The LED at P2.7 went on when P1 = 04 was reached. WO 50 read 04CE = 1230 (dec), giving d = 1230 x 0.0011 ft. = 1.353 ft. vs. EDB's reading of

1.4'. Thus alarm goes on when critical d of 1.309 ft. (in (4) above) is exceeded.

7. Set a new critical distance. We did for P1 = 06, WO 50 = 060F = 1551 (dec), giving d (critical) = 1.706 ft. vs. EDB's 1.7 ft.
8. Throw S high and bring target closer to the transducer. We now observe P1 = 04 and WO 50 = 04B7 = 1207 (dec), giving d = 1.328 ft. vs. EDB's 1.3 ft.
9. Throw S low. Move the target away from the transducer. The LED at P2.7 went on when P1 = 06 and WO 50 = 0615 = 1557 (dec) were reached. This corresponds to d = 1557 x 0.0011 ft. = 1.713 ft. vs. EDB's 1.7 ft. read-out. Critical distance (1.706 ft.) was exceeded.

CONCLUSION

The accuracy that is inherent with the use of the HSI unit in measuring time intervals is clearly demonstrated in this experiment. In the classic approach using the EDB's 178 usec. clock, distances could be measured with no better accuracy than 0.1 ft. With the HSI unit they were measured to accuracies of 0.001 ft.

PROBLEMS

1. See Problem suggested just after the Procedure section in Method (A).
2. We observed a delayed reaction of almost a second before P1's display gave the new N' (hi-byte) reading corresponding to a changed target position. This is so because the time between successive transmission bursts on the EDB is specified as 1000 x 177 usec. = 177 msec. Four such bursts will fill up the FIFO (i.e. 4 transmits, 4 echoes). That will take about 0.7 sec. Only then will the FIFO interrupt be generated to the ISR to calculate the NEW COUNT and output its hi-byte to P1. How can you remedy this? How about specifying an HSI interrupt EACH TIME THE HSI HOLDING REGISTER BECOMES LOADED WITH TRANSITION DATA? Try it, modifying the ISR accordingly.
3. Write a routine that will take the HEX N' value in COUNT and convert it to feet according to the formula d = (N') (dec.) x 0.0011 ft. Have the value displayed to 3 decimal places. Employ the relevant arithmetic. The 8096 instruction set is well suited for this but you'll need a routine to convert N' (HEX) to N' (dec).

EXPERIMENT 9-21

DIGITAL TO ANALOG OUTPUT SMOOTHING IN SIGNAL PROCESSING (INTERPOLATION).

INTRODUCTION, APPROACH, AND PROGRAM.

In signal processing, sampling of an analog input signal is performed and each sample is converted to digital form by an A/D converter for the microcomputer to process. The processing will usually involve arithmetic, logical, and data operations of one sort or another. After each sample is thus processed it is output back in new analog form by means of a D/A converter. This was illustrated in Expt. 9-17 with the digital filter. If the sampling rate is low relative to the period of the input signal, the output signal will show a finite step-wise progression from sampled point to sampled point rather than the smooth processed signal between points that should be our goal. In fact this was observed in Expt. 9-17 on the digital filter (see p. 591).

Now it is generally not possible to simply keep increasing the sampling rate to achieve greater accuracy and smoother waveforms (more but smaller steps). One can not go on to sample another point on the input waveform till the previous one has been converted and then processed. Thus A/D conversion time and instruction execution time in the processing portion of the software set the basic limitation on the number of input points that can be sampled in one period. That being the case, we are forced to rely on an interpolation between sampled points at the input to the D/A converter where the processed signal appears. The larger the number of interpolation points used, the greater the output accuracy and smoothness i.e. a greater number of steps approximates a truer waveform. However, the time AVAILABLE for interpolation, Nti, (N = number of interpolation points, ti = time between interpolation points) can be no greater than the sampling time, T, between sampled points LESS the SUM of the time it takes for A/D conversion AND the signal processing time.

In this experiment we shall sample an input sine wave (audio), convert the analog points to digital at channel ACH0, and then employ a linear interpolation scheme between sample points at the OUTPUT P1 (INPUT to the D/A converter: AD 558, see figure, p. 585) to achieve greater accuracy and smoothness. To keep things simple, our signal processing will consist merely of the storage of the sampled input-converted byte plus a short time delay i.e. a "dummy" processing. The main goal will be to show how our interpolation method leads to a SMOOTHER OUTPUT

WAVEFORM relative to the output waveform that would be observed WITHOUT interpolation for the SAME "signal processing" in both cases. Polling of switch S at P0.7 will allow this optional output selection (for demonstration purposes only).

The program has EXACTLY the same structure as the digital filter program (Expt. 9-17) with the difference that the "A/D Conversion Complete" ISR, in addition to reading the sampled input byte, rounding it, and "filtering" it (replaced by a simple "dummy processing" here), also does a linear interpolation based on a programmably specified number of interpolation steps between successive sample points. The interpolation takes place in the time available between sampled points S1 and S2 AFTER A/D conversion and processing are "out of the way".

The program starts at 3000H and is shown below. In the analysis that appears afterward, we shall not dwell on the main program at START, or the routine at HSOTAG, or the SOFTINT ISR at SOFTINT, as these are IDENTICAL to the SAME routines in the digital filter program already discussed and analyzed in Expt. 9-17 (except for the introduction of FLAG in the main program). We shall, however, analyze the "A/D Conversion Complete" ISR in some detail, as the interpolation algorithm between output sample points appears in that routine (the processing routine, as pointed out, is a simple "dummy" routine at "PROC" and is not the filter fractional multiply routine used in Expt. 9-17 at "FILTER" there. This was done for simplicity). The sampling rate is the same as in Expt. 9-17: 126 usec. i.e. Software Timer 0 (ST0) sampling interrupts are specified for every 126 usec. from the HSO unit (see HSOTAG routine below).

```
18 00        SP       EQU   18H         43 00        S2       EQU   43H
08 00        MINT     EQU   08H         50 00        FLAG     EQU   50H
09 00        PINT     EQU   09H         60 00        DIFF     EQU   60H
02 20        INVEC0   EQU   2002H       61 00        DIFFHI   EQU   61H
0A 20        INVEC1   EQU   200AH       70 00        DELTA    EQU   70H
06 00        HSOCOM   EQU   06H         80 00        TEMP     EQU   80H
04 00        HSOTIME  EQU   04H         90 00        COUNT    EQU   90H
02 00        ADCOM    EQU   02H         A0 00        DELAY    EQU   0A0H
02 00        ADRESLO  EQU   02H         B0 00        NSTEPS   EQU   0B0H
03 00        ADRESHI  EQU   03H         0A 00        T1       EQU   0AH
40 00        INPUT    EQU   40H         0E 00        P0       EQU   0EH
41 00        FOUT     EQU   41H         0F 00        P1       EQU   0FH
42 00        S1       EQU   42H

3000                        ORG   3000H

                  ;
3000  A1 C0 00 18  START:   LD    SP,#0C0H      ;Initialize SP.
3004  B1 00 0F              LDB   P1,#00H       ;Initialize D/A Converter.
3007  B1 00 50              LDB   FLAG,#00H     ;Initialize FLAG.7 = 0.
```

```
300A  FA                         DI                      ;Disable interrupts.
300B  B1 22 08                   LDB    MINT,#22H        ;Enable HSO Software Timer intr.
                                                         ;and A/D Completion interrupt.
300E  11 09                      CLRB   PINT             ;Clear any pending interrupts.
3010  A1 31 30 80                LD     TEMP,#ADCPLT     ;Load address of A/D complete
3014  C3 01 02 20 80             ST     TEMP,INVECO[0]   ;ISR into INT VECT table.
3019  A1 AC 30 80                LD     TEMP,#SOFTINT    ;Load address of SOFTINT ISR
301D  C3 01 0A 20 80             ST     TEMP,INVEC1[0]   ;into INT VECT table.
3022  EF 03 00                   CALL   HSOTAG           ;Call HSO command routine.
3025  FB                         EI                      ;Enable interrupts.
3026  27 FE             HERE:    SJMP   HERE             ;Loop HERE. ("BUSY").
                        ;
                        ;
3028  B1 38 06          HSOTAG:  LDB    HSOCOM,#38H      ;Load HSO command tag for
                                                         ;software timer to generate

                                                         ;an interrupt.
302B  45 40 00 0A 04             ADD    HSOTIME,T1,#0040H ;Program time of HSO command to
                                                         ;be 126 microseconds from "now"
3030  F0                         RET                     ;Return.
                        ;
                        ;        A/D CONVERSION COMPLETE ISR
                        ;
3031  F2                ADCPLT:  PUSHF                   ;Save flags and mask.
3032  3B 02 FD          ADBUSY:  JBS    ADRESLO,3,ADBUSY;If A/D not complete loop.
3035  B0 03 40                   LDB    INPUT,ADRESHI    ;Load high byte (BITS 9-2)
                                                         ;of A/D result into INPUT.
3038  37 02 07                   JBC    ADRESLO,7,NO_RND;If AD_LO.7 = 0, jump to NO_RND.
303B  99 FF 40                   CMPB   INPUT,#0FFH      ;Else compare INPUT with 0FFH.
303E  DF 02                      JE     NO_RND           ;If INPUT = 0FFH, jump to NO_RND.
3040  17 40                      INCB   INPUT            ;Else add 1 to input (round-up).
3042  EF 1E 00          NO_RND:  CALL   PROC             ;Call signal processing routine.
3045  3F 50 08                   JBS    FLAG,7,NOFIRST   ;If FLAG.7 = 1, jump to NOFIRST.
3048  B0 41 42                   LDB    S1,FOUT          ;Else this is first, load processed
                                                         ;sample into S1.
304B  B1 80 50                   LDB    FLAG,#80H        ;Load FLAG with 80H to set FLAG.7.
304E  20 11                      SJMP   END              ;Jump to END.
3050  B0 41 43          NOFIRST:LDB     S2,FOUT          ;Load present proc. sample into S2.
3053  3F 0E 05                   JBS    P0,7,SMOOTH      ;If P0.7 = 1, jump to SMOOTH.
3056  B0 43 0F                   LDB    P1,S2            ;Else just load proc. sample to D/A.
3059  20 03                      SJMP   SAVE             ;Jump to SAVE.
305B  EF 0F 00          SMOOTH:  CALL   INTPL            ;Call interpolation routine INTPL.
305E  B0 43 42          SAVE:    LDB    S1,S2            ;Load S2 into S1 for next iteration.
3061  F3                END:     POPF                    ;Restore flags.
3062  F0                         RET                     ;Return.
```

```
                        ;       SIGNAL PROCESSING (DUMMY)
                        ;
3063    B0 40 41        PROC:   LDB     FOUT,INPUT      ;Copy INPUT into FOUT.
3066    B1 05 A0                LDB     DELAY,#05       ;Load DELAY register.
3069    E0 A0 FD        WAIT:   DJNZ    DELAY,WAIT      ;Time delay loop.
306C    F0                      RET                     ;Return.
                        ;       INTPL - INTERPOLATION ROUTINE
                        ;
306D    B0 B0 90        INTPL:  LDB     COUNT,NSTEPS    ;Initialize step counter.
3070    98 43 42                CMPB    S1,S2           ;Compare present and past samples.
3073    D9 04                   JH      CASEA           ;If S1 > S2, jump to CASEA.
3075    DF 2E                   JE      CASEC           ;Else if S1 = S2, jump to CASEC.
3077    D1 16                   JNH     CASEB           ;Else if S1 < S2, jump to CASEB.
                        ;
3079    58 43 42 60     CASEA:  SUBB    DIFF,S1,S2      ;Find difference of S1 and S2.
307D    11 61                   CLRB    DIFFHI          ;Zero out upper byte of DIFF.
307F    9C B0 60                DIVUB   DIFF,NSTEPS     ;Divide difference by number of
3082    B0 60 70                LDB     DELTA,DIFF      ;steps to form DELTA.
3085    B0 42 0F                LDB     P1,S1           ;Load S1 to D/A.
3088    78 70 0F        LOOPA:  SUBB    P1,DELTA        ;Subtract DELTA from output and
                                                        ;load result to output.
308B    E0 90 FA                DJNZ    COUNT,LOOPA     ;Decrement COUNT, if != 0 jump to
                                                        ;LOOPA.
308E    F0                      RET                     ;Return.

308F    58 42 43 60     CASEB:  SUBB    DIFF,S2,S1      ;Find difference of S2 and S1.
3093    11 61                   CLRB    DIFFHI          ;Zero out upper byte of DIFF.
3095    9C B0 60                DIVUB   DIFF,NSTEPS     ;Divide difference by number of
3098    B0 60 70                LDB     DELTA,DIFF      ;steps to form DELTA.
309B    B0 42 0F                LDB     P1,S1           ;Load S1 to D/A.
309E    74 70 0F        LOOPB:  ADDB    P1,DELTA        ;Add DELTA to output and
                                                        ;load result to output.
30A1    E0 90 FA                DJNZ    COUNT,LOOPB     ;Decrement COUNT, if != 0 jump to
                                                        ;LOOPB.
30A4    F0                      RET                     ;Return.
                        ;
30A5    B0 42 0F        CASEC:  LDB     P1,S1           ;Load S1 to D/A.
30A8    E0 90 FA                DJNZ    COUNT,CASEC     ;Decrement COUNT, if != 0 jump to
                                                        ;CASEC.
30AB    F0                      RET                     ;Return.
                        ;
                        ;       SOFTINT ISR
                        ;
30AC    F2              SOFTINT:PUSHF                   ;Save flags and mask.
30AD    B1 08 02                LDB     ADCOM,#08H      ;Start A/D Conversion on channel 0
                                                        ;now.
30B0    2F 76                   CALL    HSOTAG          ;Call HSOTAG to reload the HSO
                                                        ;command.
30B2    F3                      POPF                    ;Restore flags.
30B3    F0                      RET                     ;Return.
```

In the main program FLAG is loaded with 00 to initialize FLAG.7 to 0. It will serve as a semaphore TO DISTINGUISH BETWEEN THE VERY FIRST SAMPLE AND ALL LATER ONES. Other than that, the main program at START and the routines at HSOTAG and SOFTINT are IDENTICAL to their counterparts in Expt. 9-17.

The A/D ISR at 3031 takes in the converted input byte (bits 9-2) from ADRESHI and loads it into INPUT. After deciding on whether rounding is necessary (as in Expt. 9-17's A/D ISR), the program flows to 3042 where the signal processing routine on the sampled input is performed after a call to "PROC" at 3063 in the A/D ISR is made. The "processing" there consists only of a loading of the sampled signal INPUT into register FOUT followed by a short time delay (about 10 usec). The program then returns to 3045 in the A/D ISR. There a test is made as to whether this was the FIRST sampled point or not. The JBS instruction with respect to FLAG.7 jumps to NOFIRST if it was not the first sampled point (FLAG.7 = 1) or falls through to 3048 if it was (FLAG.7 = 0). In the latter case, the first processed sample, FOUT, is loaded into register S1 (S1 will always hold the PRESENT processed sample that LATER becomes the PREVIOUS processed sample), and FLAG is set to 80 to indicate that future samples are NO LONGER the "first". The SJMP END instruction at 304E jumps to END at 3061 and then returns to where the A/D Conversion Complete interrupt was made.

If FLAG.7 was 1, we are dealing with a future sample and the jump to NOFIRST at 3050 causes a load of the processed sample from FOUT to S2 (S2 will always hold the PRESENT processed sample byte). The JBS instruction at 3053 then tests whether the switch S at P0.7 is low or high. If LOW, fall-through to 3056 occurs. There the present processed sample is output DIRECTLY to the DAC at P1 WITHOUT INTERPOLATION and the subsequent jump to SAVE also loads that present processed sample in S2 into S1 to become the PREVIOUS processed sample for the NEXT INTERATION. The program then returns to the main program at HERE ("busy" tasks) to await the next sampling interrupt from ST0 126 usec. later. THE OUTPUT SIGNAL FROM THE DAC WILL THUS CONTAIN THE NON-INTERPOLATED (NON-SMOOTHED), BUT PROCESSED, WAVEFORM AS LONG AS SWITCH S AT P0.7 IS LOW.

If, however, S is HIGH, the JBS instruction at 3053 jumps to SMOOTH at 305B where a call to the interpolation smoothing routine at 306D (INTPL) is made. That is the heart of the program. The number of interpolation steps desired, N, is loaded into register COUNT from register NSTEPS (the latter is specified by entering the number N into BY 0B0 at run-time). The CMPB instruction then compares S1 with S2 (PREVIOUS processed sample with PRESENT one). If S1 is HIGHER than S2, the slope is DOWN and an

S1-S2 subtract must be made in the interpolation routine. If S1 is LESS than S2 the slope is UP and an S2-S1 subtract must be made. If S1 and S2 are EQUAL no subtracts of any kind need be made (slope is 0).

If S1 is greater than S2 the JH instruction at 3073 jumps to CASEA at 3079 where the interpolation algorithm commences. S1-S2 is stored in DIFF (byte) and DIFFHI is then cleared to prepare DIFF as a word. DIVUB then divides the word DIFF by the number of steps in NSTEPS (byte). Quotient gets stored in low byte of DIFF and remainder goes to DIFF's high byte. THIS LEADS TO THE REQUIRED DECREMENT NEEDED FOR EACH STEP IN THE WAVEFORM TO GET TO S2 FROM THE PREVIOUS SAMPLE VALUE S1. The LDB instruction at 3082 loads the quotient result in DIFF (low byte) into register DELTA. DELTA is now our needed DECREMENT value. The PREVIOUS processed sample, S1 is then output to P1 (DAC) and DELTA is SUBTRACTED from P1 to give the NEXT interpolated value at P1 (DAC). The DJNZ instruction at 308B loops back to LOOPA at 3088 to keep subtracting DELTA from P1, thus outputting all the SUCCESSIVE interpolated points required to go from S1 to S2. This stops when COUNT, originally containing the desired number, N, of interpolation steps, reaches 0. Then the return at 308E takes us back to SAVE at 305E where the PRESENT processed sample in S2 is loaded into S1 to become the PREVIOUS processed sample the NEXT time the A/D Complete ISR is entered AFTER the next STO timer interrupt and start of conversion take place. (The sequence of events described above then repeats). The RET at 3062 then takes us back to the HERE loop ("busy") in the main program where the next STO sampling interrupt will again occur later.

If the CMPB instruction at 3070 shows that S1 is LESS than S2, the JE instruction is by-passed at 3075 and the JNH instruction at 3077 causes a jump to CASEB at 308F. There the algorithm for the interpolation is exactly as in CASEA, except that 1) S2-S1 this time is stored in DIFF, 2) DELTA now represents the required INCREMENT needed for each step in the waveform to get to S2 from the previous processed sample S1, 3) ADDB P1, DELTA replaces SUBB P1, DELTA for obvious reasons, and 4) the DJNZ instruction at 30A1 loops back on LOOPB at 309E until the number of steps remaining in COUNT reaches 0. The return at 30A4 returns to SAVE at 305E where again the PRESENT processed sample in S2 is loaded into S1 for the NEXT time around in the sampling process. S1 will then become the PREVIOUS processed sample. Remember, Port P1 drives the DAC. RET at 3062 returns to HERE.

If the CMPB instruction at 3070 reveals that S1 = S2, the JE instruction at 3075 causes a jump to CASEC at 30A5. There the present value of S2 (equal to S1) is output to the DAC at P1

AS IS and is CONTINUALLY output to P1 for as many times as the value of NSTEPS in COUNT requires till COUNT reaches 0 (the DJNZ instruction at 30A8 loops on CASEC at 30A5 in this case). The return at 30A4 is executed back to 305E (SAVE) when COUNT reaches 0. S2 is then loaded into S1 for next time around and a return to HERE ("busy") in the main program is executed.

Remember that, in choosing the number of interpolation steps, N, that you desire, the criterion must be met that Nti (ti = time between interpolation points) be no greater than T, less A/D conversion time, less processing time. In our case T is taken to be 126 usec., A/D conversion time is 42 usec., and the simple "dummy" processing at PROC takes about 10 or 11 usecs. This leaves about 73 or 74 usec. for Nti. Now, the time ti between steps in the P1 output is the time for ONE PASS in the SUBB (or ADDB or LDB) DJNZ loops in CASEA, (or CASEB or CASEC). The state times for those instructions leads to ti = 3 usec. This leads to a maximum value that can be taken for N in NSTEPS (REG 0B0) of N max. = about 25 dec. = 19H.

PROCEDURE

1. Enter BY 09 = 00 and BY 0B0 = 14 for NSTEPS (20 steps between samples). Connect a DAC to port P1 (see p. 585).
2. Connect a 500 Hz sine wave signal to ACH0 for conversion. KEEP SWITCH S AT P0.7 LOW.
3. Execute the program from 3000.
4. Observe the output of the DAC on a scope. This is the sampled, processed input waveform output WITHOUT interpolation. Note the large number of finite steps in the output waveform.
5. Now throw S at P0.7 high and observe the sampled, processed waveform at the output WITH interpolation. Note smoothing of the waveform compared to (4) above. Try to observe the miniscule interpolation steps (3 usec. intervals) during interpolation time by turning up the scope gain.
6. Repeat steps (4) and (5) above for BY 0B0 = 07, then for 19H, and then for 26H i.e. 7 steps, then 25 steps, then 38 steps between samples. Repeat for other input frequencies. Our sampling rate is 126 usec. (7900 Hz) so you can go up to about 4000 Hz. What do you notice when N in 0B0 is larger than 19H.

PROBLEM

How would you employ interrupts to have interpolation occur DURING the processing time to get still smoother waveforms?

EXPERIMENT 9-22

X-Y MOTION CONTROL: POSITION ENCODING WITH FEEDBACK (D.C. SERVOS).

INTRODUCTION, DESCRIPTION OF PROBLEM, INTERFACING AND SOFTWARE APPROACH.

Motion control is of paramount importance in all areas of engineering and science. Motor/motion control for cutting, drilling, robotics, stitching, tool placement, milling, plotting, disc drives and many areas in automation are just some applications that come to mind.

In this experiment, 2 d.c. servo motors on an X-Y table are used with 8096 A/D position input encoding and software feedback control to implement "smart" X-Y motion. X, Y coordinates of the desired STOP points are specified as XSTOP, YSTOP in a WORD TABLE, where XSTOP and YSTOP are digital BYTE values between 00 and FF. The X, Y motors on the X-Y table are linked to two potentiometers. As the motors drive the device in the X, Y plane the POT settings are changed by the linking mechanism from motor /device to POT. By inputting the X-POT and Y-POT analog position settings to, say, the ACH0 and ACH1 A/D conversion channels, we can at all times monitor the ACTUAL position coordinates XPOS, YPOS (as converted digital bytes). This is the POSITION ENCODING aspect of the solution. The FEEDBACK control is software implemented by comparing XSTOP with XPOS and YSTOP with YPOS and then causing the X motor to rotate CCW or CW depending on whether XPOS is less than or greater than XSTOP, and also causing the Y motor to rotate CCW or CW depending on whether YPOS is less than or greater than YSTOP. This will cause the device to move right or left in the X direction if XPOS is less than or greater than XSTOP, respectively, and cause the device to move up or down in the Y direction if YPOS is less than or greater than YSTOP. In this way, as long as the XPOS and YPOS device coordinates are CONSTANTLY updated with the A/D converter, and the compare/conditional "jump-to-position-correction" instructions are PART of the updating loops, the device will be forced to the STOP point XSTOP, YSTOP. There it stays (we employ a 5 sec. delay) before it is made to move to the NEXT STOP point in the table with NEW coordinates XSTOP', YSTOP'.

The path we have chosen for the motor-controlled device in going from ONE STOP point to the NEXT is, for purposes of simplicity, a right-triangle: XPOS goes from XSTOP to XSTOP' with YPOS = constant = YSTOP, and THEN YPOS goes from YSTOP to YSTOP' with

XPOS = constant = XSTOP'. (See PROBLEMS at end of experiment for a more realistic approach in this regard).

The output and input interfacing from the 8096 to the X-Y table via port P1 to drive the motors, and from the POT position encoders to the 8096 via the ACH0,1 A/D channels to establish present position XPOS, YPOS, is shown in the figure below. Note that P1 = 01 causes current flow through the Y axis motor from right to left in the figure producing UP Y motion, while P1 = 02 causes current flow from left to right in the figure producing DOWN Y motion. Similarly, P1 = 04 or P1 = 08 cause current flow through the X axis motor from right to left or left to right in the figure producing LEFT or RIGHT X motion. P1 = 00 causes a STOP i.e. no motor motion. Program is at 2F00, p. 625.

A table of XSTOP, YSTOP coordinate bytes is entered AFTER program execution begins, starting at address 5000H. This forms a word table of STOP positions. Also to be entered AFTER the program executes is the WORD length of the table i.e. the number, N, of STOPS to be executed, into register NSTOPS (40H). Throwing a switch S at P0.7 high starts motion. After all STOPS in the table are completed, a new (or same) number of NSTOPS is entered at 40H and the same table of STOP coordinates XSTOP, YSTOP is used or a new one is entered at 5000H. Only after the switch S at P0.7 is again thrown high does motion again begin. (See PROBLEMS at end of experiment on incorporating an external interrupt to "abort", go back to origin, and enter same or new number of NSTOPS with same or new table of STOPS).

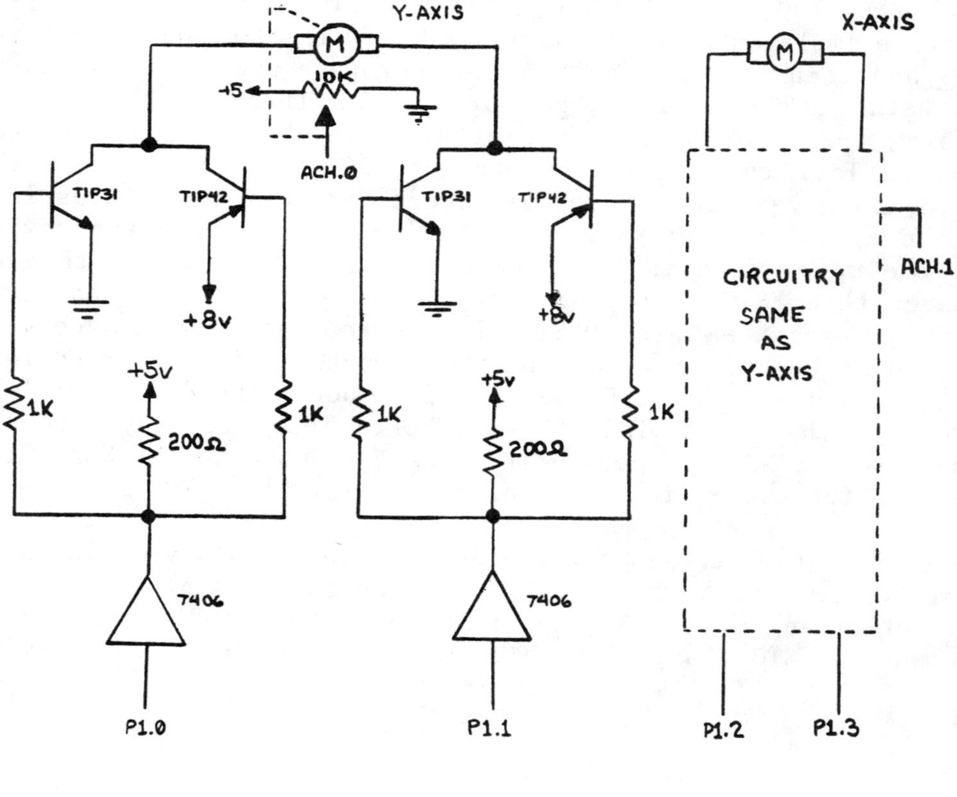

```
     70 00          XSTOP   EQU    70H          18 00          SP       EQU    18H
     71 00          YSTOP   EQU    71H          02 00          ADCOM    EQU    02H
     80 00          OFFST   EQU    80H          02 00          ADRESLO  EQU    02H
     90 00          REG1    EQU    90H          03 00          ADRESHI  EQU    03H
     A0 00          REG2    EQU    0A0H         0E 00          P0       EQU    0EH
     01 00          UP      EQU    01H          0F 00          P1       EQU    0FH
     02 00          DOWN    EQU    02H          40 00          NSTOPS   EQU    40H
     04 00          LEFT    EQU    04H          50 00          PTR      EQU    50H
     08 00          RIGHT   EQU    08H          60 00          XPOS     EQU    60H
     00 00          STOP    EQU    00H          61 00          YPOS     EQU    61H
2F00                        ORG    2F00H
                    ;
2F00 A1 C0 00 18    START:  LD     SP,#0C0H          ;Initialize SP.
2F04 FA                     DI                       ;Disable interrupts.
2F05 B1 00 40               LDB    NSTOPS,#00H       ;Initialize NSTOPS to zero.
2F08 B1 00 0F               LDB    P1,#STOP          ;Output STOP value to motor drivers
                                                     ;at P1.
2F0B EF 10 00               CALL   GETX              ;Call routine to get present X-axis
                                                     ;position and load value into XPOS.
2F0E EF 19 00               CALL   GETY              ;Call routine to get present Y-axis
                                                     ;position and load value into YPOS.
2F11 37 0E FD       WAIT:   JBC    P0,7,WAIT         ;If P0.7 = 0, loop on WAIT.
2F14 99 00 40               CMPB   NSTOPS,#00H       ;Else check if NSTOPS = 0.
2F17 DF F8                  JE     WAIT              ;If NSTOPS = 0, jump back to wait.
2F19 EF 1A 00               CALL   MOVE              ;Else call routine to move
                                                     ;device.
2F1C 27 F3                  SJMP   WAIT              ;Jump to WAIT loop.
                    ;
2F1E B1 08 02       GETX:   LDB    ADCOM,#08H        ;Start A/D conversion on channel 0.
2F21 FD                     NOP                      ;8 states times needed before test.
2F22 FD                     NOP                      ;
2F23 3B 02 FD       TESTX:  JBS    ADRESLO,3,TESTX   ;If conversion not complete, loop on
                                                     ;TESTX.
2F26 B0 03 60               LDB    XPOS,ADRESHI      ;Else load value (bits 9-2) of X-axis
                                                     ;position into XPOS.
2F29 F0                     RET                      ;Return.
                    ;
2F2A B1 09 02       GETY:   LDB    ADCOM,#09H        ;Start A/D conversion on channel 1.
2F2D FD                     NOP                      ;8 states times needed before test.
2F2E FD                     NOP                      ;
2F2F 3B 02 FD       TESTY:  JBS    ADRESLO,3,TESTY   ;If conversion not complete, loop on
                                                     ;TESTY.
2F32 B0 03 61               LDB    YPOS,ADRESHI      ;Else load value (bits 9-2) of Y-axis
                                                     ;position into YPOS.
2F35 F0                     RET                      ;Return.
                    ;
2F36 A1 00 50 50    MOVE:   LD     PTR,#5000H        ;Load address of stop table into PTR.
2F3A A1 00 00 80            LD     OFFST,#0000H      ;Initialize OFFST to 0.
2F3E B3 80 50 70    LOOP1:  LDB    XSTOP,PTR[OFFST]  ;Get XSTOP from table and load into
```

```
                                                      ;XSTOP.
2F42  98 60 70                CMPB   XSTOP,XPOS       ;Check if XSTOP = XPOS.
2F45  DF 22                   JE     YMOVE            ;If XSTOP = XPOS, no X movement needed
                                                      ;jump to YMOVE.
2F47  D9 05                   JH     RMOVE            ;If XSTOP > XPOS, jump to RIGHT.
2F49  B1 04 0F                LDB    P1,#LEFT         ;Else load LEFT move value to P1.
2F4C  20 03                   SJMP   LOOP2            ;Jump to LOOP2 (X motor is moving).
2F4E  B1 08 0F      RMOVE:    LDB    P1,#RIGHT        ;Load RIGHT move value to P1.
2F51  2F CB         LOOP2:    CALL   GETX             ;Call routine to get present X
                                                      ;position into XPOS.
2F53  99 04 0F                CMPB   P1,#LEFT         ;Check if the motor is moving LEFT.
2F56  D7 09                   JNE    MRIGHT           ;If not LEFT jump to MRIGHT.
2F58  98 60 70                CMPB   XSTOP,XPOS       ;Check if XSTOP = XPOS.
2F5B  DF 09                   JE     STOP1            ;If YPOS = YSTOP, no movt., jump STOP1.
2F5D  D1 F2                   JNH    LOOP2            ;If XSTOP < XPOS, more movt., LOOP2.
2F5F  20 05                   SJMP   STOP1            ;Jump to STOP1.
2F61  98 60 70      MRIGHT:   CMPB   XSTOP,XPOS       ;Check if XSTOP = XPOS.
2F64  D9 EB                   JH     LOOP2            ;If XPOS < XSTOP, more movement
                                                      ;needed jump to LOOP2.
2F66  B1 00 0F      STOP1:    LDB    P1,#STOP         ;Else output STOP value to P1.
2F69  07 80         YMOVE:    INC    OFFST            ;Increment OFFST to get YSTOP.
2F6B  B3 80 50 71             LDB    YSTOP,PTR[OFFST];Get YSTOP from table and load into
                                                      ;YSTOP.
2F6F  98 61 71                CMPB   YSTOP,YPOS       ;Compare YPOS to YSTOP.
2F72  DF 22                   JE     NEXT             ;If YPOS = YSTOP, no movement jump to
                                                      ;NEXT.
2F74  D9 05                   JH     UPMOVE           ;If YSTOP > YPOS, jump to UPMOVE.
2F76  B1 02 0F                LDB    P1,#DOWN         ;Else load DOWN value to P1,
2F79  20 03                   SJMP   LOOP3            ;Jump to LOOP3 (motor is moving).
2F7B  B1 01 0F      UPMOVE:   LDB    P1,#UP           ;Load UP value to P1.
2F7E  2F AA         LOOP3:    CALL   GETY             ;Call routine to get present position
                                                      ;on Y-axis and load into YPOS.
2F80  99 02 0F                CMPB   P1,#DOWN         ;Check if motor is moving DOWN.
2F83  D7 09                   JNE    MUP              ;If not moving down jump to MUP.
2F85  98 61 71                CMPB   YSTOP,YPOS       ;Compare YPOS to YSTOP.
2F88  DF 09                   JE     STOP2            ;If XSTOP = XPOS, no movt. jump STOP2.
2F8A  D1 F2                   JNH    LOOP3            ;If YPOS > YSTOP, more Y movement
                                                      ;needed, jump to LOOP3.
2F8C  20 05                   SJMP   STOP2            ;Else jump to STOP2.
2F8E  98 61 71      MUP:      CMPB   YSTOP,YPOS       ;Compare YSTOP to YPOS.
2F91  D9 EB                   JH     LOOP3            ;If YPOS < YSTOP, more movement
                                                      ;needed, jump to LOOP3.
2F93  B1 00 0F      STOP2:    LDB    P1,#STOP         ;Else load STOP value to P1.

2F96  07 80         NEXT:     INC    OFFST            ;Increment OFFST into table.
2F98  E0 40 01                DJNZ   NSTOPS,MORE      ;Decrement number of stops (NSTOPS)
                                                      ;if NSTOPS != 0, jump to MORE.
2F9B  F0                      RET                     ;Else return.
2F9C  EF 02 00      MORE:     CALL   TIME             ;Call TIME routine to delay between
                                                      ;stops.
2F9F  27 9D                   SJMP   LOOP1            ;Jump to LOOP1, need more stops.
```

```
2FA1   B1 19 90      TIME:   LDB    REG1,#0019H   ;Load outer loop with 25 (5 secs.).
2FA4   A1 FF FF A0   LOAD:   LD     REG2,#0FFFFH  ;Load inner loop with 0FFFFH.
2FA8   05 A0         AGAIN:  DEC    REG2          ;Decrement inner loop.
2FAA   D7 FC                 JNE    AGAIN         ;If inner loop != 0, jump to AGAIN.
2FAC   E0 90 F5              DJNZ   REG1,LOAD     ;Decrement outer loop reg., if != 0
                                                  ;jump to LOAD (reload inner loop reg.).
2FAF   F0                    RET                  ;Return.
                     ;
                     ;
2FB0                         END
```

The program starts by initializing SP and disabling interrupts. NSTOPS (number of STOP points in the table) is initialized to 0. #STOP = 00 is output to P1 to stop the motors (no XY motion). Two calls are then made to GETX and GETY at 2F1E and 2F2A in succession. GETX starts A/D conversion at ACH0 of POTX's setting and returns with bits 9-2 from ADRESHI in XPOS. GETY starts A/D conversion at ACH1 of POTY's setting and returns with the converted byte in YPOS. Thus the device's initial position is known. That brings us to the WAIT loop at 2F11 where the status of switch S at P0.7 is tested. The wait is in force as long as S is low. This gives user the opportunity to enter both the table of XSTOP, YSTOP byte coordinates of the desired STOP positions at 5000, and its word length, N, in register NSTOPS (40H). When S is thrown high, the CMPB and JE instructions react to the fact that NSTOPS is no longer 0 and so the CALL MOVE instruction at 2F19 is executed. Motor motion in accordance with the XSTOP, YSTOP table values for STOP positions is now to be implemented. (If S was "prematurely" high, JE WAIT at 2F17 would prevent motion from starting).

At MOVE (address 2F36) PTR is set to 5000. The OFFST register is loaded with 0 and the table indexed instruction at 2F3E fetches the XSTOP byte from the table and loads it into register XSTOP. That value is then compared with the current X coordinate value residing in XPOS (from the A/D conversion in GETX of POTX at ACH0). If they are EQUAL, we've reached XSTOP, so a jump (JE) to YMOVE is executed. There YSTOP is fetched from the table. If, however, XPOS is LESS than XSTOP, the JH instruction at 2F47 causes a jump to RMOVE at at 2F4E where a move to the right in the X direction to XSTOP is implemented. If, on the other hand, XPOS is GREATER than XSTOP, fall-through the JH RMOVE instruction occurs and #LEFT (04) is output to P1 to cause left motion in the X direction to reach XSTOP. If the RMOVE is to be implemented, we are at 2F4E where #RIGHT(08) is output to P1 to cause right motion in the X direction to reach XSTOP. In either case (a move left or a move right towards XSTOP) we find ourselves at LOOP2 (address 2F51: see SJMP LOOP2 at 2F4C).

GETX is again called to update the present X position into XPOS. A check is now made at 2F53 to see if the X motor is moving LEFT. If P1 is not equal to #LEFT (04), then it is moving RIGHT and the JNE instruction at 2F56 jumps to MRIGHT at 2F61 (more on that later). If it IS moving LEFT, the CMPB instruction at 2F58 is executed. It compares the XSTOP destination with the present XPOS. If they are EQUAL, JE at 2F5B jumps to STOP1 at 2F66 where 00 is output to P1 to cause the X motor to stop. If XSTOP is LESS than XPOS, the JNH instruction at 2F5D is executed, jumping back to LOOP2 to allow MORE movement LEFT toward XSTOP. Finally, XPOS reaches XSTOP and JE STOP1 is executed at 2F5B, causing a jump to 2F66 where 00 is output to P1 causing X motor motion to stop. NOTICE: If the JNH instruction at 2F5D is VIOLATED, then XSTOP is LARGER than XPOS (BY ONE BIT) and the fall-through to SJMP STOP1 at 2F5F will ALSO cause X motor motion to cease. Thus, we are allowing the XSTOP (and later, YSTOP) destinations to be reached WITHIN 1-BIT ACCURACY TO ALLOW FOR X OR Y OVERSHOOT (INERTIA). Notice, also, that if the motor was moving RIGHT, the JNE instruction at 2F56 causes a jump to MRIGHT at 2F61 where, again, XSTOP is compared with XPOS. If XPOS is less than XSTOP, we have not reached XSTOP and the JH instruction at 2F64 is executed, jumping back to LOOP2, allowing still further motion right toward XSTOP. When XPOS reaches XSTOP, the JH instruction at 2F64 is not executed and fall-through to STOP1 at 2F66 causes the X motion to cease. Thus, whether motion is LEFT or RIGHT toward XSTOP, the JNH LOOP2 instruction at 2F5D, or JH LOOP2 at 2F64, each gets us into the SAME loop to ENSURE that XPOS reaches XSTOP if the latter is less than XPOS (LEFT motion needed), or if the latter is greater than XPOS (RIGHT motion needed).

In any of the above situations, STOP1 at 2F66 is eventually reached. There 00 loaded into P1 causes ALL motion to cease. It is now time to implement Y motion toward YSTOP. AT 2F69 (YMOVE) OFFST is incremented and the LDB instruction at 2F6B fetches the YSTOP value from the table of stops and loads it into register YSTOP. If YSTOP = YPOS, JE NEXT at 2F72 causes a jump to NEXT at 2F96 with all motor motion stopped. There OFFST is incremented to get ready to fetch the next XSTOP value from the table i.e. ANOTHER XSTOP, YSTOP POINT WAS REACHED The DJNZ instruction at 2F98 decrements the NSTOPS counter. If it is not yet 0, the jump is taken to MORE where a delay allows the device to remain at XSTOP, YSTOP for 5 sec. before starting toward the next XSTOP', YSTOP' position (see SJMP LOOP1 instruction at 2F9F after TIME at 2FA1 is called. This jump to LOOP1 at 2F3E repeats the whole sequence of events, so far described, with respect to the NEXT XSTOP', YSTOP' point to be reached. The table pointer is all set for this). If, however, NSTOPS has been decremented to 0, fall-through to RET at 2F9B occurs. All positions have been covered. The RET to 2F1C carries us back to 2F11 where the WAIT loop (if S = P0.7 = 0) allows us to enter a new number of stops into the NSTOPS register (BY 40 entry) and also (if desired) to enter a new table of XPOS, YPOS bytes starting at 5000 (else the last table's positions wll be again traversed). If, back at 256F, 2572, YPOS does not equal YSTOP, fall-through to 2F74 occurs. From 2F74 to 2F93 in the program, the Y motion feedback control proceeds EXACTLY as the X motion feedback control just analyzed between 2F47 and 2F66 in the program, with UPMOVE, LOOP3, MUP, and STOP2 for Y motion corresponding exactly to RMOVE, LOOP2, MRIGHT, and STOP1 for X motion, respectively. Also, #DOWN, #UP, #DOWN for Y motion correspond to #LEFT, #RIGHT, #LEFT for X motion as they appear in the respective routines. The analysis, therefore, of Y motion toward YSTOP proceeds EXACTLY as that of X motion toward XSTOP already discussed.

PROCEDURE

1. Reset and enter BY 09 = 00. Connect potentiometers with 5V bias to ACH0 and ACH1, corresponding to X and Y motor motion linkages, respectively. Connect a switch S to P0.7 and keep it low.
2. Execute the program from 2F00. Enter the following STOP positions byte table starting at 5000 corresponding to positions lying on a square going from 00 to FF in X direction, then 00 to FF in Y direction, then FF to 00 in -X direction, then FF to 00 in -Y direction: BY 5000 = 00, 00, 40, 00, 80, 00, 0C0, 00, 0FF, 00, 0FF, 40, 0FF, 80, 0FF, 0C0, 0FF, 0FF, 0C0, 0FF, 80, 0FF, 40, 0FF, 00, 0FF, 00, 0C0, 00, 80, 00, 40, 00, 00.
3. Enter BY 40 = 11 corresponding to 17 (dec) stop POSITIONS in the above table (tracing out a rectangle).
4. Throw switch S at P0.7 high then low. Observe the X-Y motion start and cover all 17 points from 00, 00 to FF, 00 to FF, FF to 00, FF, back to 00, 00.
5. Then enter a new byte table at 5000 (points on a triangle) and the desired number of stop points (BY 40). Throw S high and low again and observe the motion.
6. NOTE: We were not able to verify the experiment, as several parts did not arrive before the time the book was to go to press. We shall confirm at a later date.

PROBLEMS

1. Incorporate an EXTINT routine that will abort the motion at any STOP point and cause it to proceed directly to 00, 00 for new table, NSTOPS entries.
2. Develop the algorithm to cause motion from XSTOP, YSTOP to XSTOP', YSTOP' to proceed in a "direct" straight line.
3. Have back-up STOP POSITION TABLES which can be accessed "on-the-fly" as a sensor's input may indicate new requirements i.e. a smart robot "programs itself" on-the-fly.

CHAPTER 10

EXAMPLES OF PL/M-96 AND FPAL-96. INFORMATION ON THE VLSiCE-96P IN-CIRCUIT EMULATOR.

INTRODUCTION

The development tools we have used in the book to this point have centered on the iSBE-96 Single Board Emulator and the ASM-96 assembler. There are other important software/hardware tools available for the 96 family: the high level language PL/M-96, a linker/locater, a librarian, VSLiCE-96 In-Circuit Emulator, Floating Point Arithmetic software (FPAL-96), etc. In this concluding chapter, we give two examples with PL/M-96 (one calls FPAL-96 routines) and then present some information on Intel's powerful VLSiCE-96P In-Circuit Emulator. It is a powerful tool for debugging with high level languages, among other things.

The two examples using PL/M-96 in Expts. 10-1, 10-2 were worked out and contributed by Mr. Tom Geletka of Intel's Customer Training operation in Schaumburg IL 60194 (300 No. Martingale Rd., Ste. 300, (312) 310-5751). We are greatly indebted to him for his efforts and time.

The first of the two experiments below (10-1) is a PL/M-96 version of Expt. 6-17 (p. 343). The compiler was commanded to add the ASM and object code that it produced to the listing file. Thus the PL/M-96 version of Expt. 6-17 is shown in Expt. 10-1 that follows, as well as the ASM/object code compilation. This will allow you to relate the two languages. You should also compare the PL/M-96 compiled ASM and object code shown with the original ASM program on p. 343.

The second experiment below (10-2) uses PL/M-96 and the Floating Point Arithmetic Library (FPAL-96) to compute radial distance i.e. square root of the sum of the squares of three sensor inputs (coordinates x, y, z). The PL/M-96 version and the compiled ASM/object code are presented in the experiment so as to relate the two languages. Also generated in both experiments, but not shown, were Map Files produced by the linker/locater RL96 showing which object modules were combined and where the data and code were placed.

EXPERIMENTS 10-1, 10-2

EXAMPLES OF PL/M-96. EXPT. 10-1: PL/M-96 VERSION OF EXPT. 6-17. EXPT. 10-2: A SQUARE ROOT (RADIAL DISTANCE) PROGRAM IN PL/M-96 USING FPAL-96 ROUTINES.

```
PL/M-96 COMPILER    EXPT. 6-17 PLM96


DOS PL/M-96 V1.1 COMPILATION OF MODULE PATTERN
OBJECT MODULE PLACED IN PAT.OBJ
COMPILER INVOKED BY:  C:\MCS-96\PLM-96\PLM96.EXE PAT.P96


               $ debug code title ('EXPT. 6-17 PLM96 ')

   1           pattern: do;
               /****************************************************************************/
               /*                                                                          */
               /* 8096.PLM - DEFINITION OF SYMBOLIC NAMES FOR THE I/O REGISTERS OF THE 8096 */
               /*                                                                          */
               /****************************************************************************/

 2  1      DECLARE R0           WORD AT(00H);  /* R   ZERO REGISTER  */
 3  1      DECLARE AD_COMMAND   BYTE AT(02H);  /*   W */
 4  1      DECLARE AD_RESULT    WORD AT(02H);  /* R   */
 5  1      DECLARE HSI_MODE     BYTE AT(03H);  /*   W */
 6  1      DECLARE HSO_TIME     WORD AT(04H);  /*   W */
 7  1      DECLARE HSI_TIME     WORD AT(04H);  /* R   */
 8  1      DECLARE HSO_COMMAND  BYTE AT(06H);  /*   W */
 9  1      DECLARE HSI_STATUS   BYTE AT(06H);  /* R   */
10  1      DECLARE SBUF         BYTE AT(07H);  /* R/W */
11  1      DECLARE INT_MASK     BYTE AT(08H);  /* R/W */
12  1      DECLARE INT_PENDING  BYTE AT(09H);  /* R/W */
13  1      DECLARE WATCHDOG     BYTE AT(0AH);  /*   W  WATCHDOG TIMER  */
14  1      DECLARE TIMER1       WORD AT(0AH);  /* R   */
15  1      DECLARE TIMER2       WORD AT(0CH);  /* R   */
16  1      DECLARE BAUD_RATE    BYTE AT(0EH);  /*   W */
17  1      DECLARE IOPORT0      BYTE AT(0EH);  /* R   */
18  1      DECLARE IOPORT1      BYTE AT(0FH);  /* R/W */
19  1      DECLARE IOPORT2      BYTE AT(10H);  /* R/W */
20  1      DECLARE SP_CON       BYTE AT(11H);  /*   W */
21  1      DECLARE SP_STAT      BYTE AT(11H);  /* R   */
22  1      DECLARE IOC0         BYTE AT(15H);  /*   W */
23  1      DECLARE IOS0         BYTE AT(15H);  /* R   */
24  1      DECLARE IOC1         BYTE AT(16H);  /*   W */
25  1      DECLARE IOS1         BYTE AT(16H);  /* R   */
26  1      DECLARE PWM_CONTROL  BYTE AT(17H);  /*   W */
27  1      DECLARE IOS2         BYTE AT(17H);  /* R   */
```

```
28  1      declare forever literally 'while 1=1'; /* 1 will equal 1 forever! */

29  1      declare interval word at (5000h); /* absolute location to match assembler */
30  1      declare reg1 byte;       /* a byte to load the command into to match asm
              This byte has been left relocatable as is the common practice for
              high level language. */

31  1      hsoint: procedure interrupt 3; /* the 3 says to install the interrupt vector
                                          in slot 3 of the vector table */

32  2      if not bittst(.ios0,3)  /* the bit test built-in returns true for 1
                                          or false for a bit value of 0.  */
            then
33  2         do;
34  3           reg1 = reg1 +1;
35  3           hso_command = reg1;
36  3           hso_time = timer1 + interval;
37  3         end;

38  2       else
              do;  /* ios0.3 must have been set to get here */
39  3           reg1 = 2fh;
40  3           hso_command = 6h; /*load HSO command to clear HSO.0 and 1  */
41  3           hso_time = timer1 + interval;
42  3           r0 = 0;   /* wait 8 state times before next command */
43  3           r0 = 0;   /* this is like a NOP */
44  3           hso_command = 17h; /*load HSO command to clear HSO.2 and 3  */
45  3           hso_time = timer1 + interval;
46  3         end;
47  2      end hsoint;

           /* the main program starts here. We will let PLM96 concern itself with
           setting up the stack etc. The things before this point have been data or
           procedure (subroutine) declarations.  */

48  1      int_mask=8;      /*enable only the hso interrupt */
49  1      disable; /* the interrupts */
                  /* declaring the hsoint as an interrupt procedure, caused it to
                  get its interrupt vector loaded into code memory. The "3" identified
                  which interrupt vector to use. Therefore this code does not load the
                  vector at run time.   */

50  1      reg1=30h; /* reg1 is the register that we set aside for the hso command value */
51  1      hso_command = reg1; /* "hso_command = 30h" could have been used here. */
52  1      hso_time = timer1 + interval; /* go off 2* (contents of word 5000h) Usec from now*/
53  1      int_pending = 0;  /*clear all pending interrupts */
54  1      enable; /* the interrupts */

55  1      do forever;  /* stop here forever -- just wait for interrupts */
56  2      end;
```

PL/M-96 COMPILER   EXPT. 6-17 PLM96
ASSEMBLY LISTING OF OBJECT CODE

```
                                     ;  STATEMENT    31
0000                         HSOINT:
0000  F2                             PUSHF
0001  C81C                           PUSH  TMP0
                                     ;  STATEMENT    32
0003  3B150D                         BBS   IOS0,3H,@0001
                                     ;  STATEMENT    34
0006  1700               R           INCB  REG1
                                     ;  STATEMENT    35
0008  B00006             R           LDB   HSO_COMMAND,REG1
                                     ;  STATEMENT    36
000B  470100500A04                   ADD   HSO_TIME,TIMER1,INTERVAL
0011  2019                           BR    @0002
                                     ;  STATEMENT    38
0013                         @0001:
                                     ;  STATEMENT    39
0013  B12F00             R           LDB   REG1,#2FH
                                     ;  STATEMENT    40
0016  B10606                         LDB   HSO_COMMAND,#6H
                                     ;  STATEMENT    41
0019  470100500A1C                   ADD   TMP0,TIMER1,INTERVAL
001F  A01C04                         LD    HSO_TIME,TMP0
                                     ;  STATEMENT    42
0022  0100                           CLR   R0
                                     ;  STATEMENT    43
0024  0100                           CLR   R0
                                     ;  STATEMENT    44
0026  B11706                         LDB   HSO_COMMAND,#17H
                                     ;  STATEMENT    45
0029  A01C04                         LD    HSO_TIME,TMP0
                                     ;  STATEMENT    47
002C                         @0002:
002C  CC1C                           POP   TMP0
002E  F3                             POPF
002F  F0                             RET
                                     ;  STATEMENT    48
0030                         PATTERN:
0030  A1000018           R           LD    SP,#STACK
0034  B10008                         LDB   INT_MASK,#8H
                                     ;  STATEMENT    49
0037  FA                             DI
                                     ;  STATEMENT    50
0038  B13000             R           LDB   REG1,#30H
                                     ;  STATEMENT    51
003B  B00006             R           LDB   HSO_COMMAND,REG1
                                     ;  STATEMENT    52
003E  470100500A04                   ADD   HSO_TIME,TIMER1,INTERVAL
                                     ;  STATEMENT    53
0044  1109                           CLRB  INT_PENDING
                                     ;  STATEMENT    54
0046  FB                             EI
                                     ;  STATEMENT    55
0047                         @0003:
                                     ;  STATEMENT    56
0047  27FE                           BR    @0003
0049                         @0004:
```

```
PL/M-96 COMPILER    FPAL96 EXAMPLE

DOS PL/M-96 V1.1 COMPILATION OF MODULE VECTOR
OBJECT MODULE PLACED IN VEC.OBJ
COMPILER INVOKED BY:  C:\MCS-96\PLM-96\PLM96.EXE VEC.P96


            $ CODE DEBUG TITLE ('FPAL96 EXAMPLE' )

  1         VECTOR: DO;
            /* THIS PROGRAM SHOWS HOW YOU MIGHT DO SOME FLOATING POINT WITH PLM96.
            IT USES THE FLOATING POINT ARITHMETIC  LIBRARY. */

  2   1     FP$SQRT: PROCEDURE  EXTERNAL;
  3   2     END;

  4   1     FP$LDINT: PROCEDURE (PARAM) EXTERNAL;
  5   2     DECLARE PARAM  LONGINT;
  6   2     END;

  7   1     FP$LD: PROCEDURE (PARAM) EXTERNAL;
  8   2     DECLARE PARAM  REAL;
  9   2     END;

 10   1     FP$STINT: PROCEDURE LONGINT EXTERNAL;
 11   2     END;

 12   1     FP$ST: PROCEDURE  REAL  EXTERNAL;
 13   2     END;

 14   1     DECLARE (R,X,Y,Z ) REAL;
 15   1     declare (I,J,K,RESULTANT) INTEGER;

            /*ASSUME THAT I,J,AND K HAVE THE INPUTS FROM THREE SENSORS. WE WANT
            TO COMPUTE THE RESULTANT OF THE THREE COORDINATES AS THE SQUARE ROOT
            OF THE SUM OF THE SQUARES */

            /* THE PROGRAM STARTS HERE */
 16   1     CALL SET$REAL$MODE(3FH) ; /* PLM96 BUILT-IN TO INITIALIZE FLOATING POINT */
                                         /* 3FH SPECIFIES DEFAULT ERROR HANDLER */
              /* CHANGE THE CORDINATES INTO FLOATING POINT */
              /* TO ELIMINATE OVERFLOWS AND ALLOW SQUARE ROOTS */


 17   1     CALL FP$LDINT(I); /* LOAD I AS INTEGER INTO FLOATING POINT ACCUMULATOR */
 18   1     X = FP$ST  ;  /* STORE THE VALUE AS FLOATING POINT NUMBER IN X */

 19   1     CALL FP$LDINT(J);
 20   1     Y = FP$ST  ;

 21   1     CALL FP$LDINT(K);
 22   1     Z = FP$ST  ;


 23   1     R= ( X*X + Y*Y + Z*Z );
 24   1     CALL FPLD (R);
 25   1     CALL FP$SQRT ;
 26   1     RESULTANT = FPSTINT; /* STORES THE FLOATING POINT ACCUMULATOR AS INTEGER */
             /* THE INTEGER RESULT IS BACK IN RESULTANT. AN ACTUAL PROGRAM WOULD THEN
                USE THE RESULTANT */
 27   1      END;
```

PL/M-96 COMPILER FPAL96 EXAMPLE

ASSEMBLY LISTING OF OBJECT CODE

```
                                  ; STATEMENT 16
0000                        VECTOR:
0000  A1000018          R         LD    SP,#STACK
0004  C93F00                      PUSH  #3FH
0007  EF0000            E         CALL  FPLDCW
                                  ; STATEMENT 17
000A  A0101C            R         LD    TMP0,I
000D  061C                        EXT   TMP0
000F  C81E                        PUSH  TMP2
0011  C81C                        PUSH  TMP0
0013  EF0000            E         CALL  FPLDINT
                                  ; STATEMENT 18
0016  EF0000            E         CALL  FPST
0019  C81E                        PUSH  TMP2
001B  C81C                        PUSH  TMP0
001D  EF0000            E         CALL  FPLD
0020  EF0000            E         CALL  FPST
0023  A01E06            R         LD    X+2H,TMP2
0026  A01C04            R         LD    X,TMP0
                                  ; STATEMENT 19
0029  A0121C            R         LD    TMP0,J
002C  061C                        EXT   TMP0
002E  C81E                        PUSH  TMP2
0030  C81C                        PUSH  TMP0
0032  EF0000            E         CALL  FPLDINT
                                  ; STATEMENT 20
0035  EF0000            E         CALL  FPST
0038  C81E                        PUSH  TMP2
003A  C81C                        PUSH  TMP0
003C  EF0000            E         CALL  FPLD
003F  EF0000            E         CALL  FPST
0042  A01E0A            R         LD    Y+2H,TMP2
0045  A01C08            R         LD    Y,TMP0
                                  ; STATEMENT 21
0048  A0141C            R         LD    TMP0,K
004B  061C                        EXT   TMP0
004D  C81E                        PUSH  TMP2
004F  C81C                        PUSH  TMP0
0051  EF0000            E         CALL  FPLDINT
                                  ; STATEMENT 22
0054  EF0000            E         CALL  FPST
0057  C81E                        PUSH  TMP2
0059  C81C                        PUSH  TMP0
005B  EF0000            E         CALL  FPLD
005E  EF0000            E         CALL  FPST
0061  A01E0E            R         LD    Z+2H,TMP2
0064  A01C0C            R         LD    Z,TMP0
                                  ; STATEMENT 23
0067  C80E              R         PUSH  Z+2H
0069  C80C              R         PUSH  Z
006B  EF0000            E         CALL  FPMUL
006E  EF0000            E         CALL  FPST
0071  C81E                        PUSH  TMP2
0073  C81C                        PUSH  TMP0
0075  C80A              R         PUSH  Y+2H
0077  C808              R         PUSH  Y
0079  EF0000            E         CALL  FPLD
007C  C80A              R         PUSH  Y+2H
007E  C808              R         PUSH  Y
0080  EF0000            E         CALL  FPMUL
0083  EF0000            E         CALL  FPST
0086  C81E                        PUSH  TMP2
0088  C81C                        PUSH  TMP0
008A  C806              R         PUSH  X+2H
008C  C804              R         PUSH  X
008E  EF0000            E         CALL  FPLD
0091  C806              R         PUSH  X+2H
0093  C804              R         PUSH  X
0095  EF0000            E         CALL  FPMUL
0098  EF0000            E         CALL  FPADD
009B  EF0000            E         CALL  FPADD
009E  EF0000            E         CALL  FPST
00A1  A01E02            R         LD    R+2H,TMP2
00A4  A01C00            R         LD    R,TMP0
                                  ; STATEMENT 24
00A7  C802              R         PUSH  R+2H
00A9  C800              R         PUSH  R
00AB  EF0000            E         CALL  FPLD
                                  ; STATEMENT 25
00AE  EF0000            E         CALL  FPSQRT
                                  ; STATEMENT 26
00B1  EF0000            E         CALL  FPSTINT
00B4  A01C16            R         LD    RESULTANT,TMP0
                                  ; STATEMENT 27
                                  END
```

VLSiCE™-96P In-Circuit Emulator for the MCS® -96 Family of Microcontrollers

- **Precise real-time emulation of the MCS® -96 family of components**
- **64K of mappable memory for early software debug and (EP)ROM simulation**
- **A 4K-entry trace buffer for storing a real-time execution history, including both code and data flows**
- **An 8 state event machine for establishing complex break/trace specifications**
- **Break and trace qualified on execution addresses, data addresses, and values (both external and internal RAM), opcodes, and selected PSW flags**
- **Shadow registers allow reading many 8096 write-only and writing many read-only registers**
- **Symbolic debugging allows accesses to memory locations and program variables (including dynamic variables) using program-defined names**
- **Equipped with the Integrated Command Directory (ICD) which provides**
  - **An on-line help file**
  - **A dynamic syntax menu**
  - **Dynamic command-entry error checking**
- **Serially linked to Intel Series III/IV hosts or IBM* PC-XT and AT**

The VLSiCE™-96P In-Circuit Emulator is a debugging and test tool that is used for development of the hardware and software of a prototype system based on the MCS® -96 family of microcontrollers.

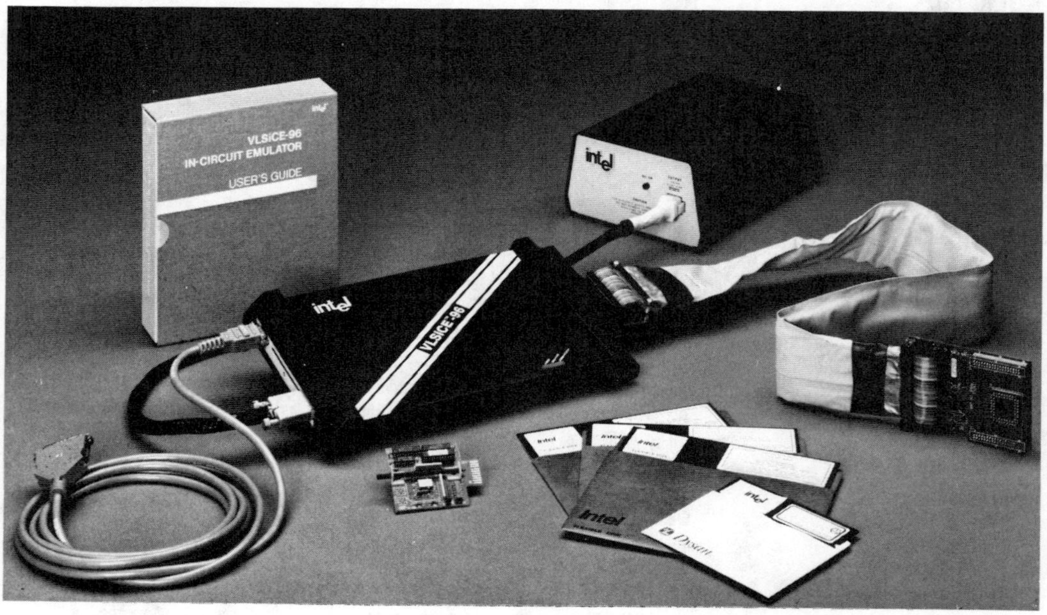

System Performance:

Mappable zero wait-state memory (zero wait-states up to 12 MHz)	Min. 0K-bytes Max. 64K-bytes	Mappable to user or ICE memory in 1K-byte blocks on 1K-byte boundaries.

Trace buffer 4K × 48 bits

Virtual symbol table — A maximum or 61K-bytes of host memory space is available for the virtual symbol table (VST). The rest of the VST resides on disk and is paged in and out as needed.

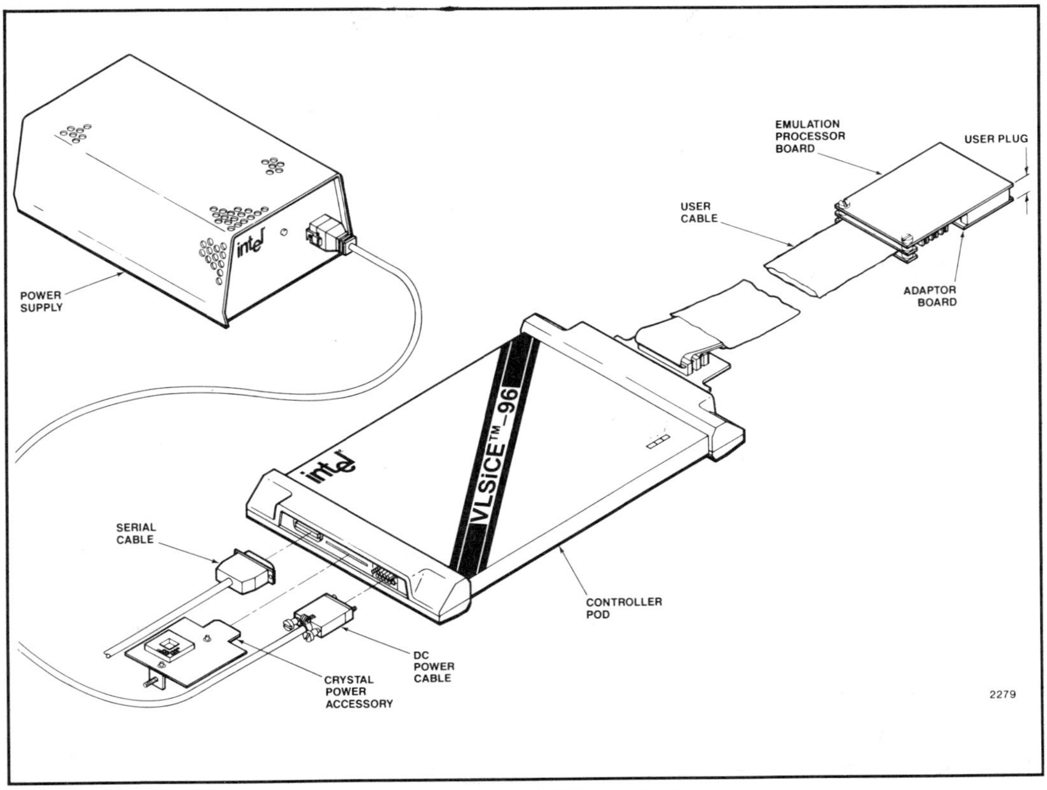

Figure 1. The VLSiCE™-96P System

```
hlt> PRINT NEWEST 8 CYCLES
FRAME ADDRESS CODE              MNEMONIC OPERANDS        TIME TIMEUNIT

(1020) 300A   C82A              PUSH 2A                    172 Micro-sec.
        [002AH]=0087H(R)  [0018H]=0028H(R)       [0018H]=0026H(W)
        [0026H]=0087H(W)

(1021) 300C   64322A            ADD  2A,32                 175 Micro-sec.
        [0032H]=0010H(R)  [002AH]=0087H(R)       [002AH]=0097H(W)

(1022) 300F   6975002A          SUB  2A,#75                180 Micro-sec.
        [002AH]=0097H(R)  [002AH]=0022H(W)
.
.
.
.
.
(1027) 3010 CC2A0002            POP  2A                    205 Micro-sec.
        [0018H]=0026H(R)  [0026H]=0087H(R)       [0018H]=0028H(W)
        [002AH]=0087H(W)
```

Figure 2. The Trace Buffer Display

VLSiCE-96 Software Package:

VLSiCE-96P emulator software
VLSiCE-96P confidence tests

```
hlt> GO
FROM  FOREVER  USING  TIL  ;  <execute>
```

```
hlt> GO FROM
<address> . : <module-name> . <symbol> # <line-number> <expr>
```

```
hlt> GO FROM 2080H
FOREVER  USING  TIL  ;  <execute>
```

```
hlt> GO FROM 2080H USING
<brkreg name>
```

```
hlt> GO FROM 2080H USING br1
, TRACE SYNCSTART FULLBUF ; <execute>
```

Figure 3. The Intregrated Command Directory for the GO Command

```
hlt> HELP ASM

The ASM command displays memory as 8096 assembler nmemonics.
The syntax is:

 ASM <partition>  [='<asm96-inst>'  [, '<asm-96inst>'*]]

where:

<partition> specifies the area of memory to be displayed and
modified.

<asm96-inst> specifies the 8096 assembly instruction to be
assembled.

Please see the VLSiCE-96 Reference Manual for more detailed
information.
```

Figure 4. HELP Screen

SPECIFICATIONS

Host Requirements:

An Intellec® Microcomputer Development System, Series III or Series IV, running under ISIS or iNDX, with at least 512K of application memory resident.

Other peripherals as desired.

Disk drives — Dual floppy or 1 hard disk and 1 floppy drive required (10M-byte Winchester optional).

An IBM PC XT or PC AT with 512K RAM and hard disk. Intel recommends PC-DOS 3.0 or later.